Neuro *ophthalmology*

Emanuel S Rosen BSc MD FRCSEd FRCOphth

Consultant Ophthalmic Surgeon
Visiting Professor Department of Vision Sciences
University of Manchester
Institute of Science and Technology
The Alexandra Hospital
Cheadle, Cheshire
UK

H Stanley Thompson MD

Professor of Neuro-ophthalmology
Department of Ophthalmology and Visual Sciences
University of Iowa
Iowa City
USA

W J Ken Cumming BSc MD FRCPI FRCP MAE MEWI

Neuroscience Unit
The Alexandra Hospital
Cheadle, Cheshire
UK

Peter Eustace MCh FRCS FRCOphth

Professor of Ophthalmology
University College Dublin
Mater Misericordiae Hospital
Dublin
Ireland

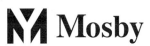 **Mosby**

London   Philadelphia   St Louis   Sydney   Tokyo

Copyright © 1998 Mosby International Limited

Published in 1998 by Mosby, an imprint of Mosby International Limited

Printed by Grafos S.A., Arte sobre papel, Barcelona, Spain.

ISBN 0 7234 1964 7

The right of Emanuel S Rosen, H Stanley Thompson, WJ Ken Cumming and Peter Eustace to be identified as authors of this work has been asserted by them in accordance with the Copyright and Design and Patents Act, 1988.

For full details of all Mosby International titles, please write to Mosby International, Lynton House, 7–12 Tavistock Square, London WC1H 9LB, England.

A CIP catalogue record for this book is available from the British Library.

Library of Congress Cataloging-in-Publication Data applied for.

Project Management:	Richard Foulsham Dave Burin
Development Editor:	Daniel Elger
Designer:	Ian Spick
Layout Artist:	The EDI Partnership: Mark Willey, Lee Smith
Cover Design:	Ian Spick
Illustration:	The EDI Partnership: Mark Willey, Lee Smith
Production:	Siobhan Egan
Index:	Laurence Errington
Publisher:	Geoff Greenwood

CONTENTS

Contents

PREFACE

A multi-authored volume is difficult to assemble but the editors are tremendously appreciative of the contributions of the experts who have produced the chapters herein.

The editors offer thanks to all the contributors and to all the other people whose contributions are essential in publishing a text. Particular thanks are due to Mrs Elizabeth King whose polite, patient and efficient assembly of the manuscript was the result of countless communications.

The editorial and production staff at Mosby together with their brilliant design and illustration department have converted tame type and rough drawings into a vibrant and brilliantly directed instruction manual. Their attention to detail has been faultless and they deserve and receive our deepest gratitude.

We believe this volume will be appreciated by novices in the field as well as seasoned practitioners. The art of education is simplicity, repetition and reinforcement and we believe we are providing a useful framework for educational purposes in the field of neuro-ophthalmology.

Emanuel Rosen
Stanley Thompson
Peter Eustace
Ken Cumming
July 1997

CONTRIBUTORS

Dr Melvin G Alper — 5454 Wisconsin Avenue N.W., Suite 950, Chevy Chase, MD 20815, USA

Mr A Ansons — Manchester Royal Eye Hospital, Oxford Road, Manchester M13 9WH, UK

Dr Jason J S Barton — Department of Neurology, Beth Israel Hospital, Deaconess Medical Center, Boston, MA, USA

Dr Roy W Beck — Jaeb Center for Health Research, 3010 East 138th Avenue, Tampa, FL, USA

Mr T Buchanan — Royal Victoria Hospital, Grosvenor Road, Belfast BT12 6BA, UK

Dr James J Corbett — Department of Neurology, University of Mississippi Medical Center, 2500 N. State Street, Jackson, MS 39216, USA

DI Flitcroft — Department of Ophthalmology, Mater Misericordiae Hospital, Dublin 7, Ireland

Prof. M A Farrell — Beaumont Hospital, P.O. Box 1297, Beaumont Road, Dublin 9, Ireland

Mr J Gillespie — Department of Radiology and Neuroscience, Manchester Royal Infirmary, Oxford Road, Manchester M13 9WL, UK

Dr Satoshi Ishikawa — Department of Ophthalmology, Kitasato School of Medicine, Kanagawa-ken, Japan

Dr Bruce James — Department of Ophthalmology, Stoke Mandeville Hospital, Aylesbury, Bucks., UK

Dr Randy H Kardon — Department of Ophthalmology, T255 GH, University of Iowa Hospitals and Clinics, 200 Hawkins Drive, Iowa City, IA 52242, USA

Dr S Kennedy — National Ophthalmic Laboratory & Registry of Ireland, Royal Victoria Eye and Ear Hospital, Dublin, Ireland

Dr Patrick Lavin — Neurology and Ophthalmology, Nashville, TN 37232, USA

Mr Brian Leatherbarrow — 10 St John Street, Manchester, M3 4DY, UK

Dr Patricia K Johnston McNussen — Carle Clinic, 602 West University, Urbana, IL 61801, USA

Dr Lois J Martyn — St. Christopher's Hospital for Children, Department of Ophthalmology, Front Street and Erie Avenue, Philadelphia, PA 19134, USA

Dr K Mukono — Department of Ophthalmology, Kitasato School of Medicine, Kanagawa-ken, Japan

Dr Michael O'Keefe — Department of Ophthalmology, Mater Misericordiae Hospital, Dublin 7, Ireland

Dr Matthew Rizzo — Department of Neurology, University of Iowa, 200 Hawkins Drive, 2007 RCP, Iowa City, IA 52242-1053, USA

Mr David Saunders — Manchester Royal Eye Hospital, Oxford Road, Manchester M13 9WH, UK

Prof. James A Sharpe — Department of Neurology, Toronto Western Hospital, 399 Bathurst Street, Toronto, Ontario, M5T 2S8, Canada

Dr Michael Wall — Department of Neurology, University of Iowa Hospitals & Clinics, 200 Hawkins Drive, Iowa City, IA 52242, USA

Dr Robert D Yee — Department of Ophthalmology, Indiana University School of Medicine, 702 Rotary Circle, Indianapolis, IN 46202-5175, USA

Prof. A Jackson — Manchester University and Manchester Royal Infirmary, Oxford Road, Manchester M13 9WH, UK

Miss Alison Spencer — Manchester University and Manchester Royal Infirmary, Oxford Road, Manchester M13 9WH, UK

Dr William N White — University Eye Specialists, 408 North Main Street, Warsaw, NY 14569, USA

CHAPTER 1

Introduction

E S Rosen

Evolution in neuro-ophthalmic practice continues inexorably. New techniques probe deeply into providing fresh insights in astonishing detail. Imaging techniques have simplified neuro-ophthalmic diagnostic detective work. Our interests are enhanced, our diagnostic acumen is embellished, and our clinical satisfaction is paralleled by improvement in patient care.

With the inderstanding of how a physiologic system works comes the gratification of seeing the pieces fall into place, and the exhilaration of getting a glimpse of the design. The urge to pass these feelings along is powerful, and provides some of the energy for the cycle of teaching and understanding that leads to progress and growth. This works just as well for the community of medical practitioners as it does for the research laboratory.

In this book we have tried to bring together clinical insights from many areas of neuro-ophthalmic practice using explanatory texts in various formats accompanied by diagrams and images. An atlas and textbook relies on the succinct didactic value of illustrations as much as it does on the text. For a deeper investigation of any aspect of neuro-ophthalmology, readers can refer to the monographs and landmark papers cited in the text. Awareness of recent advances in practice requires constant consultation with current literature. Our purpose is both to initiate clinicians into the subject as well as to provide an update and reminder for today's practitioners.

Neuro-ophthalmology is a prime example of the art and science of conventional (evidence-based) medicine. There is little tolerance here for wishful fancies like iridology, nor to those preferences for alternative medicines of plant origin.

The eye provides many clues to neurologic disorders, which is not surprising because it contains so much neural tissue and is interdependent with all cerebral functions. Ocular movements, visual acuity, color vision, visual fields, pupillary responses, and fundus appearances all provide clues to cerebral malfunction. Trained observations, supplemented by a variety of objective investigations including intracranial imaging, have consigned to history many of the mysteries that confronted former generations of practitioners. However, observation needs to be channeled. Observers need to be trained. This book serves to support these requirements and needs to be consulted in conjunction with continuing clinical experiences.

Just as the eyes provide an insight into the brain, so an understanding of the anatomy and function of the brain from chiasm to cortex, from cranial nerve nuclei to their interrelated connections, provides an insight into ocular function and disorders. Two major specialties in medical practice are thus interrelated and jointly practiced. As the bias moves toward the brain the neurologist becomes king. As the issue moves toward the territory of visual dysfunction, the ophthalmologist takes over.

This atlas and textbook is therefore designed to appeal to both medical specialties as well as to the generalist who requires competence in both aspects of medical practice. An atlas with text offers an economic expression of facts and experiences. When Shakespeare wrote of the early morning sun adorning a landscape,

Kissing with golden face the meadows green
Gilding pale streams with heavenly alchemy

he did not require illustrations, for our imagination can complete the task. But complex anatomical relationships cannot be conjured in the reader's mind with words alone; we need to see the details and we depend on diagrams and modern neuro-imaging techniques. We trust that students of all ages and experiences will profit from our labors.

CHAPTER 2

The History of Neuro-ophthalmology

H Stanley Thompson

INTRODUCTION

There have always been tumors, strokes, and inflammations that produce hemianopias, cranial nerve palsies, and sudden blindness but their relationships with each other remained mysterious until the relevant neuroanatomy and neurophysiology were understood.

Just 150 years ago it was probably possible to teach a student everything there was to know about neuro-ophthalmology in 10 or 15 minutes but in the 1990s, neuro-ophthalmology has grown into a rich and complex field of study and its history contains parts of the history of neurology, ophthalmology, and of all the related basic medical sciences. For example, the neuroanatomy of the visual pathways only fell into place late in the 19th century, with the work of Flourens, Baillarger, Gratiolet, Broca, Hitzig, Ferrier, Munk, von Gudden, Wilbrand, Henschen, Meynert, Sharpey-Schäfer, von Monakow, and many others. [1]

There is insufficient space in this chapter for a thorough review of the history of neuro-ophthalmology, so it will concentrate on some of the stories that have interested the author, starting with an account of how the decussation at the chiasm contributed to an awareness of visual-field loss and eventually led to the clinical testing of visual fields.

One of the questions that troubled ancient philosophers was 'Why, when we are equipped with two good eyes, do we not see two of everything?'. It was gradually agreed that images from the two eyes must come together somewhere in the brain and there become fused into one. It was known that the optic nerves came together at the chiasm but it was not immediately apparent that there was a decussation of the fibers at the chiasm. Galen, Vesalius, Descartes, Maitre-Jean, and Briggs said that the optic nerves did not cross; Soemmerring, Brisadecki, Mandelstamm, Kölliker, and others until 1899, said that the nerves crossed entirely; there were also several who theorized correctly, first speculating that there was a partial crossing of the optic nerves (Newton, Taylor, Wollaston) and finally demonstrating it histologically (Müller, von Gudden, and especially Cajal). [1-3]

THE ORIGIN OF THE WORDS 'DECUSSATION' AND 'CHIASM'

A brief review of the origin of these two words suggests that the first 'decussation' was at the 'chiasm'.

'DECUSSATION'

The English word 'decussation' derives from the Latin verb 'decussare' – to divide crosswise in the shape of an X. The word 'decussis' was the name of an ancient, 10 unit, Roman coin that was marked with an X to indicate its denomination. So it appears that the anatomic crossing of the optic nerves is named after the Roman numeral that resembles a cross.

In English, the word 'pound' serves as a unit of weight and also as a unit of money. The Romans had several words of this kind:
- the word 'as' (a unit)
- 'libra' (a balance for weighing), from the initial 'L' from which we get the '£' symbol
- 'pondus' (a weight used on a balance), from which the word 'pound' itself is derived

All these words eventually seem to have acquired a double meaning, referring to both weight and money.

The first Roman coinage (about 550 BC) was copper and each 'as' weighed one 'pondo', which was divided into 12 'unciae' (ounces). This coinage was very heavy and was referred to in retrospect as 'as grave', because it was too heavy to use as legal tender and was hard to transport and hard to store. This money came in several denominations, including a 'quincunx' (five ounces), a 'quadrussis' (four 'as'), and a 'decussis' (ten 'as').

These heavy copper tablets were eventually replaced (about 250 BC) by much smaller, but still substantial, round, bronze coins of which the 10-unit piece was the largest (Fig. 2.1); it was still called a decussis and it was about 4 inches (10 cm) across.

According to Columella (about AD 40), the verb 'decussare', which meant 'to make crossed lines in the form of the number ten (X)', was derived from the coin named 'decussis' that had been distinguished by the X mark. Similarly, Cicero (about 40 BC) wrote of planting trees in a 'quincunx formation' ('directi in quincuncem ordines'), that is, in straight rows with the trees spaced like the five dots on a quincunx, or on a die.

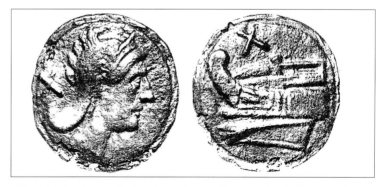

Fig. 2.1 The decussis. This large bronze Roman coin of the second century BC was marked on both sides with an 'X' to indicate that it was valued at 10 'as'. On the obverse the 'X' is behind the helmeted head of Diana and on the reverse above the prow of a ship.

'CHIASM'

The English word 'chiasm' is a contraction of the Greek word χιασμα (chiasma) – the mark of the letter X (chi). That is, the anatomic structure was clearly named after the letter of the Greek alphabet that it physically resembled. The word chiasma was used by the Greek anatomist and physician Rufus of Ephesus early in the second century to refer to the place where the optic nerves came together.

THE HISTORY OF KNOWLEDGE OF THE CHIASMAL CROSSING OF THE OPTIC NERVES

Galen of Pergamon, a generation or two after Rufus of Ephesus, saw the chiasm as a potential (hydraulic) connection between the two eyes and as the dividing point in the visual pathway that served to distribute the vital fluid from the ventricles towards both eyes.

Arab medical knowledge was based chiefly on Galen's writings and, during the European Dark Ages, it was the best medical knowledge available (*Fig. 2.2*). Arab physicians clarified many of Galen's ideas: the hollowness of the optic nerves, their merging in the chiasm 'so that their two cavities become one', the 'origin' of the optic nerves from the cerebral ventricles, and the existence of a 'pneuma', which 'constantly circulates from the ventricles to the eye in great quantity'.

René Descartes (1596–1650), the great French philosopher and mathematician, spent most of his working life in Holland. Descartes accepted most of Galen's anatomy but he conjectured that the visual 'spirits' (perhaps we would say 'impulses' today) passed from the retina, along the optic nerve (*not* decussating at the chiasm), arriving at a retinotopic array in the lateral ventricle, and from there transferred to the centrally located pineal gland ('the seat of the soul'). Descartes thought that it was in the pineal gland that each image met its fellow from the other eye, so that the two images became combined into a single visual experience. It was from the pineal that these fused images were deposited in the brain for future recall as visual memory (*Fig. 2.3*).

Thomas Willis (1621–1675) was a busy Oxford physician who undertook a major study of the anatomy of the brain. In his book 'Cerebri Anatome' (1664), Willis described the circle of vessels at the base of the brain that now bears his name (*Fig. 2.4*). In the 17th century it was not known whether the optic nerves intermingled and exchanged fibers at the chiasm or if they were just briefly bound together at the base before proceeding, each nerve to its own side of the brain.

William Briggs (1650–1704) was a fellow of Cambridge University and a physician at St Thomas' Hospital, London. He was 8 years younger than Isaac Newton and must have known of him from his days at Cambridge. Briggs described the retinal fibers as converging within the eye on the 'optic papilla' and then traveling along the optic nerve and passing through the chiasma *without any decussation* of the fibers (*Fig. 2.5*).

Isaac Newton (1642–1727), the celebrated genius, mathematician, physicist, and philosopher of Cambridge and London, reasoned that there must be a hemidecussation at the chiasm: it was the best way to get the images from the two eyes together in the brain (*Fig. 2.6*).

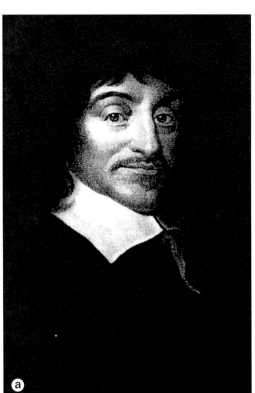

Fig. 2.3 (**a**) René Descartes (1596–1650). Engraved by W Holl from a painting by Frans Hals (in the Louvre, Paris, France).
(**b**) Descartes' Tractatus de Homine (Traité de l'homme).

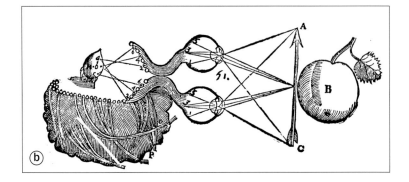

Fig. 2.2 Early Arabian illustration of the eye and its cerebral connections.

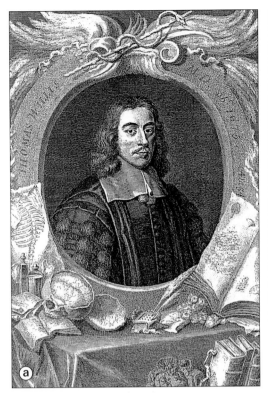

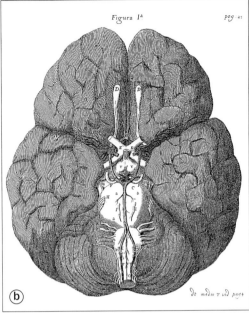

Fig. 2.4 (**a**) Thomas Willis (1621–1675). (**b**) The drawing of the base of the brain was done by Christopher Wren before he became a celebrated architect. It not only shows the circle of Willis, but also establishes as standard equipment the X-shaped 'crossing' of the optic nerves known as the chiasm.

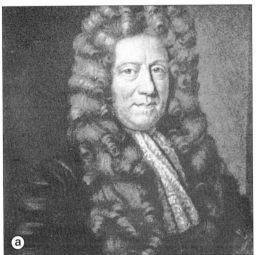

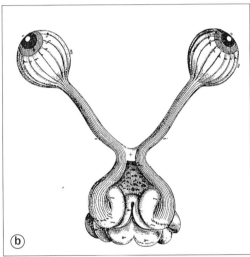

Fig. 2.5 (**a**) William Briggs (1650–1704). (**b**) The visual system as represented by William Briggs in his 'Opthalmographia' (1685). Information from certain areas of the retina went to specific areas of the hypothalamus. Briggs followed Descartes, who in turn had followed Galen, in stating that the two optic nerves remained separated at the chiasm.

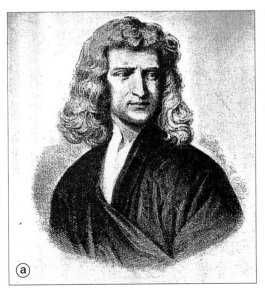

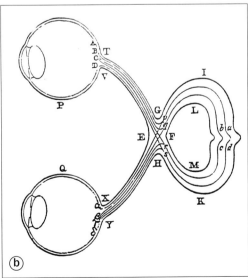

Fig. 2.6 (**a**) Isaac Newton (1642–1727). Newton lived into his 80s, having apparently breathed enough mercury fumes during his alchemy experiments to bring his IQ down to within three standard deviations of the rest of the population. (**b**) This representation of the chiasm was apparently never published by Newton. It was found among his papers and published by Brewster in his biography of Newton in 1855.[4]

After Briggs said at the Royal Society in 1682 that there was no mixing of optic nerve fibers at the chiasm,[5] Newton wrote a letter to Briggs (dated 12 September 1682) suggesting that Briggs was wrong, '... how is this coincidence [of the pictures from the two eyes] made?' Newton asked. 'Perhaps by the mixing of the marrow of the nerves in their juncture [that is, at the chiasm] before they enter the brain, the fibres on the right side of each eye going to the right side of the head and those on the left side to the left.' In 1704 (22 years later) Newton published this hemidecussation hypothesis in his book 'Opticks' as one of a series of 'Queries' and thus became the first author to indicate clearly *in print* that a partial decussation of the optic nerves in the chiasm could be the basis of single binocular vision.

Giovanni Battista Morgagni (1682–1771) was Professor of Anatomy in Bologna and Padua (*Fig. 2.7*). He has been called 'The Prince of Anatomists' and 'The Founder of Pathological Anatomy'.

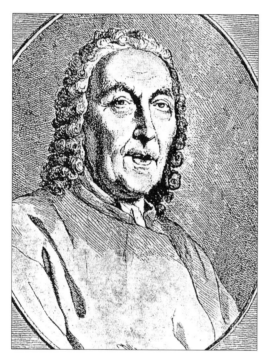

Fig. 2.7 Giovanni Battista Morgagni (1682–1771).

In 1719 Morgagni described a case of impaired vision in both eyes caused by a unilateral lesion of the brain[6]: this seems to have been the earliest correct interpretation of a homonymous hemianopia.

William Mackensie, the famous Scottish ophthalmologist, pointed out in 1830 that Abraham Vater and J Christian Heinecke (1723) published a thesis in which they described, at some length, the case of a young man who suffered the sudden onset of a homonymous hemianopia. On finding that with either eye, or with both together, he could see only half of what he was looking at '...his spirit was not a little perturbed', but it all cleared up in about an hour. (From a distance of 275 years, this sounds like a description of migraine.) The authors then argued cogently that this kind of symptom could occur only if there were a hemidecussation of the optic nerves at the chiasm. It is not too surprising that they had not noticed Newton's brief mention of this thought, because it was buried at the back of his difficult, English language, Opticks book. Chevalier John Taylor (1703–1772) was an English Ophthalmiatric 'Knight-Errant', Travelling Cataract Coucher, and Charlatan-Oculist Extra-ordinaire (*Fig. 2.8*). Posterity may not have a high opinion of Taylor's character or professional accomplishments (he is said to have blinded both Bach and Händel) but it is only fair to admit that his published views on the anatomic basis of single binocular vision were remarkably modern. Taylor, in 1738, appears to have accepted Newton's chiasmal hemidecussation (1704), Morgagni's autopsied case (1719), and Vater and Heinecke's clinical case (1723), but he gives no credit to any of them. There is some internal evidence (the discussion of chameleon's eyes) to suggest that Taylor had read Newton. In any case, Taylor went on to make the further suggestion that fibers originating at corresponding points in the two retinas meet at a single point in the brain to produce a single subjective visual experience.

William Hyde Wollaston (1766–1828) was a renowned chemist and metallurgist, famous for his work with the platinum metals. He came from an illustrious family with a longstanding interest in science (*Fig. 2.9*).

Wollaston took a medical degree and began a general medical practice in 1795. In 1800 he chose to abandon medicine ('the terra firma of physic') and devote himself to chemical research.

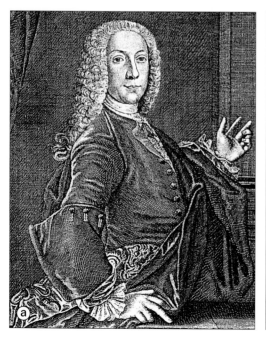 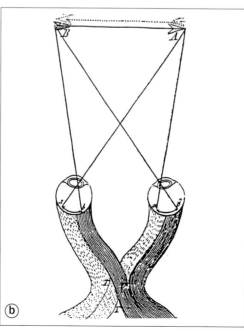

Fig. 2.8 (**a**) Chevalier John Taylor (1703–1772), taken from the frontispiece of Taylor's 1738 book 'Mechanismus'. (**b**) This appears to be the first published diagram illustrating the concept of a hemidecussation at the chiasm.

Within 5 years he had developed a process for making platinum malleable and soon discovered the new elements palladium and rhodium. He is remembered chiefly for his metallurgic contributions and as the inventor of the camera lucida. The Wollaston medal is given out periodically by the British Geological Society.

In 1824, aged 58 years, a century after Vater and Heinecke, Wollaston, apparently without knowledge of Newton's ideas or knowledge of the clinical cases of the 18th century and strictly on the basis of his own transient loss of vision to one side, conceived the idea of a hemidecussation at the chiasm. He argued persuasively that a homonymous field loss would be impossible without such a hemidecussation. Wollaston described his own transient loss of vision as follows[8]:

'It is now more than twenty years since I was first affected with the peculiar state of vision to which I allude, in consequence of violent exercise I had taken for two or three hours before. I suddenly found that I could see but half of the face of a man whom I met: and it was the same with respect to every object I looked at. In attempting to read the name JOHNSON over a door, I saw only SON; the commencement of the name being wholly obliterated to my view. In this instance the loss of sight was towards my left. This blindness was not so complete as to amount to absolute blackness, but was a shaded darkness without definite outline. The complaint was of short duration, and in about a quarter of an hour might be said to be wholly gone, having receded with a gradual motion from the centre of vision obliquely upwards toward the left. It is now about fifteen months since a similar affection occurred again to myself, without my being able to assign any cause to it whatever, or to connect it with any previous or subsequent indisposition. The blindness was first observed, as before, in looking at the face of a person I met, whose *left* eye was to my sight obliterated. My blindness was in this instance the reverse of the former, being to *my right* (instead of the left) of the spot to which my eyes were directed; so that I have no reason to suppose it in any manner connected with the former affection. In reflecting upon this subject, a certain arrangement of the optic nerves has suggested itself to me, which appears to afford a very probable interpretation of a set of facts, which are not consistent with the generally received hypothesis of the decussation of the optic nerves.'

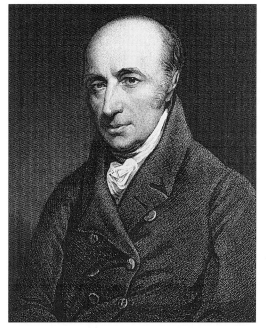

Fig. 2.9 William Hyde Wollaston (1766–1828).

In retrospect these episodes were almost certainly migrainous scotomas without headache. In fact Wollaston went on, in the same paper, to describe five other cases of a similar nature, several of which were associated with migraine. Three years later, late in 1827, Wollaston's left arm became 'numb' and in July 1828 his left pupil became fixed. He described these symptoms to a medical friend as if they were those of another person and on hearing that the medic suggested a terminal brain tumor, he went home and started to dictate papers for publication on all of his completed work; most of these papers were published posthumously. In his final weeks he remained alert and his vision and hearing were good, but he was unable to speak. He died later that year and his autopsy report described an intraventricular hemorrhage. It seems unlikely that the recurrent homonymous hemianopic scotomas that set him thinking about chiasmal hemidecussation were in any way related to his final illness.

Wollaston's publication aroused widespread interest in the chiasmal crossing of the optic nerves. Johannes Müller showed in 1826 that the lateral fibers of the chiasm do *not* cross; soon after, the 19th century microscopists (Von Gudden and Cajal especially) demonstrated that Wollaston, Chevalier Taylor, Vater and Heinecke, and Isaac Newton were right in suggesting a complete semidecussation of optic nerve fibers at the chiasm. Then, as visual-field testing came into general clinical use, it was discovered that damage to the chiasm characteristically produced a bitemporal hemianopia; some of neurosurgery's earliest successes came from removing pituitary tumors that were causing visual loss by pressing on the chiasm. This further encouraged the widespread use of visual-field testing by ophthalmologists.

THE BEGINNINGS OF CLINICAL PERIMETRY

In the middle of the 19th century, European ophthalmology was just beginning to blossom. Georg Beer, who had founded the Vienna school of ophthalmology in 1912, was succeeded by Friedrich Jaeger who was followed by Ferdinand Arlt. In Holland, Cornelius Donders was providing the scientific basis for refraction and accommodation. In Paris, the ophthalmic surgeon Desmarres was busy and productive. In London, William Bowman was at the beginning of his career. In Glasgow, William Mackenzie, was working on the fourth and final edition of his famous textbook. In Germany, Carl Ferdinand Graefe (1787–1840), who had been appointed professor of ophthalmology in Berlin aged 24 years, had a very bright son in 1828 named Albrecht von Graefe. From 1850 to 1870 Albrecht von Graefe was the superstar of ophthalmology. He started to make daily use of Helmholtz's 'Augenspiegel'. When he was still in his mid-20s, he had his own five-storey Augenklinik in Berlin and was known around the world; he gave popular lectures on ophthalmic topics; students came from many countries to work in his clinic; he was personally reshaping his specialty and single-handedly making German the language of 19th century ophthalmology. He was also publishing his own journal, writing almost everything that was published in it. He was a real sky rocket.

One of the many sparks that fell to earth after this ophthalmic explosion was the clinical testing of visual fields.

Long before Helmholtz invented the ophthalmoscope, ophthalmologists were aware that specific regions of the visual field could be lost as the result of appropriate retinal disease. For example, in 1817 Joseph Georg Beer of Vienna used terms such as 'central scotoma' and 'paracentral scotomata', 'concentric contraction of the visual field', and 'half field loss'; in 1842 Karl Himly of Göttingen wrote of 'amaurosis periphica' as opposed to 'amaurosis centralis'; and Desmarres, in 1847, in Paris, described a characteristic loss of the upper field in retinal detachment. So the field loss could be mapped and was being mapped in a rough way before von Graefe, but until Helmholtz's Augenspiegel, there was no visible proof of a retinal lesion to match the scotoma.

For some ophthalmologists, who had been struggling to make sense of scotomas and areas of field loss according to shape and location without being able to see inside the eye, the Augenspiegel freed them from the burden of wrestling with visual fields, for now they could see for themselves whether the problem was in the retina. For von Graefe, however, the ophthalmoscope brought all these observations together and gave extra clinical importance to otherwise unexplained scotomas; von Graefe became the great popularizer of visual-field testing as part of the eye examination.

Helmholtz had recommended that, in order to keep one's bearing during the examination of the ocular fundus, a numbered grid be placed in front of the patient to direct the patient's eye into certain known directions of gaze. It was a piece of blackboard marked in this way that von Graefe used as a tangent screen (*Fig. 2.10*). He worked at a distance of 18 inches and used as a test object a piece of white chalk, about 1 cm across, held in a wire.

In 1856, when von Graefe was only 28 years old, he published a paper called 'Examination of the field of vision in amblyopic disease' (*v. Graefe's Archiv* 1856;**2/2**:258–298) that made it obvious that he had been plotting visual fields on almost everybody for some years. He gave examples of ring scotomata (*Fig. 2.11*), central scotoma, concentric narrowing of the field, enlargement of the blind spot, and homonymous, bitemporal, and binasal hemianopia. He suggested that homonymous hemianopias were caused by unilateral cerebral disease and heteronymous hemianopias by growths at the base of the brain. This pioneering paper started the trend that finally put visual-field testing equipment into the ophthalmologist's clinic.

In 1857, just 1 year after von Graefe's clinical paper, Hermann Aubert and Richard Förster of Breslau began a group of papers

under the title 'Contributions to the knowledge of indirect vision'. They worked in this area for many years, at first using a tangent screen like von Graefe's (*Fig. 2.12*). The test was done in a darkened room and, to keep the fixation from wandering, the screen and the test object were only briefly illuminated by the arc from a Reis bottle. The patient watched the screen through a short tube lined with black felt so that the tested eye was not exposed to the flash.

Aubert and Förster soon decided that it was important to keep the target at a constant distance from the eye in different parts of the visual field (*Fig. 2.13*); they made a simple arc perimeter (*Fig. 2.14*) and continued their studies.

In 1869 they developed an arc perimeter for the practicing ophthalmologist; it was very popular and was known as the Förster perimeter (*Fig. 2.15a*). This perimeter was frequently improved in newer models (*Fig. 2.15b*) and the Förster perimeter dominated the field for the next 15 years.

Meanwhile, as visual-field testing became increasingly popular, various devices were tried: de Wecker, in 1871, improved von Graefe's tangent screen (*Fig. 2.16*) by equipping it with a chin rest and a stand and marking it with concentric circles, starting at 10°; a selection of colored test objects were also offered. Using colored test objects became a major preoccupation of perimetrists that lasted for another 80 or 90 years until Goldmann and Aulhorn became convinced that no new

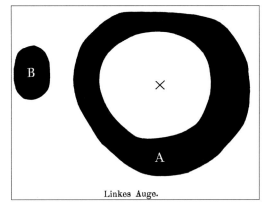

Fig. 2.11 An illustration from von Graefe's 1856 paper showing the blind spot of Mariotte and a ring scotoma in a left eye. The right eye had a similar loss.

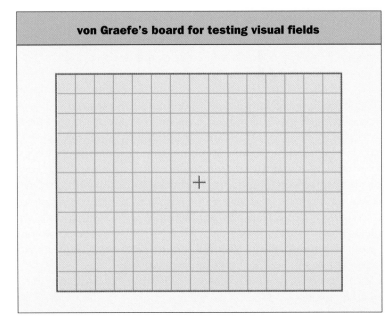

Fig. 2.10 von Graefe's board for testing visual fields.

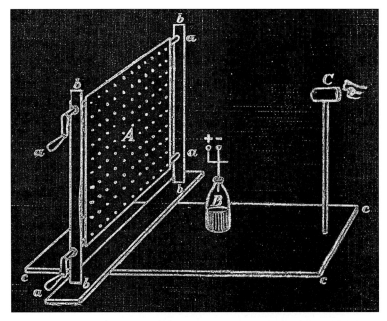

Fig. 2.12 Aubert and Förster's first apparatus for studying visual fields.

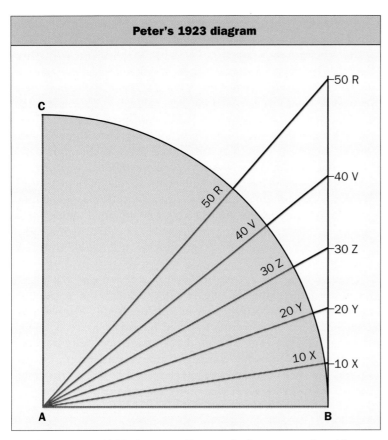

Peter's 1923 diagram

50 R
40 V
30 Z
20 Y
10 X

50 R
40 V
30 Z
20 Y
10 X

C

A   B

Fig. 2.13 Peter's 1923 diagram to illustrate the importance of equidistant targets in the arc perimeter compared with tangent screen. (Peter L. *Principles and Practice of Perimetry*. Philadelphia: Lea and Febiger, 1923.)

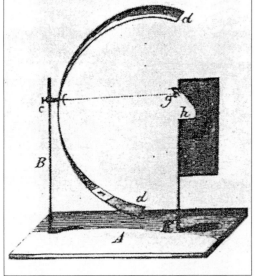

Fig. 2.14 Förster and Aubert's first 'perimeter'.

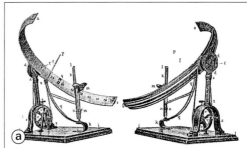

Fig. 2.15 (**a**) Förster and Aubert's first popular arc perimeter (1869). (**b**) A later self-recording version of Förster's perimeter.

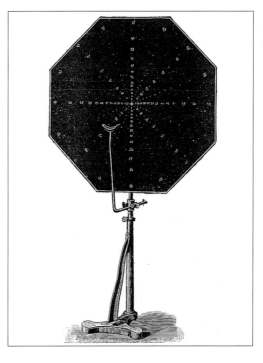

Fig. 2.16 de Wecker's improved tangent screen.

information was supplied by such test objects.

In 1872 Scherk developed a bowl perimeter (*Fig. 2.17*) to eliminate the distracting background that was always present in an arc perimeter. His problem was illuminating the surface evenly. He solved this by splitting the bowl at the zero meridian (i.e. through the blind spot) and connecting the two halves with a double hinge. This allowed him to get light onto the section that was being used. It was big, heavy, and expensive.

For the first 20 years or so after the ophthalmoscope was introduced, the custom was to plot the field on a polar projection (as

we do now) but with the blind spot as the zero mark. This was necessary to accommodate the average eye doctor who was still a very shaky ophthalmoscopist. On looking into the eye the first landmark was the optic disc and the beginner would cling tightly to this landmark as he ventured out towards the periphery. He would follow the vessels away from the disc 'four disc diameters superionasally', for example, looking for the lesion, knowing that he could always follow the vessels back to the disc. There was not much to be seen at the normal macula lutea and to ask the patient to look directly into the light was to risk getting completely lost.

The second generation of ophthalmoscopists picked up their skills during their training years; they used the ophthalmoscope every day, and felt more comfortable looking around inside the eye.

It was Brudenell Carter who stimulated the change in the standard visual-field plot. He had a Förster perimeter but he found it 'costly and cumbrous'. He asked a London instrument maker to make a simpler one with an arc of only one quadrant (*Fig. 2.18*). He wanted to map the location and size of the blind spot with more precision than had been previously attempted and he plotted its location in degrees from fixation (*Fig. 2.19*). He was also able to do what everyone else was doing, that is, plot a line marking the 'perimeter of vision' in the periphery. It was not until 1893 that Groenouw coined the term 'isopter' for a line on a perimetric chart joining points of equal sensitivity.

Carter recommended uniformity in the plotting of visual fields 'to render the charts universally intelligible'. His instrument was smaller, lighter, and cheaper than most of its competitors. It became available in 1873, and proved to be popular. Carter wanted everyone to continue to plot the visual field as seen by the patient but to record retinal locations as distances from the fovea along various radial meridians. All in all, it seemed to make better physiologic sense to plot retinal light sensitivity in this way and it soon became the universally accepted way to map visual fields. By the time Priestly Smith's perimeter arrived in 1882, there were no

more perimeters being made that adhered to Förster's old system of putting the blind spot at the center of the visual field.

The other troublesome problem with visual-field mapping was that it took some experience to decide which quadrant of the visible retina was represented by which quadrant of the field map. Helmholtz's original hand-held Augenspiegel was used as a 'direct ophthalmoscope'; that is, it was held right up to the patient's eye and it provided an enlarged, right-side-up, virtual image. The mirror caught the candlelight from the side and directed it into the patient's eye and the doctor peered through a hole scraped in the silvering on the back of the mirror to see the patient's retina. The same instrument could be used as an 'indirect ophthalmoscope' simply by backing away by about 50 cm and holding a +20 diopter lens in front of the patient's eye. This provided a significantly wider view, with less magnification and a real but *inverted* image.

When viewing the retina, the doctor and patient are face to face, but when viewing the visual field, the doctor and patient are side by side. The doctor has turned through 180°, carrying the image of the patient's retina in his mind. If he has been using a direct ophthalmoscope with an erect image, this 180° turn corrects the optical inversion in the horizontal meridian but the upper retina is still represented in the lower half of the field and vice versa. Conversely, if the mental image of the retina was formed with an indirect ophthalmoscope that provided an inverted image, the blind spot will be on the wrong side but a lesion in the upper retina will produce a defect in the upper half of the field.

The first book devoted entirely to visual-field testing was written by Wilhelm Schön and was published in 1874. The work was performed in Professor Horner's clinic in Zürich. Schön used an arc perimeter and he did not work very closely with the central 10°. He discussed the characteristic kinds of field loss found in glaucoma, retinitis pigmentosa, detachment of the retina, embolism of the central artery of the retina, retrobulbar neuritis, toxic amblyopia, and chiasmal disease.

The next book on the subject, Richard Pauli's *Beiträge zur Lehre vom Gesichtfeld* ('Contribution to the Science of Visual Fields'), was published the following year, 1875.

It is worth emphasizing here that these works were devoted only to perimetry that is, to identifying the perimeter (the very outside

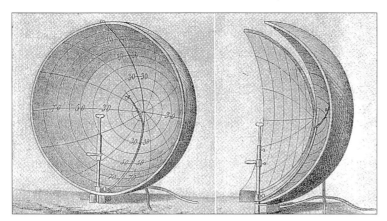

Fig. 2.17 Scherk's 1872 bowl perimeter.

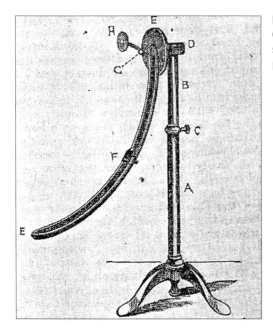

Fig. 2.18 Brudenell Carter's 1873 simplified arc perimeter.

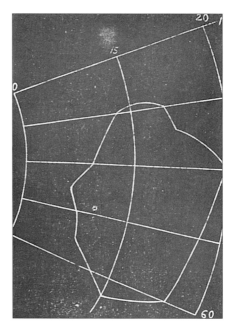

Fig. 2.19 Brudenell Carter's plot of his own blind spot, plotted in degrees from fixation.

limits) of the visual field. They used only one, fairly large, target and were not concerned with partial defects. This was 'the modern way'; von Graefe's tangent screen was considered old fashioned.

During most of the 1870s and 1880s it was generally accepted that the arc perimeter was also satisfactory for mapping central field defects. From this mistake came the idea that there were no central defects of any clinical importance and that the perimeter was the only proper way to plot visual fields. As Ralph Lloyd later pointed out, this was very much like measuring visual acuity with only a 20/40 line, which the patient would either pass or fail.

New devices kept appearing. Schweigger (*Fig. 2.20*) made a 'hand perimeter', which was held up to the patient's eye while the doctor moved the test object. After almost 100 years this is still available in optical supply catalogs. It gives no more information

than confrontation fields and it is considerably more 'cumbrous'. Wilbrand liked to use a 'bed perimeter' for patients who could not get to a regular machine. When finished, he could pack it into a box (*Fig. 2.21*).

Julius Hirschberg (*Fig. 2.22*) stubbornly stuck with a tangent screen marked with rings out to 45°. He studied his patients' visual fields very carefully with this simple device and, in 1875, coined the term 'campimetry' for the tangent screen technique to distinguish it from 'perimetry'.

In 1881, Uhthoff (*Fig. 2.23*) mounted a small campimeter screen onto his Förster arc perimeter.

In these years mechanical ingenuity was given free rein. McHardy's machine kept the patient firmly in place and at the correct distance with a bite bar and a cheek rod. It came with an accessory campimeter plate and a hot lamp overhead. The field could be plotted by pressing the plate against a moving pencil at frequent intervals. Albertotti's machine had a head-stabilizing arm and another arm that held an occluder. Under the table, movements of the arc and the test object were transmitted to a pencil holder by strings and pullies. All the patient had to do was tap. Meyerhausen's perimeter was perhaps overly clever. The cranks that moved the pencil over the chart also moved the test object at the end of a long arm.

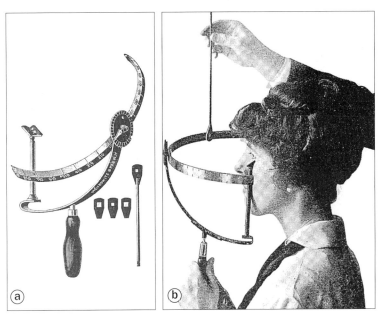

Fig. 2.20 (**a**) Schweigger's hand perimeter. (**b**) Schweigger's hand perimeter as illustrated by Luther Peter (1923).

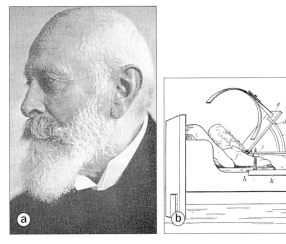

Fig. 2.21 (**a**) Herman Wilbrand (1851–1935). (**b**) Wilbrand's bed perimeter.

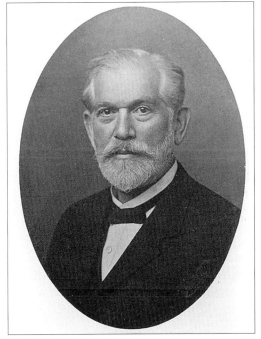

Fig. 2.22 Julius Hirschberg (1843–1925).

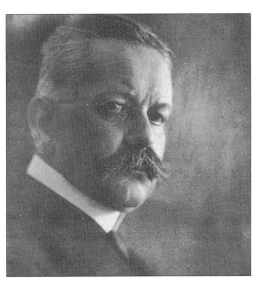

Fig. 2.23 Wilhelm Uhthoff (1853–1927).

There seemed to be a demand for something simpler; and Dana offered his 'Pocket Perimeter' (*Fig. 2.24*).

It was Jannik Peterson Bjerrum (1851–1920) (*Fig. 2.25*), Professor of Ophthalmology in Copenhagen, who reintroduced and popularized campimetry with an important paper in 1889. Bjerrum felt that mapping the subtleties of the central 30° was far more useful than the routine outlining of the perimeter of the visual field that was commonly being done. He is said to have scorned the available perimetric instruments and mounted a tangent screen on the back of his office door. Bjerrum's screen soon grew to 2 m across and it was worked at a distance of 1 and 2 m. It was of black velvet and the radial meridians were marked with inconspicuous black buttons. During the years 1909–1927 his assistant Henning Rønne (*Fig. 2.26*) emphasized the use of a graduated series of small test objects of increasing subtlety. These careful techniques restored some of von Graefe's emphasis on the central visual field. Bjerrum and Rønne were able to demonstrate the characteristics of the earliest field loss in glaucoma, with which their names are still associated. The simplicity and sensitivity of the tangent screen was very appealing and dust covers were put over a lot of arc perimeters.

In 1900, Herman Wilbrand's careful review of perimetry in volume two of the four volume work of Norris and Oliver was authoritative and made a plea for paying attention to retinal physiology and emphasized the importance of thorough quantitative perimetry.

In America, Alexander Duane, Harry Friedenwald, Clifford B Walker and Luther C Peter popularized the work of Bjerrum and Rønne. Duane and Friedenwald put their stamp of approval on the new techniques and recommended a 'tangent curtain' (*Fig. 2.27*); Peter wrote a popular book on the subject.

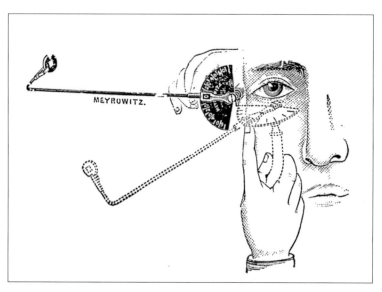

Fig. 2.24 Dana's pocket perimeter.

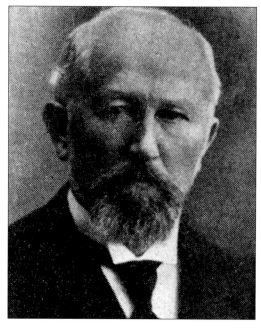

Fig. 2.25 Jannik P Bjerrum (1851–1920).

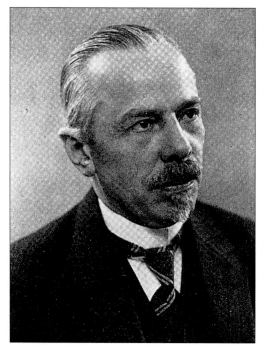

Fig. 2.26 Henning Rønne.

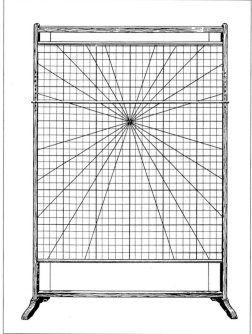

Fig. 2.27 Alexander Duane's 'tangent curtain'.

Clifford B Walker, an ophthalmologist who worked in Harvey Cushing's clinic, made many important contributions to the science of perimetry in the years 1913–1921 (*Fig. 2.28*). Walker did some remarkably careful perimetry and in his laboratory even succeeded in performing perimetry using the pupil as an indicator. He felt that Wernicke had oversimplified the pupillary pathways.

In Scotland the major innovators were AHH Sinclair (1905 and 1906) and Harry Moss Traquair (*Fig. 2.29*) of Edinburgh (from 1914 to 1949). Traquair used both an arc perimeter and a 2-m tangent screen. His many astute insights into visual-field interpretation made his book very popular.

Ralph I Lloyd, developed the stereocampimeter, a device that made it possible to fix with one eye and plot the suppression scotoma in the other, amblyopic, eye (*Fig. 2.30*).

The perimeter of Feree and Rand (1924) not only supplied its own controlled illumination but had a small campimeter attached to the arc (*Fig. 2.31*). This little tangent screen could be used for careful central field testing but could also be slipped along the arc so that free hand scotoma mapping could be done anywhere in the periphery.

The Aimark version of Maggiore's self-recording perimeter (*Fig. 2.32*) was one of the last arc perimeters offered for sale. Bowl perimeters were about to sweep the field.

Hans Goldmann of Bern devised a hemispheric bowl, with a self-illuminated, projection perimeter, in 1945, in which fixation, retinal adaptation, and stimulus size and intensity could be precisely controlled. The field could be readily recorded by means of an ingenious pantograph (*Fig. 2.33*). This dependable instrument, made by Haag–Streit of Bern, became the standard kinetic

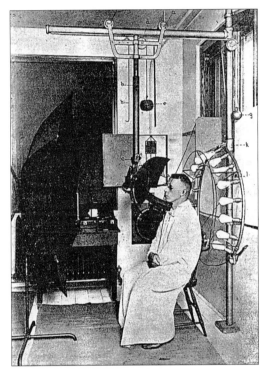

Fig. 2.28 Clifford B Walker's apparatus for perimetry research.

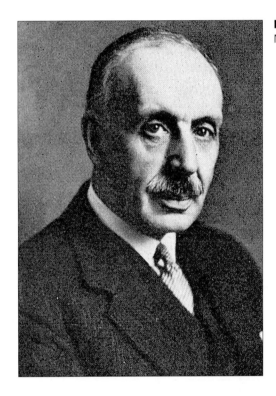

Fig. 2.29 Harry Moss Traquair.

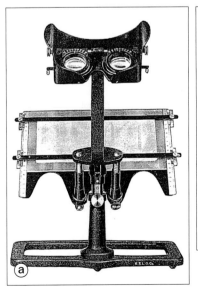

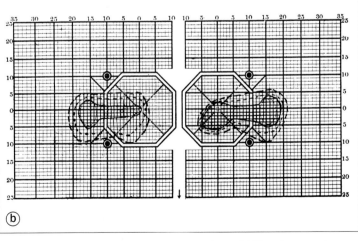

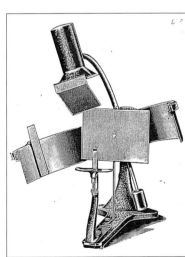

Fig. 2.30 (**a**) Lloyd's stereocampimetric slate. (**b**) The chart used on the Lloyd slate.

Fig. 2.31 Feree–Rand perimeter.

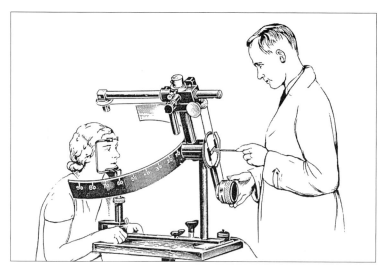

Fig. 2.32 Maggiore's self-recording arc perimeter.

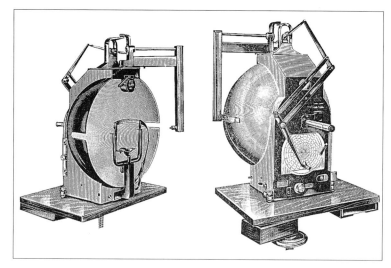

Fig. 2.33 Goldmann's perimeter.

perimeter.

David O Harrington's book *Visual Fields*, first published in 1956, emphasized careful tangent screen work and clinical interpretation. Over the next 30 years the book appeared in several new editions.

The advantages of static threshold perimetry were pointed out in 1933 by Louise L Sloan but the technique did not become popular until Harms and Aulhorn developed a perimeter specifically designed to do static threshold perimetry. This was commonly called the 'Tübinger Perimeter' and was made by Oculus in 1959. Cross-sections of the 'island of vision' could be made by finding the threshold sensitivity at various locations along a single meridian.

In 1971, Mansour Armaly and Stephen Drance developed screening tactics for glaucoma detection using suprathreshold static testing in Goldmann's perimeter.

As the technology gradually became available, computer-controlled, automated, static threshold perimetry was developed. Credit goes especially to John Lynn, Franz Fankhauser, Anders Heijl, CET Krakau, Stephen Drance, Lars Frisén, and many others. Instruments made by the Octopus and Humphrey companies are now in use in the clinics of almost every ophthalmologist and optometrist in North America.

The trouble, of course, with perimetry, automated or not, is that it is a psychophysical test, always dependent on the mood, fears, and alertness of the patient. To quote Harvey Cushing (thinking, no doubt, about Clifford Walker), 'Good perimetry depends not so much upon the perimeter, as on the man behind the perimeter.'

RECENT AMERICAN NEURO-OPHTHALMOLOGY

In the 1930s and 1940s a few American ophthalmologists began to take an interest in the borderland between neurology and ophthalmology. They started to publish papers on clinical neuro-ophthalmology. In this group were David G Cogan of Boston, Frank B Walsh of Baltimore, Donald J Lyle of Cincinnati, C Wilbur Rucker of Rochester, Minnesota, Alfred Kestenbaum in New York, and PJ Leinfelder of Iowa City. It was during these years that the word 'neuro-ophthalmology' began to appear in the titles of textbooks;for example, Rea, 1938, Lyle, 1945, Kestenbaum, 1946, Walsh, 1947.

Frank B Walsh (1895–1978) was, more than anyone else, responsible for making neuro-ophthalmology into a plausible medical subspecialty. At Johns Hopkins he brought together everything that he had learned about neuro-ophthalmology, organized it, tempered it with his own experience and, in 1947, put it into a fat, red-bound book called *Clinical Neuro-Ophthalmology*. The second edition of Walsh's book came out in 1957; it was bigger and redder. Walsh's book and his personal example led a number of young doctors to the idea that there was enough subject matter in neuro-ophthalmology to keep a person busy for a lifetime. Some neurologists and ophthalmologists (most notably William F Hoyt and J Lawton Smith) took extra training in neuro-ophthalmology and began to limit their practice to this area of medicine.[10]

Further reading

1. Polyak S. In: Klüver H, ed. *The Vertebrate Visual System*. (Chicago: University of Chicago Press, 1957) 73–116.
2   Rucker CW. The concept of a semidecussation at the chiasm. *Arch Ophthalmol*. 1958;**59**:159–171.
3. Duke-Elder S, Wybar KC. *System of Ophthalmol, vol II: The Anatomy of the Visual System*. London: Henry Kimpton, 1961, 54–64.
4. Brewster D. *Memoirs of the Life, Writings, and Discourses of Sir Isaac Newton*. 2 vols. (Edinburgh, 1855).
5. Briggs W. Nova Visionis Theoria. In: *Philosoph Collections*. 1682;**6**:167–178.

6. Morgagni GB. *Epist Anat*. 1719;**16**:art. 13.
7. Porterfield W. *A Treatise on the Eye, the Manner and Phaenomena of Vision*. 2 vols. London: A Miller; Edinburgh: G Hamilton & J Balfour, 1759.
8. Wollaston WH. On semi-decussation of the optic nerves. *Phil Tr Roy Soc London*. 1824;**114**(1):222.
9. Lloyd RI. Evolution of perimetry. *Arch Ophthalmol*. 1936;**15**: 713–732.
10. Thompson HS. The growth of American neuro-ophthalmology in the 20th century. *Ophthalmology*. 1996;**103** (suppl):S51–S65.

CHAPTER 3

Correlative Anatomy

A Jackson JE Gillespie

INTRODUCTION

The in-vivo demonstration of normal brain structure using imaging techniques became possible with the development of computed tomography (CT) in the early 1970s. Technical improvements to CT have permitted finer anatomic detail to be visualized, as well as a wide variety of pathologies. Some structures, including many of the cranial nerves and brainstem nuclei, have remained resistant to clear visualization on CT, although many of the pathologic entities that affect them are readily visualized. Magnetic resonance imaging (MRI) emerged in the 1980s as an extremely powerful diagnostic tool, capable of delineating

the anatomy and pathology of the CNS to a degree not possible on CT.

Magnetic resonance imaging not only possesses the advantage of superior soft tissue resolution compared with CT but can also acquire images in any anatomic plane without the use of ionizing radiation (*Fig. 3.1*). In this chapter, MR is used to illustrate the anatomy of the visual pathway and cranial nerves relevant to neuro-ophthalmology. This will be correlated with MRI and CT images of pathology commonly encountered in the investigation of neuro-ophthalmologic problems.

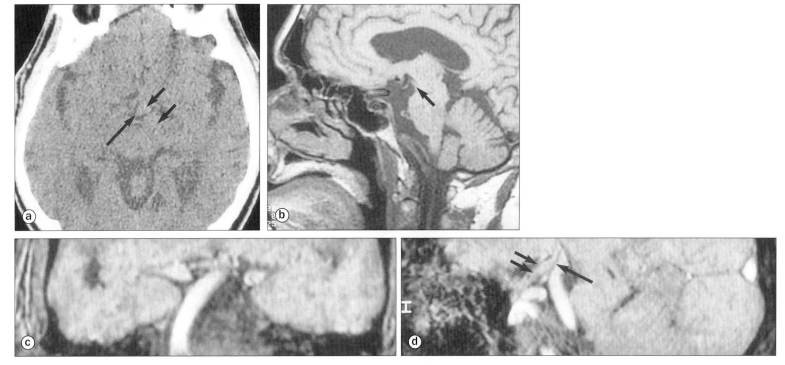

Fig. 3.1 A 75-year-old man with a right homonymous hemianopia. The diagnosis was optic tract compression by ectasia of the basilar artery. (**a**) A CT scan shows a small mass lesion (long arrow) displacing the left optic tract (short arrows). (**b**) A T1-weighted parasagittal MR scan shows an area of signal void adjacent to the left optic tract (arrow). (**c**) A T1-weighted three-dimensional MR time of flight angiogram (high-speed MRI data collection during the very moments that contrast material was flowing through the basilar artery), reconstructed in the coronal plane, clearly shows an ectatic dilated basilar artery extending up to the region of the optic chiasm. (**d**) An oblique reconstruction through the chiasm and left optic tract confirms compression of the tract (short arrows) by the basilar artery (long arrow).

SIGNAL CORRELATES OF MR IMAGES

It is well beyond the scope of this chapter to discuss the physical principles underlying MRI. Given the extensive use of MR images in this chapter, however, it is appropriate to summarize some basic principles of MR image interpretation.

Both CT and MRI are examples of digital imaging in which the numerical data obtained during scanning are represented by shades of gray, forming a recognizable anatomic image. In CT, this numerical information is based upon only one physical parameter, the X-ray attenuation coefficient of tissue. From this is derived the Hounsfield scale of CT density values, ranging from –1000 to +1000 Hounsfield units, with biologic tissues having a fairly constant position on this scale. Such a fixed scale does not exist for MRI.

In MRI the numerical data obtained represent signal intensity rather than tissue density. The MR signal is produced as the result of the interaction of mobile hydrogen protons (water) excited by radio frequency signals (pulse sequence) within a magnetic field. There are, however, several parameters contributing to MR signal intensity, the major ones being proton density, the T1 and T2 proton relaxation times, and flow (*Figs 3.1, 3.2*). Although each MR image will contain elements of all these factors, the relative contribution of any of the parameters to signal intensity can be varied by choosing an appropriate pulse sequence to give greater influence or 'weighting' to a desired parameter, for example T1- or T2-weighted images.

Altering the 'weighting' of an image can dramatically alter the appearances of the intracranial contents (*Fig. 3.3*). A classic example of this is the appearance of cerebrospinal fluid (CSF) which is dark on a T1-weighted image and bright on a T2-weighted image (*Fig. 3.2*).

Proton density is a determinant of the strength of the MR signal and structures such as cortical bone or calcification with few mobile protons will produce little or no signal. Trabecular bone produces a strong signal because of its vascular and fat component. Conversely, rapidly flowing protons within arteries and many larger veins will generate little or no signal as they do not remain within the MR slice for sufficient time to produce a detectable signal. Specifically designed gradient echo sequences may be employed to render fast-flowing blood bright for the purpose of obtaining MR angiography (*Figs 3.1c, d*).

In general terms, T1-weighted images depict anatomic detail optimally but are less sensitive to pathology. T2-weighted images are much more sensitive to pathology and will show lesions not visible on T1-weighted images. Although there are some notable exceptions, most pathology, including tumors, areas of demyelination, cerebral infarction, and edema, will have a low-signal

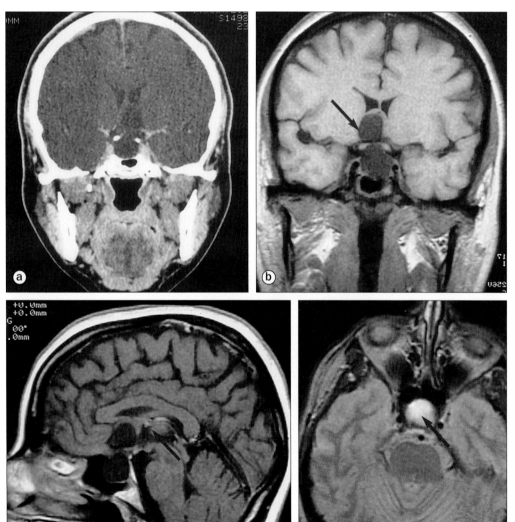

Fig. 3.2 A 54-year-old woman with progressive bitemporal hemianopia. The diagnosis was cyst of Rathke's pouch. (**a**) A coronal direct CT scan shows a low attenuation (cystic) lesion extending up from the pituitary fossa into the cisterna lamina terminalis. (**b**) A T1-weighted coronal MR scan shows a cystic lesion arising in the pituitary fossa extending into the cisterna lamina terminalis and straddling the optic chiasm (arrow). (**c**) A sagittal T1-weighted MR scan confirms the presence of a bi-lobulated cystic lesion and shows the posterior displacement of the chiasmal recess of the third ventricle (arrow). (**d**) A T2-weighted axial MR image shows a high signal within the pituitary mass confirming its cystic nature (arrow).

intensity on a T1-weighted image and a high signal on a T2-weighted image. T1- and T2-weighted images, therefore, provide complementary information.

The appearances of cerebral hematoma on MRI are more complex than on CT. Magnetic resonance signal changes reflect the biochemical composition of the hemoglobin molecule, which progresses from initially oxyhemoglobin, to deoxyhemoglobin, methemoglobin, and finally to hemosiderin, corresponding to the hyperacute, acute, subacute, and chronic stages of clot breakdown. The process is a continuum, with much overlap of the various stages but the overall signal characteristics are summarized in *Figure 3.3*.

Magnetic resonance contrast agents are gadolinium-based products which have the effect of shortening the T1 relaxation times of the tissue through which they are distributed, rendering them brighter on T1-weighted images. Although the physical mode of action of MR contrast agents differs fundamentally from the iodinated contrast agents used in CT, their clinical role is similar; that is, to cross disruptions of the blood–brain barrier and to make cerebral pathology more conspicuous (*Figs 3.9 and 3.9c*). As with CT, the pituitary gland (which does not have a blood–brain barrier) enhances normally on MR after contrast injection, as do the major venous sinuses. Fast-flowing arterial blood, however, remains dark.

THE OPTIC NERVE AND VISUAL PATHWAYS

THE OPTIC NERVE

The optic nerve carries the axons of retinal ganglion cells from the globe to synapse in the lateral geniculate body, forming a major link in the visual pathway. A small number of retinal fibers also pass directly to the tectum of the midbrain, where they play a role in the control of eye movements and pupillary function.

The Intraorbital Optic Nerve
The intraorbital portion of the optic nerve lies in the form of an elongated 'S' extending from the globe to the orbital apex, where it passes through the optic foramen to enter the cranial cavity (*Fig. 3.4*). The intraorbital portion of the nerve is 20–30 mm long

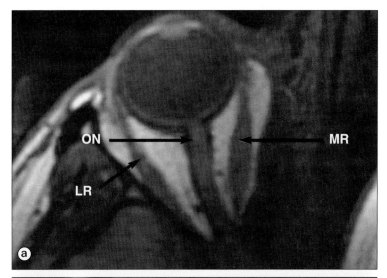
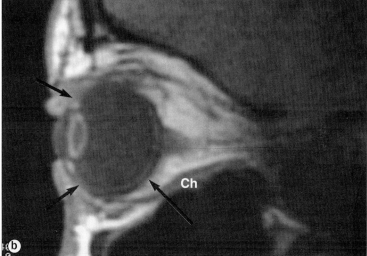
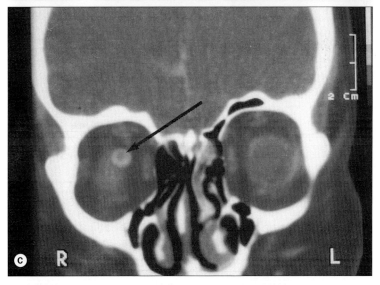

Fig. 3.4 Normal orbital anatomy. (**a**) Axial T1-weighted MR image showing the medial (MR) and lateral (LR) rectus muscles (short arrows) and the optic nerve (ON; long arrow) surrounded by CSF in the perineural space. (**b**) Parasagittal oblique T1-weighted MR scan showing the anatomy of the globe and eyelids. Note the high signal choroid (Ch) and overlying low signal sclera (long arrow). The tarsal plates are seen as areas of intermediate signal in both eyelids with the surrounding, slightly lower signal orbicularis oculi muscles (short arrows). (**c**) Coronal CT scans through the orbits after injection of radio-opaque contrast into the subarachnoid space resulting in enhancement of the perineural space of the optic nerve on the right (long arrow).

Age of clot	T1-weighted	T2-weighted
Hyperacute (hours)	Intermediate–low	High
Acute (1–3 days)	Intermediate–low	Very low
Subacute (under 14 days)	Very high	Very high
Chronic (over 14 days)	Low	Very low

Fig. 3.3 Signal changes in cerebral haematoma in MRI. (low signal, dark; high signal, bright)

and lies centrally within the extraocular muscle cone, where it is supported by fine fibrous septa, that link it to the globe and surrounding rectus muscles. As they enter the nerve at the optic nerve head, the retinal axons become myelinated and the optic nerve bundle increases in bulk so that the nerve is 3–4 mm in diameter. The nerve is surrounded by a dural sheath which fuses with the sclera anteriorly and with the orbital periosteum and ligament of Zinn at the optic foramen. In some individuals, the medial and superior rectus muscle origins extend onto the optic nerve sheath so that contractions of these may cause discomfort if the nerve is inflamed. The dural sheath is lined by arachnoid matter and the nerve itself lies in the CSF-filled subarachnoid space, where it is supported by fine fibrous arachnoid septae. The perineural CSF spaces are in direct continuity with the intracerebral subarachnoid space through the optic foramen. Approximately 10 mm behind the globe, the retinal branch of the ophthalmic artery enters the inferomedial surface of the nerve and runs forward in the center of the nerve to the optic nerve head (*Fig. 3.5*).

The Intracanalicular Optic Nerve

The optic canal is formed by the fusion of the two roots of the lesser wing of the sphenoid bone. The anterior opening of the optic canal into the orbit is known as the optic foramen. The canal runs posteriorly and medially to enter the cranial cavity below and medial to the anterior clinoid process. It contains the optic nerve, some sympathetic fibers from the carotid plexus, and the ophthalmic artery, which lies below and medial to the nerve itself. The canal is lined with dura mater, which is firmly attached to the underlying bone and fuses anteriorly with the dura surrounding the optic nerve and with the periosteum lining the orbit. The first 0.5–8.0 mm of the orbital side of the optic canal is commonly formed purely by dura with no underlying bone. The bony walls of the canal separate it from the sphenoid and posterior ethmoid air cells medially and frontal lobes anteriorly; the optic strut lying inferolateral to the canal forms the superomedial wall of the superior orbital fissure. In some individuals the roof of the canal contains a posterior extension of the frontal sinus and in 4% of patients there are small bony defects in the walls of the canal so that only the dura and sinus mucosa separate the optic nerve from the adjacent paranasal sinuses (*Fig. 3.6*).

The Intracranial Optic Nerve

The intracranial portion of the optic nerve passes posteriorly and superiorly from the optic canal to the optic chiasm (*Fig. 3.7*). The nerve lies immediately below the frontal lobes in the suprasellar cistern and the postcavernous portion of the internal carotid artery lies immediately lateral to the nerve and chiasm. The bifurcation of the internal carotid occurs immediately above the nerve and the A2 segment of the anterior communicating artery passes forward over its ventral surface, lying between the optic nerve and the more medially lying olfactory nerve. The nerve is physically connected to the carotid by the ophthalmic artery, which arises immediately above the cavernous sinus and passes forward, lateral to and below the ophthalmic nerve within its dural sheath.

Lesions commonly affecting the optic nerves are listed in *Figure 3.8* and illustrated in *Figures 3.9–3.15*.

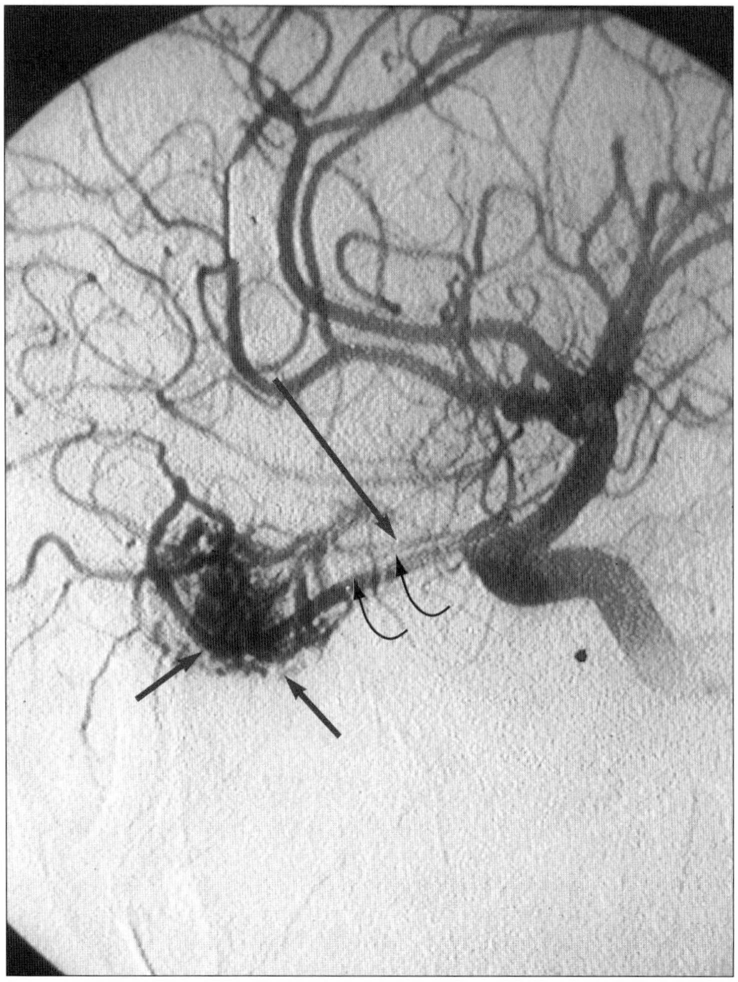

Fig. 3.5 Left-sided carotid angiogram showing a tumor blush with a paraganglionoma of the orbit (short arrows). The tumor is fed mainly by the ophthalmic artery which can be seen to arise from the postcavernous portion of the internal carotid (curved arrows); the highly vascular tumor has caused hypertrophy of the central retinal artery throughout its length (long arrow).

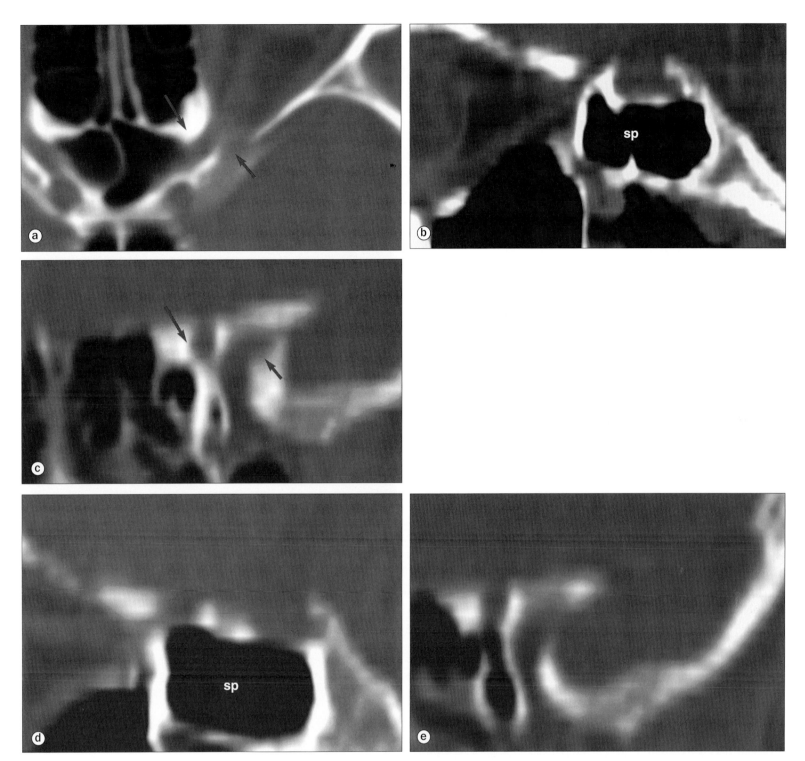

Fig. 3.6 Anatomy of the optic canal. (**a**) Axial, (**b**) parasagittal, and (**c**) curved coronal oblique reformations show the relationship of the canal (long arrow) to the superior orbital fissure (short arrow) and paranasal sinuses.
(**d**) Parasagittal and (**e**) curved coronal oblique reformations show the absence of the bony wall in the inferomedial part of the optic canal where optic nerve is separated from the sinus by only dura.
(sp=sphenoid sinus)

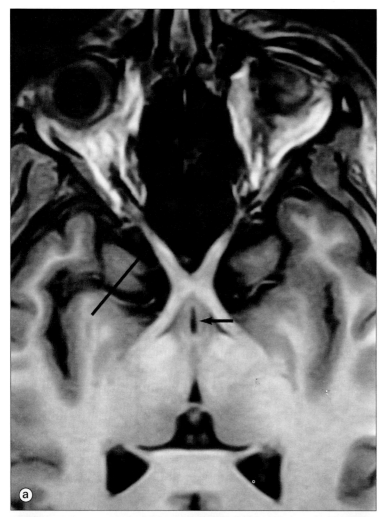

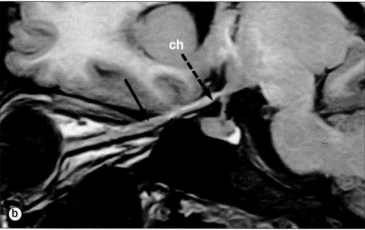

Fig. 3.7 Anatomy of the optic nerve and chiasm. (**a**) An axial oblique T1-weighted MR scan shows the optic nerves within the optic canal (long arrow) and the intracranial optic nerves and chiasm lying behind them. Note also the infundibular recess of the third ventricle extending down behind the chiasm (short arrow). (**b**) A parasagittal oblique reconstruction through the left optic nerve shows the entire length of the optic nerve. The upper long arrow points to the optic nerve in the bilateral apex. Note the perineural space extending out along the intraorbital optic nerve and the narrowing of the nerve within the optic foramen (lower long arrow). The optic chiasm is indicated by the broken arrow. The pituitary gland and pituitary stalk (infundibulum) are seen (short arrow) lying immediately below and behind the optic chiasm(ch, chiasm).

Optic nerve pathology	
A) Optic nerve and sheath lesions	
Neoplastic	Glioma Meningioma
Inflammatory	Optic neuritis Sarcoidosis
Vascular	Ischemic optic neuropathy
Traumatic	Craniofacial injuries Penetrating injuries
B) Lesions of surrounding orbital structures	
Extraocular muscles	Thyroid orbitopathy Pseudotumor Infective myositis Lymphoma Metastases
Bone	Fibrous dysplasia Meningioma Metastases
Retrobulbar masses	Hemangioma Lymphangioma Neurofibroma Schwannoma
Sinus disease	Mucocele Subperiosteal abscess Sinus tumor

Fig. 3.8 Lesions commonly affecting the optic nerves.

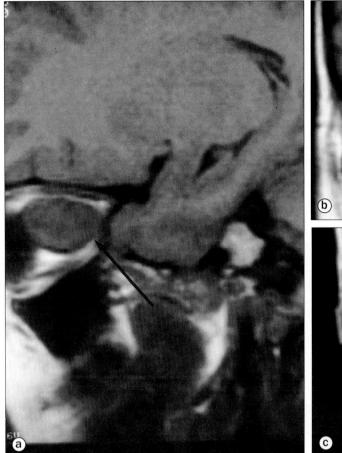

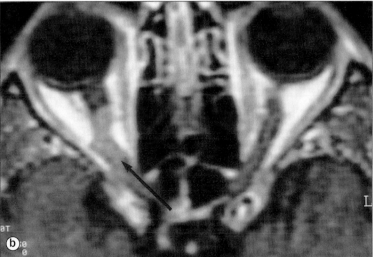

Fig. 3.9 A 6-year-old child with decreased vision in the right eye. The diagnosis was optic nerve glioma. (**a**) A parasagittal oblique T1-weighted image shows a marked enlargement of the intraorbital optic nerve with an intact surrounding perineural CSF space (arrow).

(**b**) A coronal T1-weighted MR scan confirms the location of the mass arising from the optic nerve with an intact (low-signal) perineural space (arrow). (**c**) A parasagittal oblique T1-weighted MR scan after intravenous contrast administration shows a marked increase in the signal of this optic nerve glioma, confirming its high vascularity.

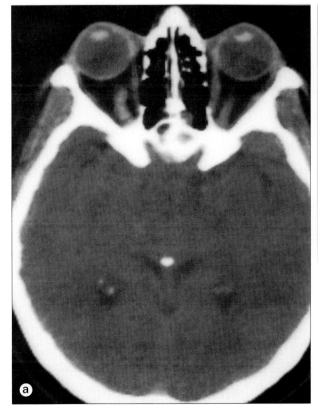

Fig. 3.10 The gradual deterioration of vision in the right eye of a 35-year-old woman. The diagnosis was intradural meningioma of the right optic nerve. (**a**) A CT scan shows an area of high attenuation conforming to the right optic nerve, in keeping with a calcified optic nerve meningioma. (**b**) A postcontrast T1-weighted MR scan confirms the presence of enhancing soft tissue within the posterior half of the right optic nerve sheath (arrow).

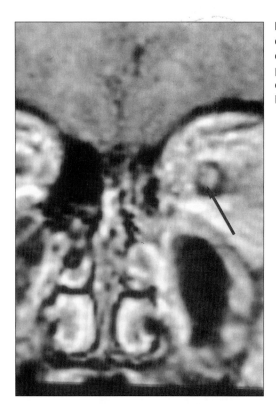

Fig. 3.11 A 21-year-old person with acute deterioration of vision in the left eye. The diagnosis was optic neuritis. A T1-weighted postcontrast MR scan shows enlargement and enhancement of the left optic nerve (arrow) in keeping with optic neuritis.

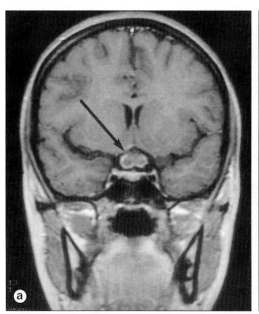
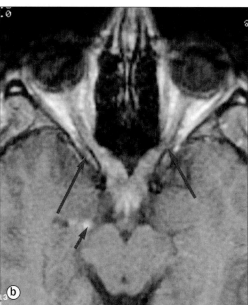

Fig. 3.12 A 13-year-old girl with gradual onset of bilateral visual deterioration. The diagnosis was meningeal sarcoidosis. (**a**) A coronal postcontrast T1-weighted MR scan shows enlargement and peripheral enhancement of the optic chiasm (arrow). (**b**) A parasagittal oblique T1-weighted MR scan after intravenous contrast confirms the enlargement and enhancement of the optic chiasm and shows the extension of this inflammatory process into the optic foramina bilaterally (long arrows). There is, in addition, basal meningeal enhancement around the right medial temporal lobe and infundibulum (short arrow).

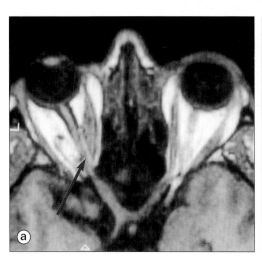
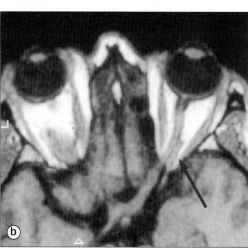

Fig. 3.13 Gradual deterioration of vision in the right eye of a patient with known thyroid eye disease. The diagnosis was orbital apex compression. (**a**) A three-dimensional axial oblique reconstructed T1-weighted MR scan shows an enlargement of the medial rectus muscle on the right and compression of the apical portion of the intraorbital optic nerve (arrow). (**b**) A reconstructed image through the left optic nerve shows less severe compression on this asymptomatic side.

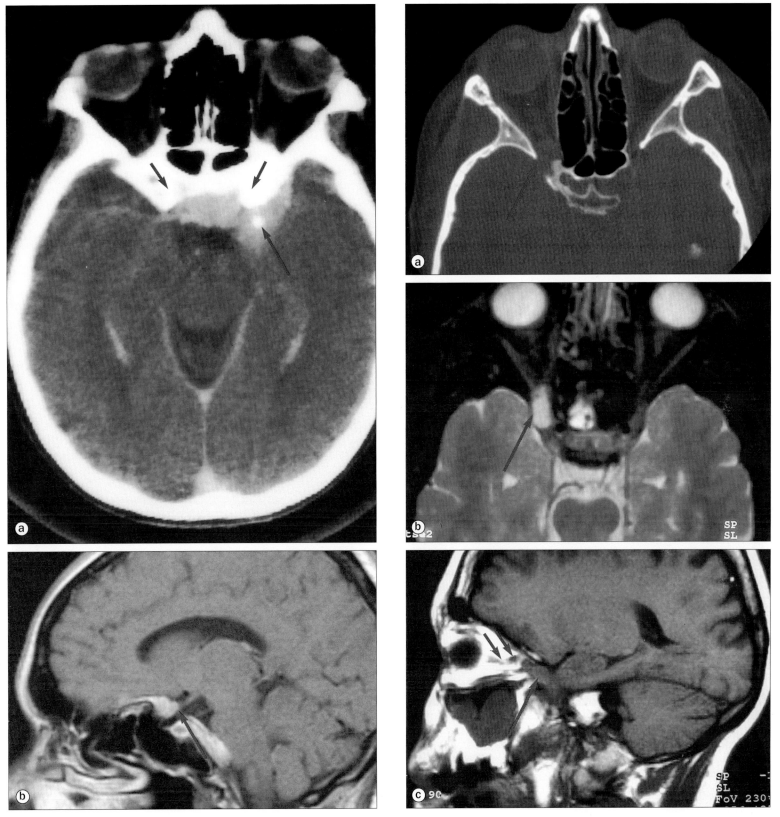

Fig. 3.14 Gradual bilateral visual deterioration in a 35-year-old woman. The diagnosis was optic nerve meningioma. (**a**) An enhancing soft tissue mass is growing across the tuberculum sellae and along the cavernous sinus and petroclinoid ligaments on the left (long arrow). The mass extends across the internal openings of the optic canals bilaterally (short arrows). (**b**) A parasagittal T1-weighted MR scan after intravenous contrast confirms an enhancing en plaque lesion growing along the clivus and across the pituitary fossa which is engulfing the intracranial optic nerves (arrow).

Fig. 3.15 A 24-year-old woman with progressive right-sided visual loss and facial dysesthesia due to a neuroma of the ophthalmic division of the fifth nerve within the superior orbital fissure. The visual loss is caused by compression of the intraorbital optic nerve by the neuroma. (**a**) A CT scan on bone windows shows erosion of the superior orbital fissure on the right by an apical soft tissue mass (arrow). (**b**) A fat-suppressed T2-weighted MR scan confirms the presence of a high-signal mass lesion within the right superior orbital fissure (arrow). (**c**) A parasagittal oblique T1-weighted MR scan shows the mass lesion within the orbital fissure extending upwards within the orbit (long arrow) to compress the optic nerve (short arrows).

THE OPTIC CHIASM

The optic chiasm lies above the body of the sphenoid, most commonly (79% of patients) lying immediately in front of, and abutting onto, the dorsum sellae. In 12% of patients it lies immediately above the diaphragma sellae, or in the sulcus chiasmaticus in 4%, when it is said to be prefixed. In 5% of individuals it lies in a postfixed position above or behind the dorsum sellae (*Fig. 3.16*). This variability in position accounts for the variability of visual field defects caused by mass lesions in the parasellar region.

The chiasm forms part of the anterior wall of the third ventricle and it is in direct contact with CSF in the subarachnoid space anteriorly and in the ventricle posteriorly. The chiasmatic cistern extends forward from the pituitary stalk, over the chiasm and optic nerves, becoming continuous with the olfactory sulcus anteriorly and with the cistern of the lamina terminalis superiorly. Below the chiasm lies the suprasellar cistern extending posteriorly from the tuberculum sellae to the dorsum sellae and communicating posteriorly with the interpeduncular cistern, which lies between the dorsum sellae and the ventral surface of the midbrain (*Fig. 3.17*).

The anterior cerebral arteries pass forward and medially over the dorsal surface of the chiasm and the anterior communicating artery commonly lies above the anterior fork of the chiasm. Immediately above the chiasm lies the optic recess of the third ventricle, which is continuous with infundibular recess that is posterior to it. The interpeduncular fossa lies within the posterior fork of the chiasm and its roof is formed anteriorly by the infundibulum and posteriorly by the mammillary bodies.

Lesions commonly affecting the optic chiasm are listed in *Figure 3.18* and illustrated in *Figures 3.19–3.22*.

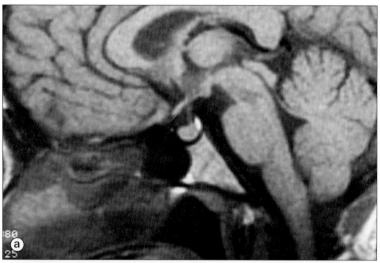

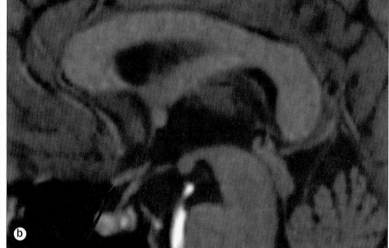

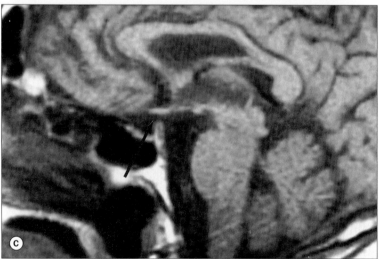

Fig. 3.16 Variations in the normal position of the optic chiasm. (**a**) A prefixed chiasm (arrow). (**b**) Normal position of the optic chiasm (arrow). (**c**) Postfixed optic chiasm (arrow).

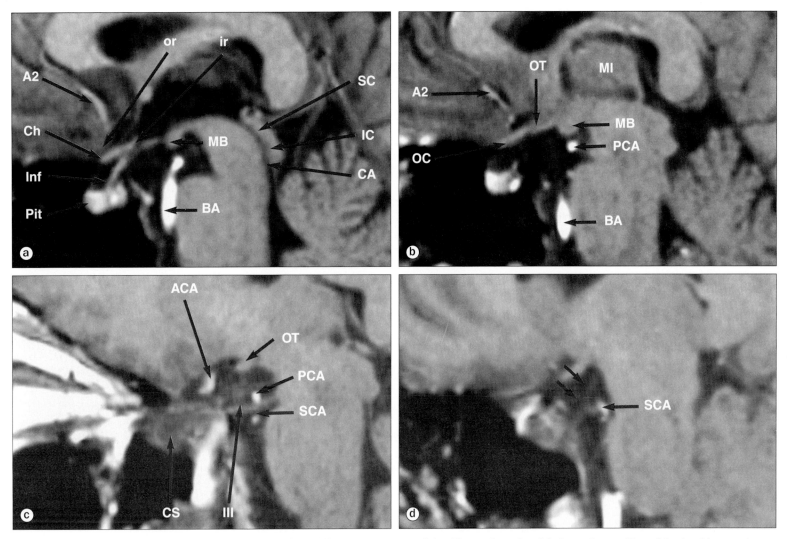

Fig. 3.17 Anatomy of the normal suprasellar cistern. (**a**) A midline sagittal T1-weighted MR shows the positions of the pituitary gland, infundibulum, and optic chiasm. Note also the infundibular and optic recesses of the third ventricle. (**b**) A parasagittal T1-weighted image just lateral to the midline shows the position of the mamillary bodies and posterior cerebral artery. (**c**) A parasagittal T1-weighted image immediately lateral to (**b**) shows the relations of the third nerve, posterior cerebral artery, and superior cerebellar artery. (**d**) A parasagittal T1-weighted image lateral to (**c**) shows the position of the trochlear nerve (short arrows). (A2, anterior cerebral artery; BA, basilar artery; CA, cerebral aqueduct; IC, inferior colliculus; SC, superior colliculus; OR, optic recess; IR, infundibular recess; Ch, optic chiasm; Inf, infundibulum; MB, mammillary body; OT, optic tract; MI, massa intermedia; PCA, posterior cerebral artery; ACA, anterior communicating artery; CS, cavernous sinus; III, third nerve; SCA, superior cerebellar artery.)

Optic chiasm pathology	
Neoplastic	Glioma Meningioma Pituitary adenoma Craniopharyngioma Rathke's Pouch cyst
Vascular	Aneurysms
Inflammatory or infective	Tuberculosis Sarcoidosis Bacterial meningitis Postoperative tethering

Fig. 3.18 Lesions commonly affecting the optic chiasm.

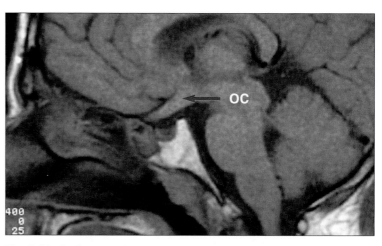

Fig. 3.19 An 8-year-old boy with neurofibromatosis type 1. The diagnosis was optic nerve glioma. A parasagittal T1-weighted MR scan shows an enlargement of the optic chiasm (arrow).

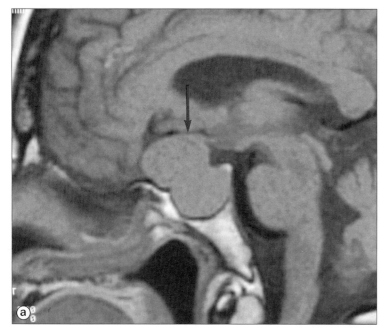

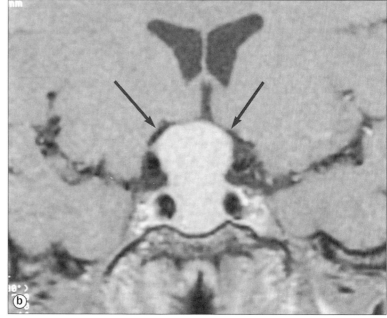

Fig. 3.20 The gradual onset of bitemporal hemianopia in a 15-year-old boy. The diagnosis was pituitary adenoma. (**a**) A T1-weighted parasagittal image shows a large bilobulated pituitary adenoma extending into the suprasellar cistern and displacing and compressing the optic chiasm (arrow).

(**b**) A postcontrast T1-weighted image shows an extensive enhancement of the pituitary adenoma, confirming its vascularity. The prechiasmal intracranial optic nerves can just be identified displaced upwards and compressed (arrows).

THE OPTIC TRACTS AND LATERAL GENICULATE BODIES

The optic tracts pass posteriorly from the chiasm, diverging to sweep around the lateral borders of the cerebral peduncles to reach the lateral geniculate bodies. The lateral geniculate bodies are a part of the posterior thalamus lying below and lateral to the pulvinar (*Fig. 3.23*). They are oval or cap-like structures, which receive the terminal synapses of all optic tract fibers subserving vision and project in turn directly onto the visual cortex via the optic radiations.

The lateral geniculate body is divided into dorsal and ventral nuclei. The small ventral nucleus receives fibers from the optic tract and projects to the midbrain, where its efferents are involved in the control of pupillary function and eye movements. The much larger dorsal nucleus is composed of alternating bands of gray and white matter. There are six gray matter laminae, which are labeled 1–6 from ventral to dorsal.

The optic tracts and lateral geniculate bodies form the roof of the anterior portion of the ambient cistern lying immediately above the posterior cerebral artery. Lateral to the lateral geniculate bodies, the optic radiation extends into the temporal isthmus and below this lies the temporal horn of the lateral ventricle. The hippocampal gyrus of the temporal lobe lies medial to the temporal horn immediately adjacent to the lateral geniculate body. Medial to the lateral geniculate body lies the medial geniculate body, which gives rise to the auditory radiation that passes laterally, above the lateral geniculate body, to the cortex in the floor of the sylvian fissure.

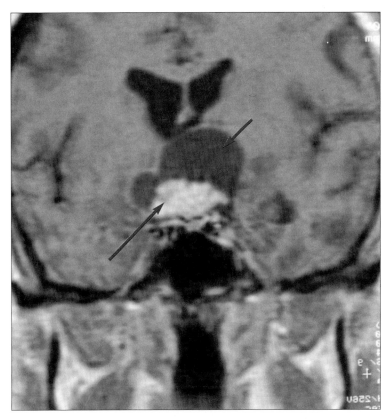

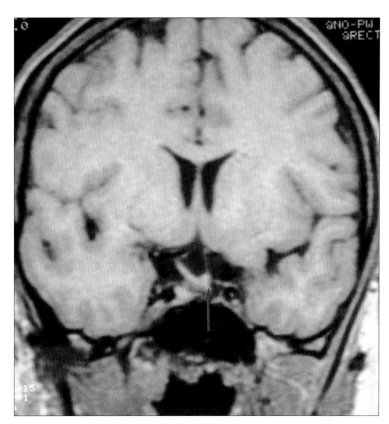

Fig. 3.21 Gross bilateral visual loss due to compression of the optic chiasm by a craniopharyngioma of the suprasellar cistern. A T1-weighted postcontrast coronal MR scan shows a large cystic (low-signal) lesion (arrow) containing a central high-signal enhancing tissue mass (long arrow). The optic chiasm and optic nerves cannot be identified because of extreme displacement and compression.

Fig. 3.22 Progressive bilateral field defects in a 45-year-old man after trans-sphenoidal pituitary surgery. A T1-weighted coronal MR shows the displacement and distortion of the optic chiasm caused by the postsurgical tethering of the chiasm to the operative site (arrow).

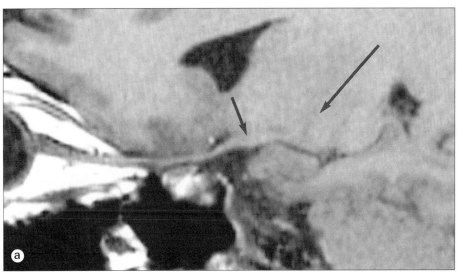

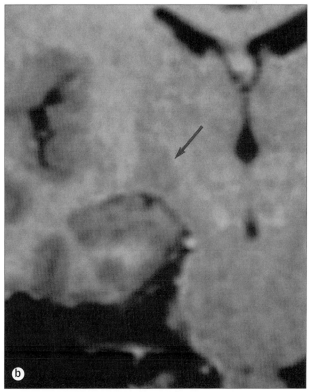

Fig. 3.23 Normal position of the lateral geniculate body. (**a**) A curved parasagittal reformation showing the optic nerve, optic tract (short arrow), and lateral geniculate body (long arrow). (**b**) A coronal T1-weighted image showing the position of the lateral geniculate body (arrow).

THE OPTIC RADIATIONS AND VISUAL CORTEX

The visual cortex, also referred to as the striate cortex or Brodmann's area 17, is situated in the posterior occipital lobe along the superior and inferior lips of the calcarine fissure (*Fig. 3.24*). Although the bulk of the visual cortex is on the medial aspect of the hemisphere it does extend around the posterior pole for a distance of 1–1.5 cm. The optic radiations connect the lateral geniculate body with the visual cortex (*Fig. 3.25*). The radiations pass out directly laterally from the lateral geniculate bodies lying adjacent to the internal capsule before splitting into three main bundles. The fibers of the dorsal and lateral bundles pass directly posteriorly to their termination in the visual cortex. The ventral bundle follows a more complex course, passing anteriorly and laterally around the temporal horn of the lateral ventricle before turning back through the sublenticular portion of the internal capsule to reach the calcarine cortex. This loop of anteriorly directed fibers is known as the 'Meyer–Archambault loop' and appears to extend as far forward as the tip of the temporal horn, accounting for the visual deficits associated with temporal lobe lesions.

Lesions commonly affecting the optic radiations and visual cortex are listed in *Figure 3.26* and illustrated in *Figures 3.27–3.32*.

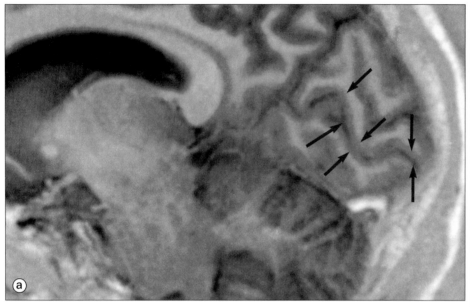
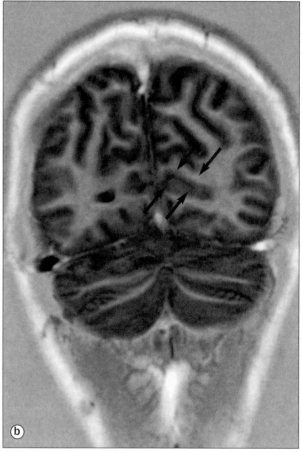

Fig. 3.24 Normal MR scan illustrating the position of the visual cortex (arrows) and calcarine fisssure. (**a**) Parasagittal T1-weighted images. (**b**) Coronal T1-weighted image through the occipital lobe. The calcarine fissure is marked with arrows in both images.

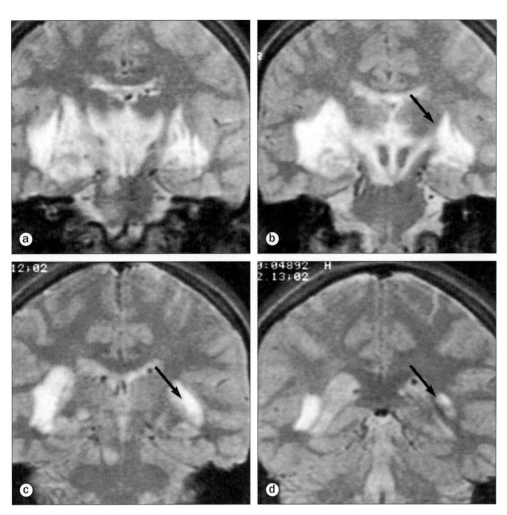

Fig. 3.25 A series of coronal images between the lateral geniculate bodies (**a**) and the occipital radiations (**d**) in a patient with neurosarcoidosis. These T2-weighted images show the extension of high signal due to edema along the optic radiations from this patient with primary optic chiasmal sarcoidosis. The optic radiations are indicated by arrows.

Optic tract and radiation pathology	
Neoplastic	Metastases
	Meningioma
	Glioma
Vascular	Infarct
	Hematoma
	Arteriovenous malformation
Inflammatory or infective	Abscess
	Demyelination
Traumatic	Contusion

Fig. 3.26 Lesions commonly affecting the optic radiations and visual cortex.

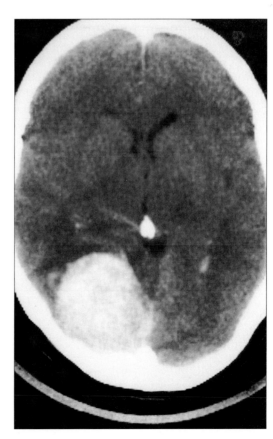

Fig. 3.27 A dense left-sided hemianopia in a 60-year-old woman. The diagnosis was right occipital meningioma. A postcontrast axial CT scan shows a large enhancing mass arising from the posterior falx and compressing the right occipital lobe and visual cortex.

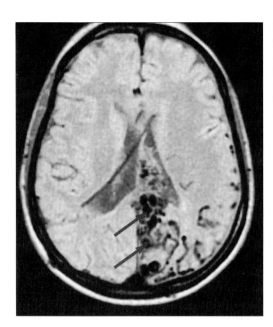

Fig. 3.28 A 23-year-old man with an extensive right-sided homonymous hemianopia. The diagnosis was occipital arteriovenous malformation. A T1-weighted axial MR scan shows numerous serpentine signal voids due to high-flow vessels and dilated and tortuous draining veins (arrows).

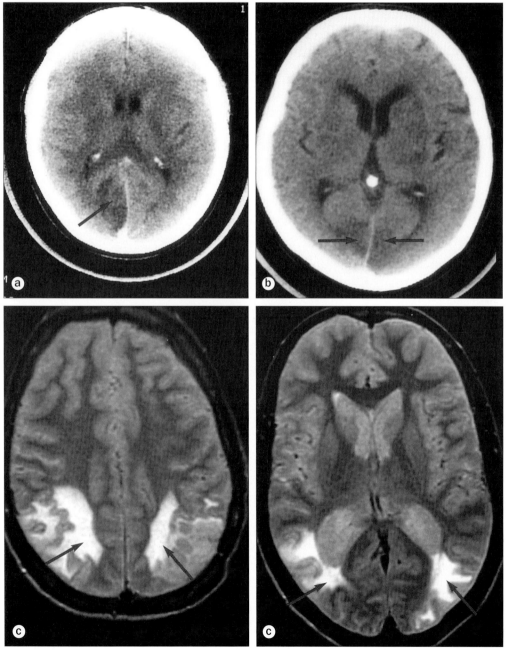

Fig. 3.29 Visual defects due to occipital lobe infarctions. (**a**) Left-sided homonymous hemianopia due to an extensive infarct in the right occipital lobe (arrow). (**b**) Bilateral extensive temporal and inframedial quadrantic hemianopia due to bilateral occipital lobe infarctions (arrows). (**c,d**) T2-weighted axial MR scans show bilateral cerebral infarctions (high signal, arrows) in the occipitoparietal regions bilaterally. The patient had some visual field defect bilaterally but suffered from simultanagnosia due to the involvement of the visual association cortices which lie in this region.

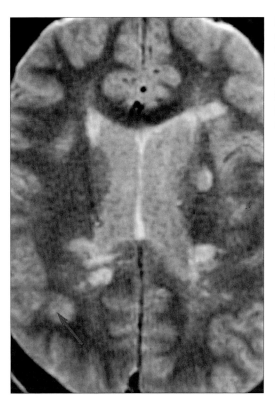

Fig. 3.30 Homonymous visual field defect due to demyelination, in multiple sclerosis. A T2-weighted axial MR scan shows multiple white matter lesions in the corona radiata and periventricular regions, in keeping with multiple sclerosis. A large lesion in the right optic radiation (arrow) corresponded to a left homonymous quandrantic field defect.

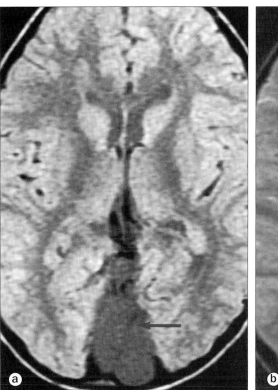
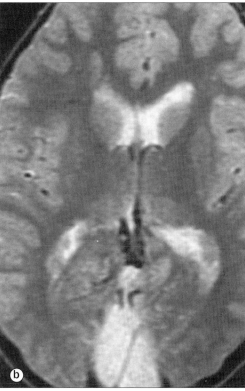

Fig. 3.31 Long-standing bilateral macular and quandrantic field defects in a 27-year-old man. The diagnosis was congenital arachnoid cyst. (**a**) A T1-weighted axial image shows a low-signal cystic mass within the interhemispheric fissure (arrow). (**b**) A T2-weighted MR image shows this lesion to be a high signal (similar to CSF), confirming its cystic nature.

TOPOGRAPHIC ORGANIZATION OF THE VISUAL PATHWAYS

The organization of fibers in the anterior optic nerve corresponds generally to the distribution of fibers in the retina (*Fig. 3.33*). Fibers from the periphery of the retina tend to lie more peripherally in the nerve, central fibers more centrally. Superior, inferior, nasal, and temporal fiber distribution also mirrors the retinal topography but is disturbed by the fibers of the papillomacular bundle. These fibers move into the nasal part of the anterior optic nerve as it nears the optic chiasm. The papillomacular bundle receives fibers from the macular retina and accounts for approximately 30% of the fibers in the nerve. At the level of the chiasm, fibers from the nasal aspect of the retina cross to enter the contralateral optic tract so that each tract carries fibers dealing with visual information from the contralateral visual field. Crossed fibers from the nasal retina begin to separate at the termination of the optic nerve. Ventral crossed fibers, particularly those from the peripheral retina, loop anteriorly into the posterior aspect of the contralateral optic nerve before passing posteriorly into the ventromedial optic tract. Dorsal retinal fibers form a similar loop more

posteriorly within the dorsal half of the chiasm before turning back into the dorsomedial optic tract. Uncrossed fibers retain their relative positions at the lateral edges of the chiasm. Fibers of the macular retina have been described as forming 'a little chiasm' lying posteriorly within the center of the chiasm itself. In the optic tract the corresponding crossed and uncrossed fibers converge so that the upper retinal fibers lie dorsomedially, the lower retinal fibers ventrolaterally, and the macular fibers dorsolaterally.

During evolutionary development the lateral geniculate body and the tract have undergone a 90° rotation so that upper retinal fibers lie medially, and lower retinal fibers laterally. This twist is corrected in the optic radiations so that in all other parts of the visual pathways the upper retinal fibers lie above, and the lower retinal fibers below. Within the lateral geniculate body, crossed fibers terminate in cell layers 1, 4, and 6, while uncrossed fibers terminate in layers 2, 3, and 5. The fibers of the macular retina terminate in the caudal two-thirds of the upper part of the lateral geniculate body. More peripheral retinal fibers are represented progressively more anteriorly within the nucleus, with upper retinal fibers terminating dorsolaterally and the lower retinal fibers more medially.

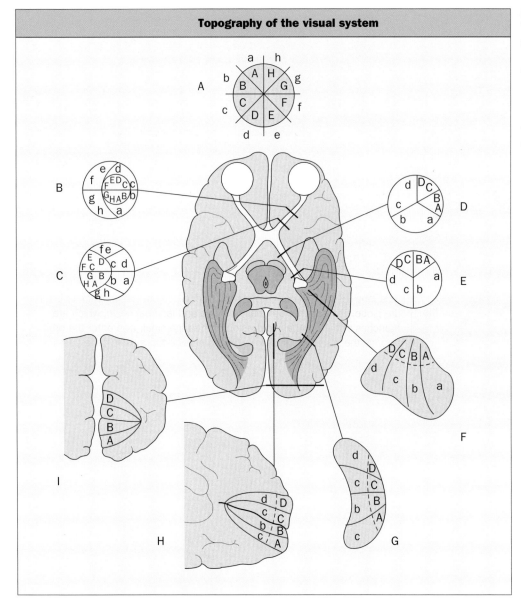

Topography of the visual system

Fig. **3.32** The topography of the visual system. The central image shows the position of each of the schematic sections (**B–I**) on a plan of the optic nerves, chiasm, optic tracts, visual radiations, and visual cortex. (**A**) The field of vision as seen by the patient. (**B–I**) The representation of that visual field in (**B**) the anterior and (**C**) posterior left optic nerve; (**D**) the anterior and (**E**) posterior left optic tract; (**F**) the left lateral geniculate body, (**G**) the left posterior optic radiation, and (**H, I**) in the left visual cortex.

In the dorsal and lateral bundles of the optic radiation the macular fibers lie laterally, with more peripheral retinal fibers located progressively more medially. Upper retinal fibers again come to lie above those from the lower retina. The topographic organization of fibers in the ventral bundle that forms the Meyer–Archambault loop remains contentious. These fibers carry the visual information concerning the contralateral upper temporal field so that lesions of the temporal lobe result in contralateral homonymous superior temporal field defects (see Fig. 3.31). It would appear that fibers from adjacent retinal elements are spatially separated in this portion of the optic radiations, with fibers from the macular retina lying medially.

Within the visual cortex the macular fibers lie posteriorly, capping the occipital pole. More peripheral retinal fibers lie progressively more anteriorly along the calcarine cortex on the medial aspect of the hemisphere. The upper retina is represented above the calcarine fissure and the lower retina below; areas of the retina furthest from the horizontal meridian are represented progressively further away from the fissure.

The Blood Supply of the Visual System

The intraorbital portion of the optic nerve receives its blood supply from the ophthalmic artery, with an extensive collateral circulation from the middle meningeal branch of the external carotid artery (see Fig. 3.5). The intracanalicular optic nerve is supplied by pial vessels from the internal carotid and the intracranial portion is supplied by multiple small perforating arteries arising from the internal carotid, anterior cerebral, and anterior communicating arteries. The chiasm has a dual blood supply with a superior group of vessels arising from the internal carotid, anterior cerebral, and anterior communicating arteries, and an inferior group arising from the internal carotid. The lateral geniculate body has a dual blood supply. The anterior pole and the optic tract are supplied by the anterior choroidal branch of the internal carotid; the posterior pole is supplied by the posterior choroidal branch of the posterior cerebral artery. The optic radiations and striate cortex receive a dual blood supply from the middle and posterior cerebral arteries.

THE ANATOMY OF THE OCULAR MOTOR SYSTEM

The Extraocular Muscles

Eye movements are produced by the four rectus and the superior and inferior oblique muscles (see Fig. 3.4). The inferior oblique muscle arises from the inferior nasal aspect of the orbit just inside its rim and passes backwards and outwards to insert in the lower portion of the globe just behind its equator. All the other extraocular muscles arise near the orbital apex from the annulus of Zinn, a ligamentous structure, which lies around the optic foramen and part of the superior orbital fissure (*Fig. 3.34*). The rectus muscles pass forward from the annulus along the corresponding wall of the orbit to reach the globe where they insert anteriorly to the equator by means of tendinous expansions which fuse with the underlying sclera. The superior rectus muscle is separated from the orbital roof by the levator palpebrae superioris muscle, which

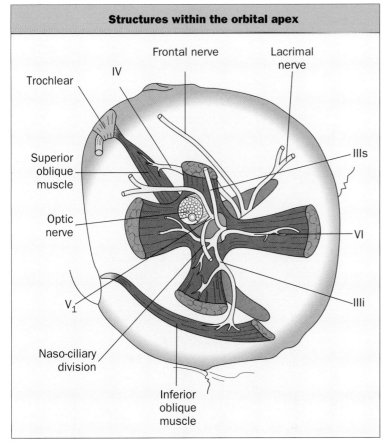

Structures within the orbital apex

Frontal nerve
Lacrimal nerve
Trochlear
IV
Superior oblique muscle
Optic nerve
V₁
Naso-ciliary division
Inferior oblique muscle
IIIs
VI
IIIi

Fig. 3.33 An outline drawing showing structures within the orbital apex. The branches of the ophthalmic division of the trigeminal nerve (V₁) are seen to pass through the superior orbital fissure and the ligament of Zinn to enter the intraconal space. The third nerve also passes through the ligament of Zinn and divides into superior (IIIs) and inferior (IIIi) divisions, which innervate the superior rectus, levator palpebrae superioris, and medial rectus muscles and the inferior rectus and inferior oblique muscles, respectively. The trochlea nerve (IV) enters the orbit through the superior ophthalmic fissure outside the muscle cone to innervate the superior oblique muscle, which passes forwards as a long tendon to hook through the trochlea before turning back to insert on the globe. The superior ophthalmic nerve and lacrimal nerve, which are branches of the ophthalmic division of the trigeminal, also enter the orbit through the superior ophthalmic fissure outside the muscle cone passing forwards along the orbital roof and lateral orbital wall, respectively. The abducens nerve (VI) enters the orbit through the superior orbital fissure and the ligament of Zinn to innervate the lateral rectus.

arises as a short tendon from the undersurface of the lesser wing of the sphenoid, adjacent to the origin of the superior rectus. It passes forward as a flat muscle belly immediately above the superior rectus until it is approximately 1 cm behind the orbital septum, where it ends in a membranous aponeurosis. This membranous expansion fans out across the upper eyelid inserting into the septa, which separate the bundles of the orbicularis oculi muscle, and into the tarsal plate itself. The superior oblique muscle passes forward only a short distance from its origin at the orbital apex, forming a long tendon that passes forwards to the supramedial aspect of the orbital rim. Here it passes through the trochlea, a U-shaped fibrocartilaginous structure that is anchored in the trochlear fossa of the frontal bone. The superior oblique tendon then turns backwards and outwards to reach the upper sclera behind the equator of the globe.

The extraocular muscles and the optic nerve are interconnected by a complex series of thin fibrous septa, which are continuous peripherally with the orbital periosteum. The rectus muscles fanning out from the orbital apex form a cone-shaped space between the orbital apex and the back of the globe, which is delineated by the septa that join the recti. The optic foramen and the lower part of the superior orbital fissure open into the apex of this cone inside the annulus of Zinn (see Fig. 3.34). The optic nerve, ophthalmic artery, superior and inferior divisions of the oculomotor nerve, abducens nerve, and the nasociliary branch of the trigeminal nerve pass into the intraconal space through the annulus of Zinn. The trochlear nerve enters the orbit through the superior orbital fissure outside the annulus of Zinn.

THE OCULAR MOTOR NUCLEI AND NERVES

The Oculomotor Nerve (Third Cranial Nerve)
The oculomotor (third cranial) nerve is the largest of the three ocular motor nerves. It carries motor fibers innervating the superior, inferior, and medial rectus muscles, the inferior oblique muscles, and the levator palpebrae superioris. It also carries parasympathetic motor fibers which innervate the ciliary muscle and the sphincter muscle of the iris.

The Oculomotor Nuclei
The oculomotor nuclei lie in the ventral periaqueductal gray matter of the midbrain, extending from the posterior commissure caudally as far as the inferior colliculus (*Figs 3.35, 3.36a*). Parasympathetic neurons involved in the control of pupillary constriction and accommodation form the Edinger–Westphal nuclei, which lie in the midline immediately rostral and dorsal to the third nerve nuclei. Similarly, neurons supplying the levator palpebrae superioris muscles lie in a single midline subnucleus, which is locat-

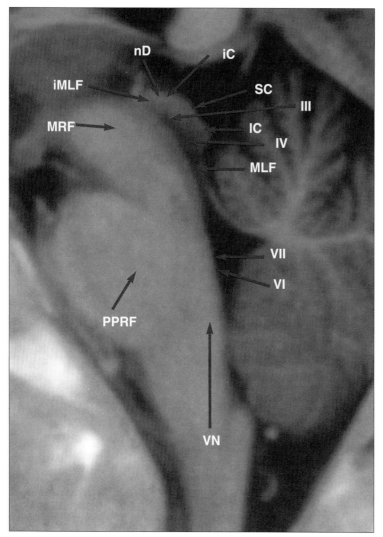

Fig. 3.34 Position of the ocular motor nuclei and their relationship to the internuclear and premotor nuclei in the brainstem. (SC, superior colliculus; IC, inferior colliculus; III, nucleus of the oculomotor nerve; IV, trochlear nerve nucleus; VI, abducens nerve nucleus; VII, fasciculus of the facial nerve; iC, interstitial nucleus of Cajal; nD, nucleus of Darkschewitz; MLF, medial longitudinal fasciculus; iMLF, rostral interstitial nucleus of the medial longitudinal fasciculus; MRF, mesencephalic reticular formation; PPRF; paramedian pontine reticular formation; VN, vestibular nuclei.)

ed dorsally in the caudal part of the nuclear complex. The remainder of the somatic motor neurons form bilateral oval-shaped cell masses extending along the periaqueductal gray matter. Cells projecting to the superior rectus muscles are located medially within the nuclei and their efferent axons cross the midline, passing through the nucleus on the opposite side, to join with axons from the other oculomotor subnuclei on that side and become the oculomotor fascicle. Neurons that project to the inferior and medial rectus muscles and to the inferior oblique muscles project ipsilaterally. The oculomotor fascicle passes ventrally into the body of the midbrain, where the axons remain widely separated, passing ventrally and laterally through the red nucleus and the medial part of the cerebral peduncle. The oculomotor fibers emerge from the interpeduncular fossa on the ventral surface of the midbrain as a series of short fascicles, which immediately form a single nerve trunk. The oculomotor nerve passes obliquely, downwards, forwards, and laterally through the subarachnoid cistern to pierce the dura

lateral to the posterior clinoid process (*Figs 3.36b, 3.36c, 3.37*). The nerve passes between the superior cerebellar and posterior cerebral branches of the basilar artery as it leaves the brainstem and lies adjacent to the medial surface of the posterior communicating artery before it penetrates the dura to enter the cavernous sinus.

The oculomotor nerve passes forwards within the lateral wall of the cavernous sinus (*Fig. 3.38*). The nerve divides into superior and inferior divisions as it passes through the superior orbital fissure to enter the orbit (*Figs 3.39a, 3.39b*). Both trunks of the nerve pass through the annulus of Zinn into the intraconal space and immediately divide into multiple small branches. The superior division supplies the superior rectus muscle and levator palpebrae superioris, whereas the inferior division supplies the medial inferior rectus and inferior oblique muscles.

Lesions commonly affecting the oculomotor nerve are listed in *Figure 3.40* and illustrated in *Figures 3.41–3.44*.

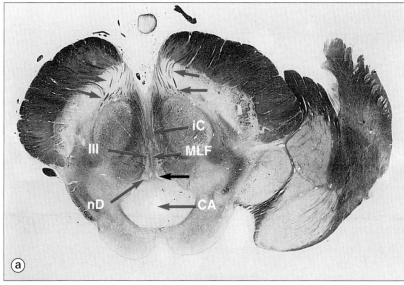

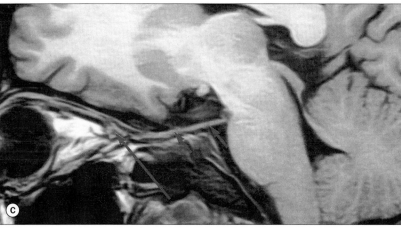

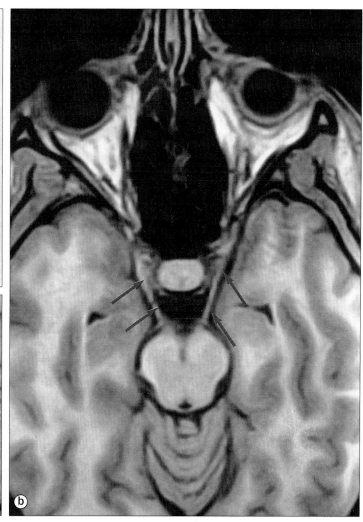

Fig. 3.35 The anatomy of the normal third nerve. (**a**) A histologic section through the brainstem of a normal human showing the position of the oculomotor nuclei (black arrow) within the brainstem ventral to the cerebral aqueduct. Labels can be identified in the legend of Fig 3.34. Note also the fascicles of the third nerve passing forward through the red nucleus to exit the anterior portion of the medial part of the cerebral peduncles bilaterally (short arrows). (**b**) An axial oblique T1-weighted MR scan showing the intracranial oculomotor nerves (arrows). The nerves exit the medial part of the cerebral peduncles at the level of the upper mesencephalon and pass forwards and laterally into the wall of the cavernous sinus bilaterally. (**c**) A parasagittal oblique T1-weighted MR scan showing the course of the third nerve (short arrows) from the midbrain through the wall of the cavernous sinus and superior ophthalmic fissure, to its bifurcation (long arrow) in the posterior orbit.

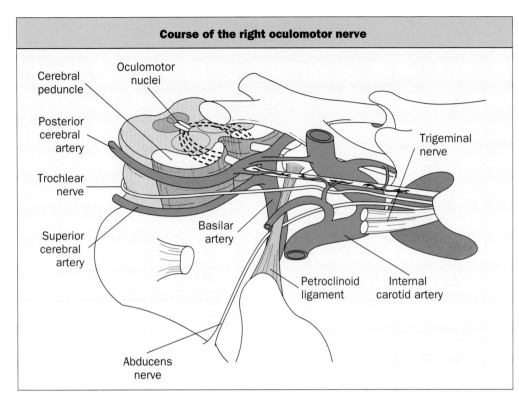

Course of the right oculomotor nerve

Cerebral peduncle

Oculomotor nuclei

Posterior cerebral artery

Trochlear nerve

Superior cerebral artery

Basilar artery

Trigeminal nerve

Petroclinoid ligament

Internal carotid artery

Abducens nerve

Fig. 3.36 A three-dimensional diagram showing the course of the right oculomotor nerve and its relationship to surrounding structures. The nerve arises in the oculomotor nuclei and passes in fascicles anteriorly through the red nucleus and cerebral peduncle to exit the medial part of the cerebral peduncle, where it passes forwards between the origins of the posterior cerebral artery and superior cerebellar artery from the basilar artery. The nerve passes forwards above the petroclinoid ligament into the wall of the cavernous sinus (not shown) to pass lateral to the internal carotid artery and into the superior ophthalmic fissure above the trochlear nerve. The abducens nerve arises in the pontomedullary junction and passes up within the prepontine cistern, pierces the dura along the clivus and passes under the petroclinoid ligament into the body of the cavernous sinus, where it passes upwards and medially to enter the orbit through the superior ophthalmic fissure. The ophthalmic division of the trigeminal nerve, carrying sympathetic fibers from the carotid plexus, also passes forwards through the inferior part of the lateral wall of the sinus.

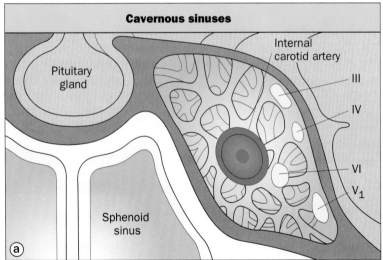

Cavernous sinuses

Internal carotid artery

Pituitary gland

III

IV

VI

V₁

Sphenoid sinus

(a)

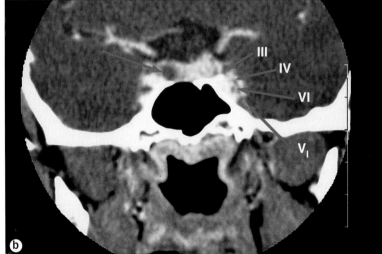

III

IV

VI

V₁

(b)

Fig. 3.37 Structures within the cavernous sinus. (**a**) The position of the oculomotor (III), trochlear (IV), abducens (VI), and ophthalmic (V₁) nerves within the carvernous sinus, relative to the internal carotid artery. (**b**) A coronal postcontrast CT scan in a patient with a small pituitary microadenoma (long arrow). On the right the scan shows the positions of the cranial nerves passing through the wall of the cavernous sinus as illustrated in (**a**).

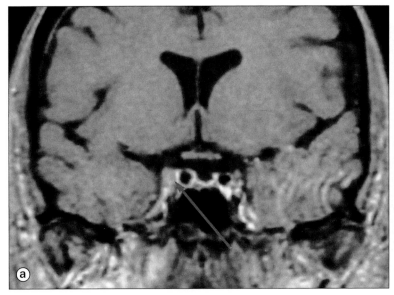

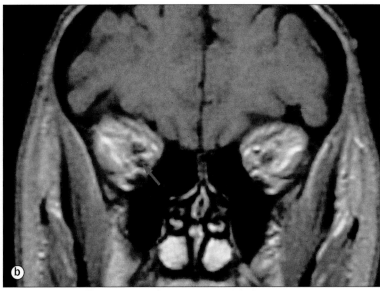

Fig. 3.38 Anatomy of the third nerve in a patient with a right third nerve neuroma. (**a**) The position of the enlarged third nerve in the upper part of the lateral wall of the right cavernous sinus (arrow) adjacent to the internal carotid artery. (**b**) A coronal T1-weighted MR scan shows the enlargement of the inferior division of the third nerve within the orbit lying immediately below the optic nerve (short arrow).

Fig. 3.39 Lesions commonly affecting cranial nerves III, IV, and VI.

Pathology of cranial nerves III, IV, and VI	
A) Brainstem	
Neoplastic	Glioma Metastases
Vascular	Infarct hematoma Arteriovenous malformation
Inflammatory or infective	Abscess Demyelination
B) CSF Cisterns	
Neoplastic	Meningioma Epidermoid Neuroma
Vascular	Aneurysm
Uncal herniation	
C) Cavernous Sinus	
Neoplastic	Meningioma Neuroma Metastases Direct spread of adjacent malignancy
Vascular	Aneurysm Cavernous sinus thrombosis
D) Superior Orbital Fissure	
Trauma Neoplastic	Superior orbital fissure syndrome Orbital apex tumors Bone tumors Meningioma

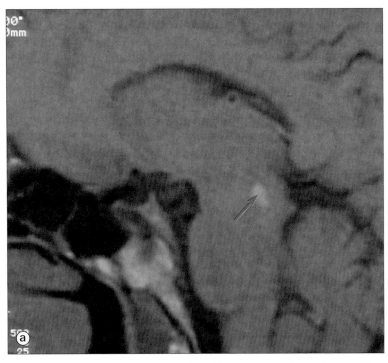

Fig. 3.40 Right-sided third nerve palsy with acute onset in a 65-year-old man. The diagnosis was brainstem hematoma. (**a**) A parasagittal T1-weighted image shows an area of high signal (hemorrhage, arrow) in the region of the periaqueductal gray beneath the tectal plate. (**b**) Axial T2-weighted scan confirms the presence of hemorrhage showing an area of high signal (arrow) in the region of the right third nerve nucleus.

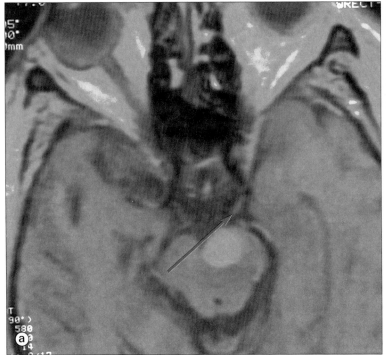

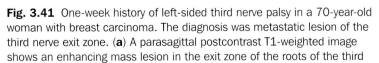

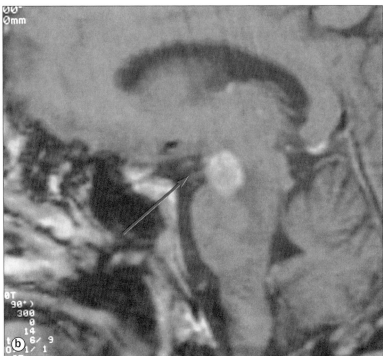

Fig. 3.41 One-week history of left-sided third nerve palsy in a 70-year-old woman with breast carcinoma. The diagnosis was metastatic lesion of the third nerve exit zone. (**a**) A parasagittal postcontrast T1-weighted image shows an enhancing mass lesion in the exit zone of the roots of the third nerve on the left. The third nerve itself can be seen to be displaced by the mass (long arrow). (**b**) A parasagittal image in the same patient shows the focal breast metastasis and its relationship to the third nerve (long arrow).

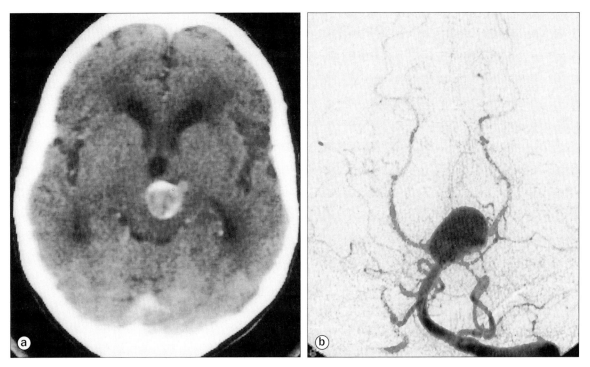

Fig. 3.42 Painful left-sided third nerve palsy in a 55-year-old woman. The diagnosis was aneurysm of the basilar artery. (**a**) A postcontrast CT scan showing a partially calcified enhancing mass lesion in the region of the interpeduncular cistern. (**b**) A left vertebral angiogram showing a basilar tip aneurysm.

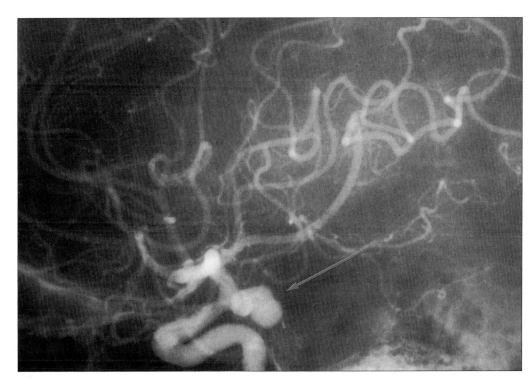

Fig. 3.43 A 58-year-old man with painful left-sided third nerve palsy. A left internal carotid angiogram shows a large posterior communicating artery aneurysm.

The Trochlear Nerve

The trochlear nerve innervates only the superior oblique muscle. The trochlear nucleus lies in the ventral periaqueductal gray matter immediately caudal to the oculomotor complex and its efferent fibers pass laterally and dorsally around the periaqueductal gray matter to converge and decussate in the anterior medullary vellum over the roof of the aqueduct at the top of the fourth ventricle (*Fig. 3.45*). The axons from each nucleus thus innervate the contralateral superior oblique muscle. The nerves exit from the dorsal aspect of the mesencephalon just below the inferior colliculi and pass forward around the lateral aspect of the midbrain in the ambient cisterns (*Fig. 3.46*). The nerves pass between the posterior cerebral and superior cerebellar arteries and around the lateral border of the cerebral peduncles to enter the lateral wall of the cavernous sinus. The trochlear nerve enters the cavernous sinus inferior and lateral to the oculomotor nerve passing forward to enter the orbit above and lateral to the annulus of Zinn in the extraconal space. As the nerve leaves the cavernous sinus it crosses over the oculomotor nerve to lie above it.

Lesions commonly affecting the trochlear nerve are listed in Figure 3.40.

The Abducens Nerve

The abducens nerve innervates the lateral rectus muscle, producing abduction of the ipsilateral eye. The abducens nucleus lies lateral to the midline just below the rostral part of the floor of the fourth ventricle and is partially encased by the fibers of the genu of the facial nerve which pass over its dorsal and lateral surfaces (*Fig. 3.47*). The fascicular portion of the abducens nerve passes ventrally, laterally, and caudally through the pons to the nerve root exit zone, which lies in the pontomedullary junction. Within the pons the fascicle has a number of important relationships, which include the motor nucleus of the facial nerve, the fascicle of the facial nerve, the motor nucleus and spinal tract of the trigeminal nerve, the superior olivary nucleus, and the corticospinal tract. The abducens nerve leaves the medulla in the pontomedullary groove immediately laterally to the pyramid. It then courses upwards along the clivus adjacent to the basilar artery to perforate the dura overlying the clivus just below the petrous ridge. The nerve runs forward below the petroclinoid ligament into the cavernous sinus, where it lies within the body of the sinus lateral to the carotid artery. The nerve is connected with both the carotid sympathetic complex and the ophthalmic division of the trigeminal nerve within the cavernous sinus and enters the orbit through the superior orbital fissure within the ligament of Zinn. The nerve usually has only a short course within the orbit before entering the lateral rectus muscle.

Lesions commonly affecting the abducens nerve are listed in Figure 3.40 and illustrated in *Figures 3.48–3.50*. Lesions producing multiple oculomotor palsies are illustrated in *Figures 3.51–3.53*.

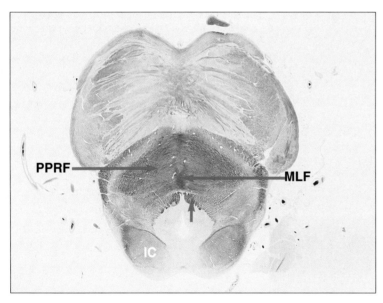

Fig. 3.44 A histologic section through the pontomesencephalic junction showing the position of the trochlear nuclei (short arrow). (IC, inferior colliculus; MLF, medial longitudinal fasciculus; PPRF, prepontine reticular formation.)

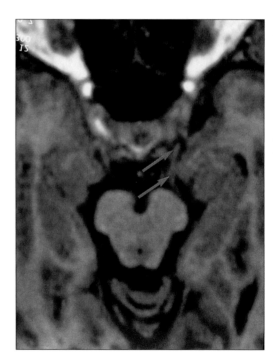

Fig. 3.45 An axial T1-weighted MR scan in a normal individual shows the position of the trochlear nerve as it leaves the ambient cistern on the left to pass forwards into the posterior wall of the cavernous sinus (arrows).

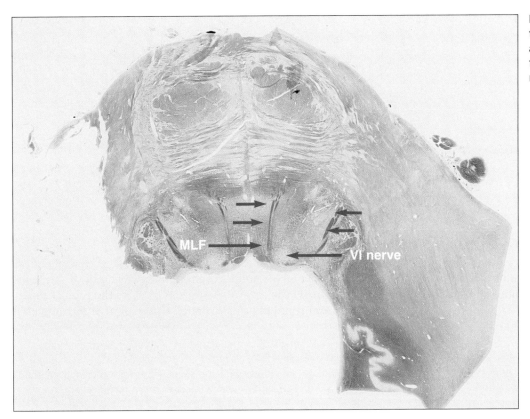

Fig. 3.46 A histologic section through the floor of the fourth ventricle showing the nuclei of the abducens nerves (long arrow) surrounded by the fascicles of the facial nerve (short arrows). (MLF, medial longditudinal fasciculus)

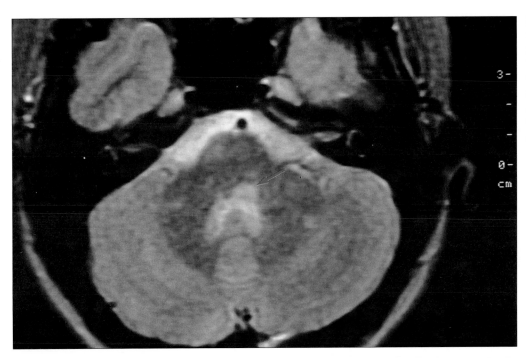

Fig. 3.47 Acute onset of left sixth and seventh nerve palsies in a 36-year-old woman. The diagnosis was multiple sclerosis. An axial T2-weighted image through the pons and fourth ventricle shows a left-sided, high-signal abnormality in the region of the abducens nucleus, where it is surrounded by the fibers of the seventh nerve (arrow), caused by local demyelination.

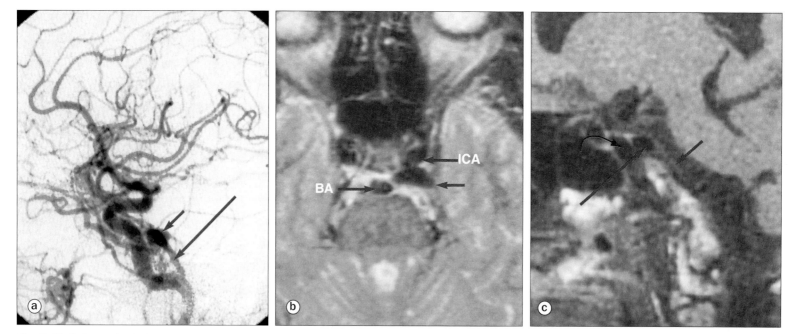

Fig. 3.48 Left-sided painful sixth nerve palsy in a 49-year-old woman. The diagnosis was dural arteriovenous malformation. (**a**) A left common carotid angiogram shows a sheath of small abnormal vessels around the postpetrous portion of the internal carotid artery. These lead to early filling of a dilated posterior cavernous sinus and inferior petrosal vein (short and long arrows, respectively). (**b**) An axial T2-weighted MR scan shows a dilated vascular structure (signal void) to the left of the basilar artery (BA) and immediately behind the internal carotid (ICA) and cavernous sinus (arrow). (**c**) A parasagittal T1-weighted MR scan again shows the dilated venous structure (long arrow) lying immediately behind the intracavernous carotid (curved arrow). On this image the sixth nerve (short arrow) can be seen passing up through the prepontine cistern and being displaced posteriorly and superiorly by the dilated cavernous sinus.

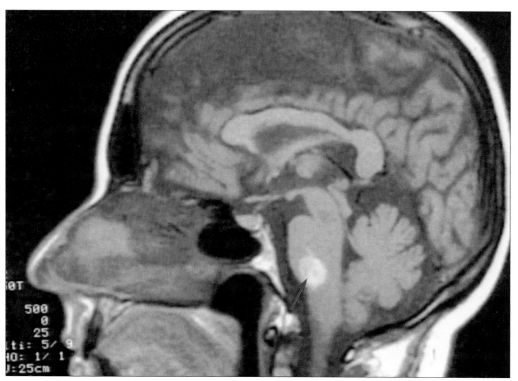

Fig. 3.49 Acute onset of a right-sided sixth nerve palsy in a 48-year-old woman. The diagnosis was brainstem hematoma. A parasagittal T1-weighted MR scan shows an area of high signal (hemorrhage, arrow) in the region of the exit zone of the right sixth nerve at the pontomedullary junction.

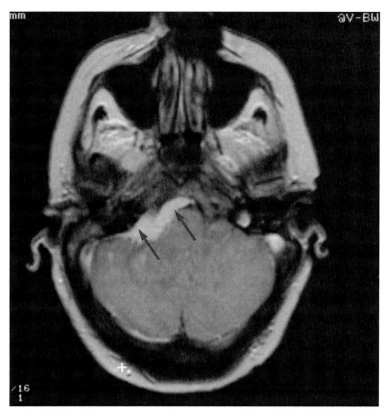

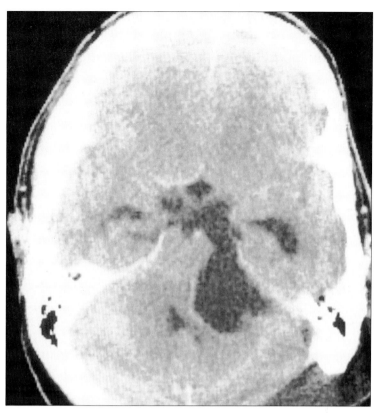

Fig. 3.50 Gradual onset of right-sided sixth, seventh, and eighth nerve lesions. The diagnosis was en plaque posterior fossa meningioma. An axial T1-weighted postcontrast MR scan shows an en plaque enhancing mass lesion of the right side of the posterior fossa at the level of the pons (arrows).

Fig. 3.51 A patient with progressive left-sided deafness, dizziness, hemifacial spasm, and loss of coordinated eye movements on left lateral gaze. The diagnosis was epidermoid tumor. A postcontrast CT scan shows a low attenuation mass lesion within the left cerebello-pontine angle. Note also the craniotomy defect on the left.

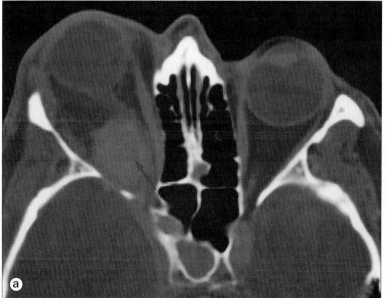

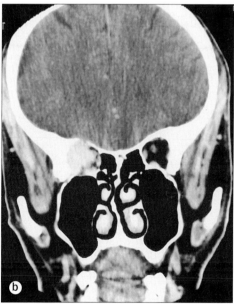

Fig. 3.52 A 52-year-old person with painful left-sided third and sixth nerve palsies and progressive visual deterioration in the right eye. The diagnosis was paraganglioma of the right orbital apex. (**a**) A postcontrast CT scan shows an enhancing mass lesion in the apex of the right orbit, expanding the superior orbital fissure and displacing the optic nerve (arrow). (**b**) A coronal postcontrast CT scan shows a marked enhancing mass lesion filling the orbital apex and eroding the orbital roof.

SUPRANUCLEAR PATHWAYS FOR CONTROL OF OCULAR MOVEMENTS

The central connections of the oculomotor nuclei are complex and a detailed description is beyond the scope of this chapter. Within the brainstem there appear to be a number of important structures involved in the immediate premotor control of eye movements, which include the medial longitudinal fasciculus, the paramedian pontine reticular formation, the rostral mesencephalic reticular formation (MRF), and the nucleus of the posterior commissure. These premotor areas provide an interface for connections with the visual association cortex, the superior colliculi, the vestibular system, and the cerebellum.

Brainstem Premotor Connections

The immediate premotor control of ocular movement can be largely divided into those structures controlling horizontal gaze, which include the abducens nuclei and paramedian pontine reticular formation, and those controlling vertical gaze, which include the MRF, the interstitial nucleus of Cajal, and the interstitial nucleus of the medial longitudinal fasciculus (see Fig. 3.35). All these pathways are connected by a single main tract known as the medial longitudinal fasciculus. This extends from the region of the oculomotor nuclei, caudally to the spinal cord. It lies close to the midline beneath the aqueduct and fourth ventricle within the brainstem and is an immediate medial and ventral relation of the

oculomotor trochlear and abducens nuclei. In the lower medulla it passes ventrally to enter the spinal cord adjacent to the ventral median fissure. Most of the fibers in the median longitudinal fasciculus come from vestibular nuclei. A large ipsilateral ascending projection from the superior vestibular nucleus supplies all the ipsilateral oculomotor nuclei, the nucleus of Darkschewitz, and the interstitial nucleus of Cajal, as well as to the contralateral third and fourth nerve nuclei. A similar ascending pathway from the rostral part of the medial vestibular nucleus crosses the midline adjacent to its origin to supply the same structures on the contralateral side. The median longitudinal fasciculus also contains descending fibers from the nucleus of Darkschewitz and the interstitial nucleus of Cajal, as well as interconnecting neurons between the oculomotor nuclei themselves.

Brainstem lesions affecting oculomotor connections are illustrated in *Figures 3.54–3.56.*

Control of Horizontal Eye Movements

A horizontal 'gaze center' appears to exist adjacent to the abducens nuclei within the paramedian pontine reticular formation. This area receives projections from the vestibular nuclei, cerebellum, superior colliculus, and frontal eye fields, and projects principally to the ipsilateral abducens nucleus. This region appears to control conjugate horizontal eye movement via its connection with the abducens nuclei and the contralateral medial rectus subnucleus of the oculomotor nuclear complex.

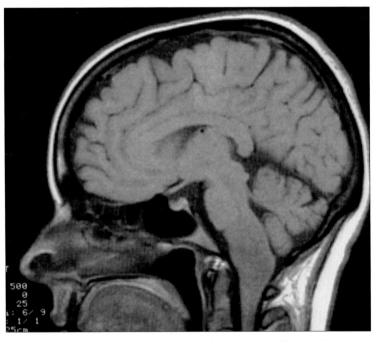

Fig. 3.53 A 33-year-old woman with gradual onset of bilateral sixth nerve palsies associated with swallowing difficulty. The diagnosis was brainstem glioma. A parasagittal T1-weighted image shows gross dilatation of the lower pons and medulla and upper spinal cord.

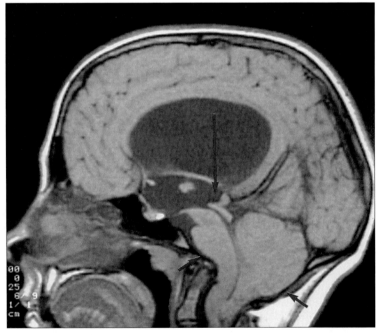

Fig. 3.54 A 17-year-old girl with severe oscillopsia, nystagmus, and loss of upward gaze bilaterally. The diagnosis was Arnold–Chiari type I malformation. A parasagittal T1-weighted image shows a severe Arnold–Chiari malformation with compression of the lower pons and medulla and impaction of the brainstem and cerebellum at the foramen magnum (short arrows). There is secondary obstructive hydrocephalus and compression of the superior colliculus by the dilated third and lateral ventricles can be seen (long arrow).

Control of Vertical Eye Movements

Immediate premotor control of vertical gaze appears to be located in the rostral MRF adjacent to the third nerve nuclei. The cells in this area form the median longitudinal fasciculus, the interstitial nucleus of Cajal, the nucleus of Darkschewitz, and the nucleus of the posterior commissure. This group has a reciprocal connection with the paramedian pontine reticular formation and receives afferent fibers from the vestibular system via the median longitudinal fasciculus and from the premotor visual cortex and superior colliculus. Its other efferent connections are to the oculomotor and trochlear nuclei for control of the vertical rectus and oblique muscles.

Cortical Control of Eye Movement

Three areas of the cortical mantle appear to be particularly involved in the control of ocular movement. These are the frontal eye fields in the frontal lobe, the internal sagittal stratum in the parieto-occipital region, and the middle temporal area in the posterior temporal lobe. There is no described topographic representation of the extraocular muscles in the cerebral cortex, where activation appears to relate to coordinated eye movements.

The Frontal Eye Fields (area 8 of Brodmann)

Stimulation of the posterior part of the second frontal convolution results in conjugate eye movements towards the opposite side; a subpopulation of neurons in this area are specifically related to visually guided saccades. This region has dense interconnections with other areas of cortex, specifically with the visual cortex and the internal sagittal stratum. Efferent fibers from the frontal eye field pass through the internal capsule, where they divide into a dorsal transthalamic pathway and a ventral pedunculotegmental pathway in the rostral diencephalon. The dorsal pathway passes into the thalamus, terminating in the dorsomedial and intralaminar nuclei and in the medial pulvinar. Some fibers pass on to the pretectal nucleus and layer 4 of the superior colliculus. The ventral pathway continues within the medial cerebral peduncle to enter the central pontine reticular formation; these fibers partially decussate to end in the ipsilateral pontine reticular formation and adjacent to the abducens and vestibular nuclei in the contralateral pons. A further branch of the ventral pathway, known as the prefrontal oculomotor bundle, projects to the ipsilateral interstitial nucleus of Cajal and bilaterally to the nucleus of Darkschewitz as well as to the oculomotor nuclei themselves.

The Internal Sagittal Striatum (area 19 of Brodmann)

Stimulation of this area also results in conjugate contralateral deviation of the eyes. Animal work has suggested that this area is related largely to pursuit movements. Efferent fibers from this area pass through the posterior internal capsule to terminate in the pulvinar and the ipsilateral superior colliculus.

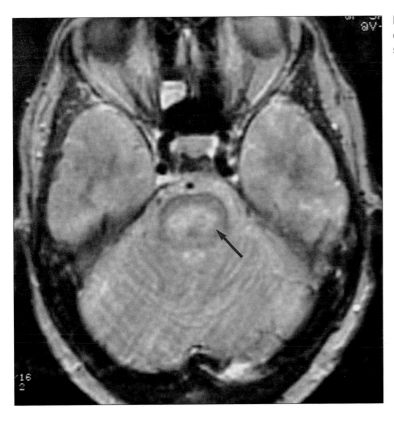

Fig. 3.55 A 41-year-old man with intranuclear ophthalmoplegia. The diagnosis was central pontine myelinosis. An axial T2-weighted MR scan shows a high-signal area of demyelination in the central pons (arrow).

The Middle Temporal Area

In subhuman primates, this area of the posterior central temporal cortex contains cells showing exquisite sensitivity to directional movement within the visual field. In humans, activation of this region has been shown *in vivo* using MRI techniques during visual stimulation. Lesions of the area impair smooth pursuit movements and cause optokinetic nystagmus.

The Superior Colliculus

Lying on the dorsal aspect of the upper midbrain, the paired superior colliculi form one of the major visually related relay nuclei. They are involved in both processing of primary visual information and control of ocular movement. The colliculi consist of seven alternating layers of gray and white matter. The three superficial layers connect strongly with the occipital cortex, whereas the four deeper layers are concerned primarily with oculomotor function. These deep layers have numerous complex afferent and efferent connections. Afferent cortical input is received from primary visual and visual associated cortex, auditory cortex, and from the primary sensory and sensory association cortices. Over 40 subcortical nuclei project to the colliculi, including the intralaminar and reticular nucleus of the thalamus,

the reticular formation of the mesencephalon, pons, and medulla, several of the pretectal nuclei, including the interstitial nucleus of Cajal, the nucleus of Darkeschwitz, the cerebellar, spinal trigeminal, and dorsal tract nuclei, and the cervical spinal cord itself. Afferent fibers from the intralaminar nuclei of the thalamus and the substantia nigra provide a direct afferent input from the basal ganglia so that the superior colliculus receives information concerning all modalities of sensory processing, as well as processed movement-related information from basal ganglia and the cerebellum.

Efferent fibers from the deep part of the superior colliculus can be divided into four pathways. The first of these ascends to terminate in the thalamus and subthalamus, the second descends ipsilaterally to terminate widely throughout the pontine and mesencephalic reticular formation. The third ascends contralaterally terminating throughout the reticular formation of the pons, medulla, and spinal cord, including a projection to the abducens nucleus and to the olivary nucleus of the medulla. The fourth and final group of efferent fibers forms a commissural tract with the contralateral, superior, and inferior colliculi.

Clinically, compression of the tectal plate (*Fig. 3.57*) results in bilateral loss of upward gaze, known as Parinaud's syndrome.

The Vestibular System

The vestibular nerve contains bipolar sensory afferent fibers which arise in the cristae ampullaris of the semicircular canals and maculae acoustica of the utricle and saccule. Their cell bodies are located in the vestibular ganglion which lies within the internal auditory meatus and their central projections terminate within the vestibular nuclei of the lower pons and medulla (*Fig. 3.58*). The vestibular nerve enters the medulla just below the pontomedullary junction and its fibers split into short ascending and long descending branches.

The vestibular nuclear complex lies below the floor of the fourth ventricle and consists of four main subnuclei: the superior nucleus of Bechterew, the inferior nucleus of Deiters, the medial nucleus of Schwalbe, and the descending nucleus (*Fig. 3.59*). There are also a number of physiologically important minor nuclear groups which have been labeled X, Y, and Z. Fibers from the semicircular canals terminate primarily in the superior nucleus and the rostral portion of the medial nucleus, whereas fibers from the utricle terminate principally in the lateral nucleus, and fibers from the saccule terminate in the Y group.

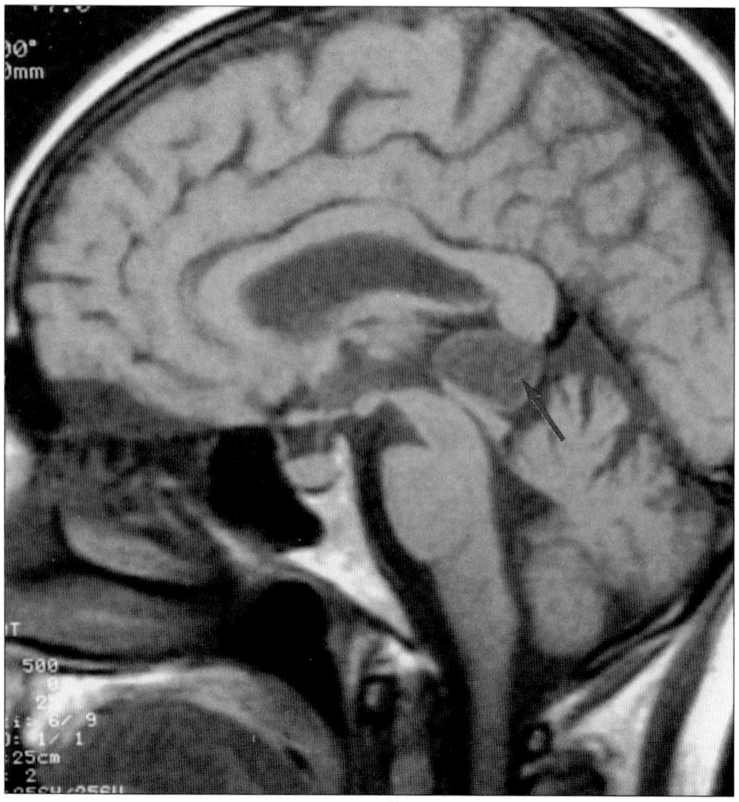

Fig. 3.56 A 23-year-old man with loss of upward gaze bilaterally. The diagnosis was pineal cyst. A T1-weighted MR scan shows a cystic pineal tumor compressing the tectal plate and superior colliculus.

The vestibular nuclei have multiple interconnections with the reticular formation, other brainstem nuclei, the thalamus, and the cerebellum. A direct three-neuron reflex loop allows vestibular input to affect ocular motility. Vestibular impulses affecting vertical gaze are mediated via direct vestibular afferents to the superior and medial vestibular nuclei. These have monosynaptic links with interneurons in the vestibular complex that give rise to contralateral excitatory and ipsilateral inhibitory fibers, which ascend in the medial longitudinal fasciculus and brachium conjunctivum to terminate in the oculomotor subnuclei. Horizontal vestibular ocular reflexes are mediated via a direct excitatory interneuronal projection to the contralateral abducens nucleus and an inhibitory ipsilateral path to the medial rectus subnucleus by fibers lying lateral to the medial longitudinal fasciculus. Relaxation of the contralateral medial rectus is also mediated by means of a crossed inhibitory pathway arising in the abducens nucleus and terminating in the medial rectus subgroup of the contralateral oculomotor complex.

In addition to the simple vestibulo-ocular reflex arcs there are also complex polysynaptic projections involving the cerebellum, paramedian pontine reticular formation, and medullary reticular formation. There are also indirect vestibulo–thalamo–cortical pathways that give rise to reciprocal connections with regions of the parietal cortex in the lateral part of the sylvian fissure.

CONTROL OF THE IRIS

The sphincter muscle of the iris is innervated by parasympathetic neurons arising in the ciliary ganglion within the orbit. The afferent parasympathetic fibers to the ciliary ganglia arise from a series of mesencephalic visceral nuclei which include the Edinger–Westphal nuclei, anterior median nuclei, and the nucleus of Perlia. All of these lie adjacent to the oculomotor nuclear complex. The Edinger–Westphal nuclei appear to give rise to the majority of parasympathetic preganglionic fibers to the iris sphincter, whereas contributions from the other nuclei are less well established. First-order parasympathetic efferent fibers originating in these nuclei pass forward with oculomotor fascicles to enter the oculomotor nerve, in which they travel to their termination in the ciliary ganglion approximately 1.5–2 cm behind the globe. From the ciliary ganglion, postsynaptic parasympathetic fibers pass forwards into the globe in the short ciliary nerves to supply the iris sphincter and ciliary body muscles. The ciliary ganglion also contains postganglionic sympathetic fibers which arise in the superior cervical ganglion and ascend in the carotid plexus to join the fifth nerve in the cavernous sinus; from here they pass forwards in the nasociliary nerves to enter the eye with the long ciliary nerves and innervate the iris dilator muscle. Some sympathetic fibers enter the orbit with the ophthalmic artery and pass through the ciliary

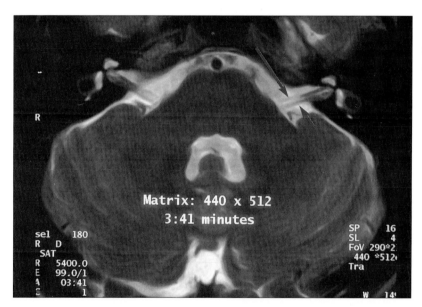

Fig. 3.57 Normal anatomy of the vestibulocochlear nerve. A high-resolution axial T2-weighted MR scan shows the vestibular (short arrow) and cochlea (long arrow) divisions of the eighth nerve leaving the brainstem and entering the inner ear through the internal auditory meatus.

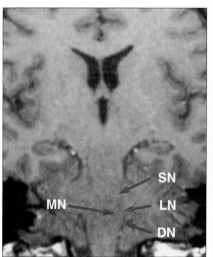

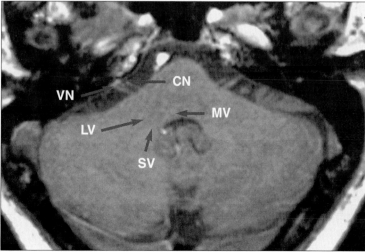

Fig. 3.58 A coronal MR scan in a normal volunteer illustrates the position of the vestibular nuclei. (SN, superior nucleus; LN, lateral nucleus; MN, medial nucleus; DN, descending nucleus.)

ganglion, without synapsing, to provide vasomotor efferents to the optic nerve and choroid. A small number of afferent sensory fibers from the eye also leave the globe in the short ciliary nerves passing through the ganglion without synapsing to join the nasociliary branch of the ophthalmic division of the trigeminal nerve. Within the ciliary ganglion it has been shown that less than 10% of the cell bodies subserve the function of sphincter contraction, whereas the vast majority give rise to motor efferents to the ciliary muscle, so that 90% or more of the mesencephalic parasympathetic outflow is concerned with accommodation rather than with pupillary constriction.

Premotor Pathways Controlling Pupillary Constriction

A number of well-known and clinically important direct reflex pathways affect pupillary constriction. These include the direct and consensual light reflex, the near reflex, and the dark reaction (these will be discussed in chapter 13).

The Light Reflex

The direct and consensual light reflex is mediated by axons of the retinal ganglion cell which bypass the lateral geniculate body to terminate within the dorsal mesencephalon. The reflex appears to be mediated by neurons in the pretectal region of the mesencephalon just rostral to the superior colliculus, the efferent fibers of which hemidecussate to pass to the visceral nuclei of the oculomotor complex. It is of interest that afferent retinomesencephalic fibers involved in the light reflex undergo a hemidecussation in the optic chiasm similar to that of primary visual afferents, so that sagittal section of the chiasm does not abolish the direct or consensual light reflexes (this is because of the mesencephalic hemidecussation).

The Near Reflex

Reflex constriction of the pupil associated with the shift of visual focus to a near object is mediated by a separate reflex pathway. The afferent link in this path consists of visual fibers to the occipital cortex, with an interneuron-mediated second pathway to the visceral nuclei of the oculomotor complex. These fibers are located more ventrolaterally in the upper midbrain than those of the light reflex pathways, with the result that pathologic lesions of the brainstem may specifically spare one of these reflex arcs.

The Dark Reaction

When a light-adapted eye is exposed to darkness for a short period the pupil dilates. This will still occur even if the sympathetic innervation to the dilator muscle has been interrupted, reflecting an inhibitory presynaptic effect on parasympathetic fibers. It is believed that complex polysynaptic pathways via the cortex, thalamus, and hypothalamus play an important role in mediating the normal parasympathetic tone of the iris sphincter muscle. A decrease in this resting parasympathetic tone is felt to be responsible for the miosis that occurs during sleep. Conversely, the mydriasis that occurs with pain or arousal is not entirely eliminated by sympathectomy and reflects, in part, an inhibition of central parasympathetic visceral neurons.

CONTROL OF THE IRIS DILATOR MUSCLE

The iris dilator muscle plays a separate role in the maintenance of pupillary size. It is innervated by sympathetic fibers originating in the hypothalamus which descend in the spinal cord to synapse with preganglionic neurons of the peripheral sympathetic pathway at C8 to T_2. Most of the fibers to the eye leave the spinal cord by the C8, T_1, and T_2 roots to the paravertebral sympathetic chain, where they ascend to pass through the stellate ganglion and the inferior and middle cervical ganglia to terminate in the superior cervical ganglion just below the base of the skull. The ganglion lies between the internal jugular vein and internal carotid artery and gives rise to postganglionic fibers that pass along the internal carotid artery into the skull (*Fig. 3.60*).

Further reading

Atlas SW, ed. *Magnetic Resonance Imaging of the Brain and Spine*. New York: Raven Press, 1991.

Bodal A. *Neurological Anatomy in Relation to Clinical Medicine*. Oxford: Oxford University Press, 1981.

Gillespie JE, Gholkar A, eds. *Magnetic Resonance Imaging and Computed Tomography of the Head and Neck*. London: Chapman & Hall, 1994.

Kretschmann H-J, Weinrich W. *Cranial Neuroimaging and Clinical Neuroanatomy*. New York: Thieme, 1992.

Newton TH, Bilaniuk LT, eds. *Modern Neuroradiology, Vol. 4: Radiology of the Eye and Orbit*. New York: Raven Press, 1990.

Rootman J. *Diseases of the Orbit: a Multidisciplinary Approach*. Philadelphia: Lippincott, 1988.

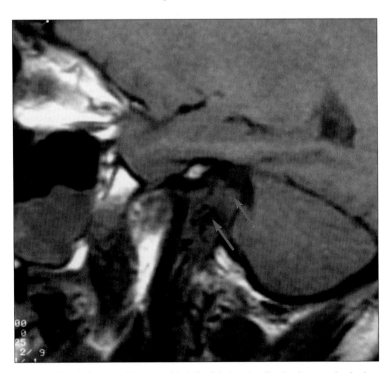

Fig. 3.59 A 56-year-old man with left-sided pulsatile tinnitus and miosis. The diagnosis was glomus jugulare tumor. A parasagittal T1-weighted image shows a typical glomus tumor of the jugular foramen (arrows).

CHAPTER 4

Ophthalmic Neuropathology

M A Farrell and S Kennedy

INTRODUCTION

This chapter describes the gross structural pathology of each of the major anatomical sites concerned with vision. Additionally, important systemic processes that lead to visual impairment are discussed and diseases of mitochondrial origin affecting the visual system have been emphasized. Where possible, a topographic approach has been adopted.

SELLAR, PARASELLAR, AND SUPRASELLAR REGIONS

An intimate knowledge of neuroanatomy is necessary to understand fully the effects of various lesions occurring in this region. Although coronal MR imaging provides almost perfect imaging of the area, it is helpful to observe the inter-relationships of the various vascular, dural, endocrine, and neural structures in a cadaver. The posterior boundaries of the sellar region, particularly the proximity of the clivus and basilar artery, are really only fully appreciated in a cadaver in which the brain has been removed, leaving the brainstem and tentorium in place. Above, the floor of the third ventricle may dip down as far as the diaphragma sella, whereas anteriorly, the sella may blend imperceptibly with the anterior cranial fossa and olfactory groove.

THE SELLA TURCICA

Intrasellar lesions do not give rise to visual symptoms. The arachnoidal cyst that fills the empty sella does not by itself cause visual loss. The associated loss of visual field is due to nerve fiber damage in a chronically swollen optic nerve head (*Fig. 4.1*). Suprasellar extension of an intrasellar lesion will invariably lead to optic nerve compression (*Fig. 4.2*). Pituitary adenomas are the most common intrasellar mass, although, rarely, tumors may arise from the posterior pituitary gland. Meningiomas and schwannomas may also

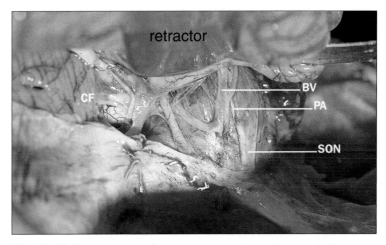

Fig. 4.2 Pituitary adenoma. Autopsy demonstration of a large pituitary adenoma showing suprasellar extension with compression of optic nerve leading to optic atrophy. Temporal lobe retracted and tentorium sectioneD. (PA, pituitary adenoma; SON, squashed optic nerve; BV, blood vessal; CF, cerebellar folia.)

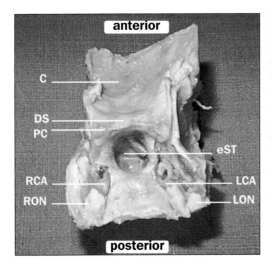

Fig. 4.1 Empty sella syndrome. Viewed from above the sella appears empty. A remnant of viable adenohypophyseal tissue is present. The patient presented with hypothermia and signs of severe hypothyroidism and died from intercurrent infection. There was no history of pituitary disease. (LCA, left carotid artery; RCA right carotid artery; LON, left optic nerve; RON, right optic nerve; DS, Dorsum sellae;PC, posterior clinoid; C, Clivus; eST, empty sella turnica).

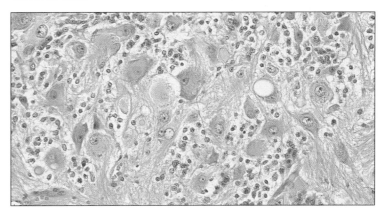

Fig. 4.3 Pituitary gangliocytoma. Microscopic examination shows numerous large ganglion cells surrounded by small deeply staining adenohypophyseal cells. The former contained corticotrophin releasing hormone whereas the latter were shown to contain ACTH. Large compressive pituitary tumor removed from patient with Cushing disease.

arise within the sella and, on occasion, a metastatic tumor may mimic a primary compressive adenoma of pituitary origin. Even with expert neuroradiology and high-quality thin slice coronal MRI, the finding of intrasellar neurenteric cysts, lymphocytic hypophysitis, and gangliocytoma (*Fig. 4.3*) may come as a surprise. An even greater surprise is the rare occurrence of an intrasellar aneurysm arising from branches of the supraclinoid carotid artery.

In neurosurgical practice, the relative incidence of endocrinologically active and endocrinologic silent adenomas and of compressive and non-compressive adenomas varies according to referral patterns with most non-functioning pituitary adenomas emanating from the ophthalmological clinic. A non-functioning pituitary adenoma may be an incidental finding at autopsy. Of the functioning adenomas, prolactin-secreting (PRL) followed by mixed PRL and growth hormone-secreting (GH) adenomas are the two most common. Adrenocorticotropic (ACTH) secreting adenomas are the next most common, whereas follicle stimulating hormone (FSH), luteinizing hormone (LH), and thyroid stimulating hormone (TSH) secreting adenomas are exceptionally rare.

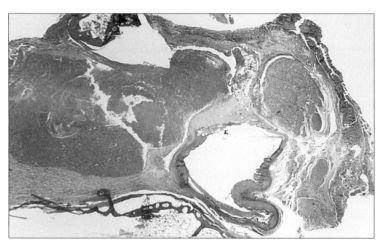

Fig. 4.4 Pituitary adenoma invading cavernous sinus. Whole-mount coronal view of sphenoid air sinus and pituitary fossa to show invasion of the cavernous sinus including the carotid artery.

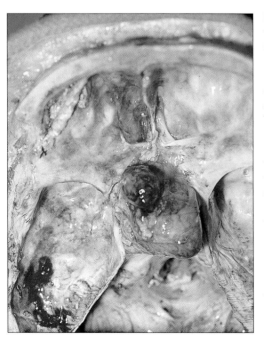

Fig. 4.5 Pituitary fossa sarcoma. Post-irradiation sarcoma replacing the entire pituitary fossa with considerable suprasellar extension. The patient underwent removal of the pituitary adenoma followed by irradiation for 10 years before onset of rapidly progressive visual failure with clinical evidence of hypothalamic insufficiency and death. The sarcoma was considered to have arisen as a result of the irradiation.

Up to 35% of adenomas may show local invasion of dura and bone, a feature that makes complete removal difficult. Lateral invasion into the cavernous sinus is uncommon but, occasionally, a third nerve palsy may herald the presence of a pituitary adenoma (*Figs 4.4, 4.5*).

Malignant pituitary tumors with intracranial and extracranial metastases are described but it is usually impossible for the pathologist to predict on the basis of the histologic features which adenomas will become malignant. From a practical viewpoint, the intraoperative role of the pathologist is to distinguish normal from adenomatous tissue. Subsequent classification of the adenoma is determined by immunocytochemistry (*Fig. 4.6*). Intraoperative difficulties in differentiating adenoma from normal or even hyperplastic pituitary tissue can also be resolved by immunohistochemistry. The presence of six hormones clearly indicates the presence of normal pituitary tissue. Obviously this is not helpful if the adenoma is non-functioning, in which case the pathologist must rely on judgment. The non-functioning adenomas are usually large with suprasellar extension and there is usually a large volume of tissue for histologic analysis. Ectopic pituitary adenomas may be found on the clivus or in the interpeduncular and suprasellar cisterns and may be functionally active.

The normal pituitary gland may be compressed by a variety of lesions, some of which may be associated with visual impairment. Rathke's cleft cysts may reach a large enough size to extend above the diaphragma and cause optic nerve compression and atrophy. The majority of patients will show improvement in visual symptoms if the cyst pressure is relieved by drainage but some patients have been reported to show a delayed chiasmal syndrome after such surgery. Lined by ciliated columnar epithelium (*Fig. 4.7*), these cysts may be difficult to distinguish histologically from neurenteric cysts or from cystic papillary craniopharyngiomas. Intrasellar arachnoid cysts are usually devoid of any identifying lining.

Lymphocytic hypophysitis is a rare cause of pituitary gland enlargement, especially in pregnancy when it may be associated with visual impairment. Of unknown etiology, the enlarged pituitary gland may show a dramatic reduction in size after treatment with steroids.

Empty sella syndrome (**ESS**; see Fig. 4.1) may result from pituitary necrosis induced by radiation, surgery, lymphocytic hypophysitis, or by spontaneous necrosis occurring in a pre-existing adenoma. The majority of patients with 'empty' sellas have no preceding intrasellar pathology but the combination of a widened

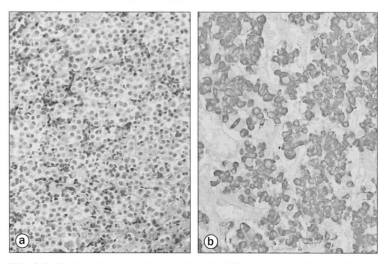

Fig. 4.6 Pituitary immunohistochemistry. (**a**) Monotonous uniform cells typical of pituitary adenoma. (**b**) Tumor immunostained with an antibody to human growth hormone. This was a large tumor with suprasellar extension in a patient with acromegaly and bitemporal hemianopia. The tumor was removed via a sub-frontal approach.

operculum in the diaphragma sella and herniation of arachnoid through the widened orifice induces enough pressure on the pituitary gland over a period of months or years to cause displacement, compression, and sometimes atrophy. Typically, patients with primary ESS have long standing headache with visual-field defects and papilledema. Patients usually have enough residual viable pituitary tissue to sustain normal endocrine function.

Intrasellar gangliocytomas (*Fig. 4.3*) are interesting and rare tumors, probably arising from clusters of hypothalamic neurons that became displaced into the sella during embryogenesis. These neurons may continue to secrete hypothalamic hormones, especially corticotrophin-releasing factor and growth hormone-releasing hormone, the presence of which may cause the pituitary tissue to become hyperplastic or even adenomatous.

Pituitary apoplexy (*Fig. 4.8*) is a life-threatening neurosurgical emergency in which an adenoma undergoes necrosis and hemorrhage. A hypofunctioning adenoma may become acutely non-functioning and lead to collapse. Swelling caused by hemorrhage and necrosis-related edema may impair the optic nerve blood supply and cause blindness. Leakage of blood into the subarachnoid space may give rise to symptoms and signs of subarachnoid hemorrhage. It is thought that an enlarging adenoma impinging on a tight diaphragmatic operculum impairs the gland's blood supply from the superior hypophyseal artery, thereby causing necrosis.

Rare gliomas (ependymoma or astrocytoma) or granular cell tumors of the posterior pituitary present with diabetes insipidus rather than with visual symptoms.

CAVERNOUS SINUS

The cavernous sinus is, in effect, a venous plexus which contains the cavernous segment of the internal carotid artery with its surrounding sympathetic sheath and the ophthalmic and maxillary divisions of the fifth cranial nerve together with the third, fourth, and sixth cranial nerves. Lesions in the cavernous sinus can produce a constellation of ophthalmic symptoms and signs, loosely referred to as the cavernous sinus syndrome. Lesions of primary

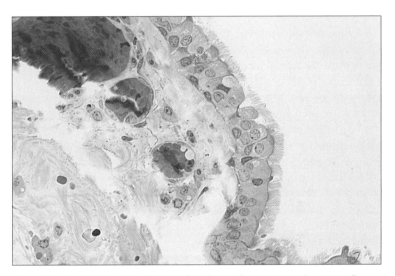

Fig. 4.7 Neurenteric cyst. Biopsy of an intrasellar neurenteric cyst wall showing ciliated columnar epithelium.

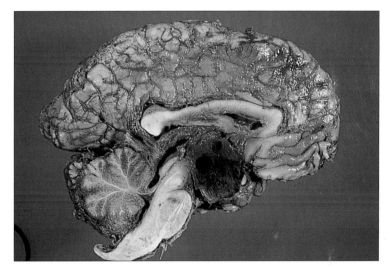

Fig. 4.8 Pituitary apoplexy. Mid-sagittal view of brain showing a large hematoma replacing the third ventricle and hypothalamus. The patient presented in coma and died shortly thereafter. The pituitary fossa contained a large non-functioning adenoma that had undergone necrosis and hemorrhage, and which extended superiorly into the third ventricle and into the subarachnoid space.

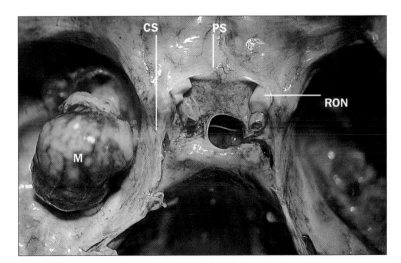

Fig. 4.9 Meningioma of middle cranial fossa. Large meningioma arising from the floor of the middle cranial fossa. There was microscopic extension into the cavernous sinus on the left side.(RON, right optic nerve; PS, planum sphenoidale; CS, cavernous sinus; M, meningioma.)

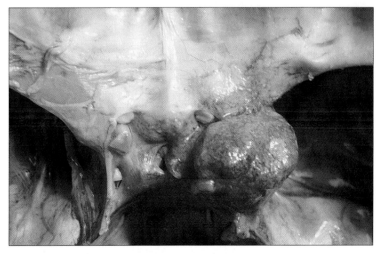

Fig. 4.10 Meningioma. Sphenoidal wing meningioma that caused unilateral optic nerve compression and atrophy.

ophthalmic interest include carotid–cavernous sinus fistulas, carotid artery aneurysms, and tumors, including meningioma (*Figs 4.9, 4.10*), pituitary adenoma, nasopharyngeal carcinoma, lymphoma, and metastases. In most series, nasopharyngeal carcinoma has been found to be the most common malignant cause of cavernous sinus syndrome, followed closely by metastases and lymphoma. Surprisingly, meningioma is infrequent.

Inflammation, especially due to mucormycosis and meningitis, is an important cause of cavernous sinus syndrome, although classic cavernous sinus thrombophlebitis is less common than it used to be. Chronic, non-specific inflammation may involve the cavernous contents and is essentially a diagnosis of exclusion. There is increasing pathologic evidence for the emergence of pathogen-free granulomatous disease, distinct from that seen in Tolosa–Hunt syndrome, which may involve any meningeal area at the skull base and which shows relentless progression, gradually affecting other cranial nerves. There may be a transient response to steroids. It may be radiologically and pathologically difficult to distinguish this process from a meningioma en-plaque.

Trauma may result in tearing or stretching of any of the structures contained within the sinus. Such trauma is usually severe enough to have produced injury to the underlying brain tissue, although in some patients the trauma may be mild. Corotid cavernous sinus fistulas (*Fig. 4.11*) may occur spontaneously or as a result of trauma, the former being due to dural arteriovenous shunts or rupture of an intracavernous aneurysm. Conditions predisposing to spontaneous carotid–cavernous sinus fistulas formation include connective tissue diseases such as Ehlers–Danlos syndrome and Marfan disease. Intracavernous aneurysms are usually of the atherosclerotic type rather than of the congenital berry type.

It is useful to consider diabetic cranial neuropathy at this point because the differential diagnosis will frequently include some of the pathologic entities mentioned above. Typical diabetic cranial neuropathy is sudden in onset, runs a limited course, improves, and most frequently involves the oculomotor nerve. The paucity of detailed neuropathologic descriptions of diabetic ophthalmoplegia using current methods for assessment of fiber size and density has fueled arguments about the relative roles of demyelination

and ischemia as causative factors. The controversy is illustrated by two single patient autopsy studies of diabetic third nerve palsy. In both there was involvement of the cavernous portion of the third nerve. However, one patient showed central loss of myelinated axons accompanied by vascular thickening and the other demonstrated focal demyelination (Dreyfus *et al.* 1957 and Asbury 1970). Detailed contemporary autopsy studies of third cranial nerves in clinically unaffected diabetic patients have shown reductions in myelinated fiber density suggestive of an atrophic process but this process may not have any great relevance to acute diabetic cranial mononeuropathy. The acute onset of most diabetic cranial neuropathies points to a vascular cause, even if good neuropathologic data are lacking. The middle segment of the extracranial third nerve – that is, that segment of the nerve just before it enters the cavernous sinus – does not receive nutrient arterioles from adjacent arteries. Consequently, there is a watershed area in this location that is potentially vulnerable to ischemia.

SUPERIOR ORBITAL FISSURE

The superior orbital fissure is a small area enclosed by the cavernous sinus posteriorly and by the orbit anteriorly. The superior orbital fissure is a relatively narrow zone in which any of the structures passing through in either direction may undergo compression. The superior orbital fissure is occasionally used for access to the contents of the cavernous sinus, particularly for embolotherapy of cavernous sinus vascular lesions. The fourth nerve and frontal and lacrimal branches of the ophthalmic division of the fifth nerve pass out through the lateral aspect of the superior orbital fissure, together with the superior ophthalmic vein. The superior and inferior divisions of the third, sixth, and nasociliary nerves plus the sensory and sympathetic roots of the ciliary ganglion pass through the central zone. Inferiorly lies the inferior ophthalmic vein.

The superior orbital fissure may be unusually large in patients with dysplasia or absence of the sphenoid bone, an uncommon but distinguishing manifestation of neurofibromatosis type 1 (NF 1). Occasionally, an accompanying arachnoid cyst may project through the fissure. Most frequently, structures in the superior orbital fissure are compressed by lesions projecting anteriorly from the cavernous sinus or posteriorly from the orbit. The pathology of these lesions is discussed elsewhere.

Dentigerous cysts and mucoceles of the maxillary sinus and enterogenous cysts of the orbit may cause a severe superior orbital fissure syndrome. Cyst drainage may result in dramatic clinical improvement but removal of the cyst wall is required to prevent recurrence. Meningiomas may arise in the superior orbital fissure and extend into the orbit or cavernous sinus. Involvement of the cavernous sinus usually prevents complete excision.

Structures in the superior orbital fissure are particularly prone to injury, especially after fractures of the zygoma when the nerves crossing the fissure are damaged by bone fragments or by compression due to increased intraorbital pressure at the time of the injury. An orbital fracture may rarely cause superior orbital fissure syndrome. Tumors, either primary or secondary, arising from the surrounding bone may result in superior orbital fissure syndrome.

Despite all that has been written about the Tolosa–Hunt syndrome, detailed pathologic descriptions of this steroid-responsive, recurrent painful ophthalmoplegia are sketchy. The inflammatory process, which is easily visualized on MRI of the superior orbital

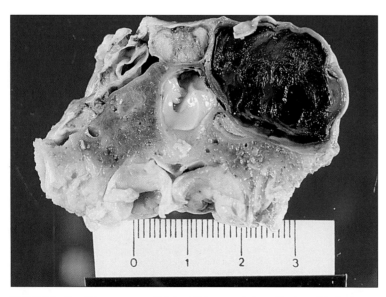

Fig. 4.11 Carotid–cavernous fistula. Mid-coronal view of sphenoid air sinus, pituitary gland, and a large enclosed area of hemorrhage in the right cavernous sinus. There was a traumatic dissection of the cavernous carotid artery which precipitated the hemorrhage and led to severe pulsating proptosis.

fissure–cavernous sinus apex region, may be non-specific or granulomatous. In some patients there may be extensive fibrosis similar to that seen in chronic idiopathic pachymeningitis, a relentlessly progressive condition that spreads across the base of the brain to produce multiple cranial nerve palsies. Clinical differentiation of Tolosa–Hunt syndrome from orbital myositis may be difficult but MRI usually shows normal intraorbital muscles in Tolosa–Hunt syndrome.

ORBITAL AND OPTIC NERVE TUMORS

Optic nerve gliomas are a heterogeneous group of tumors that become increasingly more malignant towards the chiasm. Optic nerve gliomas arising from the orbital segment of the optic nerve occur in childhood, are frequently associated with NF 1, and behave in an indolent manner with a growth pattern indistinguishable from that of a hamartoma. The nerve is fusiformly

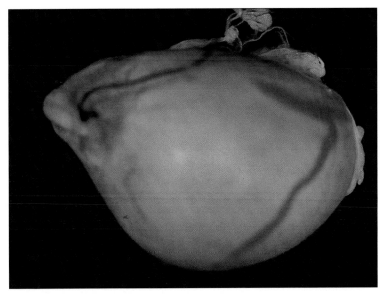

Fig. 4.12 Optic nerve glioma. Bulbous encapsulated optic nerve 3.5 × 2.5 cm at the widest dimension with dilated vessels on the surface. The diameter of the optic nerve anterior to the tumor is 5 mm.

expanded (*Fig. 4.12*), though some of the thickening is due to proliferation of meningothelial cells which are often intermixed with neoplastic astrocytes in the subarachnoid space. Microscopically, the optic nerve gliomas are composed of fibrillary astrocytes and pink carrot-shaped Rosenthal fibers (*Fig. 4.13*), features typical of a pilocytic astrocytoma. Atypia is minimal and mitoses are not present. Microcysts may be present in some cases. Occasionally, pilocytic astrocytomas may show giant cells with rare mitoses and focal vascular endothelial hyperplasia. These additional features do not confer an adverse prognosis on pilocytic astrocytomas.

Chiasmatic gliomas tend to occur more often in older patients and invariably extend through the chiasmatic sheath to involve the suprasellar cistern and hypothalamus (*Fig. 4.14*). In fact, it may be impossible for the surgeon to determine the optic nerve origin of the tumor. Microscopically, chiasmatic optic nerve gliomas may show any of the features associated with increasing anaplasia such as mitoses, necrosis, and endothelial hyperplasia. From a surgical viewpoint, the management of malignant chiasmatic gliomas is hampered by proximity to the hypothalamus. There is some evidence that treatment with oral etoposide may have the beneficial effect of slowing the rate of tumor growth.

In patients with NF 1, the presence of an orbital plexiform neurofibroma may complicate the management of optic nerve gliomas. Sphenoidal wing dysplasia and aqueduct stenosis may also be present in NF 1 patients. There are rare isolated case reports of gangliocytomas and oligodendrogliomas arising from the optic nerve.

Meningiomas occurring in this region may have a spheno-orbital, intraorbital–intracanalicular, or an optic nerve sheath origin. Bilateral optic nerve meningiomas (*Figs 4.15, 4.16*) occur sporadically as well as in association with neurofibromatosis type 2 (NF 2). Of approximately 500 primary optic nerve sheath meningiomas reported, 5% have been bilateral. Meningiomas can also be found in the orbit without attachment to the optic nerve sheath, arising from ectopic meningeal cells within the orbit. Optic nerve meningiomas occur almost as frequently as optic nerve gliomas. A circumferential growth pattern around the optic nerve is usual and makes surgical removal difficult to achieve without damage to the blood supply of the nerve. Care must be taken to ensure that the meningothelial proliferation lying outside an

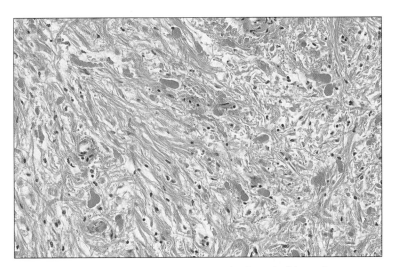

Fig. 4.13 Pre-chiasmatic glioma. Microscopic view of a biopsy from an optic nerve glioma showing numerous fibrillary astrocytes and Rosenthal fibers.

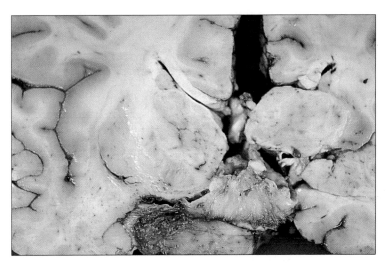

Fig. 4.14 Chiasmatic glioma. Obliteration of the optic chiasm by a large fungating mass typical of optic nerve chiasmatic glioma. There is invasion of the hypothalamus.

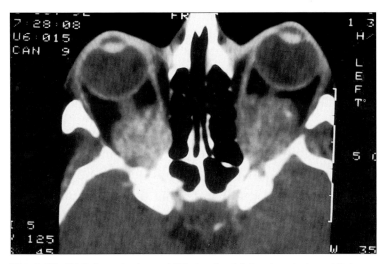

Fig. 4.15 Orbital meningioma. MRI showing bilateral posterior orbital intraconal meningiomas. No connection is seen between the two orbital tumors.

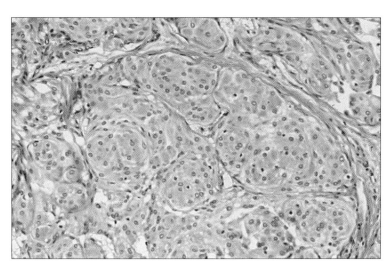

Fig. 4.16 Orbital meningioma. Low-power photomicrograph of orbital excision specimen showing whorls of bland meningothelial cells.

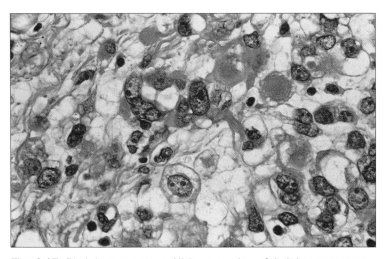

Fig. 4.17 Rhabdomyosarcoma. High-power view of rhabdomyosarcoma cells which have a high nuclear to cytoplasmic ratio, marked cellular pleomorphism, and abundant eosinophilic cytoplasm with cross striations.

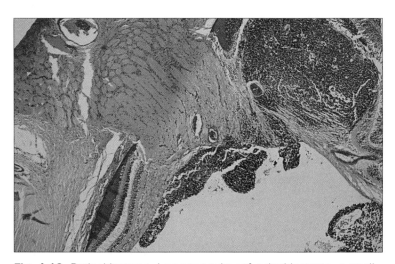

Fig. 4.18 Retinoblastoma. Low-power view of retinoblastoma, a small blue cell tumor of childhood infiltrating the optic nerve and the sclera extending into the extrascleral soft tissue of the orbit and the optic nerve canal.

optic nerve glioma is not erroneously diagnosed as meningioma by the pathologist, a mistake that may be made if a superficial biopsy is obtained. Orbital meningiomas devoid of an attachment to the optic nerve may extend through the calvarium to the scalp or extend posteriorly through the superior orbital fissure. In some patients, the bulk of the tumor may lie intracranially and removal of this component will require a combined ophthalmic–neurosurgical approach. Some subcutaneous meningiomas of the periorbital area may not have an orbital or intracranial component, although an intradiploic component is usual. In contrast to optic nerve gliomas (ONGs) and meningiomas, orbital schwannomas and neurofibromas do not have an optic nerve attachment and are usually easier to remove.

Rhabdomyosarcoma (RMS) is the most important primary orbital tumor of childhood (*Fig. 4.17*). Pathologically, it is not possible to distinguish a primary orbital RMS from one which is metastatic to the orbit. An alveolar pattern is most common. Retinoblastoma may show extensive involvement of the orbital walls either initially or at the time of recurrence (*Fig. 4.18*).

There is no consensus on the pathogenesis of orbital pseudotumor. Orbital pseudotumor is now an outdated term which encompasses a variety of conditions ranging from idiopathic chronic non-granulomatous inflammatory disease to solitary fibrous tumor (*Figs 4.19, 4.20*). In most cases, what is described as orbital pseudotumor represents an idiopathic sclerosing fibrosis which in the early stages may have a prominent lymphoid component but in the later stages consists of bland fibrous tissue. Multi-focal fibrosclerosis is the same process as other idiopathic fibrosing processes occurring in the retroperitoneum or mediastinum. The pathology is that of a steroid-responsive, pathogen-free chronic inflammatory process of varying extent which can involve some or all of the orbital contents. In the early stages of orbital pseudotumor, the lymphoid infiltrate can be distinguished from a low-grade lymphoma by means of immunohistochemistry. In contrast with lymphomas, orbital pseudotumor is an inflammatory reaction that is predominantly T cell mediated and the B cells do not show kappa or lambda light chain restriction. Another inflammatory process that appears to have a predilection

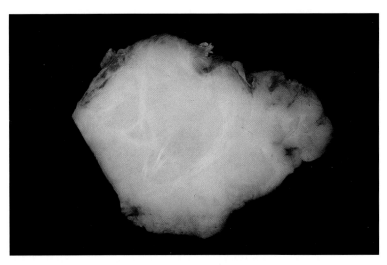

Fig. 4.19 Fibrosing variant of orbital pseudo-tumor in which there is sub-total replacement of the lacrimal gland by intersecting bands of firm white fibrous tissue.

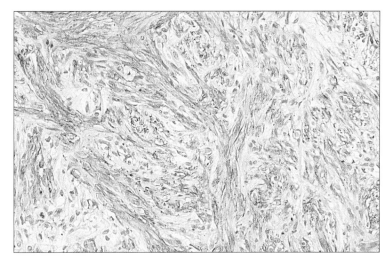

Fig. 4.20 Fibrosing variant of orbital pseudo-tumor. Immunohistochemistry of fibrosing variant of orbital pseudo-tumor in which the participating cells are immunostained by an actin antibody, thereby confirming the myofibroblastic nature of the cells.

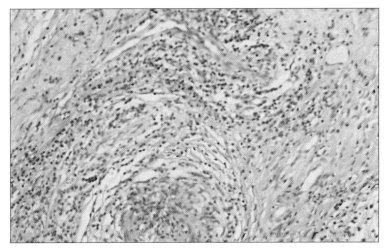

Fig. 4.21 Orbital Kimura disease. Low-power view of orbital biopsy from patient with Kimura's disease showing perivascular inflammatory infiltrate with many eosinophils and lymphocytes. Prominent aggregates and abundant eosinophils are distinguishing features from inflammatory pseudo-tumor (sclerosing fibrosis).

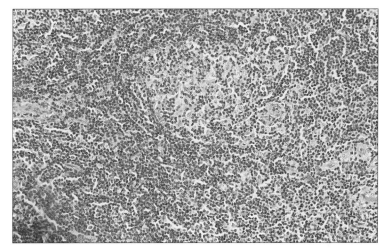

Fig. 4.22 Orbital lymphoma. Medium-power view of low-grade B cell lymphoma of MALT type. The tumor is composed of small round and small cleaved lymphocytes and a residual reactive germinal center can be seen.

for the orbit is Kimura disease, characterized by an angiolymphoid proliferation with many eosinophils, peripheral eosinophilia, and an elevated serum IgE (*Fig. 4.21*). As a rule, ocular adnexal lymphomas are non-Hodgkin's B cell lymphomas.

The newest classification of lymphomas is the REAL classification, which encompasses both nodal and extranodal tumors and includes in the extranodal group mucosal-associated lymphoid tumors (MALTs). MALT lymphomas are low-grade B cell lymphomas and are the most common type of primary orbital lymphoma. MALT lymphomas have an indolent natural history and respond well to radiotherapy (*Fig. 4.22*). They may recur and the site of recurrence may be another typical MALT site such as a bronchus or the gastrointestinal tract. Recent clinicopathologic studies, focused on identifying MALT lymphomas in the orbit, found that although a high proportion of ocular adnexal lymphomas had MALT characteristics, there was no significant difference in outcome between patients with MALT changes and those without.

Orbital lymphoma may arise as a complication of Sjögren or Felty syndromes and is an increasingly frequent complication of HIV infection.

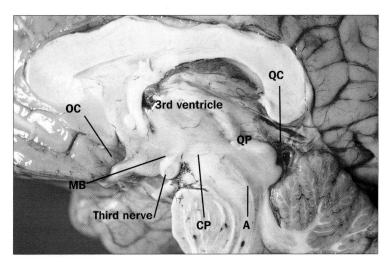

Fig. 4.23 Third ventricle anatomy. Mid-sagittal section of brain to show anatomical structures in the region of the third ventricle including aqueduct (A), optic chiasm (OC), and quadrigeminal cistern (QC), quadrigeminal plate (QP), mamillary body (MB), cerebral peduncle (CP), optic chiasm (OC).

SUPRASELLAR REGION

The suprasellar region is an anatomically complex region, bounded above by the floor of the third ventricle, optic chiasm and optic tracts, tuber cinereum, and pituitary stalk (infundibulum) and laterally by the choroidal fissure, lamina terminalis, gyrus rectus, parahippocampal gyrus, and cerebral peduncles (*Fig. 4.23*). Any lesions arising within the sellar region can extend up into the suprasellar cistern. Craniopharyngioma and germinoma are the two most important tumors in this location. Rarely, non-neoplastic lesions, including neurenteric, arachnoid and Rathke cysts, may arise here and cause pressure-related symptoms on the optic nerve and pituitary stalk. The region is also particularly prone to involvement in neurosarcoidoma (see below).

Craniopharyngiomas are epithelia-derived tumors (*Fig. 4.24*) which arise from embryonic rests. The presence of epithelial elements evokes a florid glial response around the tumor, resulting in adherence of the tumor to any or all of the suprasellar contents.

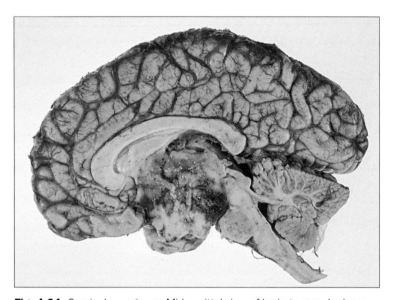

Fig. 4.24 Craniopharyngioma. Mid-sagittal view of brain to reveal a large partly hemorrhagic and partly necrotic craniopharyngioma destroying much of the third ventricle and hypothalamus.

Consequently, complete removal of a craniopharyngioma with preservation of function in the optic nerves and hypothalamus is difficult to achieve. The florid glial reaction is histologically very similar to the appearance of an optic nerve glioma, and its presence in a biopsy without epithelial elements may lead to an erroneous diagnosis of glioma. Craniopharyngiomas may be solid or cystic and may show secondary changes, including hemorrhage, calcification, cholesterol cleft formation, and necrosis. The epithelial elements consist of keratin-producing squamous cells or basaloid cells similar to adamantinomatous epithelium in adamantinomas of the jaw (*Fig. 4.25*). Adults may develop craniopharyngiomas, although these are usually papillary in type.

Although the term germinoma is used most often when referring to germ-cell tumors in the suprasellar region, it is vital to remember that any germ-cell tumor in any location may include endodermal, ectodermal and mesodermal elements, as well as tissues of extra-embryonic origin including yolk sac and chorionic derived tissues. Whereas the presence of the latter two elements invariably implies malignancy, the other elements may show varying degrees of maturity. It is crucial that these tumors be sampled extensively at surgery because an accurate prognosis can be established only by careful examination of all of the elements within a suprasellar germ-cell tumor.

THE CLIVUS

The extra-axial sixth nerve leaves the brainstem at the pontomedullary junction and travels up the clivus, on the way to the cavernous sinus. Chordomas (*Fig. 4.26*), nasopharyngeal carcinomas, meningiomas, and basilar aneurysms arising in this location may present with a sixth nerve palsy. The chordoma is a slow-growing but relentlessly progressive tumor of notochordal origin which has a lobulated soft slimy appearance and originates at the spheno-occipital synchondrosis. Microscopically, it is composed of large bubbly cells that contain a mucinous substance (*Fig. 4.27*). Mitoses are infrequent. The tumor is radioresistant and, although surgical access to this area has improved, complete removal is often impossible. Chondrosarcomas and chondroid chordomas, which share histologic features with chordomas and chondrosarcomas, may also

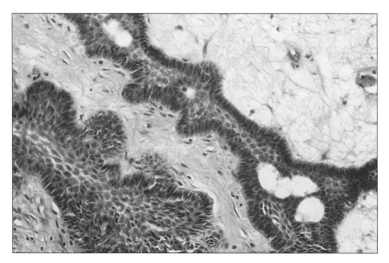

Fig. 4.25 Craniopharyngioma. Typical basaloid or adamantinomatous epithelium present in a craniopharyngioma.

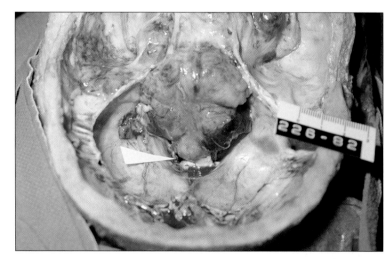

Fig. 4.26 Chordoma. Skull base exposed after brain removal to show large multi-lobulated mass arising from clivus. Tumor had a semi-soft greasy consistency. Patient presented with isolated sixth nerve palsy and progressed over several years to develop signs of brainstem compression.

occur in this location and behave in a similar manner. Nasopharyngeal carcinomas progress rapidly and usually show clival destruction on plane skull radiograph. Unruptured basilar aneurysms may present with an isolated sixth nerve palsy.

QUADRIGEMINAL CISTERN

Although the anatomy of this area is complex (*Fig. 4.28*), the key structures are the pineal gland, resting between the superior colliculi, and the inferior colliculi, which together form the anterior wall. Above lie the internal cerebral veins, the splenium of the corpus callosum, and the pulvinar of the thalamus. The superior vermis bounds the area posteriorly. Lesions in the quadrigeminal cistern may impinge on those regions of the midbrain tectum involved in control of vertical gaze, namely the nucleus of Darkschewitsch, the rostral interstitial medial longitudinal fasciculus, the interstitial nucleus of Cajal, and the posterior commissure, and, of course, the trochlear nerves. Typically, lesions in the quadrigeminal cistern result in Parinaud syndrome and, if large enough, may compress the aqueduct of Sylvius to cause hydrocephalus.

Tumors of the pineal gland include pineoblastoma, pineocytoma, and germinoma, collectively termed primitive neuro-ectodermal tumors. Pineoblastomas are very similar to medulloblastomas and retinoblastomas in histologic appearance and behavior, including the propensity to disseminate through the neuraxis. Pineocytomas, by contrast, are very similar to normal pineal tissue in appearance and are much less likely to spread via the CSF pathways. (Germ cell tumors are identical in histologic-type to those described under 'Suprasellar Region') Gliomas may arise from the quadrigeminal plate and occasionally may have a better than expected prognosis, particularly if the growth pattern is exophytic rather than the usual endophytic pattern of intra-axial brainstem growth. Arachnoid and glial cysts of the quadrigeminal cistern are usually amenable to complete cure, whereas some difficulty may be expected in achieving a complete removal of the rare lipomas and meningiomas which can also occur here. Aneurysms of the perimesencephalic or choroidal branches of the posterior cerebral artery may give rise to a Parinaud syndrome, whereas a vein of Galen aneurysm may cause hydrocephalus and or heart failure in infancy.

Progressive supranuclear gaze palsy (Steele–Richardson–Olszewski) syndrome classically involves the tectal region of the midbrain. Clinically, there is L-Dopa resistant parkinsonism of the akinetic–rigid type with bradykinesia and axial rigidity. Voluntary vertical gaze is impaired. Postural instability and falls are characteristic, the patient often falling backwards while attempting to sit. Dementia and a pseudo-bulbar palsy may be prominent. MR examination will confirm collicular atrophy. Accurate diagnosis requires a combination of the appropriate clinical symptoms and the post-mortem demonstration of neurofibrillary tangles and neuropil threads in the basal ganglia and brainstem together with an absence of other pathology such as Lewy bodies and infarcts.

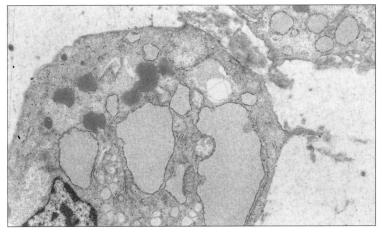

Fig. 4.27 Electron micrograph of physalipherous cell typical of chordoma. The cytoplasm is distended with mucinous material.

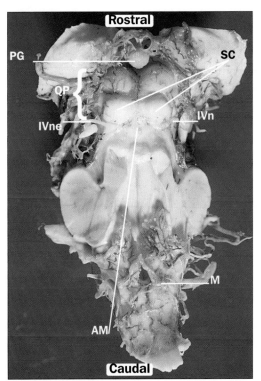

Fig. 4.28 Quadrigeminal plate anatomy. Posterior view of the brainstem to show the quadrigeminal plate (QP) above with the pineal gland (PG) lying between the superior colliculi (SC). The fourth nerve exits just below the inferior colliculi. (IVn, 4th nerve; IVne; AM, anterior medullary velum covering the aqueduct; M, medulla)

NEURO-OPHTHALMIC ASPECTS OF MITOCHONDRIAL DISEASE (SEE ALSO CHAPTER 29)

Brain, muscle, and eye are the organs most frequently affected by mitochondrial dysfunction. Mitochondria are unique in that they possess their own DNA which is distinct from nuclear DNA. Mitochondrial DNA (mtDNA) is a circular, closed, double-stranded molecule consisting of 16 569 nucleotides, which encodes protein subunits as well as the structural RNA required for their translation. MtDNA is maternally inherited through the oocyte cytoplasm. Thus, maternal inheritance is a feature of many mitochondrial diseases. There is increasing recognition, however, that defects in the nuclear control of mtDNA function may also cause mitochondrial disease. MtDNA codes for only 13 of the more than 80 polypeptides that are distributed among the five respiratory chain enzyme complexes (I–V) involved in oxidative phosphorylation. It is apparent, therefore, that the nucleus has by far the dominant role in oxidative phosphorylation.

Nuclear-encoded polypeptides are assembled in the cell cytoplasm and are imported into the mitochondrion before final assembly into a functional unit. Very little is known at present about diseases that are caused by defects in this importation process. The recently recognized autosomal dominant chronic progressive ophthalmoplegia (CPEO) is likely to have a primary nuclear basis. MtDNA has poor repair mechanisms, as a result of which mutations are frequent. Development of a new mutation results in a mixture of mutant and normal (wild type) mtDNA within a cell, a process known as heteroplasmy. The consequences for a cell or organ of this mixture of mutant and wild type mtDNA in terms of impaired oxidative phosphorylation and reduced energy output mixture will depend on the proportions of wild type and mutant mtDNA present. Organs such as brain, retina, and muscle, with high energy requirements, are particularly prone to injury in mitochondrial disease.

Ragged red fibers (*Fig. 4.29*) in muscle are the cardinal histologic feature of mitochondrial disease, although their absence does not exclude mitochondrial disease. Ragged red fibers represent accumulated and usually morphologically abnormal mitochondria. Electron microscopy is another important tool for demonstrating the presence of abnormal mitochondria. Additionally, the histochemical demonstration of cytochrome

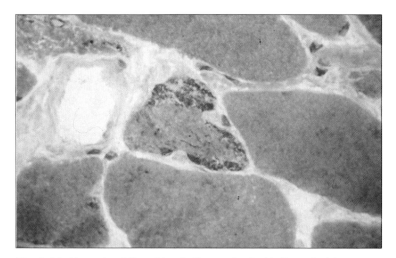

Fig. 4.29 Ragged red fiber. Muscle fiber stained with Gomori trichrome to show large red areas beneath the sarcolemmal membrane representing accumulated abnormal mitochondria, in a patient with mitochondrial myopathy.

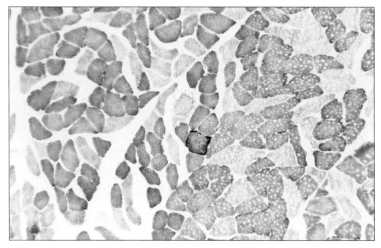

Fig. 4.30 Section of skeletal muscle stained with combined cytochrome oxidase (brown) and succinic dehydrogenase stain (blue). A cytochrome oxidase depleted fiber in the center shows enhanced blue staining consistent with increased SDH reactivity which indicates a nuclear attempt to compensate for depletion of cytochrome oxidase encoded by mitochondrial DNA.

oxidase depletion in affected muscle fibers supports a defect in mitochondrial function (*Fig. 4.30*).

A satisfactory classification system encompassing all of the genetic, biochemical, pathologic and clinical features of mitochondrial disease conditions is awaited. Currently, mitochondrial diseases are classified on the basis of particular phenotypes associated with specific mitochondrial point mutations or deletions. However, there is considerable clinical variability in disease expression. Important clinical issues, such as the ability of Leber's hereditary optic neuropathy to show improvement, remain difficult to explain on a genetic or biochemical basis.

It is likely that, in addition to those detailed below, many new mitochondrial disorders attributable to defects in nuclear control of mtDNA will be described in the near future and many of these will undoubtedly involve the visual system.

MITOCHONDRIAL MYOPATHY, ENCEPHALOPATHY, LACTIC ACIDOSIS, AND STROKE-LIKE EPISODES (MELAS)

Typically, MELAS present in young adults as stroke often with cortical blindness. Migraine and epilepsy are common. An important clue is the observation that areas of cerebral cortical infarction lie outside a major vascular territory. In some families, there may be clinical overlap with chronic progressive external ophthalmoplegia (CPEO) and myoclonic epilepsy with ragged red fibers. The ragged red fibers are variable in number with some patients having few if any in skeletal muscle. Death occurs in most patients, usually from cerebral infarction. Most cases of MELAS are associated with an A–G transition at position 3243 in the mitochondrial tRNA$^{leu\,(UUR)}$ gene. Other point mutations involving tRNA$^{leu\,(UUR)}$ genes at positions 11084, 3252, 3256, 3271, and 3291 have been reported. Deficiencies of complexes I, III, and IV have been described in MELAS patients but the mechanisms whereby the point mutation results in reduced activity of the respiratory chain enzymes remain undetermined. There is a poor correlation between the levels of mutant mtDNA and the presence or absence of disease in particular families. As in LHON, the presence of disease modifying mutations in other areas of mtDNA may explain this variability in disease expression.

The MELAS brain typically shows areas of necrosis coupled with intense proliferation of capillaries and occasional preserved neurons within the necrotic areas, a feature that distinguishes MELAS-associated necrosis from conventional vascular-based infarction.

MYOCLONIC EPILEPSY WITH RAGGED RED FIBERS (MERFF)

The complete clinical expression of myoclonic epilepsy with ragged red fibers (MERRF) includes myoclonus, epilepsy, myopathy, and ataxia but optic atrophy may sometimes be present. There may be clinical overlap with MELAS. Onset may be in childhood or adulthood. Neuropathologic descriptions are rare but there may be loss of neurons and gliosis affecting striatum and cerebellar cortex, and in some patients the pattern of involvement resembles that seen in Leigh disease. Most MERRF patients have an A–G transition in the tRNA^{lys} gene at position 8344 in mtDNA and deficiencies in enzyme complexes I and IV of the respiratory chain.

LEBER'S HEREDITARY OPTIC NEUROPATHY

The majority of patients with Leber's hereditary optic neuropathy have one or other of three G–A point mutations at positions 11 778, 3460, or 14 484 in mtDNA, with resultant biochemical dysfunction in complexes I, III, or IV. Visual loss may occur simultaneously in both eyes or sequentially, and clinical progression may be rapid or slow. The spontaneous improvement in vision in some patients has not been adequately explained on either a genetic or biochemical basis but there is evidence that the rate of disease progression and likelihood of recovery are linked to particular mutations, patients with the 11 778 mutation having the worst prognosis and those with the 14 484 mutation having the best. A multiple sclerosis-like syndrome is described in women with the 11 778 mutation. Although other optic nerve diseases may cause diagnostic confusion with Leber's hereditary optic neuropathy, the issue is resolved by detection of a Leber's hereditary optic neuropathy-associated mtDNA mutation. There is no good evidence that either excess alcohol or tobacco alters the expression of these mutations.

Not all patients with Leber's hereditary optic neuropathy have a family history of disease and not all relatives of an affected patient who themselves have a mutation will express the disease. Other missense or secondary mtDNA mutations at positions 3394, 4216, 4917, 7444, 13 708, and 15 812 may be present and influence the disease expression in an at-risk family member. The high proportion of male patients has led to a suggestion that an X-linked gene may exert an influence but no such X-linked gene has been reported. There are no effective treatments to alter disease outcome. Detailed pathologic descriptions of the disease in the early stages are not available.

NEUROPATHY, ATAXIA, AND RETINITIS PIGMENTOSA

Neuropathy, ataxia, and retinitis pigmentosa (NARP) is an extremely rare condition in which a sensorimotor neuropathy is accompanied by developmental delay, dementia, ataxia, and retinitis pigmentosa. A T–G point mutation at position 8993 in subunit six of mitochondrial ATPase is present. There are no detailed pathologic descriptions of NARP.

LEIGH'S DISEASE: SUBACUTE NECROTIZING LEUKOENCEPHALOPATHY

Leigh's disease is the prototype childhood mitochondrial disorder (*Fig. 4.31*). Clinical presentation and course vary considerably and several adult patients with onset have been reported. From an ophthalmologic viewpoint, brainstem involvement may give rise to eye movement disturbances. Optic atrophy, dystonia, pyramidal or extrapyramidal signs, or respiratory insufficiency are frequently present. Defects in the pyruvate dehydrogenase complex, cytochrome C oxidase, complex I, and complex IV activity have all been described in Leigh's disease patients. Depending on the series reported, either complex I or complex IV deficiency is the most common biochemical defect. Point mutations involving T–G and T–C transitions at position 8993 or A–G transition at position 8344 have been reported in Leigh's disease. There is no correlation between the phenotype and either the mutation or biochemical defect. Defects in nuclear DNA have been reported in isolated patients.

The clinical course is one of fairly rapid progression leading to

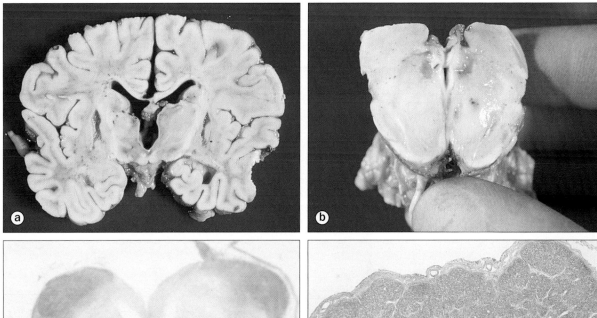

Fig. 4.31 Leigh's disease. (**a**) Coronal view of brain showing bilateral symmetric areas of cavitation in the putamen. (**b**) Horizontal section of midbrain showing severe swelling, pallor of the substantia nigra, and small areas of dark discoloration in the tectal region indicative of previous old capillary hemorrhage typical of Leigh's disease. (**c**) Transverse section of medulla showing large confluent area of myelin loss involving the pyramids and tegmentum. (**d**) Central area of myelin loss in the optic nerve.

death. Pathologically, the lesions are characterized by a relatively stereotyped pattern of distribution and by striking vacuolation, macrophage infiltration, gliosis, intense capillary proliferation, and some neuronal loss. Involvement of the periaqueductal gray matter, substantia nigra, the pontine and medullary tegmentum, and several cranial nerve nuclei is typical. The cerebellar dentate nucleus, thalamus, and striatum but not the mamillary bodies are usually involved. Gray and white matter may be involved and myelin loss may be severe in the centrum semiovale.

KEARNS SAYRE SYNDROME AND CHRONIC PROGRESSIVE EXTERNAL OPHTHALMOPLEGIA

Kearns Sayre syndrome (KSS), distinguished from chronic progressive external ophthalmoplegia (CPEO) by the presence of systemic involvement, usually occurs before 20 years of age and is characterized by external ophthalmoplegia, pigmentary retinopathy, and one of either ataxia, cardiac conduction defect, or raised CSF protein. Patients with KSS may go on to develop diabetes mellitus, deafness, or Pearson's syndrome. Deletions involving large segments of mtDNA are usual in KSS or CPEO. Some patients with autosomal dominant CPEO may have multiple deletions. All large deletions remove tRNA and protein-coding areas, with the result that mitochondrial protein translation is impaired. Loss of a 4977 bp sequence referred to as 'the common deletion' is the most frequently encountered. In KSS, high levels of mutant mtDNA are confined to brain and muscle (skeletal, cardiac, and eye), and in CPEO, high levels are probably confined only to eye muscle. Autosomal dominant CPEO has been linked to chromosome 10q in a Finnish family and to 3p in Italian kindreds, whereas a recessive form of CPEO has been characterized in related Arab families, factors that indicate a significant role for the participation of nuclear DNA.

The size and site of the deletion does not correlate with the severity of the disease. Skeletal muscle shows RRFs, together with depletion of cytochrome oxidase, and the accumulation of structurally abnormal mitochondria. In patients with pure CPEO, biopsy of skeletal muscle is unlikely to be rewarding but the orbicularis oculi muscle or other extraocular muscle will show diagnostic features. However, these muscles are not usually available for diagnosis. Detailed neuropathologic descriptions of KSS are rare but white matter vacuolation has been reported as well as spinal cord changes similar to those seen in Leigh's disease.

PEARSON MARROW–PANCREAS SYNDROME

Pearson Marrow–Pancreas syndrome (PMPS) is a rare fatal disorder of infancy in which pancytopenia is accompanied by pancreatic exocrine insufficiency and in which patients go on to develop KSS. Most patients have a 4.9 kb mtDNA deletion but deletions may range in size from 9 to 14 kb and are located between tRNA^{cyst} and the D-loop.

WOLFRAM SYNDROME

Wolfram syndrome is a rare, progressive neurodegenerative autosomal recessive disorder characterized by optic atrophy, diabetes mellitus, diabetes insipidus, neurosensory hearing loss, urinary

tract abnormalities, and neurologic dysfunction. A heteroplasmic 8.5 kb deletion in mtDNA has been reported in a family with Wolfram syndrome. Recently, this syndrome was linked to markers on chromosome 4p16, which indicates a role for nuclear-encoded genes whose products may interact with mtDNA.

MITOCHONDRIAL NEUROGASTROINTESTINAL ENCEPHALOMYOPATHY

Mitochondrial neurogastrointestinal encephalomyopathy is another rare syndrome of probable mitochondrial origin which is clinically characterized by gastrointestinal symptoms, including recurrent nausea, vomiting, and intestinal dysmotility with diarrhea. Eye movement abnormalities and peripheral neuropathy may be present. Neuroimaging reveals widespread white matter changes. Ragged red fibers may be present and a partial defect of cytochrome c oxidase activity has been demonstrated in several patients. Multiple deletions in mtDNA have been reported.

BRAINSTEM VASCULAR DISEASE

It is not our intention to describe in detail the numerous lacunar stroke syndromes associated with eye signs. Of importance is the realization that the brainstem has a vascular supply similar to that of the striatum, in that tiny perforating end-arteries branch directly from the vertebrobasilar and posterior cerebral arterial systems (*Fig. 4.32*). These vessels do not have collateral anastomoses and are particularly prone to the development of microscopic atheroma (lipohyalinosis) at their origin as well as to rupture from hypertension. Occlusion by atheroma will cause a small but critically located area of infarction which after a few months will be visible as a lacune on MRI.

In the brainstem, the perforating vessels are grouped into straight perforators which run directly into the brainstem from the basilar artery; short and long circumferential perforators pass around the brainstem. Occlusion of the different vascular groupings gives rise to medial or lateral medullary or pontine clinical syndromes. The pontine syndromes may be further subdivided depending on whether the superior, mid, or inferior pons is involved. Occlusion of the posterior paramedian thalamo-subthalamic perforating vessels produces a bilateral ischemic lesion

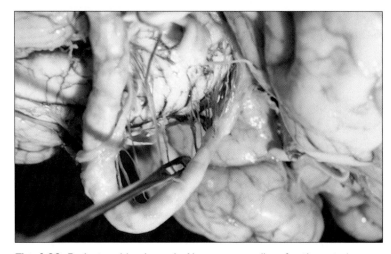

Fig. 4.32 Brainstem blood supply. Numerous small perforating arteries are seen to arise from the posterior surface of the atherosclerotic basilar artery.

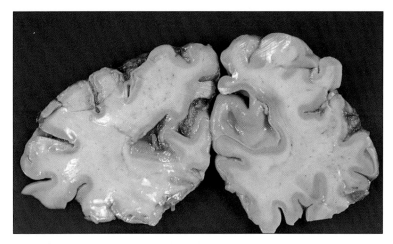

Fig. 4.33 Creutzfeldt–Jacob disease. Coronal section through the occipital lobe showing bilateral shrinkage and yellow discoloration of the calcarine cortex typical of the Heidenhain variant of Creutzfeldt–Jacob disease.

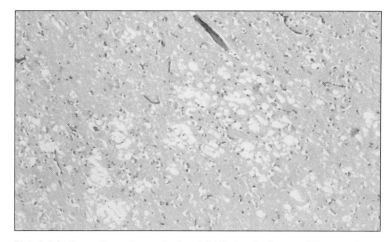

Fig. 4.34 Spongiform change in Creutzfeldt–Jacob disease. Microscopic view of calcarine cortex showing spongiform change in neocortex typical of Creutzfeldt–Jacob disease.

in the paramedian thalamic region that is associated with a complex clinical disorder, including an amnesic syndrome, dysarthria, and ataxia. It has been argued that the vertical gaze impairment in these patients occurs in the absence of midbrain involvement but there has not been definite neuropathological confirmation of this. Occlusion of both posterior cerebral arteries with sparing of the perforating branches may cause bilateral occipital cortical infarction and give rise to cortical blindness. Other pathological processes that can cause cortical blindness include trauma-induced contusions and the Heidenhain or occipital variant of Creutzfeld–Jacob disease (*Figs 4.33, 4.34*).

MULTIPLE SCLEROSIS

Optic neuritis, nystagmus, and internuclear ophthalmoplegia are the principal eye abnormalities in multiple sclerosis (MS). Optic neuritis is a frequent presenting feature of MS. Fat-suppressed fast-spin echo imaging is excellent at demonstrating plaques of demyelination in the optic nerve. All patients with optic neuritis require full cranial MRI examination, evoked responses, and CSF examination for oligoclonal bands to determine whether they fulfil the diagnostic criteria for MS. Symptoms and signs of brainstem

involvement in MS may be due to plaques encroaching on any of the surrounding structures, including the internuclear white matter connections, intra-axial segments of the cranial nerves, ascending and descending sensory and motor tracts, and the autonomic fibers and ganglia. Diplopia is usually due to involvement of the intra-axial third or sixth cranial nerve. Internuclear ophthalmoplegia (INO) is a result of the disruption of the medial longitudinal fasciculus. Involvement of the brainstem cerebellar connections in the superior, middle, and inferior cerebellar peduncles may give rise to nystagmus.

Multiple sclerosis plaques are classified pathologically into acute, chronic active, and chronic inactive (*Figs 4.35, 4.36*). Acute plaques may present with considerable edema, leading to a mistaken clinical CT or MRI diagnosis of tumor. Biopsy of acute plaques in this setting reveals an intense cellular infiltrate composed of lipid-filled macrophages, occasional lymphocytes, and infrequent plasma cells. Axons are relatively well preserved. Chronic plaques are characterized by diminution in the number of macrophages and an increasing number of astrocytes. Activity of chronic plaques is determined by the degree of lymphocytic infiltration, especially at the plaque edge. With plaque progression, axons may be lost. Axonal loss is pivotal in the development of persistent clinical disability in MS. Quantitative MRI is a useful

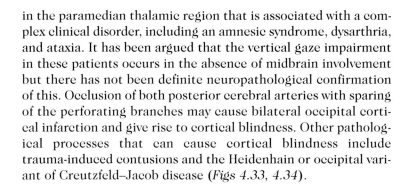

Fig. 4.35 Multiple sclerosis. Transverse sections of brainstem showing large confluent plaques characterized by brown discoloration.

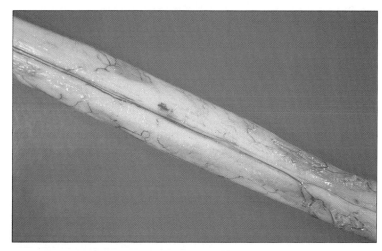

Fig. 4.36 Multiple sclerosis. Ventral surface of spinal cord showing many gray–brown multiple sclerosis plaques.

method for determining the severity of axonal loss from plaques.

The causes of MS remain as elusive as ever but the combination of an environmental trigger, such as a virus that shares antigenic epitopes with myelin basic protein, occurring in a genetically susceptible individual remains the most plausible explanation.

OCULAR MYASTHENIA

Weakness of the extraocular muscles occurs in up to 60% of patients presenting with myasthenia gravis. Most patients progress to generalized weakness but in some patients the weakness remains restricted to the ocular muscles (ocular myasthenia gravis). Myasthenia gravis is caused by an anti-acetylcholine receptor antibody but the level of antibody positivity in patients with ocular myasthenia gravis is much lower than in patients with systemic myasthenia gravis. It has been shown that the AChRs in extraocular muscles are different from those in peripheral limb muscles. Anti-acetylcholine receptors are composed of five subunits (α, β, χ, δ, ϵ) and there are higher levels of the ϵ (adult type) subunit in extraocular muscles than in peripheral muscle. When measuring anti-acetylcholine receptor antibodies in ocular myasthenia gravis, it is crucial that an antigen source rich in the adult subunit (such as adult non-denervated muscle) be used in the antibody assay. Approximately one-third of patients who undergo thymectomy for ocular myasthenia gravis will have a complete remission at a 10-year follow-up.

NEUROSARCOID AND OTHER BASAL MENINGEAL GRANULOMATOUS DISEASES

Involvement of the meninges, brain, cranial nerves, or spinal cord occurs in up to 14% of patients with respiratory tract sarcoidosis. Clinically isolated neurosarcoidosis is much less common and it is extremely difficult to establish a diagnosis of neurosarcoidosis. The pattern of pathologic CNS involvement is similar in both types (*Figs 5.37, 5.38*). Typically, there is extensive meningeal involvement, usually over the base of the brain where the optic nerves and cranial nerves II to VIII are surrounded by a non-necro-

tizing granulomatous inflammatory process. The resultant meningeal thickening may be so great as to produce extension of the chronic inflammatory process into the brain parenchyma with formation of a mass lesion. Blockage of the foramen of Luschka will cause obstructive hydrocephalus.

Very localized involvement of the optic nerve may simulate an optic nerve glioma, whereas localized involvement of any of the other cranial nerves will provide a major diagnostic challenge. A CSF pleocytosis is usually present. MRI scans will show the meningeal involvement but are not specific for neurosarcoidosis. Other basal granulomatous conditions including tuberculosis enter the differential diagnosis and must be excluded before high-dose steroid therapy is commenced. A pathogen-free granulomatous disorder involving the meninges has been described and may present with visual symptoms due to optic nerve involvement. This condition pursues a relentless clinical course, insidiously picking off cranial nerves, and is usually only transiently responsive to treatment with prednisone. Pathologically, it may be impossible to distinguish between this condition and neurosarcoidosis.

CONGENITAL SYNDROMES OF OCULOMOTOR DISTURBANCE

Duane's retraction syndrome, Moebius syndrome, and the superior oblique tendon sheath syndrome of Brown are the most important conditions in this category.

DUANE'S RETRACTION SYNDROME

It is generally thought that Duane's retraction syndrome (DRS) is best explained by anomalous or paradoxical innervation of the lateral rectus muscle, possibly by the third nerve. This results in limitation or absence of abduction and variable limitation of adduction. There is narrowing of the palpebral fissure and retraction of the globe on attempted adduction. Most cases of Duane's retraction syndrome are sporadic. A variety of conditions have been described in association with DRS including facial hemiat-

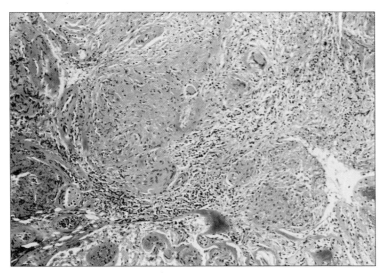

Fig. 4.37 Neurosarcoid. Coronal section of brain taken through the third ventricle to show an ill-defined area of brown discoloration obliterating the ventricle and extending up into the hypothalamic region.

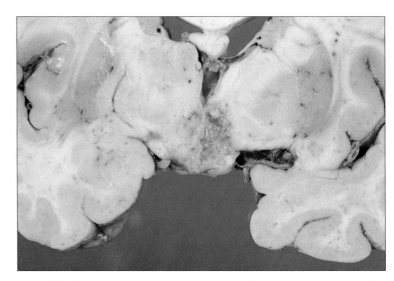

Fig. 4.38 Neurosarcoid. Numerous non-caseating granulomata typical of neurosarcoid involving the meninges (not shown).

rophy, hypogonadism, arthrogryposis multiplex, and the fetal alcohol syndrome. The occasional finding of these syndromes in association with DRS suggests that an early teratogenic event may be responsible. Up to 10% of cases may be familial and it is noteworthy that a deletion of a segment of the long arm of chromosome 4 (4q27–31) has been found in one patient with Duane's retraction syndrome. Neuropathologic studies of this condition are rare but have shown complete absence or hypoplasia of the sixth nerve with variable absence of the sixth nerve nucleus. Additionally, the trigeminal and facial nerve nuclei may appear unduly small. Clinical findings may be unilateral in some patients who are subsequently shown to have bilateral brainstem changes at autopsy.

MOEBIUS SYNDROME

The presence from birth of a non-progressive bilateral lower motor type facial weakness is typical of Moebius syndrome. A sixth nerve palsy is present in as many as 75% of affected patients. Autopsy findings include an absence or hypoplasia of the seventh and sixth

cranial nerve nuclei. In some patients there may be microscopic evidence of a perinatal brainstem hypoxic–ischemic insult in the form of focal necrosis, although such patients usually have a greater degree of cranial involvement. There is also a well-characterized association between Moebius syndrome and hypogonadotropic hypogonadism. These patients may also have hypoplasia of the optic discs.

SEPTO-OPTIC DYSPLASIA

Hypopituitarism may be associated with optic nerve hypoplasia and variable absence of the septum pellucidum. Autopsy descriptions are sparse but the optic nerve shows a reduction of myelinated fibers and variable loss of neurons in the lateral geniculate body. Both the anterior and posterior gland may be absent, as may some of the hypothalamic paraventricular nuclei. Complete absence of all functioning pituitary tissue, however, is usually incompatible with survival. The olfactory tracts and bulbs may be similarly affected.

Further reading

Achiron L, Strominger M, Witkin N, Primo S. Sarcoid optic neuropathy: a case report. *J Am Optom Assoc*. 1995;**66**:646–651.

Acierno MD, Trobe JD, Cornblath WT, Gebarski SS. Painful oculomotor palsy caused by posterior-draining dural carotid cavernous fistulas. *Arch Ophthalmol*. 1995;**113**:1045–1049.

Asbury AK, Aldredge H, Hershberg R, Fisher CM. Oculomotor palsy in diabetes mellitus; a clinopathological study. *Brain*. 1970;**93**:555–566.

Barke RM, Yoshizumi MO, Hepler RS, Krauss HR, Jabour BA. Spontaneous dural carotid–cavernous fistula with central retinal vein occlusion and iris neovascularization. *Ann Ophthalmo.l* 1991;**23**:11–17.

Bassetti C, Bogousslavsky J, Barth A, Regli F. Isolated infarcts of the pons. *Neurology*. 1996;**4**:165–175.

Bogousslavsky J, Regli F, Maeder P, Meuli R, Nader J. The etiology of posterior circulation infarcts: a prospective study using magnetic resonance imaging and magnetic resonance angiography. *Neurology*. 1993;**43**:1528–1533.

Brackett LE, Demers LM, Mamourian AC, Ellenberger C Jr, Santen RJ. Moebius syndrome in association with hypogonadotropic hypogonadism. *J Endocrinol Inves.t* 1991;**14**:599–607.

Brockington M, Alsanjari N, Sweeney MG, Morgan-Hughes JA, Scaravilli F, Harding AE. Kearns–Sayre syndrome associated with mitochondrial DNA deletion or duplication: a molecular genetic and pathological study. *J Neurol Sci*. 1995;**131**:78–87.

Cahill M, Bannigan J, Eustace P. Anatomy of the extraneural blood supply to the intracranial oculomotor nerve. *Br J Ophthalmol*. 1996;**80**:177–181.

Cannella B, Aquino DA, Raine CS. MHC II expression in the CNS after long-term demyelination. *J Neuropathol Exp Neurol*. 1995;**54**:521–530.

Cannella B, Raine CS. The adhesion molecule and cytokine profile of multiple sclerosis lesions. *Ann Neurol*. 1995;**37**:424–435.

Chaloupka JC, Goller D, Goldberg RA, Duckwiler GR, Martin NA, Vinuela F. True anatomical compartmentalization of the cavernous sinus in a patient with bilateral cavernous dural arteriovenous fistulae. Case report. *J Neurosurg*. 1993;**79**:592–595.

Charteris DG, Cullen JF. Binasal field defects in primary empty sella syndrome. *J Neuroophthalmol*. 1996;**16**:110–114.

Chew CK, Foster P, Hurst JA, Salmon JF. Duane's retraction syndrome associated with chromosome 4q27–31 segment deletion. *Am J Ophthalmol*. 1995;**119**:807–809.

Chiechi MV, Smirniotopoulos JG, Mena H. Pineal parenchymal tumors: CT and MR features. *J Comput Assist Tomogr*. 1995;**19**:509–517.

Claudio L, Raine CS, Brosnan CF. Evidence of persistent blood-brain barrier abnormalities in chronic-progressive multiple sclerosis. *Acta Neuropathol Berl*. 1995;**90**:228–238.

Conliffe IA, Moffat DA, Hardy DG, Moore AT. Bilateral optic nerve sheath meningiomas in a patient with neurofibromatosis type 2. *Brit J Ophthalmol*. 1992;**76**:310–313.

Coulter CL, Leech RW, Schaefer GB, Scheithauer BW, Brumback RA. Midline cerebral dysgenesis, dysfunction of the hypothalamic–pituitary axis, and fetal alcohol effects. *Arch Neurol*. 1993;**50**:771–775.

Crotty TB, Scheithauer BW, Young WF Jr, et al. Papillary craniopharyngioma: a clinicopathological study of 48 cases. *J Neurosurg*. 1995;**83**(2):206–214.

Delfini R, Missori P, Tarantino R, Ciapetta P, Cantore G. Primary benign tumors of the orbital cavity: comparative data in a series of patients with optic nerve glioma, sheath meningioma, or neurinoma. *Surg Neurol*. 1996;**45**:147–153.

Dorfman DN, King TO, Dickerson GR, Rosenberg AE, Pilch BZ. Solitary fibrous tumor of the orbit. *Am J Surg Path*. 1994;**18**:281–287.

Dreyfus PM, Hakim S, Adams RD. Diabetic opthalmoplegia. *Arch Neurol Psychiatry*. 1957;**77**:337–349.

Dutton JJ. Optic nerve sheath meningiomas. *Surveys of Ophthalmology*. 1992;**37**:176–183.

Eshbaugh CG, Siatkowski RM, Smith J, Kline LB. Simultaneous, multiple cranial neuropathies in diabetes mellitus. *J Neuroophthalmol*. 1995;**15**:219–224.

Fujita I, Koyanagi T, Kukita J, Yamashita H, Minami T, Nakano H, Ueda K. Moebius syndrome with central hypoventilation and brainstem calcification: a case report. *Eur J Pediatr*. 1991;**150**:582–583.

Goldberg RA, Goldey SH, Duckwiler G, Vinuela F. Management of cavernous sinus-dural fistulas. Indications and techniques for primary embolization via the superior ophthalmic vein. *Arch Ophthalmol.* 1996;**117**:707–714.

Guglielmi G, Vinuela F, Briganti F, Duckwiler G. Carotid–cavernous fistula caused by a ruptured intracavernous aneurysm: endovascular treatment by electrothrombosis with detachable coils. *Neurosurgery.* 1992;**31**:591–596.

Hammans SR, Sweeney MG, Hanna MG, Brockington M, Morgan-Hughes JA, Harding AE. The mitochondrial DNA transfer RNALeu(UUR) A—>G(3243) mutation. A clinical and genetic study. *Brain.* 1995;**118**:721–734.

Harris NL, Jaffe ES, Stein H, et al. A revised European-American classification of lymphoid neoplasms: A proposal from the international lymphoma study group. *Blood.* 1994;**84**:1361–1392.

Hennessey JV, Jackson IM. Clinical features and differential diagnosis of pituitary tumors with emphasis on acromegaly. *Baillieres Clin Endocrinol Metab.* 1995;**9**:271–314.

Hidayat AA, Cameron JD, Font RL, Zimmerman LE. Angiolymphoid hyperplasia with eosinophilia (Kimura's disease) of the orbit and orbital adenexa. *Am J Ophthalmol.* 1983;**96**:176–189.

Ikawa F, Uozumi T, Kiya K, Arita K, Kurisu K, Harada K. Cavernous sinus meningioma presenting as orbital apex syndrome. Diagnostic methods of dynamic MRI, spoiled GRASS (SPGR) image. *Neurosurg Rev.* 1995;**18**:277–280.

Kaminski HJ, Ruff RL. Ocular muscle involvement by Myasthenia Gravis. *Ann Neurol.* 1997;**41**;419–420.

Keane JR. Cavernous sinus syndrome. Analysis of 151 cases. *Arch Neurol.* 1996;**53**:967–971.

Kim JS, Kang JK, Lee SA, Lee MC. Isolated or predominant ocular motor nerve palsy as a manifestation of brainstem stroke. *Stroke.* 1993;**24**:581–586.

Kleinschmidt-DeMasters BK, Lillehei KO, Stears JC. The pathologic, surgical, and MR spectrum of Rathke cleft cysts. *Surg Neurol.* 1995;**44**:19–26.

Kovacs K, Scheithauer BW, Horvath E, Lloyd RV. The World Health Organization classification of adenohypophysial neoplasms. A proposed five-tier scheme. *Cancer.* 1996;**78**:502–510.

Macfarlane R, Levin AV, Weksberg R, Blaser S, Rutka JT. Absence of the greater sphenoid wing in neurofibromatosis type I: congenital or acquired: case report. *Neurosurgery.* 1995;**37**:129–133.

Maroon JC, Kennerdell JS, Vidovich DV, Abla A, Sternau L. Recurrent spheno-orbital meningioma. *J Neurosurg.* 1994;**80**:202–208.

Masera N, Grant DB, Stanhope R, Preece MA. Diabetes insipidus with impaired osmotic regulation in septo-optic dysplasia and agenesis of the corpus callosum. *Arch Dis Child.* 1994;**70**:51–53.

Milazzo S, Toussaint P, Proust F, Touzet G, Malthieu D. Ophthalmologic aspects of pituitary apoplexy. *Eur J Ophthalmol* 1996;**6**:69–73.

Miller DC. Pathology of craniopharyngiomas: clinical import of pathological findings. *Pediatr Neurosurg.* 1994;**21** Suppl 1:11–17.

Morris AA, Leonard JV, Brown GK, et al. Deficiency of respiratory chain complex I is a common cause of Leigh disease. *Ann Neurol.* 1996;**40**:25–30.

Moulin T, Bogousslavsky J, Chopard JL, et al. Vascular ataxic hemiparesis: a re-evaluation. *J Neurol Neurosurg Psychiatry.* 1995;**58**:422–427.

Mulhern M, Keohane C, O'Connor G. Bilateral abducens nerve lesions in unilateral type 3 Duane's retraction syndrome. *Br J Ophthalmol.* 1994;**78**:588–591.

Natori Y, Rhoton AL Jr. Microsurgical anatomy of the superior orbital fissure. *Neurosurgery.* 1995;**36**:762–775.

Ng KL, McDermott N, Romanowski CA, Jackson A. Neurosarcoidosis masquerading as glioma of the optic chiasm in a child. *Postgrad Med J.* 1995;**71**:265–268.

Nicoll JA, Moss TH, Love S, Campbell MJ, Schut WH. Clinical and autopsy findings in two cases of MELAS presenting with stroke-like episodes but without clinical myopathy. *Clin Neuropathol.* 1993;**12**:38–43.

Noonan C, O'Connor M. Greater severity of clinical features in older patients with Duane's retraction syndrome. *Eye.* 1995;**9**:472–475.

Oldfors A, Holme E, Tulinius M, Larsson NG. Tissue distribution and disease manifestations of the tRNA(Lys) A—>G(8344) mitochondrial DNA mutation in a case of myoclonus epilepsy and ragged red fibres. *Acta Neuropathol.* 1995;**90**:328–333.

Ono N, Kohga H, Zama A, Inoue HK, Tamura M. A comparison of children with suprasellar germ cell tumors and craniopharyngiomas: final height, weight, endocrine, and visual sequelae after treatment. *Surg Neurol.* 1996;**46**:370–377.

Paja M, Lucas T, Garcia-Uria J, Salame F, Barcelo B, Estrada J. Hypothalamic-pituitary dysfunction in patients with craniopharyngioma. *Clin Endocrinol Oxf.* 1995;**42**:467–473.

Parchi P, Castellani R, Capellari S, et al. Molecular basis of phenotypic variability in sporadic Creutzfeldt-Jakob disease. *Ann Neurol.* 1996;**39**:767–778.

Poulton J, Morten KJ, Marchington D, et al. Duplications of mitochondrial DNA in Kearns–Sayre syndrome. *Muscle Nerve.* 1995;**Suppl 3**: S154–158.

Powrie JK , Powell M, Ayers AB, Lowy C, Sonksen PH . Lymphocytic adenohypophysitis: magnetic resonance imaging features of two new cases and a review of the literature. *Clin Endocrinol Oxf.* 1995;**42**:315–322.

Puchner M, Ludecke DK, Saeger W, Riedel M, Asa SL. Gangliocytomas of the sellar region – a review. *Exp Clin Endocrinol Diabetes.* 1995;**103**:129–149.

Raine CS. Multiple sclerosis: immune system molecule expression in the central nervous system. *J Neuropathol Exp Neurol.* 1994;**53**:328–337.

Raine CS. The Dale E. McFarlin Memorial Lecture: the immunology of the multiple sclerosis lesion. *Ann Neurol.* 1994;**36 Suppl**:S61–72.

Riordan Eva P, Sanders MD, Govan GG, Sweeney MG, Da Costa J, Harding AE. The clinical features of Leber's hereditary optic neuropathy defined by the presence of a pathogenic mitochondrial DNA mutation. *Brain.* 1995;**118**:319–337.

Robinson DB, Michaels RD. Empty sella resulting from the spontaneous resolution of a pituitary macroadenoma *Arch Intern Med.* 1992;**152**:1920–1923.

Smith BE, Dyck PJ. Subclinical histopathological changes in the oculomotor nerve in diabetes mellitus. *Ann Neurol.* 1992;**32**: 376–385.

Thapar K, Stefaneanu L, Kovacs K, et al. Estrogen receptor gene expression in craniopharyngiomas: an *in situ* hybridization study. *Neurosurgery.* 1994;**35**:1012–1017.

Volpe NJ, Liebsch NJ, Munzenrider JE, Lessell S. Neuro-ophthalmologic findings in chordoma and chondrosarcoma of the skull base. *Am J Ophthalmol.* 1993;**115**:97–104.

Wallace DC. 1994 William Allan Award Address. Mitochondrial DNA variation in human evolution, degenerative disease, and aging. *Am J Hum Genet.* 1995;**57**:201–223.

Weiner HL, Wisoff JH, Rosenberg M. et al. Craniopharyngiomas: a clinicopathological analysis of factors predictive of recurrence and functional outcome. *Neurosurgery.* 1994;**35**:1001–1010.

Whyte WL, Ferry JA, Harris NL, Grove ES. Ocular adnexal lymphoma – A clinicopathologic study with identification of lymphomas of mucosa associated lymphoid tissue type. *Ophthalmology.* 1995;**102**:1994–2006.

CHAPTER 5

Neuro-ophthalmic History and Examination

Peter Eustace

INTRODUCTION

Taking a history is a skill developed with experience. Learn to let the patient talk, and listen! Listen! Then, gently encourage and persuade the patient to give more information. There are very few disorders in neuro-ophthalmology that are not reflected in a history obtained from carefully listening to the patient's story.

Only then should you ask leading questions, which must be done in a systematic way: first ask questions related to the visual sensory system and then to the visual motor system. It is also imperative to obtain routine information relating to general medical history, including family history, and, finally, social history.

A systematic approach to history taking requires a logical scheme (*Fig. 5.1*).

SYMPTOMS RELATING TO THE VISUAL SYSTEM

VISION

Vision is the most important part of the history for an ophthalmologist to explore and visual loss is always a catastrophe to the patient. The ophthalmologist should ascertain the following:

- Is vision normal? If not, what is wrong? Ask about each eye separately.
- If there is visual loss, ask the patient clearly to define his or her estimate of the loss.
- Exactly when was vision last normal?
- If loss of vision is transient, is it complete loss or just gray out?
- Exactly how long does the visual loss last for?
- How does vision depart?
- How does it return?

VISUAL FIELD

Most patients if asked directly will be able to state 'I have lost the vision in the center' or 'I have lost the right side of my vision'. The patient's reply is as important as performing automated perimetry with the most sophisticated perimeter. However, most patients with homonymous hemianopia believe that the eye on the side with visual loss is a blind eye. It is often necessary to show patients that they have lost half the field of vision from both eyes.

STEREOPSIS

Ask the patient directly: 'Is your sense of depth normal, can you judge distance? Can you place your feet on the stairs? Can you pour fluid into a cup?'

COLOR VISION

Direct questioning invariably reveals any defect of color vision. Patients are keenly aware of longstanding color vision defects and of any recent change, particularly any desaturation of red.

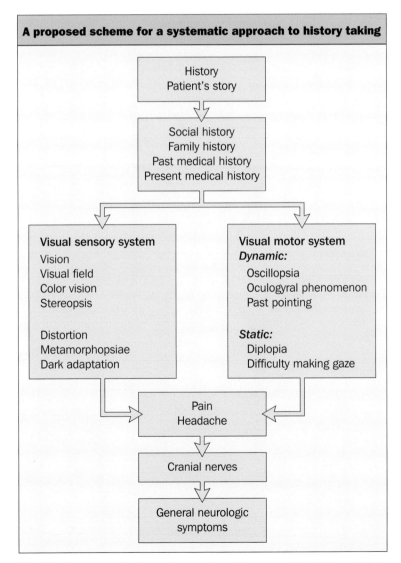

Fig. 5.1 A proposed scheme for a systematic approach to history taking.

DARK ADAPTATION

Poor dark adaptation is always described as poor night vision and is an early and significant symptom of patients with retinitis pigmentosa of any sort. Poor night driving is most frequently a result of cataract as opposed to retinal dystrophy.

METAMORPHOPSIAE

Photopsiae (flashing lights) are characteristically associated with eye movement. If this is the case, vitreoretinal pathology is likely. The episodes are usually described as being of momentary duration. A retinal tear is associated with a distinct flash, whereas vitreous traction produces a series of less distinct light flashes. Photopsiae not associated with eye movement are more likely to have a neurologic basis. Prolonged photopsiae, with shimmering heat, haze, zigzagging, and a fortification spectrum lasting 5–10 min or up to 1 hour, are the classic symptoms of a migraine aura. The aura is frequently isolated and associated with no headache or perhaps with only a slight muzziness of the mind.

Occipital cortical photopsiae proceed from very bright and disturbing flashes to frank epilepsy. Micropsiae (reduction in visual size) and teleopsia (the sense of remoteness of objects being viewed) are the result of macular pathology.

DISTORTION OF VISION

Persistent distortion is a symptom of macular disease, due to a misalignment of the normal relationship of retinal receptors. Straight lines are bent and familiar objects have distortions only when looked at directly. The visual distortion that occurs with parietotemporal lesions is always evolving, never static, and often is associated with other parietotemporal symptoms.

PAIN

Very careful direct questioning is always required to elucidate the true nature and quality of a patient's pain. Really find out what the patient means and relate it to the previous history. Reaction to pain is very relative and some patients are so stoic that they regard headache as a normal feature and will not volunteer a story of frequent headache unless asked directly.

Abnormal sensations limited to a single sensory dermatome can be assumed to be of neural origin.

SYMPTOMS RELATING TO THE VISUAL MOTOR SYSTEM

DYNAMIC

A nystagmus of recent onset may produce symptoms of oscillopsia (a wobbling to-and-fro sensation or a jumping up and down of the environment) or the oculogyral phenomenon (a rotary sensation in the opposite direction to the slow phase of the nystagmus). This is explained by the phenomenon of visual suppression during the saccadic (fast) phase of the nystagmus.

Past-pointing, by which the patient attempts to locate objects

projected further away than they really are, is associated with restrictions of eye movement.

An unusual perceptual phenomenon of 90° tilt of the environment is an unusual symptom of the lateral medullary, or posterior inferior cerebellar artery syndrome.

DIPLOPIA

Diplopia (the perception of two images of the same object) results from ocular misalignment in which the macula of the fixing eye sees the real object but the image of the misaligned eye falls on an extramacular point and is, therefore, projected to a different point in space (*Fig. 5.2*).

All patients with diplopia will have a moment in their history when they first noticed diplopia. The most important question to ask is: 'Is there any separation of the two images vertically, that is, one above the other?' If there is any vertical separation of images, even if there is also horizontal separation, the important separation etiologically is the vertical separation. Clearly show the patient that you only need to know if there is any vertical separation, even if there is also horizontal separation. It is also useful to ask if there is any torsion of the images (*Fig. 5.3*).

Diplopia is worst when the patient looks in the direction of action of the defective gaze system. With vergence problems, diplopia is present in a plane. For convergence problems, diplopia is elicited

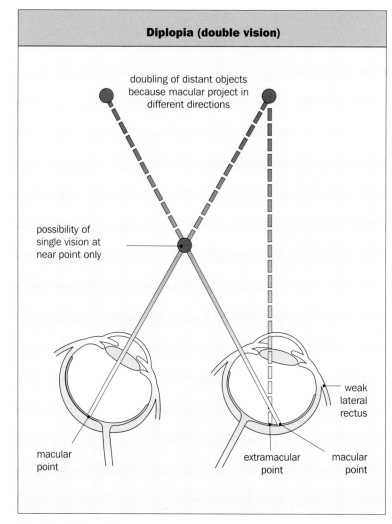

Fig. 5.2 Diplopia (double vision) is the result of the projection in space of the extramacular point.

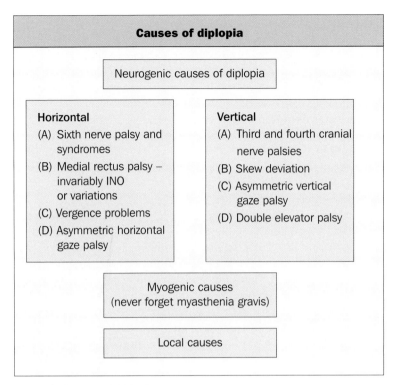

Fig. 5.3 Causes of diplopia.

at a certain distance from the patient and at that distance the image separation is constant in all directions of gaze. For divergence problems, diplopia is present when looking at distant objects, whereas for convergence, diplopia is present for near objects.

NEURO-OPHTHALMIC EXAMINATION

When examining a patient, the ophthalmologist should consider the following points:
- Get to the level of the patient. Before starting to examine the patient, make sure you are at eye level with the patient. Handle the patient's head as little as possible.
- Examine slowly. A slow examination allows the examiner to clearly identify what abnormalities are seen. This applies particularly to examination of eye movements.
- Think physiologically. When examining eye movements or the pupil you are testing a specific physiologic system.
- Then think anatomically. Make a clear mental image of the neuroanatomy relevant to the system being examined when carrying out any examination.

The scheme in *Figure 5.4* shows a systematic way to undertake a complete clinical neuro-ophthalmic examination.

VISION

The standard visual acuity charts are all of equal value in a neuro-ophthalmic assessment of vision. If the patient wears a distance-correction aid it should be worn for testing distance vision and, similarly, the patient should wear a near-correction aid for testing near vision. A pin-hole vision test is a reasonable compromise for testing distance vision but ultimately the neuro-ophthalmologist may have to refract the patient. Astigmatic or anisometropic amblyopia has often been investigated by MRI scanning; at the very least, an automated refraction must be obtained.

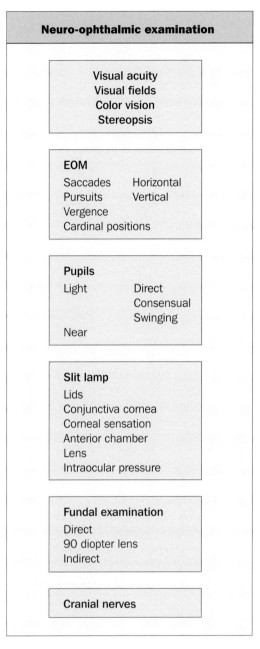

Fig. 5.4 A scheme for neuro-ophthalmic examination. (EOM, examination of movement)

VISUAL FIELDS

Confrontation testing compares the patient's field with the examiner's presumed-normal field. The nasal visual field is tested at a point midway between the examiner and the patient. The temporal, superior, and inferior fields are tested by moving the test object from behind the patient and then extrapolating into the same plane at which the nasal field was tested. The patient should be tested specifically along the vertical meridian and also the central field. The test should be from the blind field into the seeing field.

COLOR VISION

Specialized color plates (e.g. Hard–Rand–Rittler or Ishihara plates) are usually readily available. The use of a red drop bottle top, popularized by Joel Glaser, is a useful compromise but make sure the patient describes color desaturation, not target movement.

STEREOPSIS

Ask the patient to place his or her finger on the tip of a pen moved around in the visual space but within arm's reach.

Stereopsis tests using polarizing glasses are widely available, and can be used to estimate the quality of the stereopsis in minutes of arc separation. A Wirt Fly test or a similar stereoscopic test is useful to measure stereopsis more precisely. Loss of stereopsis can be a very useful clue to longstanding amblyopia.

EXAMINATION OF EYE MOVEMENTS

The types of eye movement are listed in *Figure 5.5*.

PURSUIT EYE MOVEMENTS

Horizontal and vertical pursuits are assessed in terms of character and range. Saccadic intrusions are the observable clinical sign of pursuit system dysfunction (*Fig. 5.6*).

Disturbance of gaze range may be of neurogenic, myogenic, or local cause. The pursuit system will function only if following a slowly moving target. The optimum speed is 20–30° of arc/s. Remember that the pursuit system generates a reflex eye movement, the only voluntary component being the effort of will to look at the target. It is impossible to mimic slow eye movements without a slowly moving target.

VERGENCE

Convergence is also assessed in terms of range and character. The near point at which divergence occurs is more or less constant. The nondominant eye will diverge with diplopia if stereoscopic vision is present and without diplopia if there is any suppression and the vergence problem is longstanding. Vergence eye movements are both voluntary and reflex.
- Voluntary vergence is tested by asking the patient to look into the distance and then to a new object presented suddenly at the tip of the nose.
- Reflex vergence is tested by slowly moving a target from 1 m to the tip of the nose.

The vergence system is essentially controlled in the upper brain stem. This means that in all but very large pontine lesions vergence is intact.

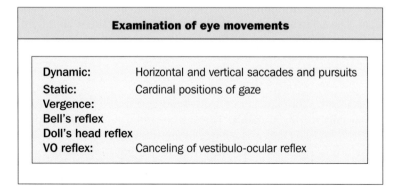

Examination of eye movements	
Dynamic:	Horizontal and vertical saccades and pursuits
Static:	Cardinal positions of gaze
Vergence:	
Bell's reflex	
Doll's head reflex	
VO reflex:	Canceling of vestibulo-ocular reflex

Fig. 5.5 Examination of eye movements.

SACCADIC EYE MOVEMENTS

Saccades are tested by directing the subject to look at two specific targets (e.g. a finger and then a pen), and asking the subject to repeat this as fast as possible. Saccades are judged clinically in the following categories:
1. Character of movement: smooth, fast, slow, louping (*Fig. 5.7*).
2. Accuracy (i.e. hypometric or hypermetric, or dysmetria) (*Fig. 5.8*).
3. Superimposed abnormalities, such as opsoclonus or flutter (*Fig. 5.9*).
4. Synchronicity of conjugate gaze (*Fig. 5.10*).

Some characteristic disturbances of eye movements are detected only when the patient is requested to make rapid shifts of fixation. The particular pattern of lag in adduction caused by medial rectus weakness ('adduction lag') is the hallmark of internuclear ophthalmoplegia and is seen only during rapid horizontal eye movements. Convergence retraction nystagmus on attempted voluntary up-gaze is the hallmark of the dorsal midbrain syndrome. It is most clearly demonstrated by the use of an optokinetic target. The eyes slowly follow the downward movement at a speed allowing a pursuit or following movement. The eyes move with an upward saccade to pick up the next target. This test is an extremely potent stimulus to the saccadic system and, in the presence of the dorsal midbrain syndrome, produces a well-sustained convergence retraction nystagmus in which the eyes beat towards each other and syn-

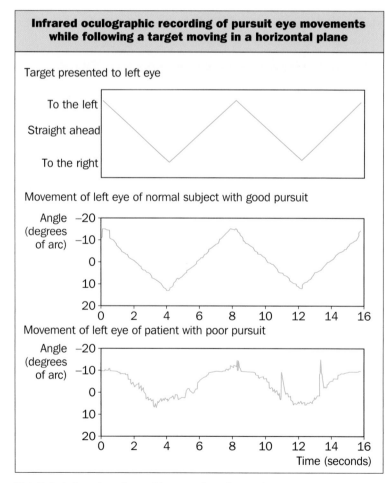

Fig. 5.6 Infrared oculographic recording of pursuit eye movements. The upper trace shows very disordered pursuits with multiple abnormal saccadic intrusions. The lower trace shows normal pursuits with small 'catch-up' saccades that occur normally.

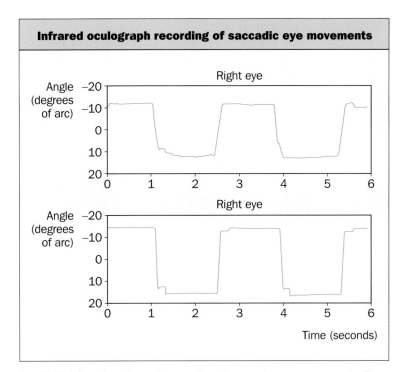

Fig. 5.7 Infrared oculograph recording of saccadic eye movements. The upper trace shows slow saccades. The lower trace shows normal saccades with an adjusting hypometric saccade, a normal feature.

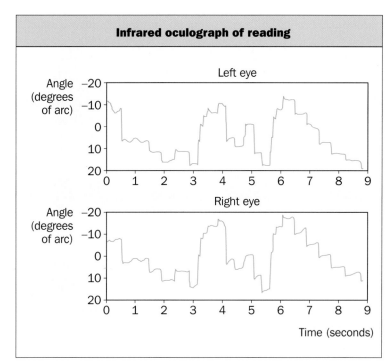

Fig. 5.8 Infrared oculography of reading, which is a saccadic function. The trace shows hypermetric saccades in a patient with thyrotoxicosis.

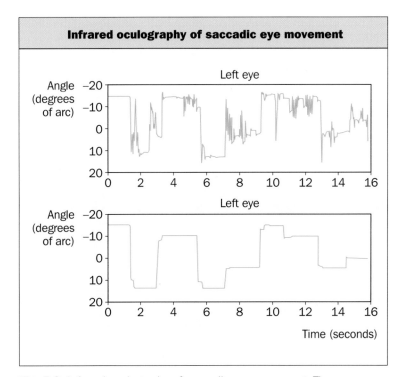

Fig. 5.9 Infrared oculography of saccadic eye movement. The upper trace shows multiple 'back-to-back' random saccades of opsoclonus and fixation 'flutter' saccades. The lower tracing is of a normal subject with hypometric saccades within a normal range.

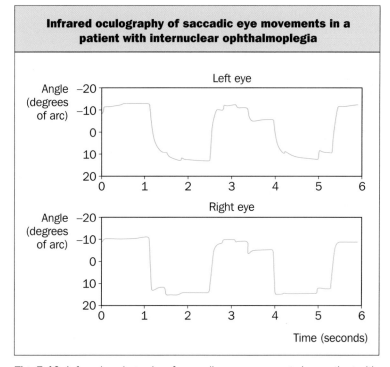

Fig. 5.10 Infrared oculography of saccadic eye movements in a patient with internuclear ophthalmoplegia. The upper trace shows adduction lag of the left eye on right gaze; the lower trace, when viewed with the upper trace, shows some gaze slowing to the left with 'abducting nystagmus' on left gaze.

chronously retract. Without using an optokinetic drum, convergence retraction nystagmus may be only a few ill-sustained beats. Optokinetic nystagmus (OKN), elicited with an OKN drum, provides a valuable clinical examination of the pursuit and the saccadic systems. OKN testing requires vision sufficient to see the drum stripes and is, therefore, a valuable test of vision. It is very difficult for a patient feigning poor vision to look through the rotating drum. OKN uses the pursuit and the saccadic systems. A dissociation of OKN is commonly seen in parietal lesions.

Having assessed the distinct physiologic systems that control eye movements the ophthalmologist should now think anatomically and examine horizontal eye movements.

When testing horizontal movements, the integrity of the medial rectus and lateral rectus muscles, and particularly the horizontal gaze system, is being tested. Similarly, when testing vertical gaze, the integrity of the vertically acting muscles and the vertical gaze mechanism is being tested. Asymmetry of vertical gaze is a common clinical finding in the dorsal midbrain syndrome and, therefore, vertical diplopia will be one of the presenting symptoms in this important disturbance of vertical eye movements.

When analyzing a horizontal diplopia, the examiner is thinking about not only whether the medial and lateral recti can contract in one direction, but whether they can relax appropriately in the other direction, and in addition is considering the possibility of an abnormality of the horizontal gaze mechanism. It is therefore helpful for the examiner to pose a routine series of questions:
• Could this diplopia be monocular rather than binocular? I.e. due to an optical irregularity of cornea, lens, or vitreous in one eye and not a matter of ocular misalignment at all?
• Is the diplopia 'crossed' or 'uncrossed'. i.e. an exotropia or an esotropia?
• How does the ocular misalignment and hence the diplopia vary when looking to the right and looking to the left?
• Is the amount of diplopia influenced by whether it is the right

eye or the left eye that is fixing?
• Does convergence produce a stronger adduction than simple horizontal gaze?
• Does manipulation of the eye with forceps demonstrate that it is free to move and not tethered?
• Might an antocholinesterase enliven the myoneural junction and eliminate the diplopia etc.? There is of course a similar set of questions for problems of vertical gaze.

If there is a horizontal gaze deficit, remember that the majority of horizontal gaze defects are asymmetric and, therefore, have the symptoms of horizontal diplopia. It is important to make a clear mental picture of the defect of the eye movement being seen. For example, is there a weakness of abduction or adduction in all four horizontally acting muscles? Similarly, consider the anatomy of the vertical muscles when examining vertical movement.

The oblique eye movements should now be tested and the ophthalmologist should consider defects of individual muscles (*Fig. 5.11*). When testing oblique eye movements only the actions of individual muscles are being tested, not recognized gaze systems.

The next stage is to examine Bell's phenomenon and the visually aided doll's head reflex.

BELL'S REFLEX

This is an extremely powerful and repetitive reflex. It is elicited clinically by forced lid opening against maximum effort to sustain closure. The normal response is an upward and outward deviation of the eyes. Cogan described the symmetric deviation of both eyes to the opposite side in some intracerebral lesions, particularly of the parietotemporal lobes. He called this lateralizing sign 'spasticity of conjugate gaze' (*Fig. 5.12*).

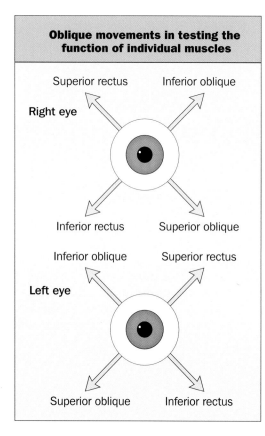

Fig. 5.11 This diagram illustrates the value of oblique movements in testing the function of individual muscles.

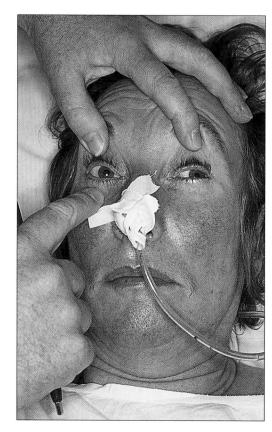

Fig. 5.12 Conjugate deviation of the eyes in an unconscious patient. Cogan's 'spasticity of conjugate gaze', the deviation of the eyes to the left with a left-sided lesion.

DOLL'S HEAD REFLEX

In some cases of apparent gaze paralysis either horizontal or vertical flexion or extension of the neck, or side-to-side movements of the head, produce normal eye movements. This clinical sign should, and usually does, mean an upper motor neuron disturbance of gaze. However, with dorsal midbrain lesions it is very common that an apparent up-gaze palsy can be overcome by vertical head movements. Perhaps the reflex is so powerful that impulses can be driven through a damaged but not destroyed gaze system. This reflex is a synthesis between the vestibulo-ocular reflex and vision; it is the visually assisted vestibulo-ocular reflex (*Figs 5.13–5.15*).

The doll's head reflex can be quantified clinically by first testing visual acuity and then measuring the decay in terms of lines on the visual acuity chart produced on side-to-side and up-and-down head movements. With a normally functioning vestibulo-ocular reflex, normal vision is maintained throughout this test.

Canceling of the reflex is tested by seeing if the patient can

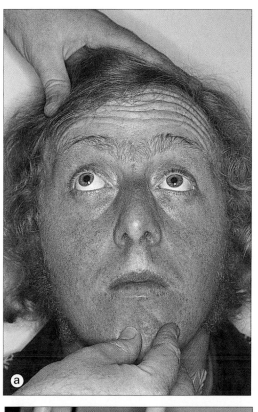

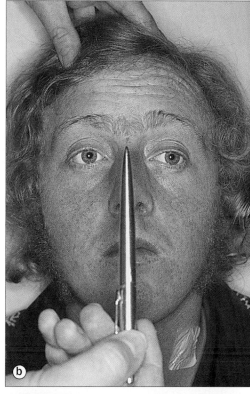

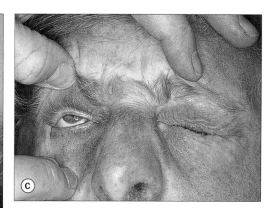

Fig. 5.13 (**a**) Impairment of vertical gaze in a patient with a pinealoma. (**b**) Loss of convergence. (**c**) Absent Bell's reflex showing a complete paralysis of reflex and voluntary vertical gaze.

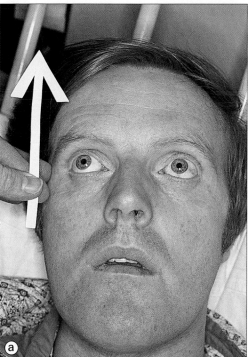

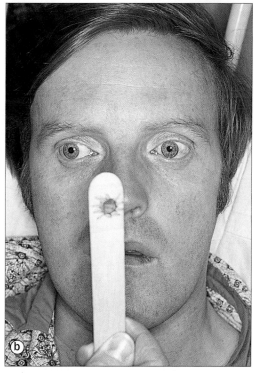

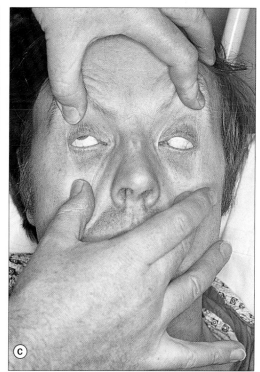

Fig. 5.14 (**a**) A patient with dorsal midbrain syndrome due to an arteriovenous malformation showing marked restriction of up-gaze. (**b**) The same patient showing convergence paralysis. (**c**) The same patient showing a normal Bell's reflex despite a demonstrable lesion of the dorsal midbrain.

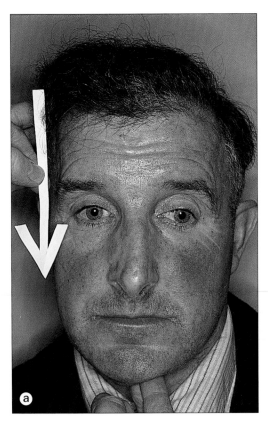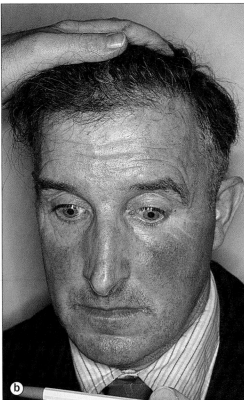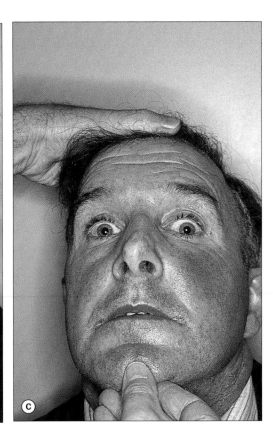

Fig. 5.15 (**a**) A patient with Steele–Richardson syndrome showing loss of voluntary down-gaze. (**b**) The same patient showing retention of down-going pursuits. (**c**) The same patient showing a well-preserved doll's head reflex.

maintain normal reading vision when keeping the head still while being rotated in a rotating chair. Inability to cancel this reflex may be the cause of ocular motor apraxia.

Since reading consists of making a saccade and then holding fixation for a moment before doing it again, rotating a patient who is reading from a book tests the quality of both the pursuit and saccadic eye movement mechanisms. A patient with poor pursuit mechanism will be unable to maintain his or her eyes on the page while a patient with defective generation of saccades (for example, a patient with congenital ocular motor apraxia) will find his or her eyes deviated away from the direction of rotation. Neither patient will be able to continue reading.

COVER AND UNCOVER TESTS

THE COVER TEST

Cover testing is used to detect manifest strabismus and uncover testing is used to detect latent strabismus. When carrying out these tests it is easier to separate the two, doing the cover test first and then the uncover test.

The right eye should always be covered first, while watching the left eye carefully in order to detect the smallest movement. The test is then repeated, covering the left eye. If there is any movement to take up fixation of the right eye, a right strabismus is present; if there is any movement of the left eye, a left strabismus is present. It there is movement to take up fixation on both tests, an alternating strabismus is present.

THE UNCOVER TEST

A phoria is shared equally between the two eyes. As a result, an alternating cover test, moving the occluder alternately from right to left and back again fairly briskly, is the most satisfactory way of detecting a latent squint. If a latent squint is present, the alternating cover test breaks it down and a small movement of either eye is readily seen.

PUPIL

It should be clear in the ophthalmologist's mind that the light reflex and the near reflex have different neurologic substrates. The light reflex has no voluntary component and does not require central vision. The reflex arc passes from the receptor cells in the retina, along the visual pathway, to the pretectal area; the automatic components of the near reflex require vision and, therefore, impulses must pass along the visual pathway to reach the occipital cortex. From there, the descending pathway passes anteriorly to the midbrain to synapse in the Edinger–Westphal nucleus. The anatomic separation of the two reflex pathways explains the mechanism of pupil disassociation seen in dorsal midbrain lesions.

The patient should be asked to look into the distance while the ophthalmologist observes the pupils of both eyes. A light is shone directly into the pupil. The light response in the eye being tested, and the consensual response in the fellow eye, should be noted. The fellow eye should then be tested in a similar way. A low level of illumination in the examination room and a bright light are prerequisites for this examination. The patient must not look at any near object and keep his or her view fixed in the distance. The ophthalmologist must not stand in front of the patient when carrying out this test.

To test the near reflex the patient should look at a distant target, which is then presented to the tip of the patient's nose; the reaction is as brisk as the light reflex. The direct light reflex and the consensual reflexes are equal.

It is often helpful to examine the pupil reaction, and the iris itself, on a slit lamp. This is particularly helpful if the patient has a tonic pupil.

AFFERENT PUPIL DEFECT

A complete lesion of the anterior visual pathway blocks all sensory input to the pretectal area. Therefore, there will be no direct light response, nor will there be a synchronous consensual response (afferent pupil defect).

If there is a partial block of the anterior visual pathway (e.g. a 50% block), there will be a 50% reduction of both direct and consensual responses. If the light is now swung into the fellow normal eye, which is 50% constricted, it will constrict fully, that is to 100%. At the same time, the pupil on the affected side now constricts to 100% because of the consensual response. If the light is then swung back to the affected side, it dilates from 100% constriction to 50% constriction again, therefore dilating despite the fact that light has been projected into the pupil. As the two pupils move in opposite directions to the swinging light, the difference is effectively magnified two-fold. This clinical sign is one of the most useful in neuro-ophthalmology.

SLIT LAMP EXAMINATION

The lids, conjunctiva, and cornea should now be examined on the slit lamp. During this examination, corneal sensation is tested. The patient is asked to elevate his or her eyes and the cornea is touched with a wick of cotton wool, just central to the limbus. The response is observed and the patient is asked to comment on a comparison between the two eyes. The tear film is assessed and tear break-up time and Schirmer tests are carried out if relevant. An intraocular pressure measurement is advisable at this stage and must never, ever, be overlooked.

FUNDUS EXAMINATION

A routine ophthalmoscopic examination is possible in the eye's undilated state. Ideally, the pupil should be dilated and the posterior pole examined with a +90 diopter lens. This is the most satisfactory way of looking at the optic nerve head and the immediately adjacent posterior pole, including the macula. The stereoscopic view obtained greatly enhances the value of this examination, which is much more informative than direct ophthalmoscopy.

The fundus examination is completed with indirect ophthalmoscopy.

CRANIAL NERVES

FIFTH CRANIAL NERVE

When testing corneal sensation, a cotton bud should be used to gently touch the cornea as the patient looks upwards. The cornea is exquisitely sensitive in the normal state and the patient will respond with a definite blink. The ophthalmologist should compare the patient's reaction to both eyes and ask the patient if there is any difference between eyes. It is important not to forget to test the motor root of the trigeminal nerve which supplies the masseter muscle and the medial and lateral pterygoid muscles.

SEVENTH CRANIAL NERVE

The muscles of the brow are represented bilaterally in the motor cortex and, therefore, are spared in cortical lesions producing a facial palsy. If the motor division is directly involved there is a complete paralysis of the facial expression muscles unilaterally. Sensation to the tympanic membrane and to the skin of the internal auditory meatus, and to a small area of skin behind the ear, is also carried in the facial nerve and should be specifically tested for numbness.

A lesion in the canal but peripheral to the nerve of the stapedius muscle leads to hyperacusis. The parasympathetic component of the seventh cranial nerve supplies the lacrimal gland and is the nerve of reflex tear secretion. It has a lengthy and complex course intracranially and extracranially (Fig. 5.16). The special sense of taste to the anterior two-thirds of the tongue is also carried with the facial nerve and should be specifically tested. Therefore, testing the nerve requires a clear understanding of neuroanatomy and a specific intent to test all four functional modalities carried in the nerve (i.e. motor and sensory function, parasympathetic, and the special sense of taste).

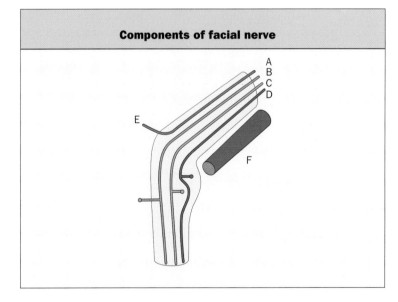

Components of facial nerve

Fig. 5.16 Components of the facial nerve. (A, parasympathetic division – N. intermedius secretomotor to the lacrimal gland; B, motor division – muscles of facial division; C, sensory division – to external auditory meatus; D special sensory division – chorda tympani – supplies tast to anterior two-thirds of tongue; E, nerve to stapedius – causes hyperacusis if damaged; F, vestibulo acoustic nerve.

EIGHTH, NINTH, ELEVENTH, AND TWELFTH CRANIAL NERVES

Clinical testing of these nerves should be carried out routinely. Examination of the mouth and palate is an essential part of any neuro-ophthalmic examination. The palate may be paralyzed or moving synchronously with the eyes; in oculopalateal myoclonus the tongue may be spastic or paralyzed and atrophic. Occasionally, nasopharyngeal tumors are visible or palpable (Fig. 5.17) and the black palate of mucormycosis once seen is never forgotten.

Further reading

Glaser JS, ed. *Neuro-Ophthalmology*, 2nd edition (Philadelphia: JB Lippincott, 1990).

Slamovits TL, Burde R, eds. Neuro-ophthalmology. *Textbook of Ophthalmology*, Vol. 6 (St Louis: Mosby, 1991).

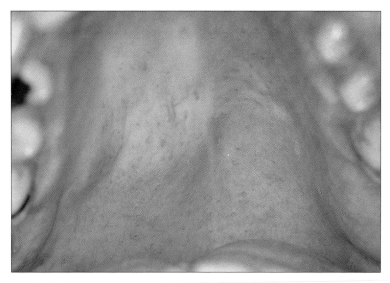

Fig. 5.17 A patient who presented with slight proptosis and recurrent corneal erosions. The lesion, an osteogenic sarcoma, was visible in the patient's mouth.

CHAPTER 6

Tests of Visual Function

David C Saunders

INTRODUCTION

There are many tests of visual function that have relevance in neuro-ophthalmology. Some of these tests should be used routinely for every patient (e.g. visual acuity), others are indicated only in certain clinical circumstances, whereas others are primarily research tools.

VISUAL ACUITY

Visual acuity is a measure of a patient's ability to resolve detail; the methods used rely on varying the minimum angle of resolution of an object on the retina until the patient is unable to resolve the detail. Best corrected visual acuity is a familiar measure of central vision. It is of great importance that vision is estimated only after any refractive error has been corrected. If corrective lenses are not available, a pinhole should be used to obtain at least an approximation to corrected visual acuity. It is meaningless to record uncorrected visual acuity alone. Vision should first be established in each eye individually, using an effective occluder. Binocular acuity may be measured subsequently.

The aim of any method is to provide the examiner with an accurate, reliable, and reproducible measure of acuity. The most widely used method is the Snellen chart which was developed in 1862 by Herman Snellen. The letters are designed using a 5 × 5 grid format

(*Fig. 6.1*) and are constructed so that appreciation of an angle of resolution of 1' of arc is needed to identify the letter, and the whole letter subtends 5' of arc. The letters are sized so that the first line letter forms this angle at a distance of 60 meters, the second line letters at 36 m, the third line letters at 24 m, and so on (*Fig. 6.2*). Patients are seated 6 m from the chart and asked to read the letters. The 'normal' patient should achieve the 6-m line of letters. This method has the advantage of being familiar to patients and quick and simple to perform.

The Snellen chart is often used in combination with a mirror to reduce the space required in the examination room, and reversed charts are available for this purpose (*Fig. 6.3*). Unfortunately, the Snellen chart measures acuity in an ordinal fashion (i.e. there is no linear relationship in the difficulty of the task between lines) (*Fig. 6.4*) and, as a result, statistical analysis of the measure is unreliable for research purposes. This does not detract from the chart's value in normal clinical practice, however. It is important to be aware of the degree of accuracy and reproducibility of any measure, so that appropriate importance is placed on any observed change. Vision is recorded in the familiar fractional fashion, the numerator representing the distance of the patient from the chart (conventionally 6 m in Europe and 20 ft in the USA) and the denominator representing the smallest line read by the patient. Thus, 6/18 represents a poor vision because at a distance of 6 m the patient can make out only the letters that a normal subject should be able to read at 18 m.

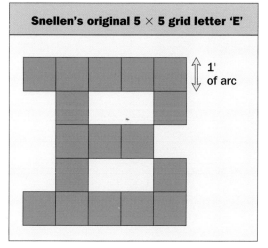

Snellen's original 5 × 5 grid letter 'E'

1' of arc

Fig. 6.1 The original 5 × 5 grid letter 'E' as described in 1862 by Herman Snellen.

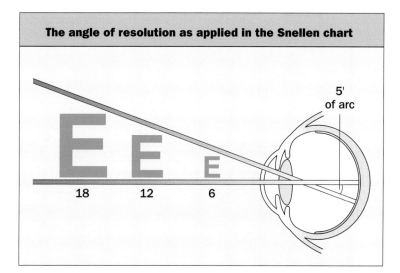

The angle of resolution as applied in the Snellen chart

5' of arc

18   12   6

Fig. 6.2 Diagrammatic representation of the angle of resolution as applied in the Snellen chart.

Various methods have been employed to test vision in illiterate patients. The Snellen 'E' chart allows patients to indicate the direction of the 'E' without the need to know the name of the letter (*Fig. 6.5*). Thus, an accurate Snellen measure may be obtained.

When assessing the pre-school child, the Sheridan–Gardner system is often very helpful. The normal Snellen chart is used but the child is given a card to hold with a selection of letters printed on it. Individual letters are indicated by the examiner and the child points to the matching letter on the hand-held card (*Fig. 6.6*). The child does not therefore need to know the letter names but merely must be able to match the shapes of the letters.

An alternative approach is a picture chart (*Fig. 6.7*) that has pictures of easily identified objects that can be named by the child. This does not provide the same degree of accuracy as the 'E' chart or Sheridan–Gardner technique because the objects do not conform to the standard Snellen grid pattern. Nonetheless, the picture chart is useful when dealing with children whose concentration may fail when performing the less-appealing tests.

When assessing infants, a number of methods can be employed to gain an approximate measure of visual acuity. The simplest methods involve tasks such as picking up 'hundreds and thousands' of cake decorations. This is especially popular when the child is allowed to eat the test objects! Alternatively, balls of progressively smaller sizes may be rolled in front of the infant at a set distance

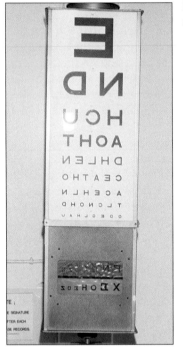

Fig. 6.3 A reversed Snellen chart for use in confined spaces with a mirror.

The nonlinear relationship between Snellen acuity lines	
Snellen acuity	Angle of resolution (")
6/6	1.0
6/9	1.4
6/12	2.0
6/18	3.3
6/60	10.0

Fig. 6.4 Table showing the nonlinear relationship between Snellen acuity lines.

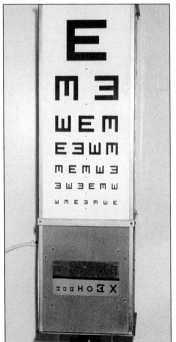

Fig. 6.5 The Snellen illiterate 'E' chart.

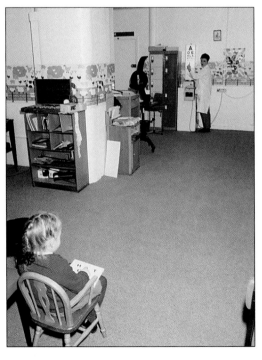

Fig. 6.6 The Sheridan–Gardner test establishing a child's visual acuity.

until the smallest size that attracts the child's interest is reached.

The Catford drum (*Fig. 6.8*) may be used to estimate visual acuity in infants. The drum moves to and fro and the child is observed for fixation and following movements (optokinetic nystagmus). Black discs of various sizes are displayed to identify the smallest disc to which the infant responds.

The preferential looking test is the most reproducible measure of an infant's acuity (*Fig. 6.9*) and relies on the observation that infants look preferentially at patterned objects rather than plain ones. The test involves placing the infant at a set distance in front of a screen and presenting two targets, one with a striped grating and one plain. The child's reaction is observed and finer gratings are presented until there is no consistent response from the infant indicating that he or she is unable to distinguish between the plain and striped targets. Considerable practice and expertise are required to obtain consistent results and preferential looking is generally confined to use by teams involved regularly in pediatric practice.

In adults, the LogMAR chart (Logarithm of the Minimum Angle of Resolution) provides a measure of acuity that is interval in nature (i.e. there is a direct relationship in the difficulty of the task between lines) and allows valid statistical analysis to be performed (*Fig. 6.10*). Each line has an equal number of letters and there is 0.1 log unit difference in the angle of resolution between lines. Ideally, the LogMAR chart could be used in routine clinical practice because it is possible to obtain both the logarithmic measure and a good approximation of the Snellen acuity from the LogMAR chart. This satisfies the dual needs of providing a measure familiar to patients, doctors, and other healthcare professionals, and a mathematically usable measure for research and audit purposes.

Near visual acuity is measured using standard typeface charts (*Fig. 6.11*). These should be used at an appropriate reading distance with good lighting and corrective lenses, if worn. This can be a useful measure for use at the bedside but it is not routinely used as the only measure of acuity because of the greater variability of viewing conditions compared with more formal chart-based measures. The smallest print visible to the patient is recorded. The print size is measured according to the printer's standard 'N' system. Letters are cut on blocks that are measured

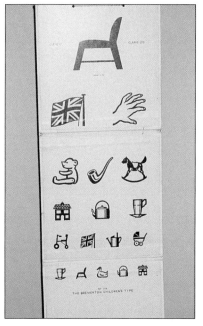

Fig. 6.7 The picture chart for testing children's visual acuity.

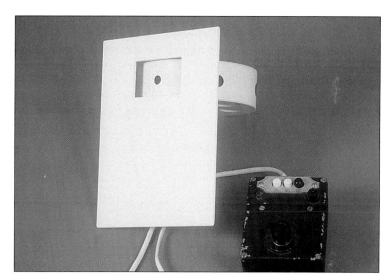

Fig. 6.8 The Catford drum used to elicit optokinetic nystagmus.

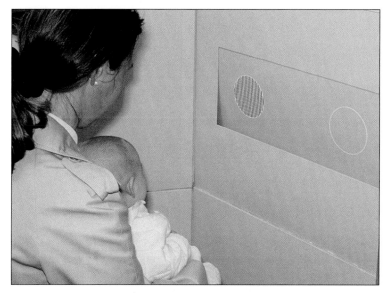

Fig. 6.9 Preferential looking test. (Courtesy of Dr IC Lloyd)

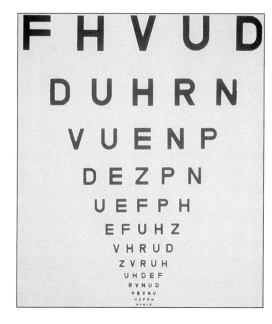

Fig. 6.10 The LogMAR chart.

in multiples of 1/72 inches. Thus, print using a block 5/72 inches in size is N5 print, whereas N48 print is produced using a block 48/72 inches in size.

Electrodiagnostic methods can be used to estimate visual acuity and are discussed below.

When measuring vision with the chart-based methods, some patients require considerable encouragement to obtain their best acuity and time should be allowed for this. Much information can be gained by close observation of the patient. For instance, a patient with a hemianopic field defect may read only the 'visible' half of the chart.

VISUAL FIELDS

The visual field has been described in three-dimensional terms by Traquair as 'an island of vision in a sea of darkness'. The central 'peak' of the island represents the highly sensitive central field, whereas the 'coastal' rim represents the relatively insensitive far peripheral field. Rather than being an island of granite, the visual field is more like an island of jelly. The visual field is a dynamic area that changes according to a large number of variables. This must always be borne in mind when assessing the results of visual field testing.

Tests of visual field should ideally provide a reliable and reproducible measure of the extent and sensitivity of the field. The development, progression, and regression of field defects can then be documented.

The simplest form of field assessment is confrontation testing. The patient is seated facing the examiner at arms' length and instructed to maintain fixation on the examiner's eye. A target is held as far peripherally as possible, midway between the patient and examiner. The target may take the form of a finger, a hat pin, a pencil with eraser, or wand. The target is moved centrally and the patient indicates when it becomes visible in the periphery of his or her field. This maneuver is repeated twice in each quadrant and a mental comparison is made between the observer's own (presumed normal) field and the patient's field. The test is performed separately for each eye. The technique may be modified for children by playing the 'finger mimicking' game. The child is instructed to copy the number of fingers held up by the examiner in each quadrant of the field (*Fig. 6.12*).

For infants the test is modified further. The appearance of an object in the peripheral field will usually result in an eye movement towards the object to take up fixation (the visually elicited eye movement). During confrontation testing the infant is observed for these visually elicited eye movements.

Confrontation testing can identify large defects in the peripheral field (e.g. hemianopia) but is unreliable in detecting subtle loss of sensitivity, especially if occurring as a paracentral scotoma. In no way is confrontation testing a substitute for formal visual field testing but it can be helpful as a gross screening test.

Goldmann perimetry is a substantially more sophisticated method of field assessment (*Fig. 6.13*). The apparatus consists of a bowl, illuminated evenly to a preset level, on to which is projected a point of variable size and brightness. The patient responds by pressing a buzzer on seeing the light. The examiner maintains sight of the patient's fixation through a lens in the center of the bowl that the patient is using as the fixation target.

Both static threshold and kinetic perimetry can be performed with the Goldmann perimeter. Static threshold perimetry involves displaying a non-moving target at varying points throughout the field and increasing its size and brightness, until the point is just seen at each location. A detailed map of the field can thus be built

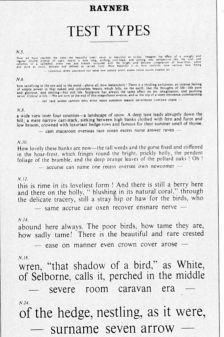

Fig. 6.11 Reading test types.

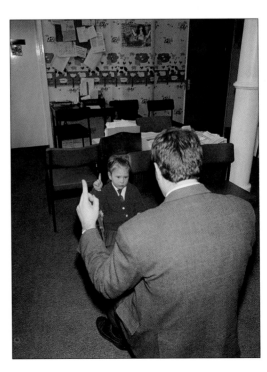

Fig. 6.12 Finger mimicking test used to screen a child's visual field.

up, albeit rather laboriously. Kinetic perimetry involves moving the target from a 'non-seeing' area into a 'seeing' area. A contour map of the island of vision can thus be established by using targets of varying size and brightness. Kinetic perimetry is usually the preferred method when using a Goldmann perimeter.

Both static and kinetic techniques will identify relative (partial) as well as complete scotomata. It must be remembered that many factors influence the size and shape of the visual field, including the patient's state of mind, previous practice at the test, refraction, pupil size, and ocular media opacities. In addition, the examiner's technique has a significant effect on the final result. In an attempt to standardize the examination protocol and thus remove one source of error, computer-assisted perimetry has become very popular.

Computer-assisted perimetry performs static threshold perimetry according to predetermined examination protocols (*Fig. 6.14*). The sophisticated techniques now available allow very detailed analysis of the island of vision. New statistical software empowers the clinician with additional means of refining the assessment and representation of the visual field (*Fig. 6.15*). It must, however, be remembered at all times that the tests are subjective and the advent of computerization has not changed this fact.

COLOR VISION

Defective color vision is often a genetically determined trait and is commonly known as 'color blindness'. Various forms of color-test plates have been produced, including Ishihara, Stilling, and Hardy–Rand–Rittler plates. Many of the available tests have been developed specifically to identify individuals with the genetic traits rather than acquired color defects associated with neuro-ophthalmic disease. Nonetheless, a normal response to the color plate tests is helpful in excluding a color-vision defect.

The color-test plates consist of dots of the primary colors on a background of dots of confusing colors. The dots are in

recognizable patterns, such as numbers or shapes. The patient is shown the plates one at a time and asked to identify the number or shape (*Fig. 6.16*). Some plates have a 'path' to follow rather than a number or shape and are useful in the examination of children.

A more sophisticated test of color vision is the Farnsworth–Munsell 100-hue test (*Fig. 6.17*). In this test, 100 discs of varying shades (numbered on the underside) are placed before the patient in a random fashion. The patient is asked to rearrange the discs into a sequence with a smooth and gradual change of color. The examiner is then able to plot graphically, on a color wheel, the results of the test, indicating the zones in which discontinuities have been introduced into this sequence. This test is not commonly used but does provide a comprehensive record of color vision.

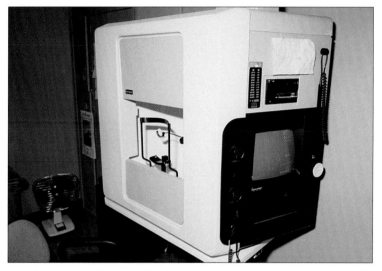

Fig. 6.14 An automated computerized perimeter.

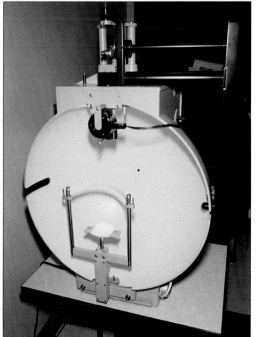

Fig. 6.13 The Goldmann perimeter.

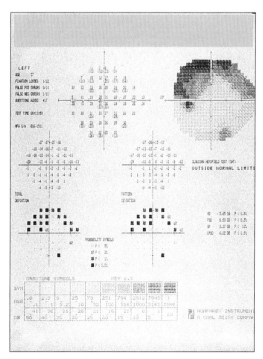

Fig. 6.15 An example of the type of sophisticated report produced by computerized perimetry.

Color desaturation is a common neuro-ophthalmic symptom. The intensity of color as seen by each eye can be compared by using, for example, a bright red pen top. The patient is asked to subjectively assess the brightness and intensity of the displayed object with first one eye and then the other. Although this test is entirely subjective, it can be valuable and is simple to perform. The test can also be used to compare color saturation between each half of the field in one eye as a screening test for hemianopic defects.

RELATIVE AFFERENT PUPILLARY DEFECT

Testing for a relative afferent pupillary defect (RAPD) is a very important part of the examination and should be performed prior to dilatation of the pupils in all patients. The test requires a bright light source that is shone first in one eye and then swung directly to the fellow eye so that the pupil reactions in each eye can be compared. Normally, the pupillary responses will be about the same in each eye. However, in an eye with sufficient retinal or optic nerve disease, the pupil of the affected eye will be seen to dilate when the light is swung from the fellow eye (*Fig. 6.18*).

LIGHT STRESS TEST

This simple test is effective in distinguishing loss of acuity caused by optic nerve disease from that caused by fundal lesions. In the presence of retinal disease there is a prolonged recovery time after exposure to bright light. In normal patients the recovery time is rapid (10–30 s). The best corrected acuity is determined and then the normal eye is subjected to a bright light for a specific time (e.g. 5 s) with the suspect eye covered. The light is extinguished and the time taken to recover acuity is recorded. The procedure is repeated for the fellow eye. The recovery period would be expected to be equal in optic nerve disease while being prolonged in an eye with retinal disease.

FUNDUS FLUORESCEIN ANGIOGRAPHY

Fundus fluorescein angiography (FFA) involves injecting sodium fluorescein intravenously and photographing the fundus repeatedly to show the passage of fluorescence through the choroidal and retinal vasculature. It is valuable in the assessment of subtle

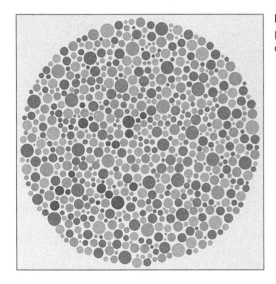

Fig. 6.16 The pseudoisochromatic color-test plate.

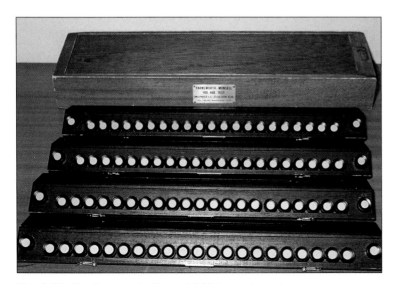

Fig. 6.17 The Farnsworth–Munsell 100-hue color-vision test.

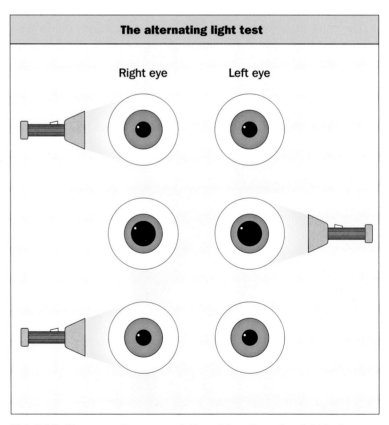

Fig. 6.18 Diagrammatic representation of the alternating light test showing a left relative afferent pupillary defect.

retinal lesions. These lesions may be responsible for defective vision that might otherwise be attributed, mistakenly, to neuro-ophthalmic disease (*Fig. 6.19*). In the specific instance of optic disc drusen mimicking papilloedema, fundus photography using the FFA filter (but without injecting fluorescein) shows the auto-fluorescence of drusen.

ELECTRODIAGNOSTIC TESTS

ELECTRORETINOGRAM

The electroretinogram (ERG) records the changes in the electrical potential of the retina after exposure to light. A contact lens electrode may be used to obtain the response. Alternatively, a flexible electrode in the lower fornix can be used. A standard method for producing an ERG was recommended by the International Standardization Committee in 1989. Sophisticated equipment is needed, along with experienced operators, to produce reliable results (*Fig. 6.20*). The ERG is therefore limited in routine clinical practice. The ERG is composed of the 'a', 'b', and 'c' waves, along with an early receptor potential and oscillatory potentials (*Fig. 6.21*). These waves are measured in millivolts (mV) and must be amplified in order to be recorded.

By varying the stimulus brightness, duration, and color, the response of various elements of the retina can be elicited. A pure cone response is produced by a stimulus flickering at 30 Hz because rods cannot respond at this rate. A rod response can be elicited by stimulating the dark-adapted retina to dim blue light below the cone threshold.

The ERG is especially valuable when investigating the possibility that one of the retinal dystrophies is responsible for defective vision. Interpretation of the ERG requires a full understanding of the factors that may influence the response. External factors include electrical artefacts, eye movements, blinking, refractive error, pupil size, and many others.

ELECTRO-OCULOGRAM

The electro-oculogram (EOG) is a recording of the corneoretinal potential measured in dark-adapted and light-adapted conditions. Skin electrodes at the medial and lateral canthi are used, along with a third electrode on the forehead. Brisk horizontal eye movements of fixed sizes are elicited using two small red fixation lights on either side of a screen (*Fig. 6.22*). This generates a modified square-wave pattern, attributable solely to the existence of the standing potential between retina and cornea (*Fig. 6.23*). The eye acts as a dipole. The potential measured is directly proportional to the angle of rotation of the globe.

The Arden index is calculated as the ratio of the average maximum light response to the average minimum dark response expressed as a percentage. A normal response is an index of more than approximately 185%. Variations in equipment mean that each laboratory should establish its own normal results.

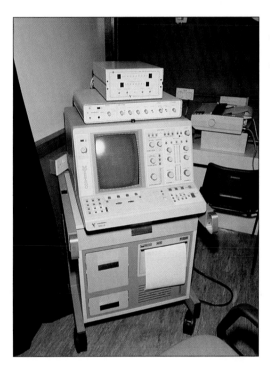

Fig. 6.20 The equipment used to record the electroretinogram (ERG).

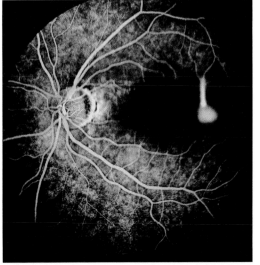

Fig. 6.19 A fluorescein angiogram showing central serous retinopathy.

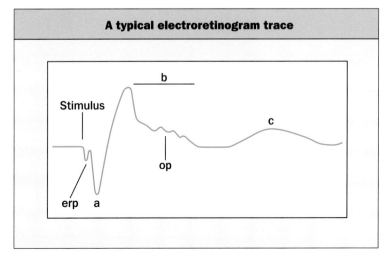

Fig. 6.21 Diagrammatic representation of a typical ERG trace.

The EOG is useful in conjunction with the ERG in the diagnosis of retinal dystrophies. Both ERG and EOG are valuable research tools. The ERG measures rapid responses of the retina to light whereas the EOG measures longer-term changes.

VISUAL-EVOKED POTENTIAL

The visual-evoked potential (VEP) is a recording of the brain's electrical activity in response to visual stimuli, that is, a 'visual electroencephalogram (EEG)'. In order to measure the VEP, four elements are required: a repeatable visual stimulus, scalp electrodes, an amplifier, and an averaging system to display the information. No internationally agreed method of producing the VEP has been agreed and results vary from center to center. The stimulus may take the form of a bright flash of light or a pattern displayed on a screen. The pattern stimulus is becoming the preferred method because it produces a larger response and is more closely related to 'seeing'. The electrodes may be placed in various positions on the scalp, depending on which aspect of the VEP is of particular interest. The VEP response is masked by background 'noise' and repeated stimuli are used so that averaging may be employed to remove the 'noise', leaving a pure trace.

The wave form of the 'normal' VEP varies enormously from one individual to another, making interpretation difficult. Fortunately, there are some typical features of the VEP that allow comparison. Positive peaks are typically produced at 10–20 ms and 150–200 ms after the stimulus. The latency of these peaks is increased by optic nerve conduction defects. This has proved clinically useful in identifying individuals who have apparently recovered from retrobulbar neuritis clinically but who still show VEP abnormalities in latency.

The VEP can be used to estimate visual acuity by varying the grating of the pattern stimulus. The VEP appears to be derived from the central 5–10° of visual field. The acuity estimate does not bear comparison with Snellen acuity but can sometimes be of value. The VEP is a valuable research tool.

In summary, electrodiagnostic testing has limited clinical availability but is proving to be a valuable tool in specific circumstances. The research value of these tests is immense and our understanding of the sense of sight is being advanced at a rapid rate with the help of these tests.

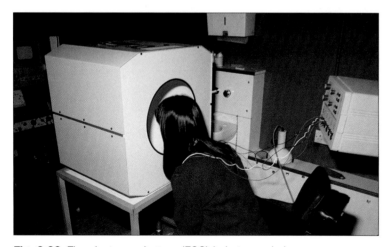

Fig. 6.22 The electro-oculogram (EOG) being recorded.

An electro-oculogram trace

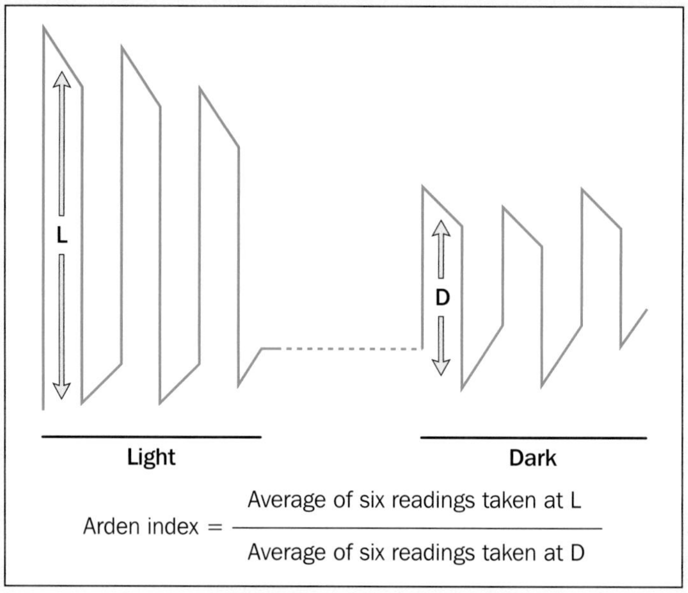

Light   Dark

$$\text{Arden index} = \frac{\text{Average of six readings taken at L}}{\text{Average of six readings taken at D}}$$

Fig. 6.23 Diagrammatic representation of an EOG trace.

Further reading

Duke-Elder S. *Visual Acuity*. In: Duke-Elder S, ed. *System of Ophthalmology, Vol. VII*. (London: Kimpton, 1972) 366–379.

Galloway NR. *Electrodiagnosis*. In: Walsh T, ed. *Neuro-Ophthalmology, 3rd edn*. (Philadelphia: Lea and Febiger, 1992) 353–396.

Glaser JS. *Neuro-Ophthalmic Examination*. In: Duane TD, Jaeger EA, eds. *Clinical Ophthalmology, Vol. 2*. (Philadelphia: JB Lippincott, 1988) 1–38.

CHAPTER 7

Tests of Ocular Motor Function

Alec M Ansons and Alison L Spencer

TESTS OF OCULAR MOTOR FUNCTION

This first half of the chapter refers to the clinical testing of the eye movement systems and their defects. For a brief review of the physiology of eye movements see Chapter 9.

TESTING SACCADIC EYE MOVEMENTS

The clinical observation of saccades in co-operative patients can readily be performed by instructing them to refixate between the examiner's out-stretched finger and nose (*Fig. 7.1*). Movements made to command are observed in all directions for prompt initiation; if delays in initiation are found, the patient is observed for head thrusts or eyelid closure – strategies that are frequently used by patients with ocular motor apraxia. A slow peak saccadic velocity is most easily identified when differences in peak saccadic velocity exists between the eyes (as in the lateral rectus slowing in sixth nerve palsy); global reductions in saccadic velocity (as in chronic progressive external ophthalmoplegia) can be harder to detect clinically. Large amplitude saccades accentuate small difference in peak saccadic velocity and make identification easier. An optokinetic drum or tape is useful in forcing the patient to make multiple saccades, which again may help accentuate differences in peak saccadic velocity or fatigable conditions, such as myasthenia gravis.

Saccadic dysmetria is identified by the nature of the corrective saccade required to reach the target. As hypometria is associated with large amplitude saccades, small saccadic amplitudes of 5–10°

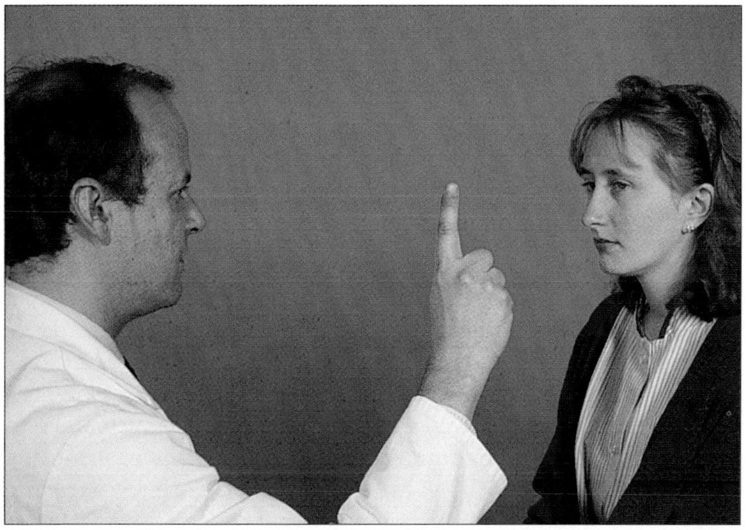

Fig. 7.1 Clinical observation of saccadic eye movements.

should be examined, care being taken to ensure that any inaccuracies identified are reproducible.

In infants and uncooperative patients, reliance is often made on observing spontaneous eye movements or eye movements made to novel or threatening stimuli. Optokinetic stimuli, along with rotational testing, can be useful in stimulating saccadic eye movements.

Inappropriate saccades can interrupt steady fixation, occurring as either bursts of horizontal back-to-back saccades (ocular flutter), or as multidirectional saccades (opsoclonus).

PURSUIT SYSTEM

FUNCTION AND ANATOMY

The pursuit system maintains stable eye tracking or combined eye–head tracking of slowly moving objects, counteracting any slow movements that may act to destabilize the retinal image. The normal stimulus for pursuit movements is image movement (retinal slip) in the parfoveal region.

The higher control centers for pursuit movement lie in the parieto-occipital cortex, the fibers descending to the brainstem paramedian pontine reticular formation (PPRF) for horizontal pursuit commands. The cerebellum is also closely associated with normal pursuit movements, signals being generated during pursuit with the head still and during combined eye–head tracking (cancellation of the vestibulo-ocular reflex [VOR]).

COMPONENTS OF PURSUIT MOVEMENT

Pursuit movements, like saccades, have a latency after the stimulus before the movement starts; this is in the order of 100 ms. For target velocities up to 50–60°/s most eyes are able to track the object accurately, with eye velocity equal to target velocity (Gain = 1). For higher target velocities the eye has increasing difficulties in matching target velocity (Gain < 1), either falling behind the target or requiring a catch-up saccade. Pursuit movements are influenced by the nature of the stimulus, how it is behaving, the attention of the patient, and by certain drugs. Combined eye–head tracking of objects requires the normal VOR associated with the head movement (eye movement equal and opposite to head movement) to be suppressed for stable object tracking. This property of the pursuit system to cancel the VOR can be tested clinically and provides a sensitive measure of the performance of the pursuit system.

TESTING PURSUIT EYE MOVEMENTS

Observing the patient tracking a slowly moving small target, attention is paid to the smoothness of the movement; regular catch-up saccades suggest a low pursuit gain. Movements are examined in all directions with the head held still.

During combined eye–head tracking, the property of the pursuit system to cancel the VOR provides a sensitive measure for pursuit performance. If a slowly moving target is tracked by moving the head, the VOR normally generates eye movements equal and opposite to the head movement. If this occurred, the eyes would move off the target with resultant loss of fixation. A normally functioning pursuit system has the property of canceling this VOR response, so maintaining stable fixation. A simple way to test for cancellation of the VOR is by using a wooden tongue depressor, which has a small fixation target mounted on the end, and getting the patient to secure this between his or her teeth (*Fig. 7.2*). The patient then slowly rotates his or her head, either from side to side or up and down, while maintaining fixation on the target. Failure of the pursuit system to cancel the VOR results in breaks of fixation because the VOR drives the eyes in the opposite direction to the head rotation. Multiple saccades are observed in the direction of head movement as the eyes attempt to regain fixation.

VERGENCE SYSTEM

FUNCTION AND ANATOMY

The vergence system functions to maintain binocular alignment, permitting stereopsis and avoiding diplopia. It provides the commands for disjugate (oppositely directed) eye movements. There are two main types of vergence eye movements: accommodative vergence generated in response to retinal blur and fusional vergence generated in response to retinal image disparity. In this respect the vergence system functions entirely differently from the saccadic and pursuit systems which generate conjugate (same direction) eye movements.

The higher center control for vergence movements is poorly understood. Striate cortex neurons responding to retinal image disparity have been identified in monkeys. Premotor signals are

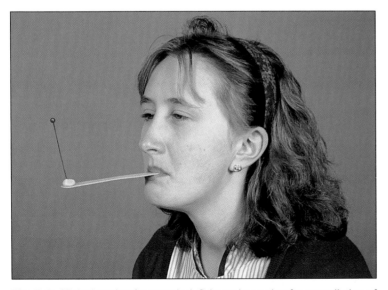

Fig. 7.2 Clinical testing for pursuit deficiency by testing for cancellation of the VOR.

thought to originate in the mesencephalic reticular formation, with separate populations of convergence and divergence cells. At the level of the medial rectus nucleus, three subnuclei (a, b, and c) have been identified, with subnucleus c thought to be involved principally with vergence movements.

COMPONENTS OF VERGENCE MOVEMENT

Pure vergence movements have a maximum velocity of approximately 20°/s; however, vergence movements are more often associated with versional saccades, in which case the velocity of the vergence is much increased. The dynamic properties (relationship between peak vergence velocity and vergence amplitude) of vergence movements are more variable than those of saccades, being influenced by type of stimulus (retinal disparity or blur), its size, and the conditions of viewing (monocular or binocular). Convergence is normally associated with accommodation and pupillary miosis, the near triad.

TESTING VERGENCE EYE MOVEMENTS

The vergence system is extremely sensitive to uncorrected refractive errors, presbyopia, and developmental or acquired deficiencies in binocular single vision. All correctable deficiencies must be rectified, in addition to recording the patient's best corrected visual acuity for both distance and near before testing.

In the clinic it is useful to separate accommodative from fusional (disparate) vergence because there are specific treatments available to improve the near point of convergence and horizontal fusional reserves.

The near rule is useful to test both the near point of convergence and accommodation. The patient views the smallest test type while the type is moved closer along the midsagittal plane until either the patient reports diplopia or the examiner observes a loss of alignment, indicating the near point of convergence (*Fig. 7.3*). The same procedure is carried out monocularly; this time a subjective response of image blur indicates the near point of accommodation. It is normal for the near point of accommodation to recede with advancing age (presbyopia). A poorly motivated patient may not cooperate fully during testing, leading to erroneous results. It is usually possible to help to identify those patients lacking motivation by their attitude and willingness during testing while observing for pupil constriction.

The fusional vergence system is tested at both 6 and 0.3 meters by producing retinal image disparity, either with prisms or with a haploscopic device such as the major amblyoscope (*Fig. 7.4*). When the limits of the patient's fusional reserves are exceeded, the patient reports diplopia or the examiner observes a loss of alignment. Normal horizontal fusional amplitudes range from 10 prism diopters base in to 35 prism diopters base out (base out and denote the position of the prism base relative to the midsagittal plane). Vertical fusional amplitudes rarely exceed 1–2 prism diopters in either direction, except in longstanding or slowly progressive vertical deviations, such as developmental superior oblique palsy or thyroid eye disease.

Accommodation is linked with accommodative convergence to maintain visual alignment at all distances, with the relationship often expressed as the AC/A ratio. The ratio is normally 4:1, with very high ratios typically in developmental concomitant strabismus such as convergence excess esotropia.

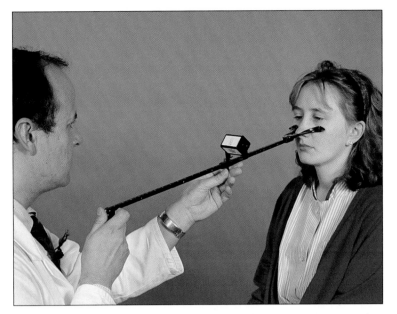

Fig. 7.3 Measuring the near point of accommodation using the near rule.

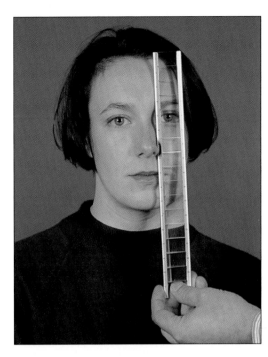

Fig. 7.4 Measuring horizontal fusional amplitudes with the prism bar.

TESTING THE VESTIBULAR AND OPTOKINETIC SYSTEMS

Observation

Vestibular Testing

Vestibular dysfunction can lead to spontaneous slow eye movements that break fixation. These movements can be horizontal, vertical, torsional, or a combination of the three. Visual fixation mediated through the pursuit system acts to dampen any slow drift of the eyes; therefore, it is not surprising that vestibular imbalance can be made more prominent by disrupting visual fixation. Visual fixation can be disrupted by using an opaque lens, a high plus fresnel lens, or by placing the patient in the dark.

The examiner should first look for any static imbalance in the vestibular system by instructing the patient to fixate a distant target and, keeping the patient's head still, observe the eyes for any primary positional nystagmus. Next, fixation should be disrupted and the examiner looks for either the appearance of nystagmus or an increase in any existing nystagmus. Small amplitude nystagmus may be easily identified by observing the optic disc using the direct ophthalmoscope; the optics of the system reverse the true direction of any movement.

The examiner should then stimulate the vestibular system and observe for any dynamic imbalance. The patient is asked to read down a distant Snellen test type, then, while standing behind the patient, the examiner rotates the patient's head from side to side at between 2–3 cycles/s and gets the patient to read down the chart again. Vestibular imbalance reflected in abnormal gain (eye velocity/head velocity) will result in failure to maintain fixation as the eyes repeatedly drift off target, requiring small saccades to recover fixation. In the presence of an abnormal vestibular gain, visual acuity will deteriorate by 1–2 lines when tested with the head rotating. Repeat the procedure, this time rotating the head in the vertical plane.

Caloric testing is useful to determine the side of a peripheral vestibular lesion. Before testing, check that no significant wax is

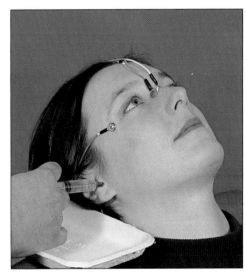

Fig. 7.5 Caloric testing of vestibular function.

present in the ears and that the tympanic membranes are intact. The test relies on using warm and cold water to set up temperature gradients across the semicircular canals, the resulting convection currents in the endolymph bending the cupula, so stimulating the hair cells. The patient's head is positioned 30° from supine, which places the lateral canal in the vertical plane, maximizing the effect from the convection currents. Cold water (30°C) is irrigated into the external auditory meatus of first one then the other side (*Fig. 7.5*). The procedure is then repeated using warm water (44°C). A normal response is for cold water to produce nystagmus with a fast phase directed to the opposite side; with warm water the fast phase is to the same side. An asymmetry in the response of greater than 25% is suggestive of peripheral vestibular imbalance. Ideally the patient should be alert during the test, with fixation disrupted either with fresnel lens or by performing the test in darkness while recording the eye movements.

Positional Testing

Positional testing is useful in patients complaining of vertigo associated with a change of posture. The patient is seated on a suitable couch, with the head central, and is rapidly placed supine on the couch, with the neck extended, resulting in the head hanging 30° below the horizontal (*Fig. 7.6*). After 30 s rapidly return the patient to the upright position. The procedure is repeated with the head turned both to the right and left shoulders. Transient nystagmus produced during these maneuvres, often in association with vertigo, is strongly suggestive of benign paroxysmal positional vertigo.

Doll's Head Test

The main uses of the doll's head test are to differentiate supranuclear causes from nuclear and infranuclear causes of eye movement limitation, and to investigate muscle function in infants and unconscious patients.

For adults the procedure is performed by gently rotating the patient's head in both the horizontal and vertical planes, while the patient fixates the examiner's face. A normally functioning VOR will result in eye movements equal and opposite to head movements. With supranuclear disorders the doll's head test results in a larger range of movement compared with duction testing. Nuclear and infranuclear disorders cause equal limitations on both doll's head and duction testing.

For infants and unconscious patients, the doll's head test can confirm the integrity of the nuclear and infranuclear pathways, confirming the presence of lateral rectus function in childhood esotropia, or identifying muscle palsies in the unconscious patient.

The presence of an intact Bell's phenomenon confirms the integrity of the infranuclear pathways serving up-gaze.

Optokinetic Testing

The small optokinetic drum or tape principally tests the pursuit system. A large field stimulus does stimulate the optokinetic system; however, the response is made up of both optokinetic and pursuit components, which are not readily separable clinically. To isolate the optokinetic response a sophisticated recording laboratory is required.

ELECTRODIAGNOSTIC ASSESSMENT OF EYE MOVEMENTS

Observation of eye movement provides a simple qualitative measure and is able to identify most abnormalities. With the advent of eye movement recorders the physician can now examine a profile of the eye movement and obtain quantitative data on its component parts. Despite there being a wide range of commercially available eye movement recorders, few are used regularly in the clinical setting. Clearly, more work is necessary before eye movement recording becomes part of day-to-day clinical eye movement assessment.

A wide range of eye movement recorders are now available. The electro-oculography technique of recording eye movements is the most widely available and is reliable for moderate to large amplitude movements (*Fig. 7.7*). Unfortunately, its resolution is poor for small amplitude movements. The infra-red techniques have the advantage of improved resolution for small angle movements. Both techniques can suffer from eyelid blink artifacts when recording vertical movements. The scleral search coil is the only technique that can reliably record torsional eye movements; however, the need for the patient to wear a contact lens and the size of the equipment means that its clinical use is limited.

A range of videographic recorders are now available. These combine the benefits of high resolution and being noninvasive; some of the newer products are able to record torsional eye movements. This type of recorder may well finally find a place in clinical practice.

ELECTROMYOGRAPHY

The electrical activity of a muscle can be recorded using suitable recording equipment. The procedure is performed using topical anesthesia in adults or ketamine anesthesia in children. Two silver–silver chloride skin electrodes are fixed to the patient, one acting as an indifferent electrode, the other as the negative electrode (*Fig. 7.8*). A needle, which is insulated except for its tip, acts as the active (positive) electrode and is inserted into the extraoc-

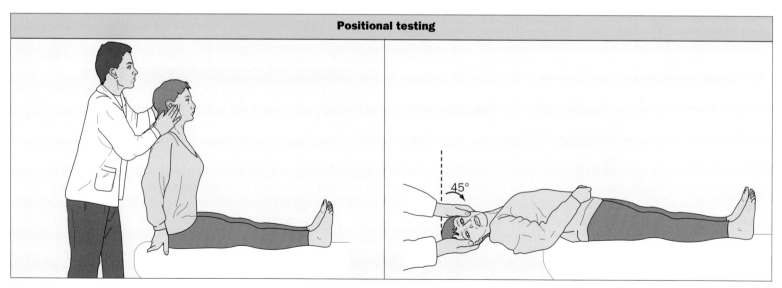

Positional testing

Fig. 7.6 Vestibular function assessment. Testing for positional nystagmus. (Modified from Leigh RJ, Zee DS. *The Neurology of Eye Movements* ,2nd edn. Contemporary Neurology Series.)

ular muscle. The electrodes are connected to an amplifier providing visual or auditory output. By instructing the patient to look in the direction of the muscle being tested the increased electrical activity can be detected. Electromyography can be used to differentiate between neurogenic and myogenic muscle palsies, in addition to assessing for residual muscle function in cases of lateral rectus muscle palsies. Its main use in ophthalmology is for assisting the delivery of botulinum toxin into the extraocular muscle.

ASSESSMENT OF THE RANGE OF OCULAR MOVEMENT

The first half of the chapter discussed the assessment of the qualitative or dynamic aspects of ocular movement. This half will discuss assessment of the extent of the movement.

An understanding of both the laws relating to ocular movement and the direction of ocular rotation is essential before proceeding with a discussion of the techniques involved in testing ocular movement.

LAWS AND DEFINITIONS RELATING TO EYE MOVEMENT

HERING'S LAW OF EQUAL INNERVATION

Equal neural innervation is directed to a muscle and its contralateral synergist (yoke muscle) in order to ensure coordinated binocular eye movements. A paralyzed muscle requiring extra innervation for it to contract results in overaction of its normal synergist.

SHERRINGTON'S LAW OF RECIPROCAL INNERVATION

When a muscle contracts, its antagonist relaxes to the same extent, permitting a full range of smooth eye movement.

Primary Position

This is the eye position when viewing an object at infinity on the horizon with the head erect and facial plane vertical. Both visual axes are parallel and the corneal vertical meridians are also vertical and parallel.

Comitant and Incomitant

A concomitant deviation between the eyes is one in which the deviation remains the same in all directions of gaze. This is usually seen in developmental strabismus and also in longstanding extraocular muscle palsies. Incomitance is when the deviation changes in different positions of gaze; this is the hallmark of acquired paralytic and mechanical strabismus.

DIRECTIONS OF OCULAR MOVEMENT

VERSION EYE MOVEMENTS

The pair of yoke muscles responsible for eye movement in a given direction of gaze are shown in *Figure 7.9*. These directions of movements are called the cardinal positions of gaze and are the positions of gaze for which one muscle (as shown) from each eye is the principal mover. Testing the cardinal positions of gaze is important in identifying weakness of isolated extraocular muscles. Direct up-gaze (supraversion) and down-gaze (infraversion) should also be tested to identify A, V, and X patterns. The cardinal positions, along with direct up- and down-gaze, and straight ahead, are termed the nine positions of gaze.

Testing Version Eye Movements
Versions are tested by making the patient fixate and follow a small hand light through the nine positions of gaze. A hand light is useful as it can be readily seen when visual acuity is reduced, subjective diplopia appreciation can be enhanced by using colored filters over the eyes (diplopia test), and the corneal reflections can be observed, which not only ensures that the light source is visi-

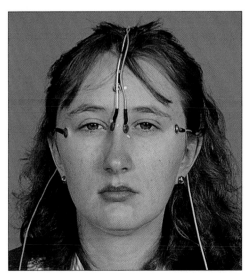

Fig. 7.7 Electro-oculographic assessment of eye movements.

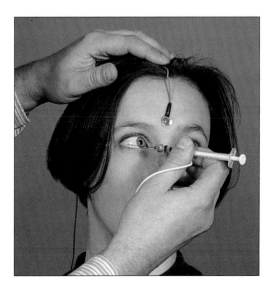

Fig. 7.8 Electromyographic control in the delivery of botulinum toxin to the lateral rectus muscle.

ble to the patient but also permits estimations of the amount of under and overactions. Underactions are graded on a scale of –1 to –4 (–4 = no movement past the midline into a particular field of action), and overactions are graded +1 to +4.

These scales may also be shown diagrammatically, readily indicating which muscles are involved (*Fig. 7.10*).

Cycloversions are involuntary and their evaluation is discussed in a later section.

DUCTION EYE MOVEMENTS

Ductions are monocular eye movements taking place around the three principal axes of ocular rotation. Ductions are tested in the same way as versions, except each eye is tested separately. Restrictions are graded using the same scale as is used for versions.

Principal muscles acting in the cardinal positions of gaze	
Cardinal positions	Principal muscles acting
1. Right lateral gaze (Dextroversion)	Right lateral rectus Left medial rectus
2. Right and up (Dextroelevation)	Right superior rectus Left inferior oblique
3. Right and down (Dextrodepression)	Right inferior rectus Left superior oblique
4. Left lateral gaze (Levoversion)	Left lateral rectus Right medial rectus
5. Left and up (Levoelevation)	Left superior rectus Right inferior oblique
6. Left and down (Levodepression)	Left inferior rectus Right superior oblique

Fig. 7.9 Principal muscles acting in the cardinal positions of gaze.

Quantifying Ductional Eye Movements

Limbus Method
The range of both horizontal and vertical movements can be quantified for either eye in the cooperative patient. One eye should be occluded and the other eye fixated on a target in the primary position. The examiner holds a transparent ruler in front of the fixing eye. To measure the range of abduction and adduction the ruler is held horizontally. The range of abduction can be measured by aligning the zero point at the nasal limbus and instructing the patient to follow the target until the limits of abduction are reached. The amount of abduction (measured as the movement of the nasal limbus), usually measured in millimeters, is measured from the scale. To measure the range of adduction the rule is aligned this time with the temporal limbus. The range of upward and downward movement can be measured in the same way by orienting the ruler vertically. Care must be taken not to allow the patient to move his or her head during the assessment.

FIELD OF UNIOCULAR FIXATION

The full extent of eye movement can be plotted using a perimeter. Each eye is tested separately by occluding the other eye. The patient is aligned so that the eye to be tested is opposite the center of the perimeter. A 2–3 mm letter is used for fixation, ensuring the letter can be clearly seen by the patient. The patient is instructed to keep his or her head still and track the target until the limit of permitted movement is reached and fixation can no longer be maintained. At this point the patient will be aware that the target is blurred. This point is recorded on the chart and other points are tested in a similar fashion.

It is important that the examiner observes the eye movement closely as occasionally the patient will not report blurring of the image, despite clearly not fixing the target. In this situation an approximation of the range of eye movement can be made from observing when the patient's eye movement stops.

TESTS FOR MECHANICAL RESTRICTIONS OF OCULAR MOVEMENT

Limitation of ocular movement may be caused by neurogenic, myogenic, or mechanical factors. As mechanical causes of ocular movement restrictions reside within the confines of the orbit,

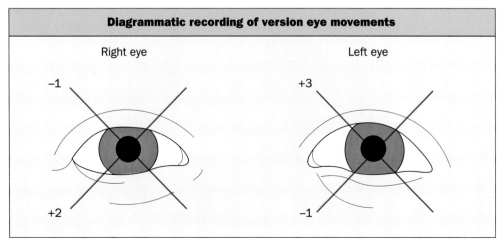

Diagrammatic recording of version eye movements

Right eye   Left eye

–1   +3

+2   –1

Fig. 7.10 Diagrammatic recording of version eye movements. Patient with a left superior oblique palsy (–1 underaction) with +3 overaction of the ipsilateral inferior oblique (ipsilateral antagonist), +2 overaction of the contralateral inferior rectus (synergist), and –1 underaction of the contralateral superior rectus (contralateral antagonist).

identifying such causes is extremely important when considering further investigations and carrying out treatment.

There are often clues available during the examination showing that a mechanical cause for the limitation of ocular movement is likely. Certain conditions are known to cause primarily mechanical restrictions, such as thyroid eye disease and blow-out fracture of the orbit. During ocular movement testing, retraction of the globe may be observed when looking in the direction of a mechanical restriction, in addition to the patient complaining of pain. When comparing version and duction eye movements, a finding of duction movements limited to the same degree as version eye movements is typical of mechanical limitations.

Saccadic eye movements have normal velocities when tested within the confines of the permitted movement in mechanical restrictions.

Forced Duction Testing

Forced duction testing (FDT) or traction testing is the definitive test to confirm the presence of mechanical restrictions. The procedure can be performed under local anesthesia for a cooperative patient. The purpose of the test is to see if the eye can be rotated further than the limitation shown by ductional eye movement assessment. In primary neurogenic or myogenic muscle palsies, forced duction testing should reveal a full range of movement is possible. If the limitation of movement is primarily mechanical, FDT will not be able to rotate the eye beyond the limitation shown by ductional eye movement testing.

The eyes are first anesthetized using topical local anesthetic drops. The patient is positioned so that the head is supported and instructed to look in the direction of the limited movement (*Fig. 7.11*). Traditionally, fine-toothed forceps are applied to the limbal conjunctiva and an attempt is made to rotate the globe beyond the limitation. A less traumatic approach is to use a cotton-tipped bud to push the globe beyond the limitation. Care needs to be taken not to push the globe back into the orbit, as this is likely to mask any mechanical restrictions.

Mechanical restrictions confirmed by FDT can reside not only in the extraocular muscles but also in the connective tissue and bulbar conjunctiva.

Rise in Intraocular Pressure

Mechanical restrictions caused by tight extraocular muscles can result in the tight muscle indenting the globe as the eye attempts to look in the direction of the restricted movement. By measuring the intraocular pressure (IOP) in the primary position and in the direction of the restricted movement, any globe indentation will cause a rise in IOP. A rise in IOP of greater than 5 mmHg is significant and suggests mechanical restriction.

Muscle Force Generation Test

In patients with longstanding muscle palsies, changes in the elasticity of the horizontal extraocular muscles takes place. These changes affect contraction of the ipsilateral antagonist and contralateral antagonist. In the case of a lateral rectus muscle palsy, contraction can occur in the ipsilateral antagonist (medial rectus) muscle and contralateral antagonist (contralateral lateral rectus) muscle. When assessing for residual function in the paralyzed lateral rectus muscle, an important sign is the ability of the eye to abduct beyond the midline. An eye with a partially paralyzed lateral rectus muscle may be prevented from abducting beyond the midline because of contraction in the ipsilateral medial rectus muscle.

Under local anesthesia the eye is gripped with forceps at the temporal limbus and the patient is instructed to look in the direction of the paralyzed muscle; in the presence of active lateral rectus muscle contraction, the force generated is readily apparent. The procedure can also be performed with a cotton-tipped stick, and is often combined with forced duction testing (*Fig. 7.12*).

ASSESSMENT OF THE ANGLE OF STRABISMUS

Misalignment of the visual axes (strabismus) is either latent or manifest. A latent deviation is held in check by the fusion reflex. If the fusion reflex is disrupted by dissociating the eyes (covering one eye), misalignment of the eyes occurs and the non-fixing eye deviates. This deviation is a latent deviation (heterophoria) with recovery back to binocular single vision taking place once dissociation ceases. A manifest deviation occurs either in the setting of

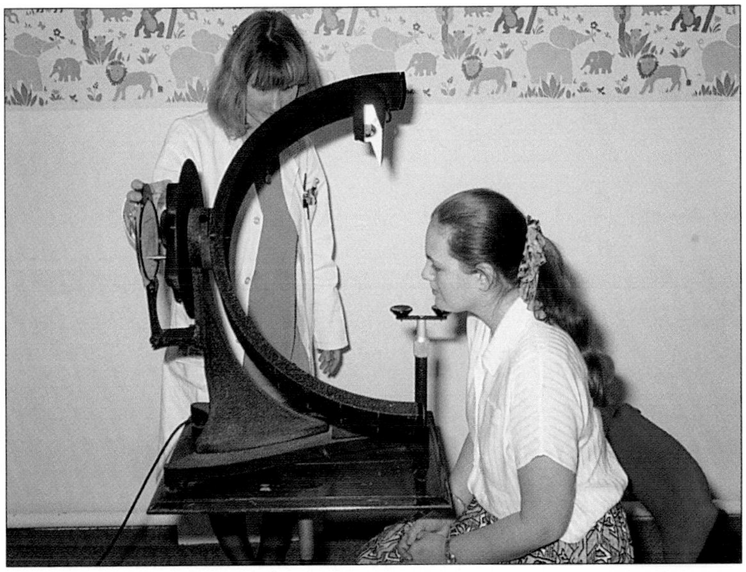

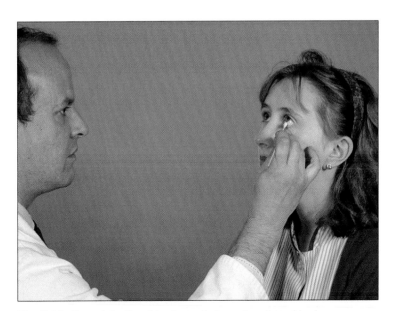

Fig. 7.11 Assessment of the field of uniocular fixation with the Lister arc perimeter.

Fig. 7.12 Forced ductional testing using a cotton-tipped bud.

absent BSV or when fusion is unable to keep the deviation in check (heterotropia).

Both subjective and objective methods can be used to detect strabismus. If the patient can recognize diplopia, subjective assessment using the diplopia tests and plotting the diplopia fields is useful to identify isolated extraocular muscle palsies.

Summary of cover and uncover test outcomes	
Cover test	
Movement of uncovered eye	Interpretation
No movement	Eye was fixating
Horizontal outwards	Esotropia
Horizontal inwards	Exotropia
Vertical downwards	Hypertropia
Vertical upwards	Hypotropia
Uncover test (no manifest deviation identified with cover test)	
Movement of eye under cover as cover removed	Interpretation
No movement	Orthophoria
Horizontal outwards	Esophoria
Horizontal inwards	Exophoria
Vertical downwards	Hyperphoria
Vertical upwards	Hypophoria
Uncover test (manifest deviation identified with cover test)	
Movement of eye under cover as cover removed	Interpretation
No movement either eye	Alternating strabismus (either eye used for fixation)
Both eyes move	Unilateral strabismus (covered eye used for fixation)

Fig. 7.13 Summary of the outcomes of cover and uncover tests.

THE COVER TEST

The cover test is the definitive objective test for investigating strabismus. The test requires accurate fixation reflexes so it may not be useful in patients with poor visual acuity or grossly eccentric fixation. Testing is performed for both distance and near, using accommodative targets appropriate to the level of vision and age of the patient.

The test is performed in three stages (*Fig. 7.13*):

1. Cover Test
The patient is instructed to fixate the target and the cover is placed over one eye while the examiner observes the fellow eye for any movement (*Fig. 7.14*). A movement of the fellow eye identifies a manifest deviation, while no movement signifies that the fellow eye was fixating the target. The test is then repeated this time covering the fellow eye.

2. Uncover Test
If a manifest deviation was not present when the cover was in place, the examiner then closely observes the eye behind the cover

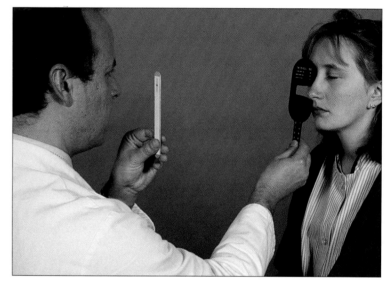

Fig. 7.14 The cover test.

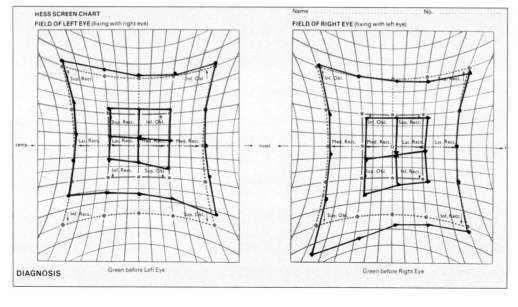

Fig. 7.15 A Hess chart showing a left inferior rectus palsy with overaction of the contralateral superior oblique muscle (synergist).

as the cover is removed. A movement of the eye to take up fixation indicates a latent deviation is present. If a manifest deviation was identified by the cover test, the behavior of the covered eye when the cover is removed can be no movement, signifying that fixation is being maintained by the fellow eye, or it may move to take up fixation.

The cover–uncover test is used to identify both latent and manifest deviations.

3. Alternate Cover Test

The aim of the alternate cover test is to disrupt the fusion reflex by dissociating the eyes by swiftly moving the cover from one eye to the fellow eye. The cover should remain over each eye for 3 s to ensure the eyes are fully dissociated. It can be seen that the alternate cover test does not differentiate between a latent and a manifest deviation. Its purpose is to expose the maximum size of any deviation by fully disrupting the fusion reflex. It is particularly useful to perform the alternate cover test in the nine positions of gaze to identify whether the deviation is incomitant or concomitant. The alternate cover test combined with prisms (prism cover test) is also used for measuring the angle of deviation.

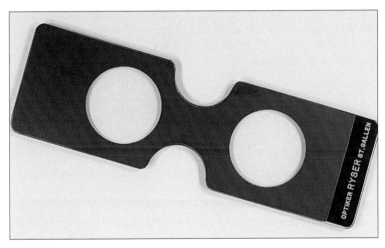

Fig. 7.16 Bagolini glasses.

HAPLOSCOPIC TESTS

Haploscopic tests rely on presenting dissimilar targets to each eye. They are valuable in showing the alignment of the eyes in the nine positions of gaze as well as providing a dependable and reproducible record of the condition.

THE LEES–HESS CHART TEST

The most popular tests in use are the Lancaster red–green test and the Hess test, which use red and green goggles to dissociate the eyes, and the Lees test, which uses a mirror.

The amount of horizontal and vertical deviation is recorded on a chart, facilitating the identification of muscle underactions, overactions, and mechanical restrictions (*Fig. 7.15*).

SENSORY TESTING AND RECORDING OF BINOCULAR SINGLE VISION

Binocular single vision (BSV) results in a single visual image from the simultaneous use of both eyes. In normal situations it arises from the use of both foveas (corresponding retinal points) without the presence of manifest strabismus. Anomalous binocular vision is present when non-corresponding points are used (the fovea of one eye and an extrafoveal point of the other eye) and a manifest strabismus is present.

The correct interpretation of many tests used in the assessment of strabismus relies on knowing the level of BSV. A vast assortment of tests are available to investigate the state of BSV. It is important to understand that different aspects of BSV exist, with tests designed to explore retinal correspondence (Bagolini glasses, *Fig. 7.16*), simultaneous perception of both eye (Worth 4 dots), sensory fusion (Major amblyopscope), and levels of stereopsis (TNO *Fig. 7.17* Frisby, *Fig. 7.18* Wirt Fly) or Randot. Certain tests are intended to be used for either distance or near viewing, or are more suitable for young children.

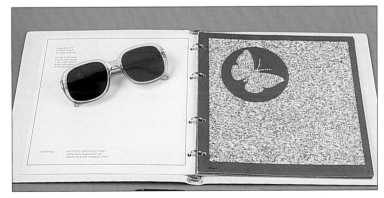

Fig. 7.17 The TNO stereo test, using red and green goggles to dissociate the eyes.

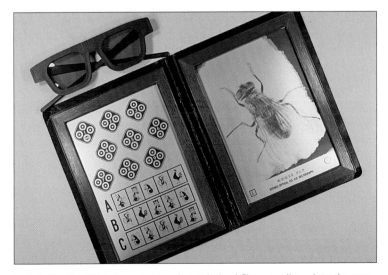

Fig. 7.18 The Wirt stereo test, using polarized filters to dissociate the eyes.

DIPLOPIA TESTS AND DIPLOPIA CHART

Red and Green Filter Test

The patient wears red and green goggles (convention states that the red filter should be over the right eye). Filters fitted into trial lenses are unsuitable because the patient's visual axis in eccentric gaze will extend beyond the limits of the trial lens. The patient fixates a linear light source, first in the primary position and then in the cardinal positions of gaze, as well as up- and down-gaze (*Fig. 7.19*). The patient is questioned about the diplopia in each of the positions, specifically if the red image is to the right or left and above or below the other image, as well as if one image is tilted (torsion).

The results are drawn (diplopia chart) usually in terms of what the patients sees using the patient's right and left eyes. A note is made of the eye projecting the red image. The amount of image separation in each field of gaze should be expressed, otherwise no valid comparison can be made with future assessments.

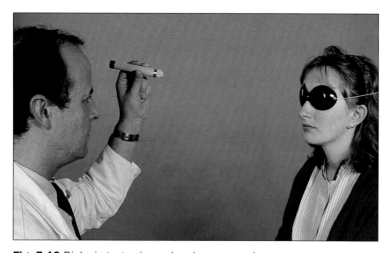

Fig. 7.19 Diplopia test using red and green goggles.

Maddox Rod Test

The Maddox rod is made up of a series of closely spaced parallel glass rods forming high-powered plus cylindrical lens. A distant point source of light is refracted by the cylinders and appears to the patient as a line image at 90° to the axis of the cylinders.

To examine for horizontal deviations the Maddox rod is placed in a trial frame in front of the patient's non-fixing eye, with the axes of the cylinders horizontal (*Fig. 7.20*). The patient fixes on the point source of light and is questioned about the position of the vertical line. With the Maddox rod in front of the patient's right eye, the line appears to the left of the point source of light in exodeviations and to the right in esodeviations. When testing vertical deviations the Maddox rod is rotated through 90° to project a horizontal image to the patient. Torsional deviations are best assessed by using double Maddox rods (*Fig. 7.21*), one in front of either eye, with the axes of the cylinders vertical, so projecting horizontal line images when viewing a distant spot of light. The patient is asked whether one or both images appear tilted and is instructed to rotate one of the rods until both images are seen to be parallel. The amount of cyclotropia is measured in degrees from the scale on the trial frame.

The Maddox rod test is more dissociative than the red and green filter test and, therefore, measures both latent and manifest deviations. Prisms can be used to neutralize any deviations detected using the diplopia tests, accurately quantifying the misalignment. Both diplopia tests are unreliable when abnormal retinal correspondence exists, a condition encountered in certain types of childhood strabismus.

OBSERVATION OF CORNEAL REFLECTIONS

By observing the reflection of a hand-held light from the cornea of each eye, a rough approximation of the angle of manifest strabismus can be made. It is important to remember that with the patient fixing the light source, the reflection from the cornea is usually located a few degrees off its center, either nasally or temporally. In some patients the reflection is displaced sufficiently to

Fig. 7.20 The patient's observation during Maddox rod testing. The Maddox rod is in front of the patient's right eye.

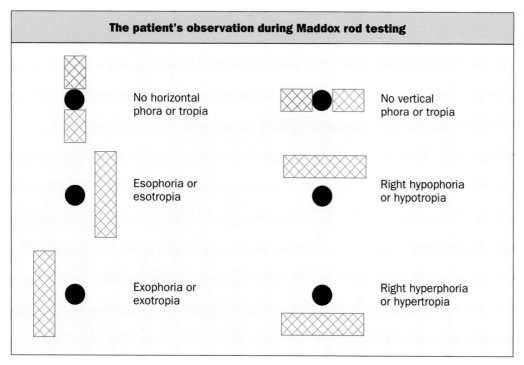

The patient's observation during Maddox rod testing

No horizontal phora or tropia

No vertical phora or tropia

Esophoria or esotropia

Right hypophoria or hypotropia

Exophoria or exotropia

Right hyperphoria or hypertropia

lead to an erroneous impression of strabismus, a situation called pseudostrabismus. Observation of the corneal reflections is principally indicated whenever other tests cannot be performed (cover test, diplopia tests), as in cases of unilateral or bilateral poor vision and in very young children. It is useful in detecting only moderate to large angle strabismus.

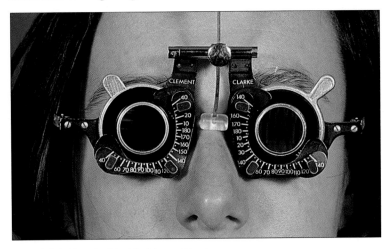

Fig. 7.21 The double Maddox rod test.

Further reading

Ansons A, Wylie J, Trimble R. Establishing a place for eye movement saccades in disorders of ocular motility. *Trans 6th Intern Orthop Cong.* 1987;222–226.

Büttner-Ennever JA, Akert K. Medial rectus subgroups of the oculomotor nucleus and their abducens internuclear input in the monkey. *J Comp Neurol* 1981;**197**:17–27.

Enright JT. Changes in vergence mediated by saccades. *J Physiol* 1984;**350**:9–31.

Collewijn H, Van der Steen J, Ferman L, Jansen TC. Human ocular counterroll: assessment of static and dynamic properties from electromagnetic scleral coil recordings. *Exp Brain Res.* 1985;**59**:185–196.

Poggio GF, Fischer B. Binocular interaction and depth sensitivity in striate and prestriate cortex of behaving rhesus monkey. *J Neurophysiol* 1977;**40**:1392–1405.

CHAPTER 8

Neurophysiology of Eye Movements

D I Flitcroft

INTRODUCTION

An appreciation of the neurophysiology of eye movements is made easier by breaking down the mechanisms that control eye movements into three functional stages:

Sensory Guidance
A variety of sensory cues, both visual and non-visual, are used to guide eye movements. Input from body movement, isolated head movement and changes in the visual world all influence eye movement.

Premotor Co-ordination
Signals from different physiologic control systems converge within the brainstem, with separate centers involved in horizontal, vertical, and vergence eye movements.

Motor Response
The motor mechanisms controlling eye movements are represented by three cranial nerve nuclei (third, fourth, and sixth) which supply the six extraocular muscles in each eye.

SENSORY GUIDANCE MECHANISMS

Eye movements perform the five key functions listed in *Figure 8.1*. These functions are achieved by the operation of the six largely independent guidance systems, namely saccades, pursuits, vergence, optokinetic responses, vestibulo-ocular responses, and ocular fixation.

VESTIBULO OCULAR REFLEXES

Characteristics and Features of Interest
The vestibular reflexes have the shortest latency of any eye movement, less than 16 ms from head movement to the start of the compensatory eye movement. Although often referred to as a single vestibulo-ocular reflex (VOR), in reality the VOR represents a set of reflexes. All these reflexes produce compensatory changes in eye position on head movement to stabilize the retinal image as the head moves. The reflexes involve the connection of the three semicircular canals of the inner ear, which detect head rotation, and the utricle and saccule, which respond to head position and linear movement, to the motor neurons supplying the extraocular muscles. There are therefore at least five VORs, one arising from each of these paired vestibular sense organs, each of which has an excitatory component and an inhibitory component that relaxes the corresponding antagonist muscles. Both sets of sense organs respond

to acceleration but not sustained movement.

There are three semicircular canals in each inner ear, lying in three different planes to allow three-dimensional detection of rotation (*Fig. 8.2*). The inputs from the semicircular canals result in what is often referred to as the dynamic VOR (*Fig. 8.3*). In contrast, the static VOR takes its input from the otolith organs in the

Five key functions of eye movements and the systems involved	
Function Of Eye Movement	**Eye Movement System**
1) To stabilize the retinal image during head or body movement and movement of the visual world	Vestibulo-ocular reflexes Optokinetic system
2) To maintain fixation on moving objects	Smooth pursuit system
3) To change fixation to new areas of interest	Volitional saccades Reflexive saccades
4) To maintain binocular alignment at different distances	Vergence system
5) To maintain fixation on stationary objects	Fixation/gaze holding system

Fig. 8.1 The five key functions of eye movements and the systems involved.

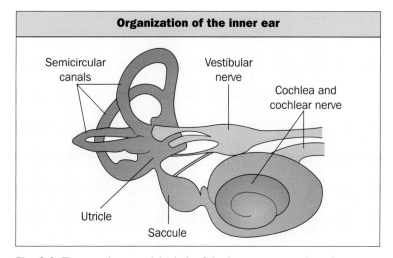

Fig. 8.2 The membranous labyrinth of the inner ear comprises three semicircular canals, two otolith organs within the utricle and saccule, and the cochlea. Information from these sensory organs is relayed centrally via the eighth cranial nerve.

utricle and saccule. These organs respond to linear acceleration and, because they are therefore affected by gravity, they provide information on the angle of the head. Movement of the eyes on tilting of the head results from the activity of the static VOR but is also referred to as the ocular tilt reaction.

Neuroanatomic Pathways
The short latency of the VOR results from a simple three-neuron reflex arc (*Fig. 8.4*), involving a sensory neuron carrying the signal from the hair cells within the membranous labyrinth, a synapse within the medial, lateral, or superior vestibular nucleus onto an interneuron which projects, in most cases via the medial longitudinal fasciculus (MLF), to the corresponding motor neuron within the third, fourth, or sixth nucleus.

Although the short latency of the VOR is in keeping with the classic description of reflexes as three-neuron arcs, this reflex differs markedly from spinal cord reflexes in that it can be entirely inhibited by voluntary effort and that the strength of the reflex is subject to alteration depending on visual experience. Voluntary inhibition of the VOR occurs whenever the head moves to follow a moving target or to change fixation. The modifiability of the VOR involves the cerebellar flocculus (*Fig. 8.5*) and allows alteration of the gain of the VOR. The VOR is therefore far more sophisticated than a simple three-neuron arc.

The adaptive capabilities of the VOR represent a mechanism by which the accuracy of the reflex can be continually regulated by detecting movement of the entire retinal image during head movements. In addition to ensuring the accuracy of the reflex, this recalibration of the VOR also occurs every time someone puts on spectacles. The magnification or minification of the retinal image by spectacle lenses requires an adaptive change in the gain of the VOR to prevent the world appearing to move during every head movement.

OPTOKINETIC REFLEXES

Characteristics and Features of Interest
The optokinetic system fulfils a similar role to that of the VOR to prevent the retinal image slipping across the retina during head movements. Whereas the vestibular system can detect only acceleration, the optokinetic system can detect any form of retinal image slip and therefore assists the VOR during sustained movements.

Neuroanatomic Pathways
In animals, the optokinetic responses are generated by the subcortical pathways of the accessory optic system. In primates and humans, both the accessory optic system and the main geniculostriate pathways contribute to optokinetic responses (*Fig. 8.6*). Within the visual cortex, areas MT (middle temporal), MST (medial superior temporal), and the posterior parietal cortex are thought to be involved in detecting movements of the visual world that trigger optokinetic responses. In primates, rudimentary optokinetic responses can be generated even in the absence of a functional geniculostriate visual system.

Special Physiologic Features: Optokinetic After Nystagmus
True optokinetic responses are unusual in having a slow onset after the start of the image movement and also continuing for several seconds after the movement has stopped. Under normal circumstances, the continued optokinetic movements can be suppressed by active fixation but in the absence of any fixation target the result is optokinetic after nystagmus (OKAN). This form of optokinetic nystagmus represents a true measure of the optokinetic system. The more rapid onset of nystagmus to a moving target (such as occurs when looking out of the window of a moving train), which is also referred to as optokinetic nystagmus, is largely driven by smooth pursuit mechanisms.

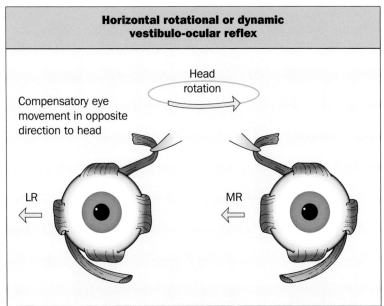

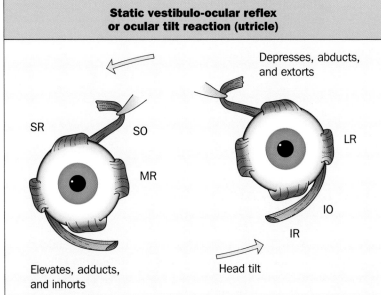

Fig. 8.3 The compensatory actions of the dynamic and static vestibulo-ocular reflexes (VORs). Although the dynamic VOR can provide almost perfect compensation for head rotation, the static VOR is largely vestigial in primates and provides only partial compensation for head tilt. The static VOR is perhaps of most significance when disturbance of otolith pathways centrally leads to skew deviation, a pathologic vertical misalignment of the eyes. (LR, lateral rectus; MR, medial rectus; SR, superior rectus; IR, inferior rectus; SO, superior oblique; IO, inferior oblique)

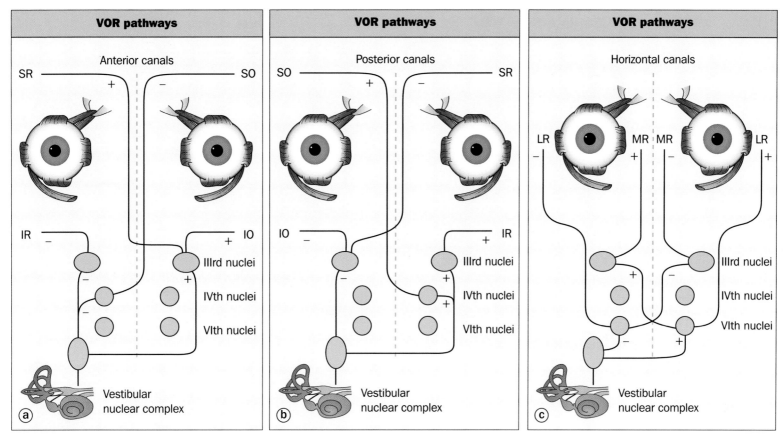

Fig. 8.4 The connections of the three semicircular canals to the motor neurons innervating the ocular muscles. Both excitatory (indicated by +) and inhibitory pathways (indicated by −) are shown.

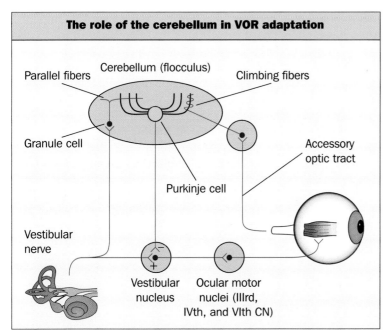

Fig. 8.5 Ito's scheme for the role of the cerebellum in modifying the gain of the VOR. In this scheme, the cerebellum receives vestibular information and visual information which converge on the cerebellar Purkinje cells. If the gain of the VOR is inappropriate, there will be a slip of the retinal image during head movement. It is proposed that this slip is used by the Purkinje cells to alter the gain of the VOR by projections to the vestibular nucleus.

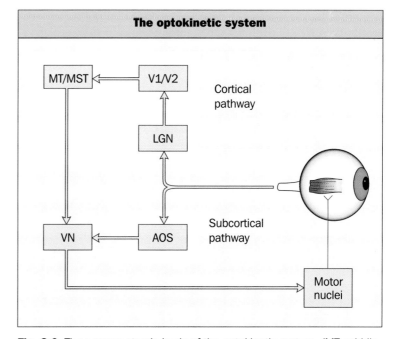

Fig. 8.6 The neuroanatomic basis of the optokinetic system. (MT, middle temporal cortical area; MST, medial superior temporal cortical area; V1/V2, primary and secondary visual cortex; LGN, lateral geniculate nucleus; VN, vestibular nucleus; AOS, accessory optic system)

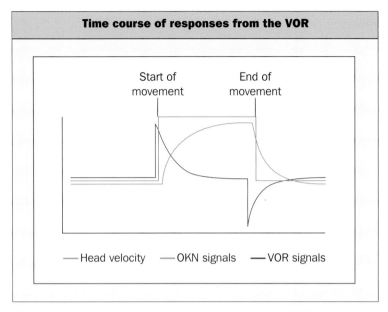

Fig. 8.7 Time course of responses from the vestibular (VOR) and optokinetic (OKN) systems during sustained head rotation. The VOR component is transient, in response to acceleration and deceleration at the start and end of head movement. The OKN component shows slow onset and slow decay.

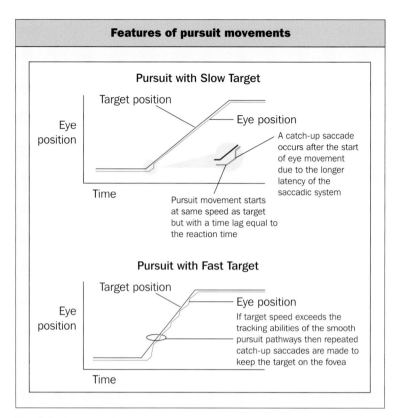

Fig. 8.8 Features of pursuit eye movements for slow and fast (>30 degrees/second) target movements.

The slow onset and decline of optokinetic responses closely matches the time characteristics of the vestibulo-ocular system, as shown in *Figure 8.7*. During the start and finish of a head movement, the head undergoes accelerations and decelerations which can be detected by the vestibular system. In the middle of a sustained response, the lack of any acceleration or deceleration results in no vestibular stimulation and, hence, no VOR responses. Optokinetic responses increase over the first few seconds of movement as the vestibular response declines and maintain compensatory eye movements during steady movement. At the end of the movement both the vestibular and optokinetic responses occur simultaneously, with the vestibular sense organs detecting deceleration and the optokinetic response declining over time with the sudden cessation of retinal image movement. These two responses are in opposing directions and hence tend to cancel each other out, ensuring stable eye position at the end of sustained head movements.

PURSUIT EYE MOVEMENTS

Characteristics and Features of Interest
Like optokinetic movements, pursuit eye movements are involved in stabilizing a moving image on the retina. The pursuit system responds to small central objects, however, in contrast to the large field stimuli that trigger optokinetic responses. Pursuits are dependent on the visual cortex and have a latency of 125 ms. Pure pursuit can be maintained at only comparatively low speeds of movement, that is, up to 30°/s; above this speed, pursuit movements are assisted by catch-up saccades (*Fig. 8.8*).

Neuroanatomic Pathways
Pursuit movements are dependent on motion detection pathways (*Fig. 8.9*) that project via the geniculostriate system to two pre-striate visual areas involved in motion detection: the MT (middle temporal) and MST (medial superior temporal) areas. The posterior parietal cortex also contributes to pursuit movements and is thought to be involved in selective attention to the moving target that is being tracked. These areas are responsible for generating pursuit movements to the ipsilateral side. The frontal eye fields (FEF) also contribute to pursuits, particularly for predictable target movement. The frontal eye fields and MT and MST areas have independent projections that converge on the dorsolateral pontine nuclei. Pursuit signals reach the motor neurons by a contralateral projection to the flocculus within the cerebellum and from there to the vestibular nucleus which projects contralaterally to the motor nuclei.

Special Physiologic Features: Predictive Pursuits
Although the pursuit system has a latency or delay of 100 ms, if a target moves in a predictable fashion then pursuit movements can appear to have no delay at all or even anticipate the movement of the target. This ability to make pursuit movements along the predicted path of a moving object is thought to be dependent on the frontal eye fields.

SACCADIC EYE MOVEMENTS

Characteristics and Features of Interest
Saccadic movements exist in many different forms representing a spectrum from the purely reflexive fast components of nystagmus, through visually guided reflexive and voluntary saccades, to purely voluntary saccades (*Fig. 8.10*).

Saccadic eye movements are extremely fast and can exceed 600°/s. In contrast to other forms of visually guided eye movement, saccades are not subject to feedback control during the

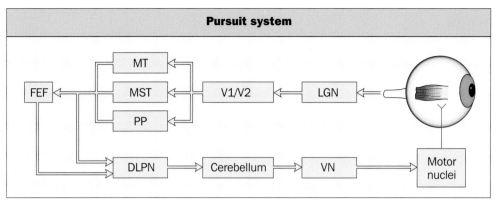

Fig. 8.9 The neuroanatomic basis of the pursuit pathways. (LGN, lateral geniculate nucleus; V1/V2, primary and secondary visual cortex; MT, middle temporal cortical area; MST, medial superior temporal area; PP, posterior parietal cortical area; FEF, frontal eye fields; DLPN, dorsolateral pontine nuclei; VN, vestibular nucleus).

Fig. 8.10 The spectrum of saccadic eye movements.

The spectrum of saccadic eye movements

Type of Saccade	Description	Voluntary/Reflexive
1) Quick phases	Fast component of nystagmus movements	Entirely reflexive
2) Reflexive saccades	Saccades to novel stimuli	Reflexive but can be voluntarily suppressed
3) Reading saccades	Refixational movements during reading	Voluntarily controlled but part of a semiautomatic reading strategy
4) Change of fixation	Refixation to a new area within the visual field	Voluntary
5) Memory saccades	To a remembered location within the visual field	Voluntary
6) Predictive saccades	To the anticipated location of a stimulus	Voluntary
7) Antisaccades	Experimental paradigm that requires a saccade away from a presented stimulus	Voluntary combined with suppression of a reflexive saccade

movement. The magnitude and direction of the movement are calculated before the eye starts moving and for this reason saccades are often termed ballistic, indicating that, like a ball being thrown, the path of the movement is predetermined from the start. This may account for the fact that saccades have a much longer latency than pursuits. Although there is evidence that, under experimental conditions, alterations can be made during a saccade and therefore saccades are not truly ballistic, most saccades are too short to allow any change in trajectory if the visual scene changes. They can, therefore, be considered effectively ballistic.

Any inaccuracies in direction or magnitude are not corrected during the movement but by small corrective saccades 100–130 ms after the original movement has been completed (*Fig. 8.11*).

The speed of a saccade increases with its amplitude (*Fig. 8.12*). This relationship is referred to as the "main sequence" and applies to all forms of saccades, indicating that all forms of saccade share a common premotor generator.

Neuroanatomic Pathways

In keeping with the various types of saccade, a variety of neuroanatomic pathways contribute to saccade control, each con-

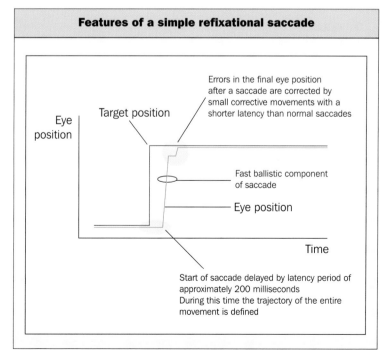

Features of a simple refixational saccade

Eye position

Target position

Errors in the final eye position after a saccade are corrected by small corrective movements with a shorter latency than normal saccades

Fast ballistic component of saccade

Eye position

Time

Start of saccade delayed by latency period of approximately 200 milliseconds
During this time the trajectory of the entire movement is defined

Fig. 8.11 Features of a simple refixational saccade.

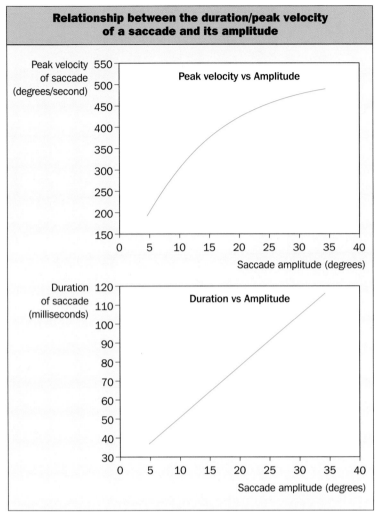

Fig. 8.12 Relationship between the duration and peak velocity of a saccade and its amplitude. This relationship is consistent for any type of saccade. (Derived from Collewijn, Erkelens, Steinman, 1988.)

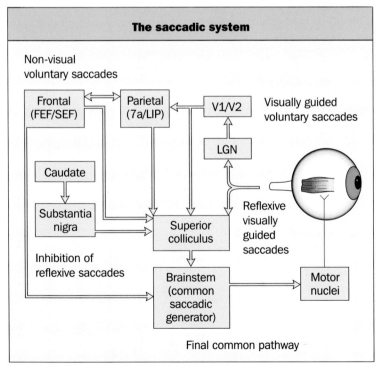

Fig. 8.13 The neuroanatomic basis of the saccadic control system. The functions of different parts of this complex pathway are shown.

tributing to a specific form of saccade (*Fig. 8.13*). The two key areas involved in the control of saccadic movements are the superior colliculus and the frontal eye fields.

Superior Colliculus
The superior colliculus appears to be important in visually driven reflexive saccades, and contributes to the accuracy of other forms of saccades. Visually reflexive saccades can be inhibited by projections originating in the frontal eye fields that reach the superior colliculus via the caudate nucleus and substantia nigra pars reticulata.

The superior colliculus is a multilayered structure that has a visual sensory map in the dorsal layers and a motor map in the ventral layers. These ventral layers contain a map of saccadic size and duration, with each point representing a saccade of a given size and direction.

Frontal Eye Fields
The classic frontal lobe eye movement area, the frontal eye field, is located mainly in Brodmann area 8 but also includes portions of the adjacent areas 6, 4, and 9. This area contributes to visually guided saccades, predictive saccades, and saccades to remembered targets. It is also involved in suppressing voluntary saccades generated by the superior colliculus via an inhibitory pathway involving the caudate nucleus and substantia nigra.

Other Cortical Areas Contributing to Saccadic Control
The supplementary eye fields are situated anterior to the supplementary motor area. Their precise role in saccadic control is unclear. Lesions in this area affect the ability to perform a sequence of memory-guided saccades.

The dorsolateral prefrontal cortex is involved particularly in producing saccades to remembered positions and in suppressing reflexive saccades.

The parietal lobe, especially area 7a and the lateral intraparietal area (LIP), also contributes to saccades with regard to target localization and controlling visual attention.

These areas generate the control signals that encode the length and direction of a saccade. The signals converge on the premotor nuclei (in particular the paramedian pontine reticular formation, rostral interstitial nucleus of the medial longitudinal fasiculus, and the interstitial nucleus of Cajal) within the brainstem responsible for generating the appropriate firing pattern within the motorneuron pool (see below).

Special Physiologic Features: Saccadic Suppression
During saccades, the retinal image moves across the retina at speeds that would be expected to generate large amounts of motion blurring. That such blurring is not detected perceptually can be attributed in part to the phenomenon of saccadic suppression. This is the term given to the reduction in visual sensitivity that occurs during saccades. This phenomenon is assisted by the effects of visual masking, the term used to describe the ability of a sharp image to suppress awareness of a preceding or subsequent blurred image.

VERGENCE EYE MOVEMENTS

Characteristics and Features of Interest
Vergence eye movements ensure the alignment of the visual axes of the two eyes on targets at different viewing distances. Objects at different distances project to different points on the retina

in the two eyes. This difference in relative retinal location in the two eyes is termed retinal disparity. Vergence eye movements ensure that the object under fixation is projected onto the fovea of the two eyes irrespective of viewing distance. This alignment is not absolute. There are small errors in alignment during fixation which are referred to as fixation disparity. Within a small range of vergence errors, the visual cortex can re-align the images from the two eyes to ensure perceptual fusion, that is the perception of a single image. The range over which this re-aligment occurs is called Panum's area of single vision (*Fig. 8.14*).

As vergence eye movements aim to minimize retinal disparity, it is not surprising that retinal disparity represents a major stimulus for vergence movements. The vergence system is, however, closely integrated with the accommodation system, which also responds to images at varying distances by altering the tone of the ciliary muscle, thereby focusing the crystalline lens to ensure a clear retinal image. Stimuli to accommodation (predominantly retinal image blur) influence vergence responses, producing accommodative convergence responses. Conversely, stimuli to vergence (predominantly retinal disparity) influence accommodation, producing convergence accommodation responses. The strength of these two interactions can be quantified and expressed as two ratios: the AC:A (accommodative convergence/accommodation) ratio, and the CA:C (convergence accommodation/convergence ratio). The relationship between the two systems can be represented as two interacting feedback loops, as shown in *Figure 8.15*.

Neuroanatomic Pathways

Although it is known that disparity plays an important role in the sensory guidance of vergence eye movements, the cortical pathways for vergence control are the least well defined of any eye movement system. Animal studies in non-primates indicate that areas associated with motion are important for vergence control, implying a role for middle temporal and medial superior temporal areas, but this has not been shown definitively in primates. The cerebellum is also important for vergence eye movements, although the relationships between potential cortical areas and the cerebellum

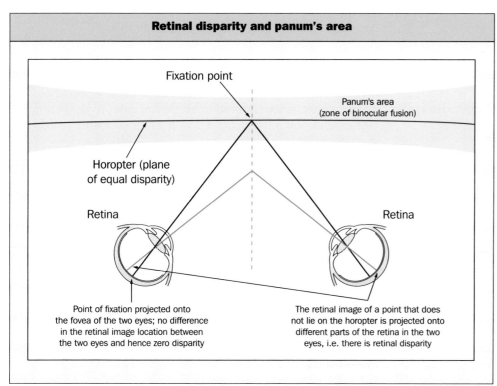

Fig. 8.14 The relationship of the fixation plane, retinal disparity, and Panum's area. All visual targets on an imaginary curved plane called the horopter have no retinal disparity. Objects in front of and behind this plane display retinal disparity, that is, are projected onto non-corresponding parts of the retina in the two eyes. Retinal disparity is used by the brain to generate depth perception (stereopsis) and to control vergence eye movements. Objects within Panum's area, an area of space in front of and behind the plane of fixation, are perceived as single. Outside this area retinal disparity is too large, resulting in physiologic diplopia.

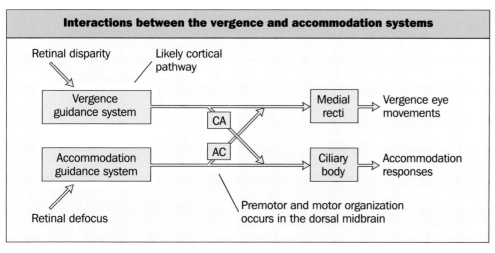

Fig. 8.15 The reciprocal interactions of the vergence and accommodation systems. (CA, convergence accommodation crosslink; AC, accommodative convergence cross-link)

are not well defined. As discussed in the section on premotor organization (below), the only neuroanatomically well-defined part of the vergence system is the location of premotor neurons in the pretectal area. These neurons carry signals for vergence and vergence velocity but do not fire during eye movements in any direction that does not involve a change in binocular alignment.

Special Physiologic Features: Saccadic Vergence Interactions
Classically, vergence responses have been considered to be relatively slow movements, and in the absence of saccades this is true. Changes in fixation associated with saccadic movements are frequently associated with a change in viewing distance as well as direction. It has been found that during such combined movements the vergence component of the movement occurs more rapidly. Animal studies indicated that this represents a facilitation of vergence responses by the saccadic system at a premotor level, rather than an ability of the saccadic system to perform vergence responses.

FIXATIONAL EYE MOVEMENTS

Characteristics and Features of Interest
Fixation on a target does not abolish all eye movements. Fixation is associated with constant low amplitude (0.1°) movements, which comprise both fast microsaccades and slow drifts (*Fig. 8.16*). There is also a fine tremor with a much lower amplitude than microsaccades and slow drifts (0.005°, comparable with the angular subtense of a foveal cone photoreceptor), which is of little physiologic significance.

Visual fixation has two physiologically and neuroanatomically separate components: firstly, an attention-dependent, visually guided process that allows us to choose what we wish to fixate on; and secondly, a set of mechanisms within the brainstem that constitute the neural integrator. A unifying feature of premotor eye movement signals in the saccadic, pursuit, and vestibular system is that these signals encode eye velocity and not eye position. For the eye to be held in its new position after a movement, a velocity signal must undergo a transformation that is described mathematically as integration.

Neuroanatomic Pathways
The visually guided attentional aspects of visual fixation do not have a well-defined neuroanatomic basis but the most likely area is within

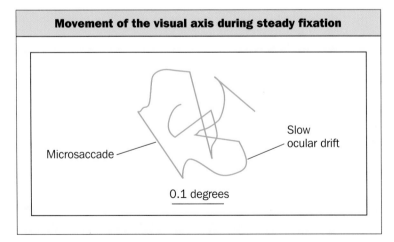

Fig. 8.16 Fixational eye movements showing linear microsaccades and curvilinear drifts. Microtremor movements are an order of magnitude smaller than these two components of fixational instability.

the parietal cortex where neurons have been found that respond to visual stimuli only when the stimuli are being attended to.

The neuroanatomic basis of the neural integrator has been well defined and is represented by neuronal connections within the medial vestibular nuclei and the nucleus prepositus hypoglossi (part of the perihypoglossal complex) within the brainstem.

Special Physiologic Features: Troxler Fading
The small microsaccadic movements and slower low amplitude drifts characteristic of fixation perform a useful physiologic function. A completely stabilized retinal image rapidly fades and becomes undetectable, a phenomenon termed Troxler fading. This results from the fact that retinal ganglion cells show phasic responses, responding best to changing stimuli and rapidly habituating to any constant stimulus. The shadows cast by retinal blood vessels are rendered invisible by this process.

PREMOTOR ORGANIZATION

COORDINATION OF THE ACTIVITY OF THE EYE MOVEMENT NUCLEI

The activity of the motor neurons controlling the eye muscles is coordinated by a number of premotor nuclei within the brainstem (*Fig. 8.17*). These nuclei integrate the activity of all the motor nuclei and separate centers are involved in horizontal gaze, vertical gaze, and convergence eye movements. Oblique eye movements represent a vector combination of appropriately sized vertical and horizontal components. The interconnections of these nuclei are largely carried within the medial longitudinal fasciculus, although other pathways are also involved including the brachium conjunctivum.

HORIZONTAL GAZE

All signals for horizontal eye movements converge on the sixth nerve nucleus. For the saccadic system, the horizontal gaze center is located within the paramedian pontine reticular formation (PPRF). Vestibular eye movement signals project directly to the sixth nucleus, whereas pursuit signals project from the medial vestibular nucleus (MVN) and nucleus prepositus hypoglossi (NPH) either directly or via the PPRF. The motor neurons supplying the two muscles involved in horizontal eye movements (medial and lateral recti) are linked by interneurons situated within the sixth nerve nucleus. These interneurons cross the midline, pass along the medial longitudinal fasciculus, and synapse on the motor neurons of the medial rectus within the third nerve nucleus, the corresponding yoke muscle (see below) of the lateral rectus (*Fig. 8.18*).

VERTICAL GAZE

Vertical eye movements are dependent on premotor nuclei situated in both the midbrain and medulla which are connected via the MLF (*Fig. 8.19*). The premotor signals for vertical saccades are generated within the rostral interstitial nucleus of the MLF (riMLF) which is situated rostral to the third nerve nucleus within the dorsal midbrain. Vertical pursuit movements and vertical gaze holding (fixation) are dependent on premotor signals generated within the so-called neural integrator that is situated within

Key brainstem nuclei involved in eye movement control

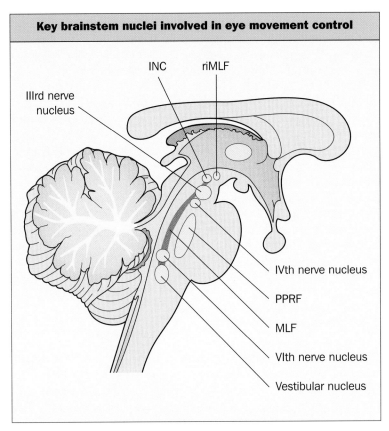

Fig. 8.17 Location of key brainstem nuclei controlling the eye muscles. (riMLF, rostral interstitial nucleus of the MLF; INC, interstitial nucleus of Cajal; MLF, medial longitudinal fasciculus; PPRF, paramedian pontine reticular formation)

Horizontal gaze pathways

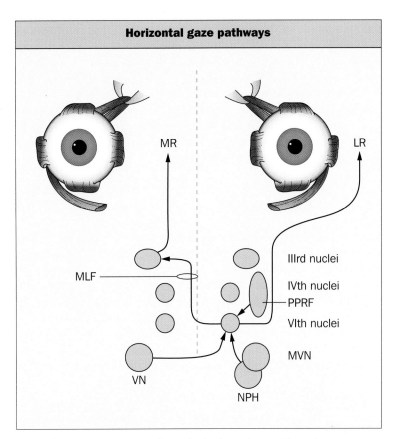

Fig. 8.18 Final common pathway for horizontal gaze. There is a convergence of signals on the sixth nerve nucleus. Interneurons in the sixth nucleus relay signals onto the motor neurons innervating the medial rectus (MR) via the medial longitudinal fasciculus (MLF). (PPRF, paramedian pontine reticular formation; MVN, medial vestibular nucleus; NPH, nucleus prepositus hypoglossi; LR, lateral rectus)

Down-gaze pathways

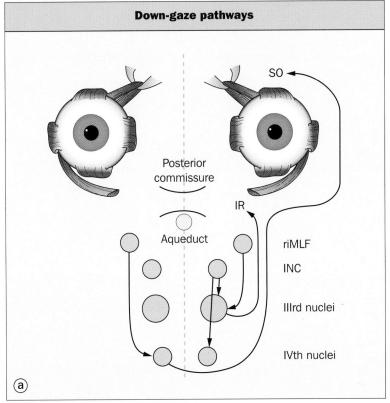

Up-gaze pathways

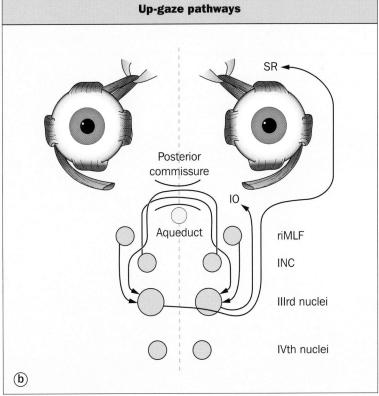

Fig. 8.19 Premotor pathways for up-gaze and down-gaze. For simplicity, the connections resulting in the innervation of the elevators or depressors of only one eye are shown. (SO, superior oblique; SR, superior rectus; IO, inferior oblique; IR, inferior rectus)

the brainstem in the medial vestibular nuclei and the nucleus prepositus hypoglossi. Signals from these nuclei are carried superiorly within the MLF to the interstitial nucleus of Cajal (INC), which contributes to the final premotor commands for vertical eye movements and has a particular role in vertical gaze holding. The bilateral connections of the riMLF and INC mean that vertical gaze is affected by lesions only if they are bilateral or midline. Unilateral lesions in these nuclei lead to torsional abnormalities and a relative sparing of vertical gaze.

VERGENCE EYE MOVEMENTS

The premotor commands for vergence eye movements are generated within the midbrain, dorsal to the third nerve nucleus within a region of the reticular formation that has not been associated with a specific midbrain nucleus. These neurons carry pure vergence or vergence velocity signals independent of the direction of conjugate gaze. Most neurons increase their firing with increasing convergence, with a smaller group increasing their firing during divergence movements. Inhibition of pause neurons (see below) during combined saccadic and vergence eye movements results in an increase in the activity of vergence premotor neurons and an associated increase in the velocity of vergence movements.

SPECIFIC FEATURES OF SACCADIC PREMOTOR SIGNALS

Motor neurons supplying the extraocular muscles have a charac-

teristic burst–tonic firing pattern. Eye fixation and slow movements are achieved by changes of the tonic firing rate of motor neurons. The rapid eye movements characteristic of saccades are achieved by intense bursts of action potentials which rapidly accelerate the eye toward the chosen position. This position is then maintained by an increase in the tonic firing rate. The combined burst–tonic signal is generated by a well-defined pattern of neural interconnections (*Fig. 8.20*). The rapid firing pattern is generated by burst cells that are tonically inhibited by pause cells. During a saccade, the pause cells are inhibited by signals generated within the saccadic control pathways (see above); the burst cells are therefore activated by release of the inhibitory influence of the pause cells. The burst cells are located within the horizontal and vertical saccade gaze centers in the pons and midbrain. The pause cells for both vertical and horizontal gaze are located within the pons in the nucleus raphe interpositus.

TONIC MOTOR NEURON RESPONSES AND THE NEURAL INTEGRATOR

The holding of the eyes in a certain position (gaze holding) is achieved with the aid of the neural integrator. It is called the integrator because this describes the mathematical process of converting a velocity or movement signal into a position signal. The neural integrator effectively stores the signals generated during eye movements to hold the eye in its final position. The neuroanatomic substrate for this mechanism is located in the medial vestibular nucleus and perihypoglossal nuclear complex.

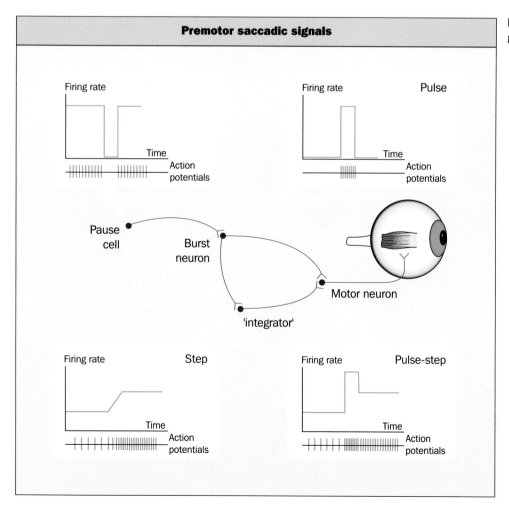

Fig. 8.20 Burst–tonic firing patterns and their generation.

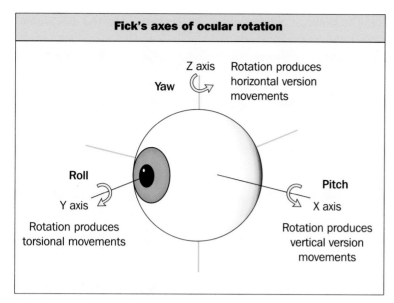

Fig. 8.21 Fick's axes of ocular rotation.

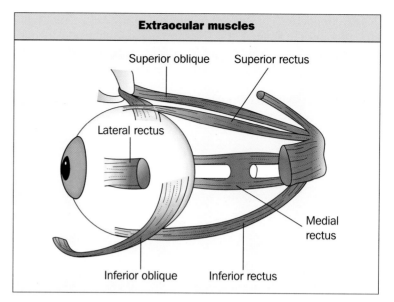

Fig. 8.22 Lateral view of the extraocular muscles.

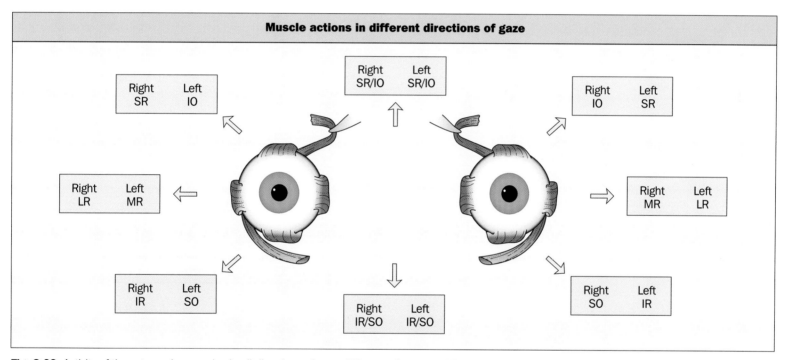

Fig. 8.23 Activity of the extraocular muscles in all directions of gaze. (SR, superior rectus; LR, lateral rectus; MR, medial rectus; IR, inferior rectus; SO superior oblique; IO, inferior oblique)

MOTOR ORGANIZATION

EXTRAOCULAR MUSCLES

The eyes are moved by six extraocular muscles, which can move the eye in any direction allowing rotation around three independent axes (Fick's x, y, and z axes; *Fig. 8.21*). Movements where both eyes move in the same direction are termed versions and result from rotation about the z or x axis. Rotations about the y axis are called torsional movements and occur as reflexes during head tilt.

The extraocular muscles are shown above (Fig. 8.22). Only the medial and lateral recti have a simple mechanical action producing a horizontal movement of the eye. The superior and inferior recti along with the superior and inferior obliques have a more complex mechanical action which varies with the direction of gaze (Fig. 8.23).

In adduction, the oblique muscles elevate and depress and the vertical recti produce torsion. In abduction, the oblique muscles produce torsion and the vertical recti elevate and depress the eye (FIg. 8.23). The muscles in the two eyes that move the eyes in the same direction, for example, the lateral rectus of one eye and the medial rectus of the other, are termed yoke muscles and under most conditions their activity is linked, a condition often referred to as Hering's Law.

CRANIAL NERVE NUCLEI

The six extraocular muscles of the eye are controlled by three cranial nerves, the third nerve (oculomotor nerve), the fourth nerve (trochlear nerve), and the sixth nerve (abducens nerve).

The connections of these three nerves to the extraocular muscles are shown in *Figure 8.25*. The third nerve supplies the medial, superior, and inferior recti along with the inferior oblique. The fourth nerve supplies only the superior oblique and the sixth nerve supplies only the lateral rectus. The connections from the nuclei to the eye are ipsilateral for all muscles except the superior rectus

and the superior oblique which are innervated by the motor neurons in the contralateral third and fourth nerve nuclei, respectively.

In summary, *Figures 8.26* and *8.27* provide an overview of the neuroanatomy of eye movements, illustrating the key cortical and subcortical centers involved in eye movement control.

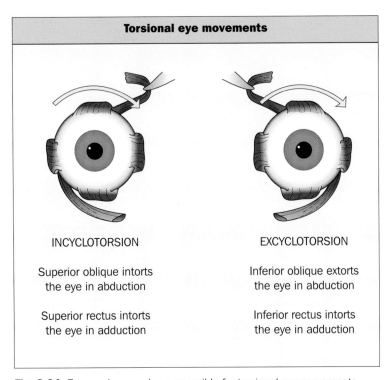

Torsional eye movements

INCYCLOTORSION

Superior oblique intorts the eye in abduction

Superior rectus intorts the eye in adduction

EXCYCLOTORSION

Inferior oblique extorts the eye in abduction

Inferior rectus intorts the eye in adduction

Fig. 8.24 Extraocular muscles responsible for torsional eye movements. Both superior muscles intort and both inferior muscles extort. The obliques exert a predominantly torsional action in abduction and the vertical recti exert a predominantly torsional action in adduction.

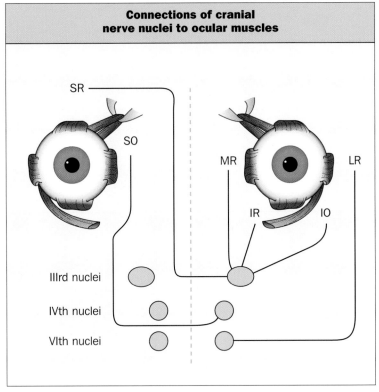

Connections of cranial nerve nuclei to ocular muscles

Fig. 8.25 Diagram of the pattern of innervation of the extraocular muscles by the third, fourth, and sixth cranial nerves.

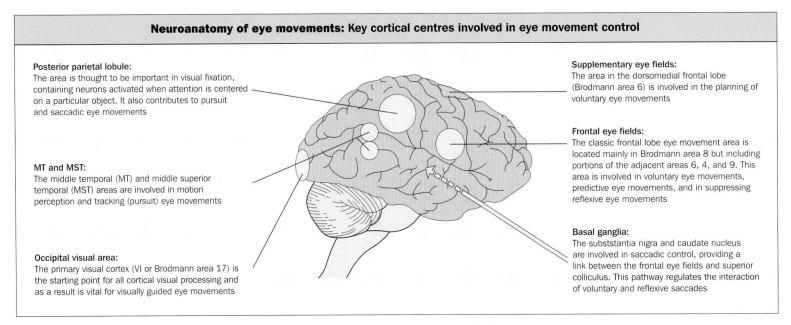

Neuroanatomy of eye movements: Key cortical centres involved in eye movement control

Posterior parietal lobule:
The area is thought to be important in visual fixation, containing neurons activated when attention is centered on a particular object. It also contributes to pursuit and saccadic eye movements

MT and MST:
The middle temporal (MT) and middle superior temporal (MST) areas are involved in motion perception and tracking (pursuit) eye movements

Occipital visual area:
The primary visual cortex (VI or Brodmann area 17) is the starting point for all cortical visual processing and as a result is vital for visually guided eye movements

Supplementary eye fields:
The area in the dorsomedial frontal lobe (Brodmann area 6) is involved in the planning of voluntary eye movements

Frontal eye fields:
The classic frontal lobe eye movement area is located mainly in Brodman area 8 but including portions of the adjacent areas 6, 4, and 9. This area is involved in voluntary eye movements, predictive eye movements, and in suppressing reflexive eye movements

Basal ganglia:
The subststantia nigra and caudate nucleus are involved in saccadic control, providing a link between the frontal eye fields and superior colliculus. This pathway regulates the interaction of voluntary and reflexive saccades

Fig. 8.26 Overview of the neuroanatomy of eye movements, showing the key cortical areas involved in eye movement control.

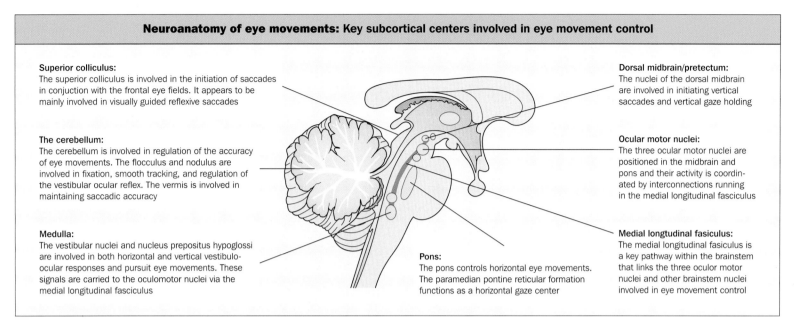

Neuroanatomy of eye movements: Key subcortical centers involved in eye movement control

Superior colliculus:
The superior colliculus is involved in the initiation of saccades in conjuction with the frontal eye fields. It appears to be mainly involved in visually guided reflexive saccades

The cerebellum:
The cerebellum is involved in regulation of the accuracy of eye movements. The flocculus and nodulus are involved in fixation, smooth tracking, and regulation of the vestibular ocular reflex. The vermis is involved in maintaining saccadic accuracy

Medulla:
The vestibular nuclei and nucleus prepositus hypoglossi are involved in both horizontal and vertical vestibulo-ocular responses and pursuit eye movements. These signals are carried to the oculomotor nuclei via the medial longitudinal fasciculus

Dorsal midbrain/pretectum:
The nuclei of the dorsal midbrain are involved in initiating vertical saccades and vertical gaze holding

Ocular motor nuclei:
The three ocular motor nuclei are positioned in the midbrain and pons and their activity is coordinated by interconnections running in the medial longitudinal fasciculus

Pons:
The pons controls horizontal eye movements. The paramedian pontine reticular formation functions as a horizontal gaze center

Medial longtudinal fasiculus:
The medial longtudinal fasiculus is a key pathway within the brainstem that links the three oculor motor nuclei and other brainstem nuclei involved in eye movement control

Fig. 8.27 Overview of the neuroanatomy of eye movements, showing the key subcortical areas involved in eye movement control.

Further reading

Buttner-Ennever JA, ed. *Neuroanatomy of the oculomotor system*. Amsterdam:Elsevier, 1988.
Carpenter RHS. *Movement of the eyes. 2nd edition*. London:Pion, 1988
Collewijn H, Erkelens CJ, Steinman RM *J Physiol* 1988;**404**:157–182.
Leigh RJ, Zee DS. *The Neurology of Eye Movements. 2nd edition*. Philadelphia:Davis, 1991.

Robinson DA. Control of eye movememts. In Brooks VB ed. *Handbook of Physiology , vol II, Part 2, The Nervous System*. Baltimore:Williams and Wilkins, 1981. pp.1275–1320.

CHAPTER 9

Cerebellar Control of Eye Movements and Eye Movement Abnormalities

Robert D Yee

INTRODUCTION

The cerebellum plays an important role in the control of eye movements. Although it does not generate the eye movements, it contributes significantly to their accuracy and to their adaptation to changes in the visual environment. A recent review described the cerebellum's general role in the control of body movements as part of a negative feedback system that uses sensory information to produce movements that interact with the environment (sensorimotor integration). The cerebellum controls the force, range, rate, and rhythm of movements and is part of an adaptive mechanism that alters movements in response to new sensory information. The recognition of characteristic eye movement abnormalities improves the localization of lesions and helps in the diagnosis and management of cerebellar disorders.

ANATOMY

Neurophysiologic and anatomic studies in animals and electronic eye movement recordings in patients have delineated the ocular motor pathways of the cerebellum. These pathways have recently been reviewed. The midline structures of the cerebellum have numerous connections with brainstem areas that serve eye movements. Many of these areas are part of the central vestibular pathways or receive afferent fibers from visual association areas in the parietal, temporal, and frontal lobes. The visual association areas process information about motion in the visual environment.

The vestibulocerebellum is located on the ventral surface of the cerebellum. Its subdivisions are the flocculus, paraflocculus, nodulus, and uvula (*Fig. 9.1a*). The vermis is a midline structure (*Fig. 9.1b*). Lobules IV to VII of the dorsal vermis participate in eye movement control. The vestibulocerebellum interconnects with central vestibulo-ocular pathways in the lower brainstem. Inputs include projections from neurons in the vestibular nuclei (VN). In primates, these are second-order neurons of the vestibulo-ocular response. In addition, projections from the inferior olive and from the nucleus prepositus hypoglossi (NPH) reach the vestibulocerebellum. These afferent fibers synapse as mossy fibers and climbing fibers (from the inferior olive) on neurons in the granular layer of the cerebellar cortex, which in turn provide input

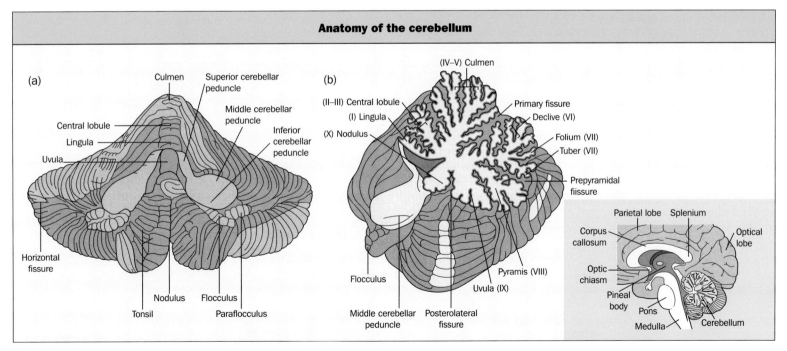

Fig. 9.1 Anatomy of the cerebellum. (**a**) Ventral view. (**b**) Sagittal view, with the numbering of vermian lobules according to Larsell. The insert shows a midline, sagittal section of the human brain illustrating the anatomic relationships of the cerebellum.

to the Purkinje cells. Purkinje cell axons are the output of the cerebellar cortex. They project to the fastigial nucleus, superior VN, medial VN, and to the γ group of the VN.

The vermis also receives inputs from the VN, NPH, and inferior olive. Brainstem areas controlling saccadic eye movements and smooth pursuit eye movements send axons to the vermis. These areas include the paramedian pontine reticular formation (PPRF), nucleus reticularis tegmenti pontis (NRTP), and dorsolateral pontine nucleus (DLPN). The vermis sends efferent fibers to brainstem areas concerned with saccades and smooth pursuit. The outputs include projections to the fastigial nucleus, PPRF, rostral interstitial nucleus of the medial longitudinal fasciculus (riMLF), NPH, DLPN, and superior colliculus.

SYMPTOMS OF CEREBELLAR DISORDERS

Characteristic patterns of abnormal eye movements are associated with cerebellar disorders. These patterns are discussed in detail below. Nystagmus and saccadic oscillations can cause blurred vision. Abnormal vestibulo-ocular responses (VOR) produce blurred vision during rapid movements of the head and body. In these instances, images on the retina are not stable. They move across the fovea at speeds greater than a few degrees per second and decrease visual acuity. Oscillopsia is an illusion of jumping of stationary visual objects. It can be caused by nystagmus, saccadic oscillations, or abnormal VOR during head movements. A skew deviation is a nonparalytic, vertical tropia that can cause vertical diplopia. It is associated with disorders of the brainstem and cerebellum.

In addition to these eye movement problems patients with cerebellar disorders almost always complain of other symptoms that reflect the cerebellum's role in other types of sensorimotor function. These include vertigo, imbalance, incoordination, and gait disturbance. The most frequently found sign is ataxia of gait, limbs, or trunk. Other signs include dysarthria, hypotonia, and dyssynergia.

PATTERNS OF CEREBELLAR EYE MOVEMENT ABNORMALITIES

Cerebellar disorders usually cause abnormal eye movements. For example, a study of patients with cerebellar lesions found that 79% had nystagmus. They have highly characteristic patterns of abnormal eye movements, including: unstable fixation (nystagmus and saccadic oscillations); inaccurate saccades; impaired smooth pursuit and optokinetic nystagmus; and abnormal VOR (*Fig. 9.2*). Recognition of the patterns can help clinicians localize lesions to the cerebellum. As with non-ocular signs associated with cerebellar disorders, however, lesions outside of the cerebellum can produce similar abnormal eye movements. This is not surprising in view of the extensive interconnections of the cerebellum and the brainstem.

GAZE HOLDING

Cerebellar lesions commonly produce fixation instabilities such as nystagmus and saccadic oscillations. Gaze-paretic nystagmus in horizontal or vertical gaze is the most frequently found form of nystagmus. Neurons within the VN and NPH form a neural integrator circuit that maintains eccentric gaze. Damage to connections between this circuit and the flocculus may impair normal gaze holding.

Rebound nystagmus is a form of gaze-paretic nystagmus that is highly characteristic of cerebellar disorders. During sustained eccentric gaze, the gaze-paretic nystagmus, which has fast phases in the direction of gaze, gradually decreases. On return to center gaze, there are several beats of jerk nystagmus with fast phases in the opposite direction.

Nystagmus in primary gaze occurs in patients and animals with cerebellar lesions.

Downbeat nystagmus that increases in frequency or amplitude in horizontal gaze is characteristic of damage to the midline structures of the cerebellum. In a study of 91 patients with downbeat nystagmus, 91% had other signs or symptoms consistent with localization to the cerebellum. Lesions of the flocculus and paraflocculus produced downbeat nystagmus in animals. Damage to the cerebellum and lower brainstem can produce upbeat nystagmus.

Periodic alternating nystagmus (PAN) that shows consistent and relatively symmetrical periodicity of phases (null, right-beating, left-beating) may be pathognomonic of cerebellar disorders. In animals, damage to the nodulus and uvula causes PAN. Baclofen can decrease PAN in most patients with these disorders.

Saccadic oscillations include macro-square-wave jerks, ocular flutter, and opsoclonus. Patients with these fixation instabilities commonly have signs and symptoms of cerebellar dysfunction. Normally, pause cells in the pons tonically inhibit burst cells in the PPRF until a saccade must be made. Loss of this inhibition may create unintentional saccades and saccadic oscillations.

SACCADES

Refixation saccades are normally very accurate in placing the target's image on the fovea. Burst neurons in the brainstem suddenly increase their firing rate to very high levels. This produces a 'pulse' increase in innervation to the ocular motor neurons of sufficient duration and amplitude to place the eyes on the target. A sustained 'step' increase in innervation then maintains the new gaze position. Cerebellar lesions cause saccadic dysmetria or inaccuracy of saccades (*Fig. 9.3*). The 'pulse' and 'step' are too large and the eyes overshoot the target (hypermetria) or they are too small and the eyes undershoot the target (hypometria).

Patterns of cerebellar eye movement abnormalities	
Gaze holding	nystagmus saccadic oscillations
Saccades	saccadic dysmetria postsaccadic drift
Smooth pursuit and optokinetic nystagmus	cogwheel pursuit impaired optokinetic nystagmus
Vestibulo-ocular responses	abnormal visual–vestibular interactions

Fig. 9.2 Patterns of cerebellar eye movement abnormalities.

Connections between the vermis and the PPRF, superior colliculus, and riMLF may underlie the cerebellum's role in maintaining the accuracy of saccades. In animals, lesions of the vermis and fastigial nuclei produce hypermetria of centripetal saccades (eccentric gaze toward primary gaze) and hypometria of centrifugal saccades (primary gaze toward eccentric gaze). Macrosaccadic oscillations result from severe saccadic hypermetria in which the initial saccade and several corrective saccades

overshoot the target. In animals, cerebellectomy can produce these oscillations.

Normally, the pulse and step are matched in duration and amplitude, such that the new position reached by the eyes at the end of the pulse is maintained by the step. Patients with cerebellar lesions can have a pulse–step mismatch in which the step does not keep the eyes precisely at the same postion. A postsaccadic drift results. At the end of the pulse, a smooth eye movement carries the eye towards or away from the target. In animals, lesions of the flocculus and paraflocculus produce postsaccadic drift.

SMOOTH PURSUIT AND OPTOKINETIC NYSTAGMUS

The visual association areas in the parietal, temporal, and frontal lobes send axons to brainstem structures that serve smooth pursuit eye movements. These structures, including the DLPN, send axons to the flocculus, paraflocculus, and dorsal vermis (lobes VI–VII). Cerebellar output to the VN may be part of the smooth pursuit pathways.

Patients with cerebellar disorders usually have impaired smooth pursuit. The velocity of the eye movement cannot match the velocity of the target and the eye falls behind the target. The position error is detected and the eye makes a 'catch-up' saccade towards the target. A combination of smooth pursuit and saccadic movements (jerky or cogwheel pursuit) replaces the normal smooth pattern of eye movements (*Fig. 9.4*). Lesions of the flocculus, paraflocculus, and vermis create impaired smooth pursuit in animals. Unilateral lesions of the flocculus and paraflocculus cause ipsilateral impairment.

Patients with cerebellar disorders also have impaired optokinetic nystagmus (OKN). The velocity of the slow phases is abnormally low and the frequency of the jerk nystagmus can be irregular (see Fig. 9.4). The motion of large patterns in the visual field stimulates the central areas of the field, as well as the peripheral areas. Therefore, optokinetic stimuli activate the smooth pursuit system. In humans, the dominant response is that of the smooth pursuit system. Impairment of OKN in patients usually parallels the defect in smooth pursuit. In animals without well-developed foveas, the accessory optic system primarily generates OKN. This system uses projections from the optic tracts to relay nuclei in the midbrain. These midbrain structures project to the VN, NPH, and cap of the inferior olive to generate smooth eye movements. The accessory optic system probably persists in primates. Some patients with cerebellar disorders can have a weak OKN response that has characteristics of the subcortical system.

VESTIBULO-OCULAR RESPONSE

The function of the vestibulo-ocular response (VOR) is to maintain the direction of gaze relative to the environment during head and body motion. For example, rotation of the head toward the right produces compensatory eye movements toward the left in the orbits. The result is that the eyes continue to be directed straight ahead in space. Although the vestibulocerebellum is not part of the basic three-neuron reflex of the VOR, it plays an important role in modifying the VOR (adaptation of the VOR) in response to visual stimuli. In primates, second-order neurons in

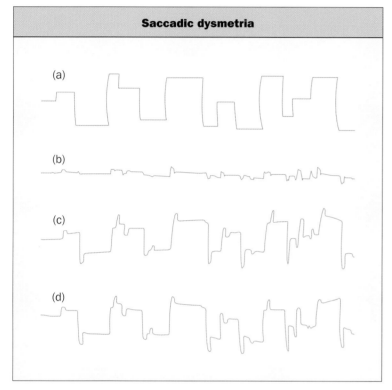

Fig. 9.3 Saccadic dysmetria. Eye movement recordings showing (**a**) target, (**b**) vertical eye movements, (**c**) left eye horizontal, and (**d**) right eye horizontal. Rightward and leftward saccades overshoot the target and small corrective saccades are made.

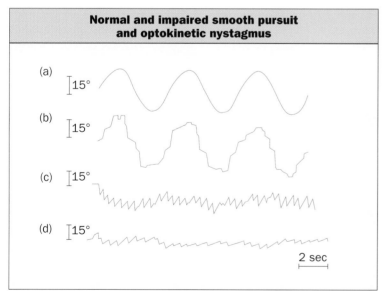

Fig. 9.4 Normal and impaired smooth pursuit and optokinetic nystagmus. Eye movement recordings showing (**a**) normal pursuit;, (**b**) impaired (cogwheel) pursuit, (**c**) normal optokinetic nystagmus, and (**d**) impaired optokinetic nystagmus. Small, catch-up saccades are made during impaired pursuit.

the VN send mossy fibers to the granular cells of both flocculi. Granular cell axons provide afferent information about vestibular stimulation to the Purkinje cells. Purkinje cells may receive information about retinal image motion from the accessory optic system via climbing fibers from the cap of the inferior olive. Purkinje cells axons project ipsilaterally to the VN.

Cerebellar disorders in patients usually do not affect the VOR during rotation in the dark. For example, the VOR gain (slow phase eye velocity/head velocity) is often within the normal range (less than 1.0). Rarely, the VOR gain is unusually high. However, some patients do show abnormal VOR during visual–vestibular interactions. Tests of these interactions present visual stimuli during rotation of the head and body.

Synergistic interactions occur when rotation takes place in a stationary visual surround. Head rotation to the right induces a VOR to the left. Simultaneously, the head rotation causes movement of objects in the visual surround toward the left relative to the eyes. Visual tracking movements (smooth pursuit and OKN) to the left result. The summated leftward eye movements are faster than VOR in the dark. Doll's eye movements in a conscious individual result from similar interactions. The VOR gain during synergistic visual–vestibular interactions is greater than the VOR gain in the dark, and is about 1.0 (*Fig. 9.5 b,c*). Patients with cerebellar disorders often show no increase in VOR gain when the lights are turned on.

Instructing an individual to fixate on a visual target that rotates simultaneously and equally with the head produces antagonistic visual–vestibular interactions. For example, the examiner instructs the person to fixate a finger while being rotated in a chair (*Fig. 9.6*). Head rotation towards the right induces VOR to the left. However, leftward eye movement in the orbit causes motion of retinal images and loss of fixation. Information about retinal image motion received by the cerebellum via the inferior olive may be used to inhibit the VOR. Normal individuals can inhibit the VOR almost completely (*Fig. 9.5d*). However, patients with cerebellar lesions cannot inhibit the VOR normally (*Fig. 9.7*).

The cerebellum also participates in long-term adaptation of the VOR. Fitting animals and human with inverting prisms or mirrors that reverse directions horizontally causes dramatic changes in the VOR. The normal compensatory VOR is in the wrong direction to maintain gaze direction in space. Within minutes of wearing the optical devices, the VOR gain in the dark decreases. After a few weeks, the direction of the VOR can actually reverse. VOR adaptation to spectacle lenses is a common phenomenon. Plus and minus lenses produce prismatic effects during eye movements called rotational magnification. When looking through the lenses, individuals must make larger (plus lenses) or smaller (minus lenses) eye movements during head movements than they would without the lenses in order to maintain their direction of gaze. The VOR gain in the dark changes after several minutes of wearing the lenses. An elderly patient's difficulty in adjusting to high-powered, plus lenses after cataract surgery may be due in part to rotational magnification. Destruction of the flocculus and paraflocculus in animals severely impairs VOR adaptation.

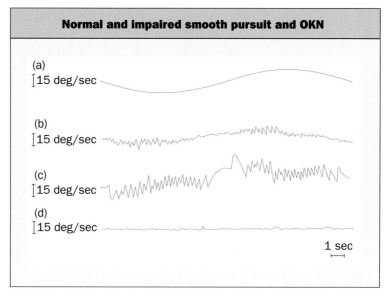

Fig. 9.5 Normal visual–vestibular interactions. Eye movement recordings showing (**a**) velocity of rotating chair, (**b**) vestibulo-ocular response (VOR) during rotation in dark, (**c**) VOR during rotation in visible, stationary surroundings, and (**d**) VOR during rotation and fixation of a target moving with the chair. Rotation in light increases VOR and rotation with fixation almost completely inhibits VOR.

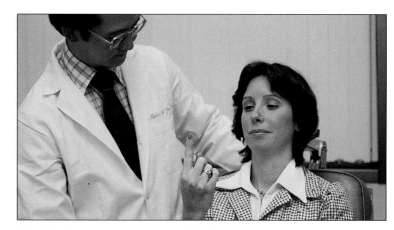

Fig. 9.6 Fixation suppression of VOR. The individual fixates a finger while the examiner rotates the chair rapidly to-and-fro and watches the person's eyes.

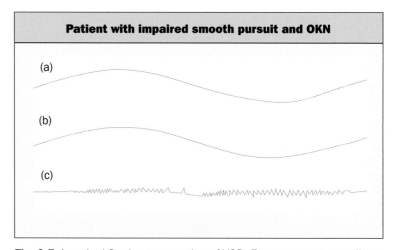

Fig. 9.7 Impaired fixation suppression of VOR. Eye movement recordings showing (**a**) velocity of rotating chair, (**b**) fixation target moving with chair, and (**c**) patient's eye movements. The patient cannot suppress the VOR and beats of vestibular nystagmus break through.

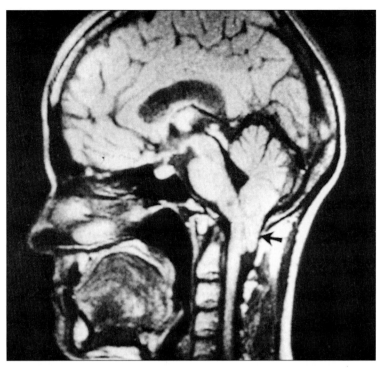

Fig. 9.8 Arnold–Chiari malformation. A sagittal MRI shows cerebellar tonsils herniating into the foramen magnum (arrow).

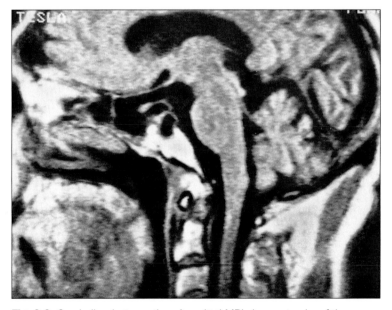

Fig. 9.9 Cerebellar degeneration. A sagittal MRI shows atrophy of the vermis.

LABORATORY TESTS

MR and CT scanning have replaced other forms of imaging structures in the posterior fossa. In general, anatomic details are better seen with MR than with CT because bones do not interfere with imaging the cerebellum, brainstem, and cranial nerves. MR studies are usually obtained both with and without intravenous gadolinium. They can clearly show herniation of the cerebellar tonsils into the foramen magnum in the Arnold–Chiari malformation (*Fig. 9.8*) and atrophy of the vermis in primary cerebellar degeneration (*Fig. 9.9*). Examination of the cerebrospinal fluid is required when inflammatory, neoplastic, infectious, and/or demyelinating disorders may be present.

CAUSES OF CEREBELLAR DISORDERS

Common causes of cerebellar disorders are listed in *Figure 9.10*. Although abnormal eye movements occur frequently in these disorders, they do not usually differentiate the causes. The patient's history (e.g. age, mode of onset, and course), family history, physical examination (e.g. signs of brainstem, spinal cord, and cranial nerve dysfunction), and laboratory tests point to the probable cause of the disorder.

Common cerebellar disorders	
Primary cerebellar degenerations	isolated cerebellar atrophy olivopontocerebellar atrophy spinocerebellar atrophy
Malformations	Arnold–Chiari malformation
Demyelinating disorders	multiple sclerosis
Toxins and drugs	alcohol heavy metals
Nutritional deficiencies	Wernicke's encephalopathy (thiamin)
Metabolic diseases	Wilson's disease
Vascular disorders	cerebellar artery syndromes (inferior, anterior, superior) cerebellar infarction, cerebellar hemorrhage
Neoplasms	cerebellopontine angle tumors primary tumors
Paraneoplastic syndromes	neuroblastoma, carcinomas
Infections	cerebellar abscess cerebellitis
Trauma	closed head injury

Further reading

Dow RS, Kramer RE, Robertson LT. *Disorders of the Cerebellum*. In: Joynt RJ, ed. *Clinical Neurology*, **Vol 3**. Philadelphia:JB Lippincott Company. 1992 1–143.

Leigh RJ, Zee DS. *The Neurology of Eye Movements, 2nd edn.* (Philadelphia: FA Davis Company, 1991) 40–43; 106–110; 156–157; 202–205; 424–428.

Yee RD. Downbeat nystagmus: characteristics and localization of lesions. *Trans Am Ophthalmol Soc.* 1989; **87**:984–1031.

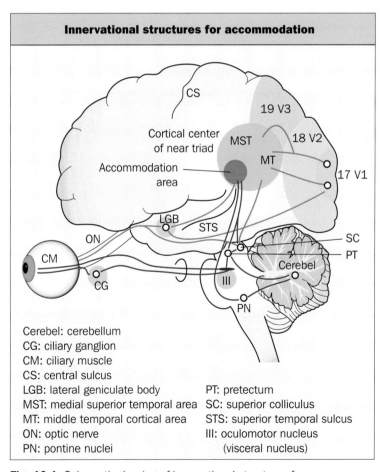

CHAPTER 10

Pupils and Accommodation

Satoshi Ishikawa and Kazuo Mukuno
(in collaboration with T Namba, K Ukai, and K Tsuchiya)

INTRODUCTION

Accommodation is the term used to describe the ability of the eye to focus and maintain a clear retinal image. Contraction of the ciliary muscle relaxes tension on the lens zonules so that the refractive power of the eye is increased. Accommodation reduces with age, reaching significant weakness by the mid-40s. In patients over 50, abnormalities of accommodation are rare. Accommodation weakness may be linked with many other neuro-ophthalmologic disorders. Recently, both functional and anatomical research on accommodation have progressed greatly and this has helped the understanding of accommodative disorders.

ANATOMIC AND PHYSIOLOGIC EVIDENCE OF ACCOMMODATION

CORTICAL CONTROL

In the 1960s, Jampel found that stimulating the cerebral cortex in Brodmann areas 19 and 22 (the upper bank of the superior temporal sulcus) of the cortex in the monkey produced an increase in accommodation, usually associated with convergence of the eyes and pupil constriction. The impulses project to the pretectal olivary and sublenticular nuclei, and to the Edinger–Westphal (E–W) nuclei, probably by way of the cortico-tectal tract.

These cortical areas in the monkey almost correspond in humans to the superior temporal sulcus (STS), especially the middle superior temporal area (MST), at the parieto-occipital junction, and also to areas 19 and 39 of the human parieto-occipital junction. In cats, the lateral suprasylvian area has been proposed as the cortical center (*Fig. 10.1*).

In the monkey, Mays *et al.* and Judge *et al.* found supranuclear near response neurons in the mesencephalic reticular formation (dorsolateral to the third nucleus) and dorsal midbrain just rostral to the superior colliculus and pretectal areas. Some of the neurons directly projected to motorneurons that related to vergence and accommodation. In the cat, a similar near triad center in the midbrain was demonstrated by Hiraoka and Shimamura.

By measuring the refractive power of the lens during stimulation of the cerebellum, Hosoba *et al.* found the area giving responses that were shorter than 160 ms in latency and larger than 0.15 diopters (D) in amplitude. The authors suggested that accommodative responses were modified by stimulation of the cerebellar cortex. Stimulation in the region of the interpositus nucleus has been shown to produce accommodation and not pupil constriction. These areas, when stimulated, cause activation of accommodation motor neurons in the E–W nucleus.

The accommodation-related neurons were mostly located later-

Innervational structures for accommodation

Cerebel: cerebellum
CG: ciliary ganglion
CM: ciliary muscle
CS: central sulcus
LGB: lateral geniculate body
MST: medial superior temporal area
MT: middle temporal cortical area
ON: optic nerve
PN: pontine nuclei

PT: pretectum
SC: superior colliculus
STS: superior temporal sulcus
III: oculomotor nucleus
    (visceral nucleus)

Fig. 10.1 Schematic drawing of innervational structures for accommodation.

ally and dorsally to the E–W nucleus according to physiologic study of the cat. Neuroanatomic study also showed a direct projection from the fastigial nucleus to the neighboring area of the E–W nucleus and dorsal central gray of the third nucleus. The dentate nucleus projects to a contralateral area similar to the fastigial nucleus slightly further away from the E–W and third nuclei.

Recently, Maekawa and Ohtsuka suggested that in the cat an accommodation-related cortical area controls the premotor circuit in the brainstem through the superior colliculus.

EDINGER–WESTPHAL NUCLEUS

It is generally assumed that the third nerve nucleus is divided into five parts composed of two main lateral nuclei – the unpaired central nucleus of Perlia, which unites the main nuclei, and the paired small-celled E–W nucleus and anteromedian nucleus situated anteriorly. However, there is still some controversy over whether the Perlia and E–W nuclei are separate entities. In monkeys, after iridectomy, Warwick observed degeneration of only 3% of the cells in the ciliary ganglion of macaque monkeys, whereas surgical removal of the short ciliary nerves produced chromatolysis in 97% of the cells in the ciliary ganglion. Warwick interpreted this as 97% of the ciliary ganglion cells relate to the ciliary muscle and 3% to the iris sphincter. It was originally thought that the ciliary ganglion received all parasympathetic fibers from the third nerve nucleus into the eye, those going to the ciliary muscle and to the sphincter muscle of the iris, synapsing in the ciliary ganglion. During the past few years evidence has been accumulating to suggest that there may be a difference between pupillary and ciliary parasympathetic innervation. Thus, studies by Westheimer and Blair conflicted with Warwick's concepts. These authors suggested that the innervation of the ciliary muscle reached the eye without synapsing at the ciliary ganglion. Loewenfeld argued strongly against this view, and Ruskell and Griffiths have recently presented anatomic evidence for a synapse of accommodative fibers. However, Jaeger and Benevento have re-opened the question by injecting horseradish peroxidase (HRP) into the ciliary muscle and iris of monkeys and finding HRP-labeled cells in the oculomotor nucleus. Loewy *et al.* also found HRP-labeled neurons in the E–W nucleus, a periaqueductal gray and ventral tegmental area, by direct application of HRP to the preganglionic part of the oculomotor nerve or to the ciliary ganglion. The authors felt that the connections of the E–W nucleus might be considerably more complex than had been previously thought. Kimura and Ishikawa applied HRP to the ciliary body of cats and monkeys 1 month after iridectomy. A direct non-synaptic pathway from midbrain structures was clearly shown. This was composed of Perlia and the rostral half of the E–W nucleus in the cat, and the AM nucleus, medial visceral columns of the E–W nucleus, and the Perlia nucleus in the monkey. These facts strongly indicate there are two innervational pathways to ciliary muscle: indirect with a synapse and direct without a synapse on accommodation.

CILIARY MUSCLE

Ciliary muscle has a parasympathetic innervation, in which the transmitter substance is acetylcholine and the receptor molecules are of the muscarinic type; sympathetic agents are said to have an effect on it. β_2 and α_1 adrenoreceptors were shown in the ciliary

muscles. Recently it has been assumed that an inhibitory sympathetic innervation is manifest when a visual task requires a substantial level of parasympathetic innervation.

ACCOMMODATIVE FUNCTIONS AND ACCOMMODOMETRY

AMPLITUDE OF ACCOMMODATION AND CLASSIC ACCOMMODOMETRY

The amplitude of accommodation is defined as the difference in refraction (D) and is the reciprocal of the distance (meters) between the far point and the near point of accommodation. The far point is the furthest position of the object that will produce a sharp image on the retina without accommodation. In the emmetropic eye, the far point is infinity (0 D), such that the amplitude of accommodation is equivalent to the dioptric expression of the near point of accommodation. In ametropic eyes the same situation can be introduced when the patients wear their best correction lenses for distance. Thus, accommodation is usually measured in terms of the near point, as the shortest distance from the eye where the object can be focused. The amplitude of accommodation (A) can be calculated by $A = 100/P - 100/r$ D, where P = near point (cm) and r = far point (cm).

Accommodation decreases its amplitude with age (*Fig. 10.2*). The variation between individuals in this aging is very large. In the clinical application of the accommodation test, the most important problem is uncertainty of the 'normal value'. To avoid this problem some care in checking interocular difference is required.

Accommodation is measured by showing the patient a test card or test letters at a distance and slowly moving the card

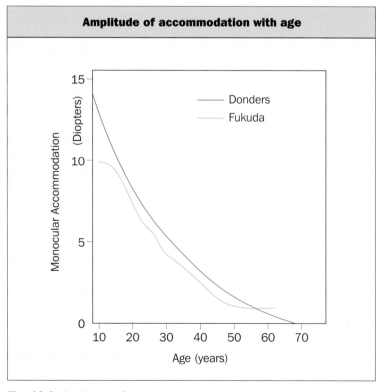

Fig. 10.2 Amplitude of accommodation with age.

towards the patient, who tries to keep the print as clear as possible. If the card passes inside the patient's near point, the print becomes blurred. This procedure is called the 'push-up method'. Near point rules by Costenbader, Gulden, or Ishihara are commercially available. In the push-up method each eye is measured separately and then both eyes together, so that a comparison can be made. The two monocular amplitudes should be equal, taking into account measurement error.

In general, accommodation measured by the above classic method includes not only the changes in focus due to the change in refractive power of the lens, but also the detection and recognition of blur.

STATIC FUNCTIONS, TONIC ACCOMMODATION, ACCOMMODATIVE ADAPTATION, AND THEIR MEASUREMENTS

The accommodative stimulus versus response (AS–AR) curve (*Fig. 10.3*) represents the static function. The theoretical line (AR = AS) indicates the value expected if accommodation corresponds to the target distance. However, the stimulus–response curve (1) exhibits an accommodative lag, which is produced by overaccommodation to far stimuli and underaccommodation to near stimuli. The slope of the AS–AR plot is less (2) when illumination, higher spatial components, or pupil size are reduced. This relationship reflects the mechanism of the control system of accommodation.

How does accommodation respond when illumination diminishes to total darkness, the target has no spatial structure (empty field), or the pupil reduces to the size of a pin hole? Under these situations the accommodative system shows no responses, as shown in the horizontal line (AR/AS = 0) in *Figure 10.3*. This accommodative state is called the 'intermediate accommodative resting point', 'functional rest', or 'tonic accommodation' (TA).

Tonic accommodation, defined as the accommodative state in the absence of an accommodative stimulus, is a theoretic concept. It can be measured as the accommodative state in total darkness (i.e. dark focus of accommodation) or under a bright uniform visual field (i.e. empty field accommodation). The accommodative state when looking through a small pin hole, or looking at a laser speckle pattern (in which the contrast is always high irrespective of defocus), is another example of tonic accommodation. However, it has recently been reported that the dark focus of accommodation and empty field accommodation are different under some circumstances.

Recent studies have shown that the resting point shifts towards the myopic direction after a near visual task. This phenomenon is called accommodative hysteresis (Ebenholtz), adaptation of tonic accommodation, or, simply, accommodative adaptation. Post-task accommodative adaptation has been investigated after short or long periods of near stimuli at various exposure distances. The rate of decay of accommodative adaptation appears to depend on the pre-task level of tonic accommodation and the visual circumstances operating after the near task. Recently, Wong *et al.* found that the accommodative adaptation in late onset myopia was significantly higher than in the emmetrope.

Static functions can be measured using a conventional refractometer (coincident optometer of Fincham) or a laser optometer. A conventional refractometer can be used in objective measurement and the accommodation of the eye contralateral to the stimulated eye is measured. An infra-red automated refractometer can be used for this purpose. In this case, the ipsilateral eye can be measured. Historically, the laser optometer had an important role in the static study of accommodative functions in the 1970s and early 1980s, as it was inexpensive and easy for the researcher to construct. However, this type of optometer is rarely used because it requires the examiner's judgment and takes a long time to complete the experiment compared with the more up-to-date objective optometer (see below).

Accommodative tonic rest can be measured by any method that does not stimulate the accommodative system. Dark focus of accommodation should be measured in total darkness. Recently an infra-red optometer (described below) that can measure accommodation without stimulating the visual system has been developed.

DYNAMIC FUNCTIONS AND THE HIGH-SPEED INFRA-RED OPTOMETER

The dynamic function of accommodation, accommodative response versus time, involves the accommodative responses to the step and sinusoidal stimuli. Measurements such as those listed in *Figure 10.4* have considerable clinical value. The response time (latency) is about 400 ms. The reaction times vary in combination with target distance, and other factors. Maximum velocity is up to 12 D/s but this value changes widely under differing stimulus conditions and the age of the patient.

The accommodative response to a stationary near target exhibits accommodative microfluctuations (average amplitude 0.1 D, with a frequency band width ranging from 0 to 5 Hz). There is still controversy over whether this fluctuation is merely the noise originated from the muscle and the lens or whether it is under central nervous control which takes a role producing

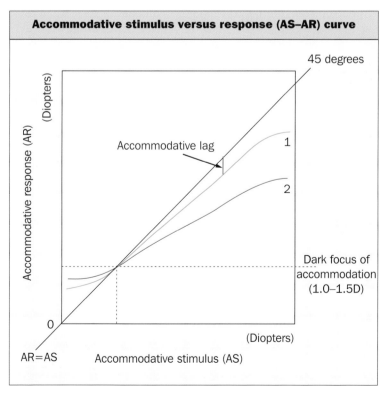

Fig. 10.3 Accommodative stimulus versus response (AS–AR) curve.

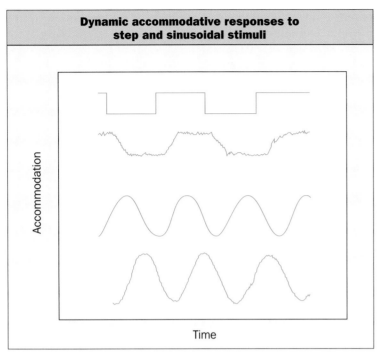

Dynamic accommodative responses to step and sinusoidal stimuli

Fig. 10.4 Dynamic accommodative responses to step stimuli (upper) and frequency responses to sinusoidal stimuli (lower).

accommodation to maintain a clear retinal image. The microfluctuations are characterized by two dominant components of activity, a low-frequency component (less than 0.5 Hz) and a high-frequency component (1.0–2.2 Hz). Recent work has shown that the control of steady-state accommodation may be mediated through the low-frequency component of accommodation microfluctuation.

Campbell first developed an instrument that can measure dynamic functions of accommodation. This instrument is based on Scheiner's principle, the separation of two retinal images that are made by incident infra-red light beams passing through different positions of the pupil plane. Although the machine had many restrictions, such as the requirement of a dental bite board to fix the patient and difficulties in calibrating the output value, it showed the difference between individuals and conditional changes in accommodative fluctuations. Later, Cornsweet *et al.* reported an improved instrument, a high-speed infra-red optometer, using the null method. The machine has a servo-controlled mechanism to minimize the separation of the two retinal images. Theoretically, this principle does not require calibration for each patient. In the 1980s many automated refractometers were developed and became commercially available. The principle of the automated refractometer is similar to the high-speed infra-red optometer. Commercially available refractometers have an easy set-up facility and modifications to enable stable measurement. Almost all studies of accommodation are currently carried out using a modified version of these automated refractometers. Modification is not so difficult because of the machines' common principles. Sometimes automated refractometers have a built-in target for fogging. It is useful for accommodation studies if the movement of the target can be controlled by a computer.

All the machines based on Scheiner's principle have two beams, separated by approximately 3 mm at the pupil plane. If the pupil diameter is less than this value, the recorded data are unreliable.

QUASISTATIC STUDY OF ACCOMMODATION

To obtain the AS–AR chart quickly, quasistatic recording has been reported by Ukai and Ishikawa, using a modified commercially available infra-red automated refractometer (Nidek Accommodometer AA-2000). While accommodative stimulus is slowly increased from –12.5 D to +12.5 D and slowly decreased from +12.5 D to –12.5 D with a constant velocity, accommodative response is continuously measured using an infra-red optometer and can be recorded on an x–y recorder (*Fig. 10.5a*). The target velocity was set at 0.2 D/s to avoid dynamic delay of the accommodative response. This recording includes measurements of the objective far point, the near point, the amplitude of accommoda-

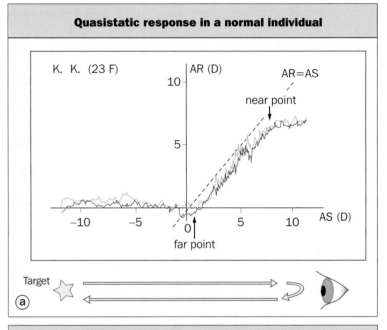

Quasistatic response in a normal individual

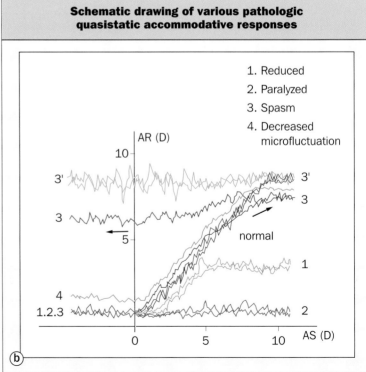

Schematic drawing of various pathologic quasistatic accommodative responses

1. Reduced
2. Paralyzed
3. Spasm
4. Decreased microfluctuation

Fig. 10.5 (**a**) Quasistatic response in a normal individual. (**b**) Schematic drawing of various pathologic quasistatic accommodative responses.

tion, the lag of accommodation, and the slope of AR–AS.

Various pathologic quasistatic accommodative responses are shown in *Figure 10.5b*.

The left side of the graph (see Fig. 10.5a) shows the position corresponding to the addition of a plus lens. If the lens is strong enough the patient cannot see any patterns. Thus, tonic accommodation before and after the near vision can be measured and accommodative adaptation can be calculated. If the illumination of the target is turned off, the dark focus of accommodation can be measured. This machine also has the ability to measure dynamic functions. The step responses and the fluctuation of accommodation can be measured.

The major advances of this machine are:
• Set-up is easy and no calibration is required.
• It takes only 4 min to measure one eye.
• There is no need for ametropic correction if ametropia is not strong but in this case one must pay attention that the recording shifts along the line of AR=AS.

ACCOMMODATION AND THE PUPIL

Alpern *et al.* reported that the relation between pupillary constriction (mm) associated with accommodation (D) is linear. Tsuchiya *et al.* confirmed that this relationship is applicable in some people but there is much variation between individuals. They also reported that the pupil constriction during near vision sometimes outlasts the release from near vision.

ACCOMMODATION AND VERGENCE

Physiologic parameters of accommodative convergence have also been measured. The latency times for target shifts from far to near and from near to far are almost equal in normal individuals (i.e. 160–200 ms). The results are virtually the same under binocular and monocular conditions. The eye movement of the fixating eye during asymmetric accommodative vergence has been analyzed. The amplitude of the induced saccadic eye movement is about 0.41°. This may be used for the fixation-holding reflex to keep the target at the fovea.

Binocular eye alignment has been measured in 2- to 6-month-old infants under both binocular and monocular viewing conditions. Corneal photography was used. A target was presented at a viewing distance of 15 cm. All infants had reliable convergence under both conditions. The presence of convergence, even during monocular viewing, indicated that an accommodative convergence link is present at an early age. The technique of 'photorefraction' has been used to investigate the refractive state of freely accommodating infants, presenting the targets at distances up to 150 cm. Most of the infants had the ability at 2–3 months to accommodate accurately on targets at 150 cm or closer. Newborn and 1-month-old infants could accommodate more accurately at 75 cm and closer than they could at 150 cm. Many infants who did not consistently accommodate 150-cm distant targets had a significant degree of astigmatism. The accommodative errors of the infants may have been due to a limited ability to process the retinal image and perhaps also to the limitation of visual attention on targets set further than 1 m away.

Vergence or phoria adaptation (i.e. control of binocular eye positions to maintain the heterophoria position regardless of any induced changes of vergence by prisms) is well known. The relationship between accommodation adaptation and vergence adaptation has been studied. Both adaptations are considered to be independent. Recently, a complex relation was reported: individuals whose AC to A ratio is lower than normal people exhibit a higher CA to C ratio, higher accommodation adaptation, and lower vergence adaptation than normal people.

CLINICAL ASPECTS OF ACCOMMODATION

SPASM OF ACCOMMODATION

Accommodative spasm is defined as an involuntary overactivity or spasm of ciliary muscle which may be continuous or intermittent, unilateral or bilateral, or asymmetric. Refraction examined by dry retinoscopy without cycloplegia may exhibit a myopic state. Symptoms are blurred vision, especially with a distant target, discomfort or pain in the brow region, and, occasionally, micropsia. Various parasympathomimetic drugs (pilocarpine, physostigmine, and other anticholinesterases) cause spasm of accommodation either directly or indirectly.

Spasm of the near reflex is a distinct clinical entity characterized by attacks of convergence with or without esotropia, accommodative spasm, and miosis. The spasm may respond to cycloplegics and be diminished by the use of a pair of glasses in which the medial third of each lens has been made opaque. Bilateral sixth nerve palsy should be differentiated. The clinical features of accommodation are described below.

ACCOMMODATIVE INERTIA

Poor accommodative flexibility is noticed by a conscious awareness of difficulty in focusing from far to near (positive accommodation) or near to far (negative accommodation). It is distinguished from accommodative insufficiency by clearing eventually being achieved. The diagnosis is made by timing the ability to clear a –1.00 D compared with a + 1.00 D sphere through the distance correction; such lenses can be conveniently mounted in a binocular 'flip' frame. Furthermore, quantitative analysis of this flexibility is carried out accurately and easily by a high-speed infra-red optometer.

Loss of accommodative flexibility is caused by early presbyopia, early cataract, Adie's syndrome, migraine, systemic medication with mild cycloplegic effects, diabetic eye, and other less common disorders.

ACCOMMODATIVE INSUFFICIENCY

Accommodative insufficiency means that the amplitude of accommodation is less than normal for the patient's age. Accommodative inertia is usually also present. Other findings may include a large lag of accommodation, low positive relative (with constant convergence) accommodation, high physiologic exophoria, and an associated convergence insufficiency.

The differential diagnosis and causes of the accommodative insufficiency should consider the following mechanisms:
• Refractive (uncorrected hyperopia, loss of miotic depth of focus, myopia corrected with contact lens).

- Premature presbyopia.
- Drugs (cycloplegics, phenothiazines, tricyclic antidepressants, iridosyncratic reactions).
- Trauma (crystalline lens, ciliary body, suspensory ligaments, ciliary nerves).
- Inflammation (ciliary ganglionitis, uveitis).
- Toxins (endogenous, oat cell carcinoma; exogenous, diphtheria, botulinum).
- Functional (poor acuity, binocular motility imbalances).

PARALYSIS OF ACCOMMODATION

Accommodative palsy can be associated with internal ophthalmoplegia or without pupil involvement. Patients notice blurred near vision, especially in the case of bilateral involvement. The most common cause of accommodative palsy is the cycloplegics effect; less common is internal ophthalmoplegia caused by midbrain lesions, encephalopathy, Wilson's disease, myasthenia gravis, trauma to the ciliary ganglion and nerves after muscle surgery (especially inferior oblique myectomy), panphotocoagulation, and Adie's syndrome. Diabetes, alcoholism, lead poisoning, herpes, diphtheria, and other conditions can also cause palsy.

There are several case reports of paralysis of accommodation. Paralysis and spasm of accommodation are well-known complications of hysteria. Usually, these conditions do not last more than a year. One young man with psychologic problems manifested bilateral accommodation palsy for about 2 years. Various etiologies have been proposed for paralysis of accommodation. Nine young patients showed failure of accommodation. Eight of them had a febrile illness preceding the onset of symptoms. Convex lenses were prescribed for eight patients and surgery diminished the symptoms in the remaining patient. The origin of this problem is unknown and although the authors consider the role of infection, fever, or antibiotic therapy, it is most probably a functional weakness of the near effort. A benign type of persistent paralysis of accommodation in four young people has been described. An almost complete, bilateral, symmetric accommodation paralysis with normal pupillary responses appeared in young and healthy individuals with no change during a follow-up study of at least 1 year. Topical application of pilocarpine or carbachol induced a significant refractive change. Absence of hypersensitivity to 2.5% methacholine chloride excluded peripheral denervation. A possible central lesion at the E–W nucleus was proposed. These conditions were treated by prescribing bifocal lenses.

Lesions of the cervical sympathetic outflow are said to produce a defect of accommodative control in which the patient is unable to relax accommodation fully from near to far. A unilateral increase in amplitude of accommodation with Horner's syndrome was described by Cogan. A case has been reported of a 12-year-old girl with Horner's syndrome and an accommodative paresis for near vision. Intravenous administration of edrophonium chloride diminished the accommodative defect on several occasions, suggesting a possible relationship to myasthenia gravis or a pupil-sparing Adie's syndrome.

DISTURBANCE OF THE DYNAMICS OF ACCOMMODATION

Disturbances of dynamic responses evoked by a step stimulus are evaluated by latency, velocity, and amplitude of contraction, that is positive accommodation (far to near), and of relaxation, that is negative accommodation (near to far). Various dynamic accommodation responses are shown in *Figure 10.6*. Adaptation to frequency analysis by phase lag or decreased responses evoked by sinusoidal stimulus would be further applications.

Disturbances of quasistatic responses evoked by a ramp stimulus are evaluated by velocity, amplitude of contraction (i.e. positive accommodation), and of relaxation (i.e. negative accommodation). Resting point (spasm or not) and microfluctuation are also evaluated (see Fig. 10.5b).

CLINICAL APPLICATION

CORTICAL LESION (PALSY AND SPASM)

Paresis (insufficiency) and palsy of accommodation and convergence with left middle cerebral artery occlusion have been reported by Ohtsuka *et al*. Accommodation was monitored by an

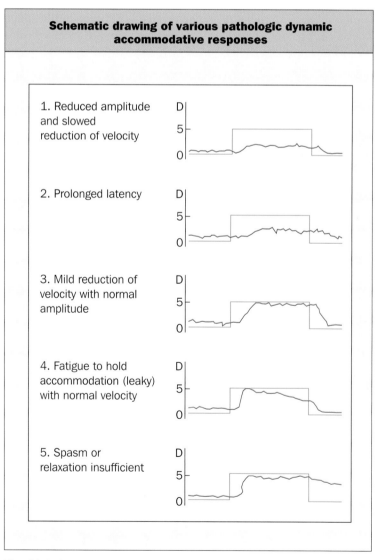

Fig. 10.6 Schematic drawing of various pathologic dynamic accommodative responses.

infra-red high-speed optometer and showed that the amplitude of accommodation was reduced and accommodation velocity to far-to-near and especially near-to-far was markedly lowered. The baseline of accommodation could not return to the previous resting position. A lesion of the superotemporal sulcus area was probably related to these abnormalities in the patient.

Spasm of near reflex is characterized by transient attacks of accommodative spasm manifesting pseudomyopia. Spasms of convergence, alone or in combination with miosis in both the attack phase and silent phase, are shown in *Figure 10.7*. These can usually be observed in young adults, especially girls, and are considered functional. These disorders may continue for several years, for example, after head trauma. Spasm of near reflex has been associated with organic diseases (e.g. cerebellar tumor, Arnold–Chiari malformation, pituitary tumors, and vestibulopathy).

It mimics sixth nerve paresis, pseudoabducens palsy, and myasthenia gravis but is frequently combined with miosis on attempted horizontal gaze, spasm of accommodation, or both. Dramatic temporary reversal of pupillary miosis when either eye is occluded is a sign of non-organic spasm of the near reflex. However, accommodative relaxation with monocular occlusion as a sign of spasm of the near reflex has not been described.

Cerebellar Lesions

Cerebellar control of accommodation of the eye in the cat has been proposed; however, little is known about its human situation. According to a study in patients with cerebellar diseases (i.e. olivopontocerebellar atrophy [OPCA], vermis tumor; and fourth ventricle tumor), a quasistatic and dynamic accommodative response was impaired in almost all patients examined. The dynamic response was paralyzed in most patients. These abnormalities were not detected by a conventional measurement of the near point of accommodation. A patient with a subtentorial

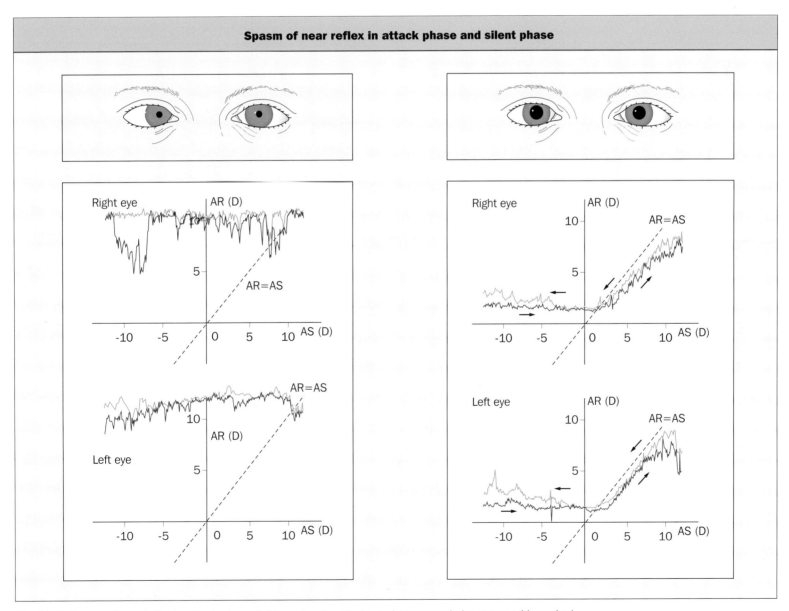

Fig. 10.7 Spasm of near reflex in attack phase (left): esotropia, miosis, and accommodative spasm with marked myopia; and silent phase (right): orthophoria, normal pupil, normal refraction, and normal quasistatic response.

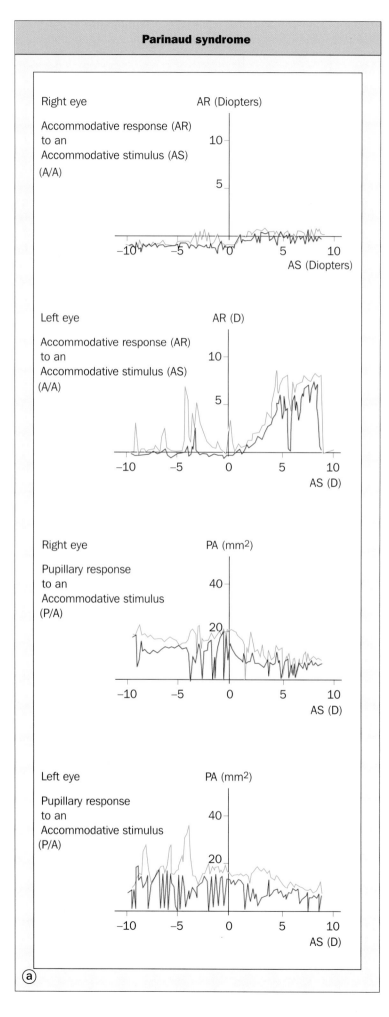

Parinaud syndrome

Right eye — AR (Diopters)

Accommodative response (AR) to an Accommodative stimulus (AS) (A/A)

Left eye — AR (D)

Accommodative response (AR) to an Accommodative stimulus (AS) (A/A)

Right eye — PA (mm²)

Pupillary response to an Accommodative stimulus (P/A)

Left eye — PA (mm²)

Pupillary response to an Accommodative stimulus (P/A)

arachnoid cyst showed normal accommodation responses for linear loads examined by the infra-red optometer. In contrast, dynamic responses to repetitive step stimulation were bilaterally impaired and there was a deficit of relaxation, possibly caused by accommodative spasm. The cerebellum seems to control accommodation more than it controls the pupil system.

BRAINSTEM LESION

Parinaud syndrome is characterized by vertical gaze palsy, convergence palsy, retractory as well as convergence nystagmus, and tectal pupil (dilated and light–near dissociation). This is caused by pineal tumors or rostral midbrain infarction (*Fig. 10.8a*). However, abnormality of accommodation in these lesions needs to be examined. Four patients were examined quantitatively. In accordance with progression of the lesion, static responses were diminished or abolished with preservation of accommodative pupillary response. Both dynamic responses and velocity were reduced. Long-term follow-up of these patients indicated that the responses were valuable indicators of progress. A schematic drawing of the possible innervation of the sympathetic and parasympathetic pathways is shown in *Figure 10.8b*.

Fisher syndrome is characterized by ophthalmoplegia, ataxia, and areflexia. The site of lesions has been considered to be either supranuclear, nuclear, or peripheral. Pupillary involvement has

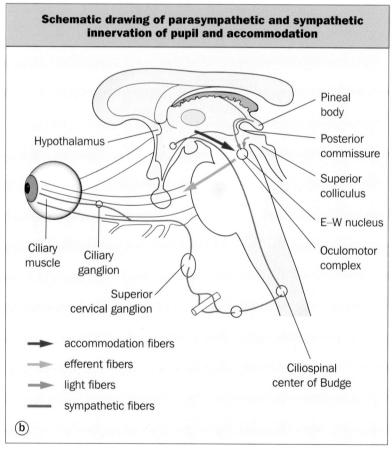

Schematic drawing of parasympathetic and sympathetic innervation of pupil and accommodation

- accommodation fibers
- efferent fibers
- light fibers
- sympathetic fibers

Fig. 10.8 (**a**) Parinaud syndrome: bilateral pupillary light–near dissociation (P/A) and accommodation (A/A) palsy of the right eye. Accommodation (upper) and accommodative pupil reaction (lower). (P/A, pupil response to an accommodative stimulus; PA, pupil area; A/A, accommodative response to accommodative stimulus [quasistatic response]). (**b**) Schematic drawing of parasympathetic and sympathetic innervation of pupil and accommodation.

Fisher's syndrome

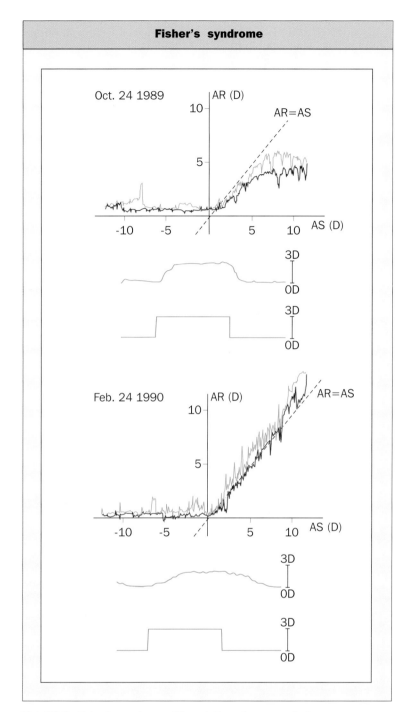

Fig. 10.9 Fisher's syndrome. Dissociation of recovery between quasistatic (upper) and dynamic responses (lower).

Tonic pupil

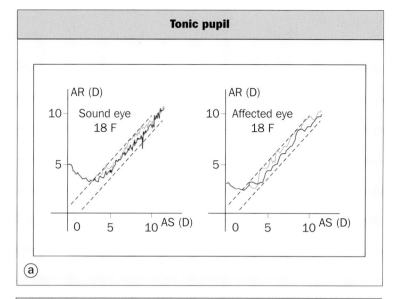

Slow in contraction and relaxation in the affected eye

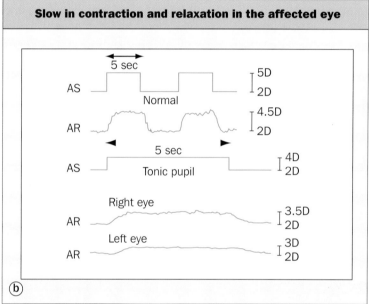

Fig. 10.10 (**a**) Tonic pupil. Quasistatic response shows decrease of microfluctuation of the affected eye (right). (**b**) Dynamic response shows decreased, prolonged, slow in contraction and relaxation in the affected eye (lower).

been observed in many patients; however, their accommodation was not well studied. Three typical patients showed apparent dissociation of pupil and accommodative functions. Static (left) and dynamic responses (right) were not impaired in parallel. Dissociation of static and dynamic involvement was noted in a patient with a lesion in the rostral midbrain (*Fig. 10.9*). Accordingly, the accommodative control system may be composed of fast and slow components.

OCULOMOTOR LESION

Aberrant regeneration of the third nerve palsy produced the pseudo-Argyll Robertson pupil. Light–near dissociation and

marked accommodative reduction by static recording were shown in a patient with traumatic third nerve palsy.

TONIC PUPIL

Tonic pupil is characterized by light–near dissociation of the pupil. On the other hand, accommodative paresis was noted in two-thirds of patients (Thompson). There was reduction of amplitude of accommodation, diminution of microfluctuation, and reduced velocity during positive and negative accommodation. Myopic deviation of the resting point of accommodation by 2.5% mecholyl or dilute pilocarpine has been reported (*Fig. 10.10*).

DIPHTHERIA

In the days when diphtheria was common, an isolated paralysis of accommodation was often mentioned. It was generally thought to be an expression of a post-diphtheritic neuropathy.

MYASTHENIA GRAVIS

The extraocular muscles were impaired in about 90% of patients with myasthenia; however, intraocular muscle involvement was rare. In addition to pupillary involvement, reduction of amplitude of accommodation was reported in 30% of 33 patients examined by Ishihara's accommodometer and also the AC to A ratio examined by the gradient method (Sloan's method) was markedly reduced in most of the patients (average value 1.8 ± 2.1 Δ/D in myasthenic patients, compared with 3.7 ± 2.1 Δ/D in normal control individuals) (*Fig. 10.11a*). 'Pseudomyopia' was reported by Romano *et al.* in 1973. By quantitative recording of static and dynamic responses, the patients showed a disturbance of relaxation under repetitive loading of accommodative effort causing transient myopia (*Fig. 10.11b*). Dynamic responses were reduced in both positive and negative accommodations. Edrophonium chloride (Tensilon) improved the reduced response.

BOTULISM

Botulinum exotoxin interferes with acetylcholine synthesis resulting in acetycholine depletion throughout the nervous system. This produces dilated nonreactive pupils and accommodative paralysis, and also associated with blurred vision, diplopia, ptosis, headache, and swallowing and respiratory disturbances.

HYPOTHYROID AND THYROID DYSFUNCTION

The pupils of patients with dysthyroid ophthalmopathy were analyzed by the edge-light pupillary oscillation method. Basic research on skeletal muscles and eye muscles showed fiber alteration from fast to slow in human and animal experiments. Furthermore, receptor distribution of the rat pupillary muscle changed under different thyroid functions. Accommodation functions remain to be analyzed in the future.

ANTICHOLINESTERASE DRUGS

The AR to AS ratio becomes larger than unity after the topical use of an anticholinesterase drug, such as the organophosphate of diisopropyonyl phosphate, phospholine iodide, or the carbamates of neostigmine and distigmine bromide. This is because of the potentiating action of impulses at the myoneural junction. These studies were performed in esotropic patients and in animal eyes. However, actual cases of environmental exposure to anticholinesterase drugs are more severe. As the examination of accommodation of these patients was made quantitatively, it is worthwhile to describe it here. Two male patients had extensive exposure to the organophosphate pesticides parathion and malathion. The patients were emmetropic before exposure. However, after extensive exposure to these anticholinesterase pesticides over 3–5 years, severe myopia of about 10–15 D developed.

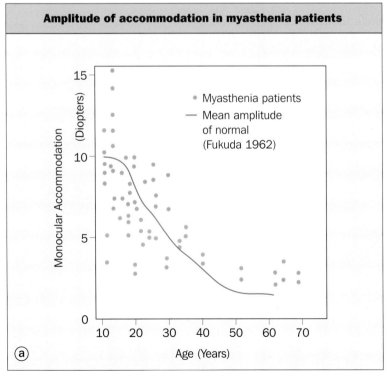

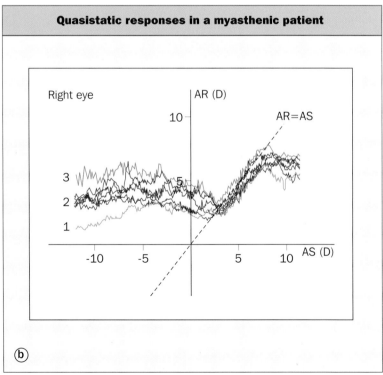

Fig. 10.11 (**a**) Amplitude of accommodation in myasthenia patients. (By permission of Sato Y, *Acta Soc Ophthalmol Jpn.* 1969;**73**:666–676.)
(**b**) Quasistatic responses in a myasthenic patient show disturbance of relaxation (spasm) after three repetative trials.

Topical use of 1% atropine methylsulfate reduced this myopia by only 1.5–2.0 D. Both men may have had ciliary spasm of central origin and the amplitude of their accommodation was reduced. At this time, the AR to AS ratio was greater than unity, which represented potentiation of the accommodative response. After a prolonged period of treatment with atropine methylsulfate, prifinium bromide, and pralidoxime methiodide, the pathologically induced myopia returned to almost 0 D, despite a residual elevation of acetylcholinesterase activity in the blood. This persistent myopia was reported as 'Saku disease' and has been called 'optico-autonomic peripheral neuropathy'. These visual problems are the most serious neuro-ophthalmic problem associated with chronic organophosphate pesticides.

AMBLYOPIA

The static response (quasistatic) of accommodation was studied in 28 monocular amblyopic patients, and the results were compared with the findings from their normal eyes. A reduced amplitude of accommodation and reduced accuracy of accommodation were seen in amblyopic eyes. In about one half of the amblyopic eyes, the magnitude of fluctuations of accommodation increased. This increase may be associated with a loss of sensitivity to change in retinal contrast. When the amblyopic eye was stimulated, the time constants of the response were normal but latencies were increased, amplitudes were smaller, and variability of responses was greater. When the dominant eye was stimulated, static and dynamic response properties of accommodation were within normal limits. These results suggest that the motor control of accommodation is normal because the responses were not affected during dominant eye stimulation. The processing delay resides in early sensory or more central areas of the pathways in amblyopia.

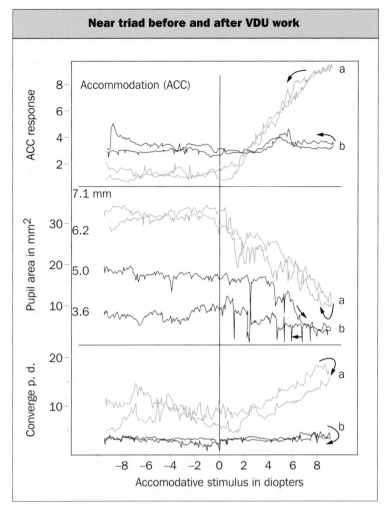

Fig. 10.12 Near triad before (**a**) and after (**b**) VDU work. (By permission of Ishikawa S, *Ergonomics*. 1990;**33**:787–798.)

WHIPLASH AND TRAUMA

Symptoms suggestive of accommodative and convergence insufficiency appear after cerebral concussion and the cervicocranial hyperextension injury known as whiplash syndrome. These symptoms may be from 1 week to years in duration and are completely relieved and disappear after litigation is settled. It may be very difficult to separate the patient with true organic post-traumatic accommodative–convergence insufficiency from the patient with functional overlay and from the dissembler unless objective signs are present or a positive response to therapy excludes the latter possibility.

VDU WORK

Recent studies have shown that the resting point shifts towards the myopic direction after visual display unit (VDU) work (*Fig. 10.12*). A part of this phenomenon corresponds to accommodative hysteresis or adaptation of tonic accommodation.

HORNER'S SYNDROME

Compared with parasympathetic innervation, sympathetic innervation to ciliary muscle is very small. The mode of action is an

inhibition of accommodation that is relatively small as well as slow and is mediated through β-adrenoreceptors. In functional terms, the role of this inhibitory sympathetic input may be to minimize the risk of accommodative hysteresis in manifest myopia after prolonged and demanding near tasks.

Measurement of dark focus is the best parameter to evaluate the effect of sympathetic innervation on ciliary muscle. Horner's syndrome shows spasm of accommodation in certain cases.

DIABETES MELLITUS

Patients with diabetes sometimes complain of early presbyopia. Precise evaluation of the amplitude of accommodation (*Fig. 10.13a*) showed a reduction of amplitude of accommodation in the 20th year in early onset diabetes mellitus patients. This is comparable to the miosis seen in young people with diabetes, especially with high blood-sugar levels. The dynamic responses of far-to-near accommodation and near-to-far accommodation were examined (*Fig. 10.13b*). The latter were markedly disturbed and slowed, especially in patients with high blood-sugar levels compared with those with lower blood-sugar levels. These abnormalities caused inertia, especially in negative accommodation.

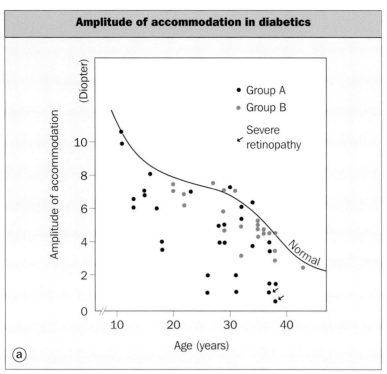

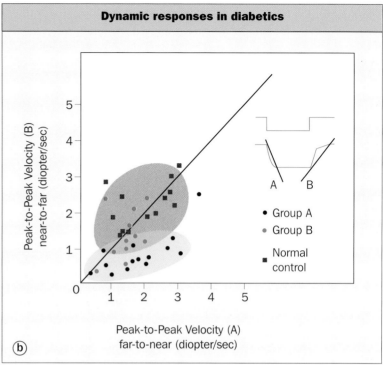

Fig. 10.13 (**a**) Amplitude of accommodation in diabetes measured by accommodogram. Group A: high blood glucose level; Group B: well-controlled blood glucose level. Decreased amplitude in Group A. (**b**) Dynamic responses in diabetes. Reduced velocity of near to far response in Group A.

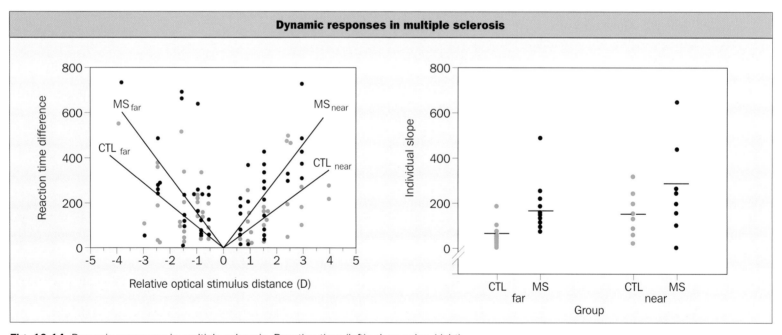

Fig. 10.14 Dynamic responses in multiple sclerosis. Reaction time (left); slope value (right). (By permission of Ogden NA *et al.*, *Invest Ophthalmol Vis Sci*. 1992;**33**:2744–2753.)

AFFERENT ACCOMMODATIVE DEFECT

Multiple sclerosis (MS) patients showed a significantly greater increase in reaction time for stimuli viewed at relative near and far optical distances, especially extreme near or far optical distances. However, MS patients did not differ significantly from healthy control individuals in near point, far point, accommodative range, and tonic accommodation (*Fig. 10.14*). These patients, as a group, showed a significant reduction in the ability to sustain resolution for stimuli viewed at distances closer to or further from the individual tonic accommodative position. Dynamic factors may make an important contribution to the spatial visual losses (episodes of blurred vision) that have been reported previously in MS patients, and the appropriate application of refractive correction may minimize this particularly disruptive visual aspect of MS and diabetes mellitus previously described.

TREATMENT OF
ACCOMMODATION ABNORMALITY

Weak cholinergic eye drops such as anticholinesterase are sometimes helpful. Control of the patient's general health, especially alcoholism and diabetes, is important; and management of refractive error, offending drugs and toxins, and ocular inflammations will often remove the underlying cause.

Functional causes may require orthoptics, such as focusing on a swinging ball (accommodative rock), as described by Griffin (1976).

Biofeedback can be supplied by converting accommodation into a continuous audible tone. With just a few hours of practice, normal patients have learned to control their own accommodation. This may prove to be applicable to patients with accommodative paresis or spasm.

Further reading

Jampel RS. Convergence, divergence, pupillary reactions and accommodation of the eyes from faradic stimulation of macaque brain. *J Comp Neurol.* 1960;**115**:371–400.

Bando T, Toda H, Awaji T. Lens accommodation-related and pupil-related units in the lateral suprasylvian area in cats. *Prog Brain Res.* 1988;**76**:231–236.

Mays LE. Neural control of vergence eye movement: convergence and divergence neurons in midbrain. *J Neurophysiol.* 1984;**51**: 1091–1108.

Judge SJ, Cummings BG. Neurons in the monkey midbrain with activity related to vergence eye movement and accommodation. *J Neurophysiol.* 1986;**55**:915–930.

Zhang Y, Mays LE, Gamlin PDR. Characteristics of near response cell projecting to the oculomotor nucleus. *J Neurophysiol.* 1992;**67**:944–960.

Hiraoka M, Shimamura M. The midbrain reticular formation as an integration center for the near reflex in the cat. *Neurosci Rec.* 1989;**7**:1–12.

Hosoba M, Bando T, *et al.* The cerebellar control of accommodation of the eye in the cat. *Brain Res.* 1978;**153**:495–505.

Bando T, Ishihara A, Tsukahara N. Interpositus neurons controlling lens accommodation. *Proc Jpn Acad.* 1979;**55** ser B153–156.

Maekawa H, Ohtsuka K. Afferent and efferent connections of cortical accommodation area in the cat. *Neurosci Res.* 1993;**17**:315–323.

Ishikawa S, Sekiya H, Kondo Y. The center for controlling near reflex in the midbrain of the monkey. A double labeling study. *Brain Res.* 1990;**519**:217–222.

Warwick RB: The ocular parasympathetic nerve supply and its mesencephalic sources. *J Anat (London).* 1954;**88**:71–93.

Westheimer G, Blair SM. The parasympathetic pathway to internal eye muscles. *Invest Ophthalmol.* 1973;**12**:193–197.

Jaeger RJ, Benevento LA. A horseradish peroxidase study of the innervation of internal structures of the eye. *Invest Ophthalmol Vis.* 1980;**19**:575–583.

Kimura S. The parasympathetic direct pathway from the midbrain to the ciliary muscle in cats and monkeys. *Acta Soc Ophthalmol Jpn.* 1991;**95**:1031–1036.

Gilmartin B, Bullimore MA. Sustained near-vision augments inhibitory sympathetic innervation of ciliary muscle. *Clin Vision Sci.* 1987;**1**:197–208.

London R. Amplitude of accommodation. In: Eskridge *et al.*, eds, *Clinical Procedures in Optometry* (Philadelphia: JB Lippincott, 1991) 69–71.

Schor CM, Kotulak JC, Tsuetaki T. Adaptation of tonic accommodation reduces accommodative lag and is masked in darkness. *Invest Ophthalmol Vis Sci.* 1986;**27**:820–827.

Woung L-C, Ukai K, Tsuchiya K, Ishikawa S. Accommodative adaptation and age of onset of myopia. *Ophthal Physiol Opt.* 1993;**13**:366–370.

Leibowitz HW, Owens DA. Night myopia and the intermediate dark focus of accommodation. *J Opt Soc Am.* 1975;**65**:1121–1128.

Alpern M, Manson GL, Jardinico RE. Vergence and Accommodation, 5. Pupil size changes associated with changes in accommodative vergence. *Am J Ophthalmol.* 1961;**52**:662–767.

Tsuchiya K, Ukai K, Ishikawa S. A quasistatic study of pupil and accommodation after effects following near vision. *Ophthal Physiol Opt.* 1989;**9**:385–391.

Yoshida T. Control system of accommodation and convergence—a review. *Neuro-Ophthalmol Jpn.* 1988;**5**:150–155 (in Japanese; cited in reference 48).

Campbell FW, Robson JG, Westheimer G. Fluctuations of accommodation under steady viewing conditions. *J Physiol.* 1959;**145**: 579–594.

Charman WN, Heron G. Fluctuations in accommodation: a review. *Ophthal Physiol Opt.* 1988;**8**:153–164.

Gray LS, Winn B, Gilmartin B. Accommodative microfluctuations and pupil diameter. *Vision Res.* 1993;**33**:2083–2090.

Cornsweet TN, Crane HD. Servo-controlled infrared optometer. *J Opt Soc Am.* 1970;**60**:548–554.

Ukai K, Tanemoto Y, Ishikawa S. Direct recording of accommodative response versus accommodative stimulus. In: Breinin GM, Siegel IM, eds, *Advances in Diagnostic Visual Optics* (Berlin: Springer-Verlag, 1983) 61–68.

Sethi B. Vergence adaptation: a review. *Doc Ophth.* 1986;**63**:247–263.

Owens D, Leibowitz H. Accommodation, convergence, and distance perception in low illumination. *Am J Optom Physiol Opt.* 1980;**57**:540–550.

Schor C. Imbalanced adaptation of accommodation and vergence produces opposite extremes of the AC/A and CA/C ratios. *Am J Optom Physiol Opt.* 1988;**65**:341–348.

Michaels DD. Accommodation, vergences, and heterophorias. In: *Visual Optics and Refraction. A Clinical Approach* (St Louis: Mosby, 1985) 369–373.

Ohtsuka K, Maekawa H, *et al.* Accommodation and convergence insufficiency with left cerebral artery occlusion. *Am J Ophthalmol.* 1988;**106**:60–64.

Cogan DG, Freese CG. Spasm of the near reflex. *Arch Ophthalmol.* 1955;**54**:752–759.

Dagi LR, Chrousos GK, *et al.* Spasm of the near reflex associated with organic disease. *Am J Ophthalmol.* 1987;**103**:582–585.

Namba T, Kimura S, *et al.* Cerebellar control of human accommodative function. In: Yoshikawa M, Uono M, Tanabe H, Ishikawa S, eds, *New Trends in Autonomic Nervous System Research Ams Excerpta Medica* (Int Congr Ser)1991;**951**:151.

Kawasaki T, Kiyosawa M, Fujino T, Tokoro T. Slow accommodation release with a cerebellar lesion. *Br J Ophthalmol.* 1993;**77**:678.

Mukuno K, Ukai K, *et al.* Clinics of accommodation and convergence. *Neuro-ophthalmol Jpn.* 1988;**5**:138–149 (in Japanese).

Hara N, Ishikawa S, *et al.* Accommodation in Fisher's syndrome – Dissociation of quick and slow responses. Presented at the VIIIth International Neuro-ophthalmology Symposium, Winchester, June, 1990.

Mukuno K, Ishikawa S. Pupil and autonomic nervous system. *J Women Med Co.* 1993;**63**:88–99 (in Japanese).

Yamazaki A, Ishikawa S. Abnormal pupillary responses in myasthenia gravis. A pupillographic study. *Br J Ophthalmol.* 1976;**60**:575–580.

Sato Y. Myasthenia gravis with special reference to the function of intraocular muscles. *Acta Soc Ophthalmol Jpn.* 1969;**73**:666–676.

Higashi JT, Ishikawa S, Mukuno K, *et al.* Pupillary analyses in Graves' disease. *Jpn J Ophthalmol.* 1982;**26**:213–323.

Ishikawa S, Miyata M. Development of myopia following chronic organophosphate pesticide intoxication. An epidemiological and experimental study. In: Merrigan WH, Weiss B, eds, *Neurotoxicity of the Visual System* (New York: Raven Press, 1980) 233–254.

Ishikawa S. Chronic optico-neuropathy due to environmental exposure of organophosphate pesticides (Saku Disease). Clinical and experimental study. *Acta Soc Ophthal Jap.* 1973;**10**:1835–1886.

Dementi B. Ocular effects of organophosphates: a historical perspective of Saku disease. *J Appl Toxicol.* 1994;**14**:135–143.

Hamernik KL. Proposed protocols for the determination of potential ocular effects of organophosphorous pesticides. *J Appl Toxicol.* 1994;**14**:131–134.

Ukai K, Ishii M, Ishikawa S. A quasistatic study of accommodation in amblyopia. *Ophthal Physiol. Opt* 1986;**6**:287–295.

Ciuffreda KJ, Kenyon RV. Accommodative vergence and accommodation in normals, amblyopes and strabismics. In: Shor C, Ciuffreda KJ, eds, *Vergence Eye Movements: Basic and Clinical Aspects* (Boston: Butterworths, 1983) 101–173.

Ishikawa S. Examination of the near triad in VDU operators. *Ergonomics.* 1990;**33**:787–98.

Gilmartin B. A review of the role of sympathetic innervation of the ciliary muscle in ocular accommodation. *Ophthal Physiol Opt.* 1986;**6**:23–7.

Namba T, *et al.* Accommodation abnormalities in young diabetics. *Rinsho Ganka (Clinical Ophthalmology)* 1985;**39**:654–655.

Ogden NA, Raymond JE, Seland TP. Visual accommodation and sustained visual resolution in multiple sclerosis. *Invest Ophthalmol. Vis Sci* 1992;**33**:2744–2753.

Cornsweet TN, Crane HD. Training the visual accommodation system. *Vision Res.* 1973;**13**:713–715.

CHAPTER 11

Neuro-ophthalmic Signs: Eyelid Malpositions

Brian Leatherbarrow

The malpositions of the eyelids associated with neuro-ophthalmic disorders are ptosis, eyelid retraction, and lower eyelid ectropion.

PTOSIS

Ptosis of the upper eyelid can affect all age groups and may be congenital or acquired. The causes of ptosis are numerous. It is important to recognize that ptosis itself is merely a physical sign and before therapeutic decisions are made it is essential to make every effort to determine the underlying cause. In considering the causes it is useful to use a classification of ptosis that is based on etiologic factors (*Fig. 11.1*); this classification of ptosis aims to provide some insight into the pathologic processes involved.

Pseudoptosis refers to a condition that mimics a true ptosis. True ptosis may result from neurologic disorders (*Fig. 11.2*) or from specific defects in the innervation of the levator palpebrae superioris muscle, from disorders affecting the levator muscle itself, from defects in the levator aponeurosis or in the attachment of the aponeurosis to the tarsal plate, or from mechanical factors that restrict normal movement of the eyelid. These etiologic mechanisms may be found in all age groups but with varying frequency. Congenital dystrophic ptosis and involutional aponeurotic ptosis are by far the most common types of ptosis to be encountered.

It is particularly important that a pseudoptosis is clearly recognized and that a neurologic cause of ptosis requiring further evaluation or an alternative therapeutic approach is excluded before ptosis surgery is embarked on.

BLEPHAROSPASM

Blepharospasm may be voluntary or involuntary. Essential blepharospasm is characterized by an idiopathic bilateral involuntary contraction of the orbicularis oculi muscles (*Fig. 11.3*). Frequently, the corrugator superciliaris muscles are affected, causing a furrowing of the eyebrows. In addition, dystonic movements of the lower facial musculature may be seen. In the early stages of the disorder, patients are frequently misdiagnosed and may even be dismissed as having a functional problem. Blepharospasm may also be seen in neurologic conditions, such as Parkinson's disease. The majority of patients respond very well to local injections of botulinum toxin. Surgery, in the form of orbicularis oculi excision and selective facial nerve avulsion, for this condition is very rarely required.

Classification of ptosis
Pseudoptosis
Neurogenic
Myogenic
Aponeurotic
Mechanical

Fig. 11.1 Classification of ptosis.

Pseudoptosis in neurologic disease
Blepharospasm
Hemifacial spasm
Aberrant reinnervation of the facial nerve
Spastic paretic facial contracture
Apraxia of eyelid opening
Duane's retraction syndrome

Fig. 11.2 Pseudoptosis in neurologic disease.

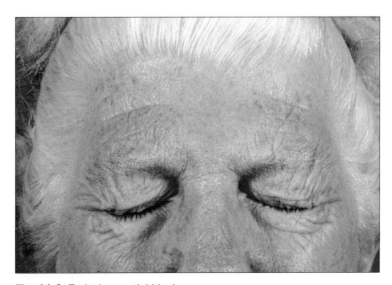

Fig. 11.3 Typical essential blepharospasm.

HEMIFACIAL SPASM

This condition is characterized by unilateral involuntary intermittent irregular contractions of the muscles of facial expression (*Fig. 11.4*). The orbicularis muscle is usually the first facial muscle to be involved. In some cases the cause is compression of the facial nerve in the posterior fossa by an aberrant artery. In these cases neurosurgical decompression of the nerve may be successful. Local injections of botulinum toxin can be very successful in controlling the associated blepharospasm.

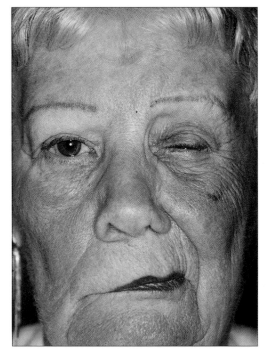

Fig. 11.4 Typical left-sided hemifacial spasm.

ABERRANT REINNERVATION OF THE FACIAL NERVE

Aberrant reinnervation may occur after a peripheral lower motor neuron facial nerve palsy. This condition is characterized by involuntary eyelid closure stimulated by the use of other facial muscles (e.g. on smiling or whistling) (*Fig. 11.5*). The involuntary eyelid closure may be controlled by local injections of botulinum toxin (*Fig. 11.6*).

SPASTIC PARETIC FACIAL CONTRACTURE

This condition may mimic hemifacial spasm but is characterized by ipsilateral facial weakness. It may be associated with disorders located within the pons (e.g. demyelination or glioma).

APRAXIA OF EYELID OPENING

This is a rare condition in which there is impairment of eyelid opening in the absence of active blepharospasm and without paralysis of the eyelid retractors. Blepharospasm may, however, co-exist. The condition has been described in Huntingdon's disease, Parkinson's disease, and bilateral cerebral hemisphere disease.

DUANE'S RETRACTION SYNDROME

Narrowing of the palpebral fissure may be associated with ocular movements. Patients may present with a complaint of ptosis but a careful examination of the ocular motility will reveal the true diagnosis.

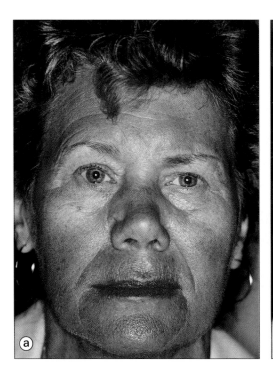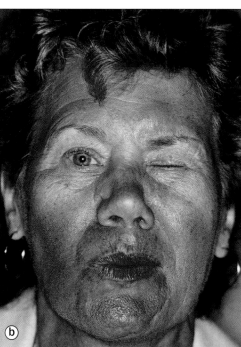

Fig. 11.5 Aberrant reinnervation of the facial nerve after a peripheral lower motor neuron facial nerve palsy. (**a**) Patient at rest showing mild left brow ptosis and slightly narrowed left palpebral fissure. (**b**) Patient pursing lips with simultaneous contraction of the orbicularis oculi and closure of the left eye.

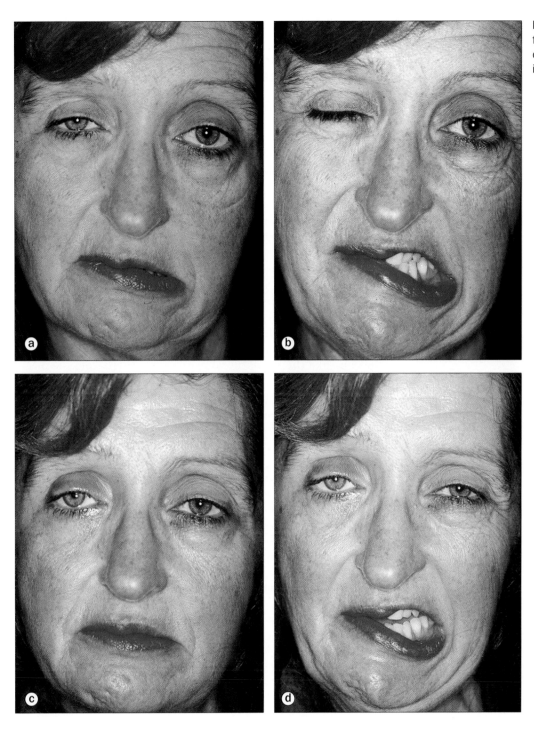

Fig. 11.6 (**a,b**) Aberrant reinnervation of the facial nerve demonstrating closure of the right eye on smiling. (**c,d**) The same patient after periorbital injections of botulinum toxin.

PTOSIS IN NEUROLOGIC DISEASE

The neurologic diseases that can cause ptosis are listed in *Figure 11.7*.

OCULOMOTOR NERVE PALSY

Oculomotor nerve palsy is characterized by a variable degree of ptosis associated with deficits of adduction, elevation, and depression of the eye caused by weakness of the levator muscle, the superior, inferior, and medial rectus muscles, and the inferior oblique muscle (*Fig. 11.8*). The pupillary fibers of the oculomotor nerve may be affected or spared depending on the underlying cause. Lesions confined to the superior division of the oculomotor nerve result in only a ptosis and weakness of the superior rectus muscle. Myasthenia may mimic an oculomotor nerve palsy when the pupil is spared. The Bell's phenomenon is typically absent or poor.

Cyclic oculomotor nerve palsy is a rare phenomenon characterized by alternating paresis and spasm of the extraocular and intraocular muscles. These cyclic phenomena are usually noted in early childhood and may be evident at birth.

An oculomotor nerve palsy may be caused by neoplastic, inflammatory, vascular, or traumatic lesions, any of which may affect the nerve in its course from the midbrain to the orbit. Associated symptoms and signs help to localize the underlying lesion.

Ptosis in neurologic disease

Oculomotor nerve palsy
Horner's syndrome
Myasthenia gravis
Synkinetic ptosis
• Marcus Gunn jaw wink
  phenomenon
• Aberrant reinnervation of the
  oculomotor nerve
Myotonic dystrophy
Chronic progressive external
  ophthalmoplegia
Cerebral ptosis
Botulism

Fig. 11.7 Ptosis in neurologic disease.

Treatment of the ptosis is problematic because of the impaired Bell's phenomenon, with a risk of exposure keratopathy. A frontalis suspension procedure may be undertaken after strabismus surgery has been performed to realign the globe in the primary position. A frontalis suspension procedure may be undertaken before strabismus surgery in infants to treat amblyopia.

HORNER'S SYNDROME (OCULOSYMPATHETIC PARESIS)

Horner's syndrome is characterized by a ptosis of 1–2 mm, with good levator function and a raised skin crease, miosis, an apparent enophthalmos, and is occasionally associated with facial anhydrosis (*Fig. 11.9*). The features of Horner's syndrome are due to interference with the sympathetic nerve supply to Muller's muscle in the upper eyelid and to its smooth muscle counterpart in the lower eyelid, and to the dilator pupillae muscle. The resultant anisocoria is accentuated in dim illumination. The apparent enophthalmos is due to the decrease in size of the palpebral aperture.

Horner's syndrome may be caused by a lesion that interrupts the course of the sympathetic neurons anywhere from the origin in the hypothalamus to the orbit. There are three neurons carrying the sympathetic innervation to the orbit. The first (central) neuron commences in the hypothalamus and synapses with the second neuron in the intermediolateral cell column of the lower cervical and upper thoracic spinal cord. The second (preganglionic) neuron travels from the thorax across the neck of the first rib and ascends behind the cartoid sheath, synapsing with the third neuron in the superior cervical ganglion, which lies in front of the lateral mass of the atlas and axis. The third (postganglionic) neuron travels along the internal carotid artery to innervate the smooth muscle of the upper and lower eyelids, the dilator pupillae muscle, and the sweat glands, hair follicles, and blood vessels of the head and neck (*Fig. 11.10*).

The diagnosis of Horner's syndrome is made clinically but may be confirmed by the instillation of 5% cocaine solution into both eyes. Cocaine blocks the re-uptake of catecholamines by the nerve endings. The Horner's pupil, in contrast to the normal pupil, will fail to dilate as there is less free noradrenaline present at the synapse. The use of hydroxyamphetamine solution can assist in

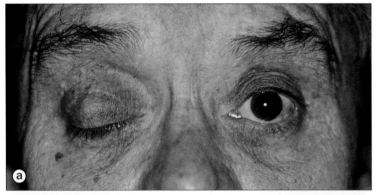

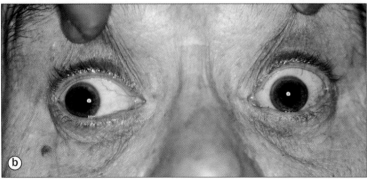

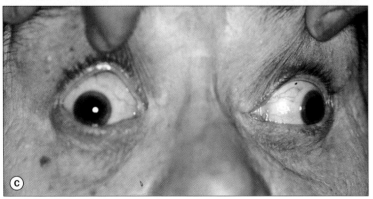

Fig. 11.8 Complete right oculomotor nerve palsy. (**a**) Patient at rest showing complete right ptosis. (**b**) Patient at rest with right upper lid elevated manually showing right globe in a typical position of slight abduction and depression due to the unopposed actions of the lateral rectus and superior oblique muscles. (**c**) Patient attempting levoversion.

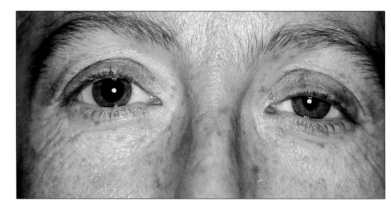

Fig. 11.9 Typical left Horner's syndrome. Note that the ptosis of the left upper lid is moderate, and that the left lower lid is slightly elevated. Both of these effects are due to palsy of the sympathetically innervated retractor fibers of the lids.

the differentiation of a preganglionic lesion from a postganglionic lesion. Hydroxyamphetamine displaces catecholamines from the nerve terminal. It will therefore dilate the pupil only if the third neuron is intact. In a postganglionic lesion, therefore, the pupil will fail to dilate. The differentiation between a first- and second-order neuron lesion is based on the neurologic signs associated with a first-order neuron lesion. The instillation of a weak solution of phenylephrine (1%) may show denervation hypersensitivity, resulting in the temporary resolution of the ptosis and restoration of a normal skin crease (*Fig. 11.11*).

It is important to differentiate a preganglionic from a postganglionic Horner's syndrome because lesions that result in a postganglionic Horner's syndrome are usually benign, in contrast to those resulting in a preganglionic Horner's syndrome (*Fig. 11.12*).

The ptosis may be treated surgically either by means of a Fasanella–Servat procedure or by means of a levator aponeurosis advancement procedure.

MYASTHENIA GRAVIS

Myasthenia gravis is an autoimmune disorder caused by antibodies to the acetylcholine receptors of the motor end plate of voluntary muscle. The antibodies block access of the neurotransmitter acetylcholine to the receptors. The hallmarks of the disorder are variable muscular weakness and fatigue on exercise. Myasthenia may be generalized and threaten the muscles of respiration or it may be localized to the eyes (ocular myasthenia). Approximately 30% of patients with myasthenia gravis complain first of ocular problems (ptosis and diplopia), whereas 80–90% of myasthenia patients have ocular signs at the time of diagnosis. If the symptoms and signs remain confined to the eyes for 3 years, progress to generalized myasthenia is unlikely. Ptosis is the most common clinical manifestation of myasthenia. It may be unilateral or bilateral. Exercise of the levator or sustained up-gaze may provoke or worsen a ptosis. Attempted rapid saccades from down-gaze to the primary position may provoke an overshoot of the upper eyelid above the superior limbus, with a gradual fall of the lid to its original position (Cogan's twitch sign). There may be an associated weakness of the orbicularis oculi muscle and the Bell's phenomenon may be poor.

The diagnosis of myasthenia should be contemplated in any patient with an acquired ptosis and normal pupils. The diagnosis may be confirmed by means of a Tensilon test (edrophonium

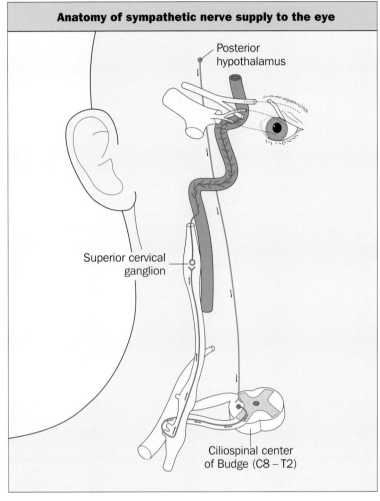

Fig. 11.10 Anatomy of the sympathetic innervation of the eye and eyelids.

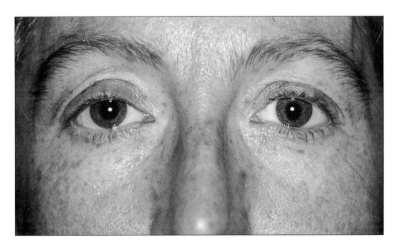

Fig. 11.11 Horner's syndrome after instillation of 1% phenylephrine in the left eye.

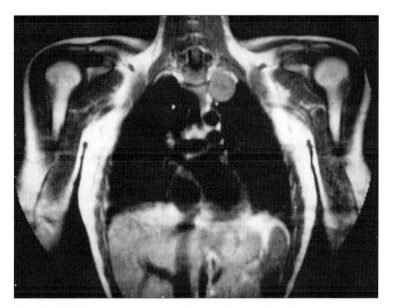

Fig. 11.12 CT scan showing an apical carcinoma of the left lung in a patient who presented with Pancoast's syndrome.

chloride). Tensilon is a short-acting anticholinesterase agent which, when given intravenously, increases the amount of acetylcholine available at the motor end plate. In the majority of patients it will temporarily overcome the muscle weakness of myasthenia (*Fig. 11.13*). Failure to do so, however, does exclude the diagnosis. Other confirmatory tests can be performed, such as an acetylcholine receptor antibody assay or repetitive stimulation electromyography showing decremental responses.

Precautions should be taken before performing the Tensilon test. Resuscitation equipment should be available and an intravenous cannula placed for venous access. Monitoring of vital signs should be performed before and during the test. Atropine should be drawn up ready to counteract any adverse systemic cholinergic effects. A small intravenous test dose of Tensilon (2 mg) should be given and the response observed. If there is no improvement in myasthenic signs nor any adverse side effects, the remaining 8 mg should be slowly injected.

The treatment of the patient with myasthenia is best undertaken by the neurologist. The treatment may involve the use of anticholinesterase agents, systemic steroids, immunosuppressants, or plasmapheresis. Thymectomy may be beneficial in some cases. The ophthalmologist plays a role in the management of ptosis and diplopia unresponsive to medical therapy. The ptosis may be treated by the use of ptosis crutches if the Bell's phenomenon is absent and if the orbicularis function is poor. Patients with normal orbicularis function rarely tolerate ptosis crutches. The surgical management depends on the levator function; if this is better than 4–5 mm, a levator aponeurosis advancement procedure may be used. If the levator function is less than 4 mm, a frontalis suspension

procedure will be required. The risk of exposure keratopathy must be considered carefully before embarking on such surgery.

SYNKINETIC PTOSIS

A synkinesis is simultaneous movement of muscles supplied by different nerves or by separate branches of the same nerve. It can be congenital or acquired.

MARCUS GUNN JAW WINK PHENOMENON (CONGENITAL TRIGEMINO-OCULOMOTOR SYNKINESIS)

In this disorder there is a central anomalous innervational pattern between the oculomotor and trigeminal nerves. The phenomenon is characterized by eyelid synkinesis with jaw movement (*Fig. 11.14*). Characteristically, a unilateral ptosis of variable degree is noted shortly after birth. The ptotic eyelid is noted to open and close as the infant feeds. The phenomenon accounts for approximately 5% of congenital ptosis patients, and may be associated with amblyopia, anisometropia, and strabismus. It may also be associated with a superior rectus palsy or a double elevator palsy (*Fig. 11.15*).

There are two major groups of trigemino-oculomotor synkinesis:
* External pterygoid–levator synkinesis, in which the lid elevates when the jaw is thrust to the opposite side, when the jaw is projected forward, or when the mouth is widely opened (*Fig. 11.16*).
* Internal pterygoid–levator synkinesis, in which the lid elevates on teeth clenching (*Fig. 11.17*).

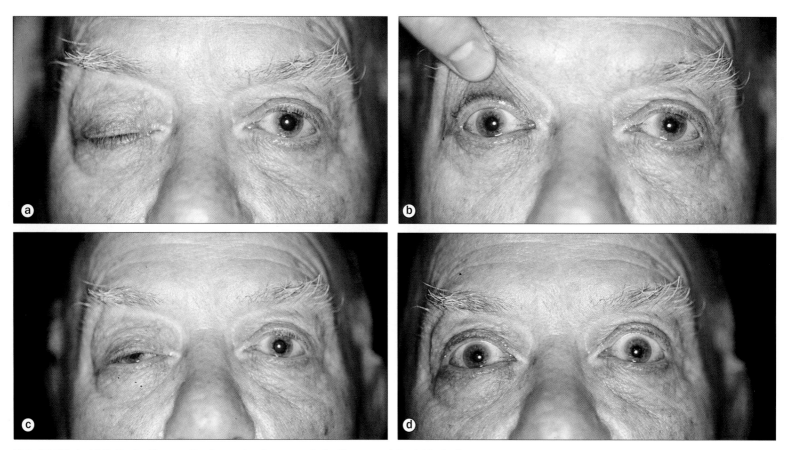

Fig. 11.13 (**a,b**) Patient with myasthenia gravis who presented with a complete right ptosis. (**c,d**) Appearance after the injection of Tensilon.

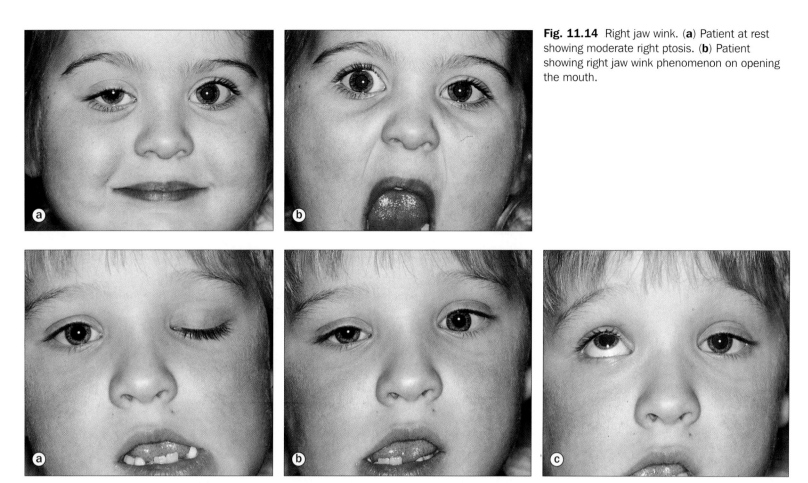

Fig. 11.14 Right jaw wink. (**a**) Patient at rest showing moderate right ptosis. (**b**) Patient showing right jaw wink phenomenon on opening the mouth.

Fig. 11.15 Left jaw wink phenomenon and left double elevator palsy. (**a**) Patient thrusting jaw to left with complete ptosis. (**b**) Patient thrusting jaw to right showing left jaw wink phenomenon and left hypotropia. (**c**) Patient attempting upgaze demonstrating left double elevator palsy.

Fig. 11.16 External pterygoid levator synkinesis. (**a**) Patient at rest showing moderate left ptosis. (**b**) Patient demonstrating left jaw wink phenomenon on opening the mouth.

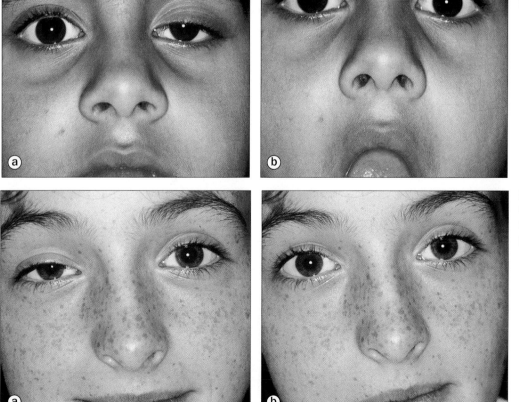

Fig. 11.17 Internal pterygoid levator synkinesis. (**a**) Patient at rest showing moderate right ptosis. (**b**) Patient demonstrating right jaw wink phenomenon on clenching the teeth.

In some patients the abnormal movements are only provoked by sucking (*Fig. 11.18*).

A rare condition in which the lid falls as the mouth opens has been referred to as the inverse Marcus Gunn jaw wink phenomenon.

The treatment of this phenomenon is very complex and a discussion of such treatment is beyond the scope of this text.

ABERRANT REINNERVATION OF THE OCULOMOTOR NERVE

In this disorder there is an innervational anomaly within the neural sheath between the eyelid and other targets of the oculomotor nerve. It is characterized by inappropriate eyelid and extraocular muscle synkinesis (*Fig. 11.19*). The disorder typically follows trauma or compression of the oculomotor nerve.

MYOTONIC DYSTROPHY

Myotonic dystrophy is a rare myopathic process which may be associated with a mild degree of symmetric ptosis (*Fig. 11.20*) with a fair to poor degree of levator function. It is characterized by pro-gressive symmetric external ophthalmoplegia, myopathy with atrophy affecting the musculature of the face, neck, and limbs, and classic cataracts. The latter consist of small, colored crystalline opacities or posterior, subcortical, and spoke-like opacities. Classically, these patients show myotonia, a delayed relaxation after contraction, which is most noticeable on hand shaking. Men may show frontal balding and testicular atrophy. Affected patients typically have a poor Bell's phenomenon (*Fig. 11.21*). Other ocular signs of myotonic dystrophy include pupillary light–near dissociation, ocular hypotonia, dry eyes, and a retinal pigmentary degeneration. The management of the ptosis is similar to that of ptosis complicating myasthenia (see above).

CHRONIC PROGRESSIVE EXTERNAL OPHTHALMOPLEGIA

This condition is characterized by progressive symmetric paralysis of the extraocular muscles, which do not respond to oculocephalic movements nor to caloric stimulation. The levator muscle is also affected, resulting in a degree of ptosis related to the degree of severity of the disorder. The levator function is usually poor, as is the Bell's phenomenon (*Fig. 11.22*). The orbicularis function is usu-

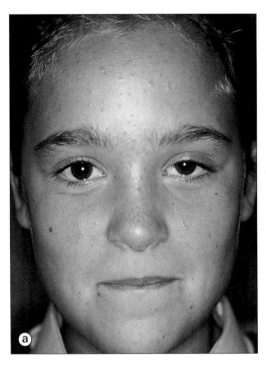
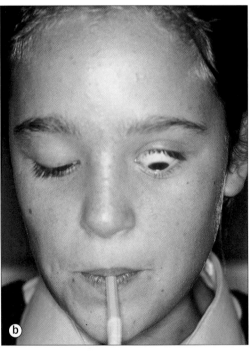

Fig. 11.18 A further variant of the Marcus Gunn jaw wink phenomenon. (**a**) Patient at rest showing mild left ptosis. (**b**) Patient demonstrating marked left jaw wink on sucking.

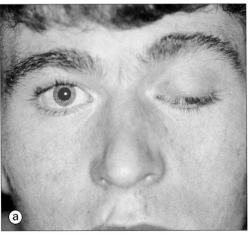
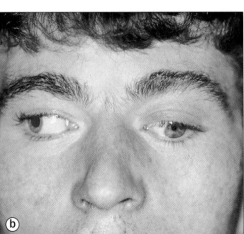

Fig. 11.19 Aberrant reinnervation of the oculomotor nerve. (**a**) Patient at rest showing marked left ptosis. (**b**) Patient demonstrating left eyelid elevation on attempted dextroversion.

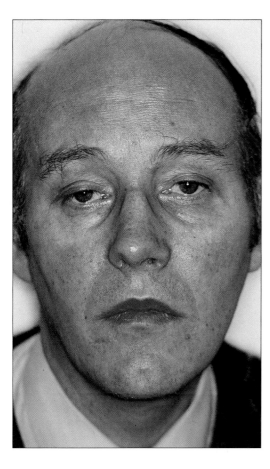

Fig. 11.20 The typical myopathic facies of myotonic dystrophy.

ally good.

Muscle biopsy material may reveal characteristic 'ragged-red' muscle fibers on light microscopy; electron microscopy typically shows strikingly abnormal mitochondria.

The term 'ophthalmoplegia plus' has been used to refer to a range of abnormalities that may be found with chronic progressive ophthalmoplegia. These abnormalities may be manifestations of associated neurodegenerative disorders. The Kearns–Sayre syndrome refers to a condition characterized by chronic progressive ophthalmoplegia, a retinal pigmentary degeneration, cardiac conduction defects often leading to complete heart block, and elevated levels of cerebrospinal fluid (CSF) protein. It is important to identify the cardiac conduction defect by means of an electrocardiogram because a cardiac pacemaker may be lifesaving. Oculopharyngeal muscular dystrophy is a hereditary condition, with affected individuals typically showing ptosis, difficulty swallowing, and a progressive external ophthalmoplegia. A large number of such patients are of French–Canadian descent.

The management of the ptosis is similar to that of ptosis complicating myasthenia (see above). A levator aponeurosis advancement procedure is best performed via a posterior lid approach; this affords a greater control of the final eyelid position and offers greater protection of the cornea in the early postoperative period because the eyelid is initially low and the degree of lagophthalmos less than with an anterior approach.

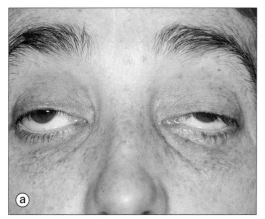
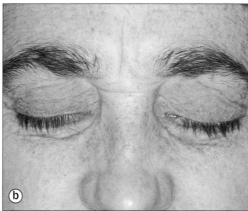
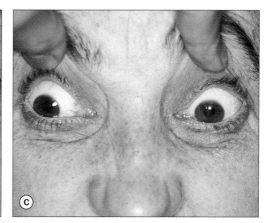

Fig. 11.21 A patient with myotonic dystrophy. (**a**) Patient at rest showing bilateral markedt ptosis. (**b**) Patient attempting forced eyelid closure demonstrating poor orbicularis function. (**c**) Patient attempting forced eyelid closure against resistance demonstrating a poor Bell's phenomenon.

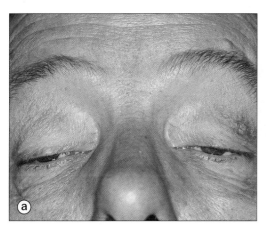
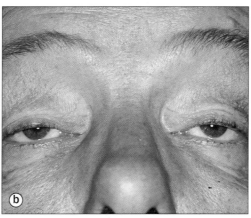

Fig. 11.22 A patient with chronic progressive external ophthalmoplegia. (**a**) Patient at rest showing bilateral marked symmetric ptosis and frontalis overaction. (**b**) Patient attempting upgaze showing poor ocular elevation and poor levator function.

ACUTE POST INFECTIOUS POLYNEUROPATHY (GUILLAIN–BARRÉ SYNDROME)

This rare disorder normally presents as a generalised illness with acute loss of muscle strength and minor sensory symptoms. Bulbar and respiratory involvement can occur. Ptosis which is usually of mild degree is symmetric and occurs in the context of a rapidly progressive bilateral ophthalmoplegia and facial diplegia (Miller–Fisher variant). This is associated with ataxia and areflexia but no peripheral weakness. Classically, the CSF shows a raised protein level in the absence of a cellular response.

CEREBRAL PTOSIS

A moderate to severe bilateral ptosis may be seen after acute damage to the right cerebral hemisphere. The ptosis may be asymmetric. A conjugate ocular deviation is also seen in this condition.

BOTULISM

Botulinum toxin blocks neuromuscular transmission and is commonly used therapeutically in the treatment of essential blepharospasm. Botulism, acquired through food poisoning, is a very rare neurologic disorder characterized by ptosis and ophthalmoplegia, followed by dysarthria and dysphagia and then by weakness of the extremities.

EYELID RETRACTION

There are a number of conditions that cause retraction of the upper eyelid (*Fig. 11.23*), the most frequently encountered being thyroid eye disease (*Fig. 11.24*). Additional non-neurologic causes are the instillation of sympathomimetic drugs, the prolonged use of systemic corticosteroids, upper lid scarring, and contracture or entrapment of the inferior rectus muscle.

Bilateral upper eyelid retraction is a common finding in dorsal lesions of the rostral midbrain (Collier's sign). The associated neuro-ophthalmic signs consist of pupillary light–near dissociation, paralysis of up-gaze, and convergence–retraction nystagmus on attempted up-gaze. Hydrocephalus in infancy is also thought to produce upper eyelid retraction via involvement of the rostral midbrain.

The synkinetic ptoses have been described above. A contralateral partial ptosis may give rise to an ipsilateral upper eyelid retraction because of Hering's law of equivalent innervation. The

upper lids are 'yoked' and, in the primary position, Hering's law of equivalent innervation is applicable. A patient exerting maximum effort to overcome a partial ptosis will, therefore, demonstrate retraction of the opposite upper eyelid (*Fig. 11.25*).

A patient with a chronic lower motor neuron facial palsy will demonstrate retraction of both the upper and lower eyelids, owing to the unopposed action of the eyelid retractors (*Fig. 11.26*). The

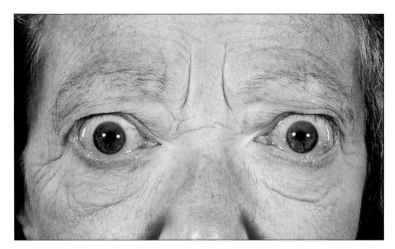

Fig. 11.24 Thyroid eye disease showing bilateral upper lid retraction.

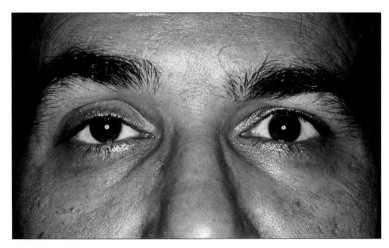

Fig. 11.25 Right ptosis showing contralateral upper lid retraction.

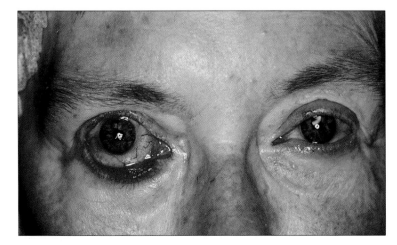

Fig. 11.26 Right chronic complete lower motor neuron facial palsy showing retraction of the right upper eyelid and a severe ectropion of the lower eyelid.

Eyelid retraction in neurologic disease
Dorsal midbrain (Parinaud's) syndrome: Collier's sign
Hydrocephalus
Synkinetic ptosis
Contralateral ptosis
Facial palsy

Fig. 11.23 Eyelid retraction in neurologic disease.

retraction will further aggravate the lagophthalmos that results from the palsy of the orbicularis oculi muscle. Surgical treatment is directed at recessing the lid retractors, either alone or in addition to the use of other treatment modalities aimed at reducing the degree of lagophthalmos (e.g. the implantation of an upper lid gold weight or the use of a lateral tarsorrhaphy).

LOWER LID ECTROPION

Ectropion of the lower eyelid is a frequent complication of a lower motor neuron facial palsy (*Fig. 11.27*). The ectropion is caused by a combination of factors, including paralysis of the orbicularis oculi muscle, the transmitted weight of the face from an untreated midfacial ptosis, and contractural changes in the lower lid skin caused by constant epiphora. The treatment of choice depends on a number of factors, including the underlying cause of the facial palsy, the age and general health of the patient, and the major contributing factor to the cause of the ectropion. A detailed description of the treatment modalities is beyond the scope of this chapter.

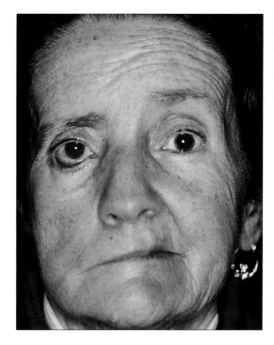

Fig. 11.27 Recent onset right complete lower motor neuron facial palsy showing a typical lower lid paralytic ectropion.

ACKNOWLEDGMENT

To Mr JRO Collin, MA, FRCS, DO, Consultant Ophthalmic Surgeon, for allowing me to use the photographs of some of his patients in this chapter, my sincere thanks.

Further reading

Boerner M, Seiff S. Etiology and management of facial palsy. *Current Opinion in Ophthalmology.* 1994;**5**(V):61–66.

Dutton JJ, Buckley EG. Long-term results and complications of botulinum A toxin in the treatment of blepharospasm. *Ophthalmology.* 1988;**95**(11):1529–1534.

Frueh BR. The mechanistic Classification of Ptosis. *Ophthalmology.* 1980;**87**:1019–1021.

Patel BCK, Anderson RL. Blepharospasm and related facial movement disorders. *Current Opinion in Ophthalmology.* 1995;**6**(V):86–99.

Sommer N, Melms A, Weller M, Dichgans J. Ocular myasthenia gravis. A critical review of clinical and pathophysiological aspects. *Doc Ophthalmol.* 1993;**84**(4):309–333.

Wilhelm H, Ochsner H, Kopyeziok E, Trauzettel-Klosinski S, Schiefer U, Zrenner E. Horner's syndrome: a retrospective analysis of 90 cases and recommendations for clinical handling. *GER J Ophthalmol.* 1992;**1**(2):96–102.

CHAPTER 12

Orbital Disease and Proptosis

Melvin G Alper

INTRODUCTION

Proptosis is the hallmark of orbital disease. The cause usually lies behind the globe in the orbit, hidden from routine ophthalmic examination (*Fig. 12.1*). The history and certain physical signs suggest clues to the clinical diagnosis. These guide the physician in further techniques for special evaluation and point to the area to be examined. It is the goal of this chapter to present a variety of orbital conditions, to define a method of clinical evaluation, and to correlate the findings with the results of medical imaging.

HISTORY

Diagnosis of orbital disease begins with a careful history of symptoms, characteristics of onset, and nature of progression. Specific inquiry should be made regarding pain, diplopia, visual loss, and systemic disease.

Expanding orbital masses may be localized on the basis of the history. If the onset is associated with early painless proptosis and late visual loss, the mass probably lies within the anterior or mid-third of the orbit (*Fig. 12.2*). On the other hand, if there is early painless loss of vision and late exophthalmos, the mass

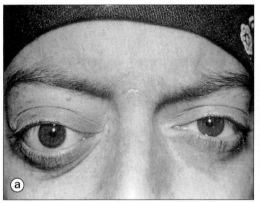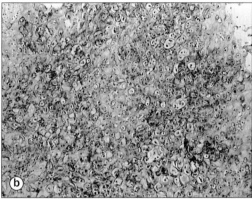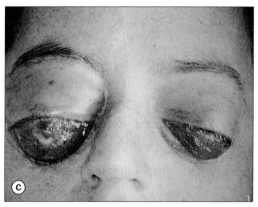

Fig. 12.1 (**a**) Painless right monocular proptosis in a 26-year-old woman. Note baring of sclera by the right lower eyelid, a sign of true proptosis. CT images are not available since this patient was seen in the pre-CT era. Excisional biopsy demonstrated an extraskeletal mesenchymal chondrosarcoma. (**b**) Low-power photomicrograph shows a characteristic picture of two cellular elements; namely, undifferentiated round mesenchymal cells with hyperchromatic nuclei and islets of differentiated cartilaginous tissue. (**c**) Same patient after 2 years of progressive tumor growth despite surgery, and radio- and chemotherapy. Note exposure damage to eyes with ulceration of the right cornea.

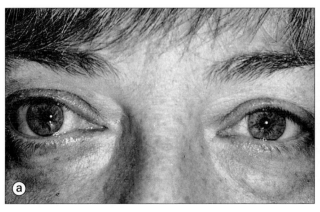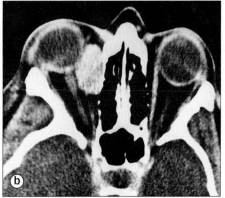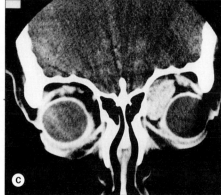

Fig. 12.2 (**a**) Right monocular proptosis without visual loss in a 42-year-old woman. Horizontal diplopia occurred upon levoversion. (**b**) Axial CT scan shows a large enhancing mass lying in the anterior one-third of the right orbit within the central and peripheral surgical space. Note location adjacent to the right globe which is both proptopic and slightly exotropic. There was no visual loss. (**c**) Coronal CT scan of same patient, demonstrating medial location of the tumor mass which has molded to the globe and to the medial orbital wall. Excision of tumor revealed a cavernous hemangioma.

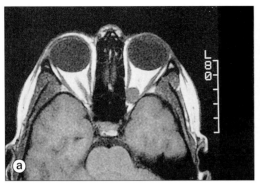
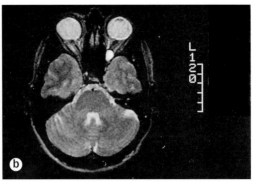

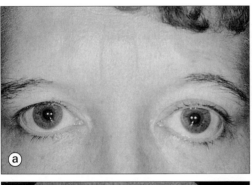
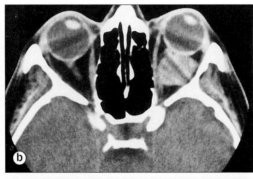

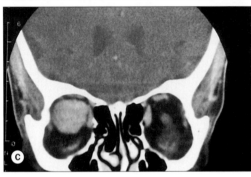
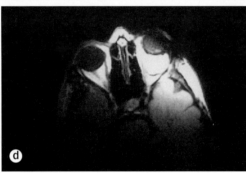
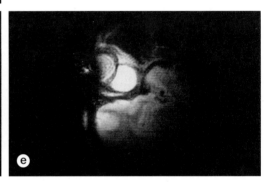

Fig. 12.3 (**a**) MR T-1 weighted image of a 37-year-old woman with recent onset of blurred vision in her left eye. No proptosis was present. Note the tumor in apex of left orbit. It is hypointense to orbital fat. (**b**) MR T-2 weighted image of same patient. Note that tumor is hyperintense in this fat suppressed image. Removal of tumor by transcranial skull-base approach revealed a cavernous hemangioma.

Fig. 12.4 (**a**) Left monocular proptosis in a 45-year-old woman with horizontal diplopia and visual distortion present. Again, sclera is visible above left lower eyelid, a sign of 'true' proptosis. Diagnosis was cavernous hemangioma. (**b**) CT scan of same patient. A large enhancing mass fills central surgical space. Diagonal shadow overlying mass is superior ophthalmic vein. (**c**) Coronal view of CT image demonstrates large enhancing mass in central surgical space of the patient. Diagnosis was cavernous hemangioma. (**d**) T-1 weighted MR image. Large mass slightly hyperintense to orbital fat fills central surgical space. (**e**) T-1 weighted MR image in sagittal section demonstrated large mass hyperintense to orbital fat filling the central surgical space. Hyperintensity of orbital fat is characteristic but not diagnostic of cavernous hemangiomas.

probably lies in the posterior third of the orbit (*Fig. 12.3*). Anterior lesions usually affect horizontal gaze with horizontal diplopia, whereas apical or posterior lesions cause impairment of upward gaze with vertical diplopia (*Fig. 12.4*).

A history of proptosis with deviation from the anteroposterior axis (A-P axis) may be caused by a mass arising in the paranasal sinuses or lacrimal fossa. Tumors arising within the orbit usually,

although not invariably, cause axial proptosis, which may be due to a variety of well-known expanding masses. The differential diagnosis involves the more common cavernous hemangioma, schwannoma, neurofibroma, fibrous histiocytoma, hemangiopericytoma, and metastatic disease. If there is associated sudden spontaneous subconjunctival hemorrhage or ecchymosis, with axial proptosis, lymphangioma should be suspected (*Figs 12.5–12.9*).

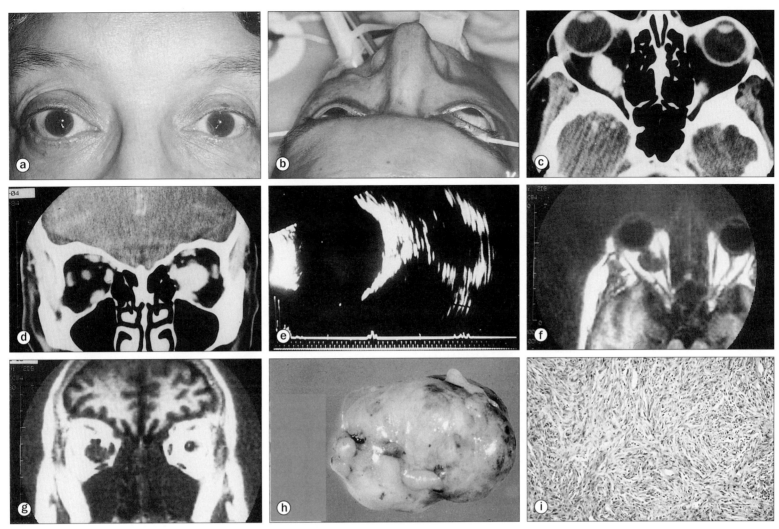

Fig. 12.5 (**a**) Frontal view of a 54-year-old woman with painless right monocular proptosis present for 2 years. There was no visual deficit. Diagnosis was fibrous histiocytoma. (**b**) Over-the-brow view of the patient demonstrates the degree of right monocular proptosis. (**c**) Transaxial CT scan demonstrates an enhancing fusiform-shaped mass filling the central surgical space. Compare with (**a**) and (**b**) in which the mass is more rounded and globular in shape. Either morphologic characteristic may be found in cavernous hemangioma and/or fibrous histiocytoma. (**d**) Coronal CT image in mid-orbit of same patient shows mass in left orbit to be globular shaped. Note optic nerve is elevated by the mass. (**e**) Ultrasonogram, B mode of the same patient. Note that the mass is homogeneous and anechoic with no interfaces. This is more characteristic of fibrous histiocytomas than cavernous hemangiomas. (**f**) T-1 weighted MR image demonstrates that mass is hypointense to orbital fat in this transaxial view, indicating rapid blood flow through the tumor. (**g**) T-1 weighted MR coronal image shows that mass fills central surgical space, and has pushed the optic nerve upward and slightly medially. Mass has a nodule on its upper surface next to the optic nerve. (**h**) Gross specimen of the tumor removed from right orbit of patient noted in (**a**). Note nodules on surface of tumor which correspond to MR images. (**i**) Photomicrograph of tumor shown in (**h**). Note storiform or cartwheel pattern of spindle-shaped cells interspersed with rounded 'histiocytic' cells. These tumors are usually benign in their growth pattern but can be malignant with both local and distant metastases.

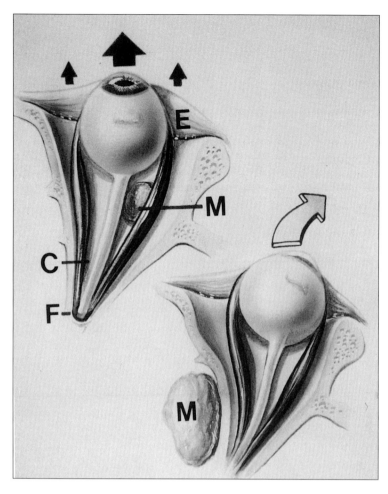

Fig. 12.6 Artist's conception of effect of intraorbital and extraorbital mass (M) on globe and vision. A mass within muscle cone pushes globe and eyelids (E) forward in an axial fashion. If the mass (M) is in anterior orbit as shown here, proptosis occurs early in its course and vision is usually unaffected. If it occurs at the apex near the optic foramen (F) or canal (C), vision is affected early and proptosis occurs late. If the expanding mass occurs in the paranasal sinus, the exophthalmic eye is deviated. (From *Highlights of Ophthalmology*, Silver Anniversary Edition, p. 583. Reprinted with permission of publisher and artist.)

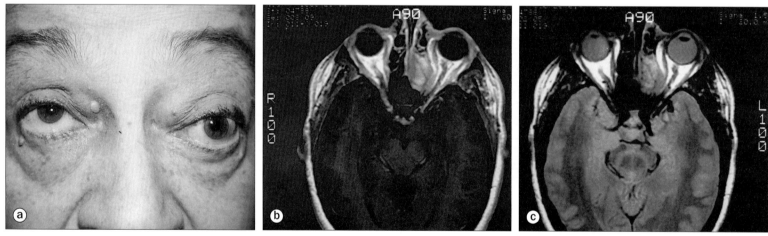

Fig. 12.7 (**a**) Full face of 67-year-old woman with left monocular proptosis, vertical diplopia, and left exotropia. Diagnosis was carcinoma of left fronto-ethmoid sinus. (**b**) T-1 weighted MR image of patient described in (**a**). Note left extropia and proptosis. The tumor is slightly hyperintense to orbital fat. (**c**) T-2 weighted MR image of same patient seen in (**a**). The tumor noted in the ethmoid sinus is hypointense to the fat in the left orbit.

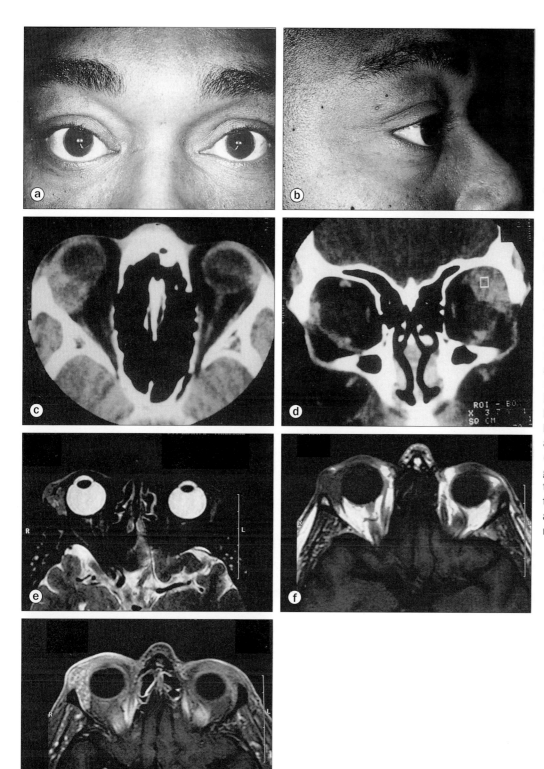

Fig. 12.8 (**a**) Full face photograph of a 32-year-old man with right painless proptosis of 2 years' duration. Vision was normal but vertical diplopia developed on gaze up and right. Note fullness in upper outer quadrant of right upper eyelid and baring of sclera above right lower eyelid. Diagnosis was mixed cell tumor of right lacrimal gland (benign pleomorphic adenoma of the lacrimal gland). (**b**) Lateral view. Note fullness in upper outer quadrant of right upper eyelid. A mass was palpable through the eyelid. (**c**) Transaxial CT scan. Note that an enhancing mass replaces lacrimal gland in right orbit (to reader's left). Compare to left orbit. The mass has a smooth contour, encroaches on the globe, and occupies both the peripheral and central surgical space. (**d**) Coronal CT scan in mid-orbit demonstrates globular shape and non-homogeneous character of the mass. Note that the bone is smooth indicating no bony invasion. (**e**) T-2 weighted MR image. Note that lacrimal mass in right orbit is hyperintense to orbital fat, moulds to globe, and lies in both the peripheral and central surgical space. Bone is uninvolved. (**f**) T-1 weighted MR image. Note that the lacrimal gland tumor in the right orbit involves both lobes of the lacrimal gland and is hypointense to orbital fat. It moulds to the globe and does not involve the lateral bony orbital wall. (**g**) T-1 weighted MR image enhanced by gadolinium-DTPA with fat suppression (compare to (**f**)). Note the non-homogeneous character of the tumor, which occupies both the peripheral and central surgical space. Enhancement of nasal mucosa is normal.

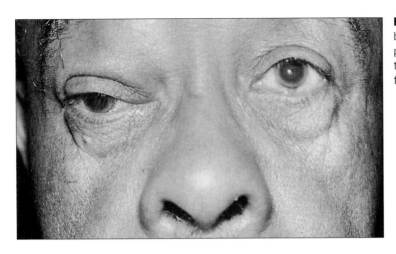

Fig. 12.9 Full face view of 72-year-old man with right exophthalmos. There is both right exotropia and hypotropia. Vertical diplopia was present in primary position increasing on up-gaze. Note fullness overlying the medial aspect of the right upper lid extending into the right supra-orbital area. Diagnosis was fronto-ethmoid mucocele.

A history of increasing proptosis with raised intra-abdominal pressure (Valsalva maneuver) or change of position may indicate an orbital varix or mucocele. Swishing noises in the head may implicate a caroticocavernous fistula, especially if synchronous with the pulse beat (*Figs 12.10, 12.11*)

Onset of exophthalmos with retraction of one or both upper lids may implicate thyroid disease. If unilateral, the patient may complain that one upper lid is drooping, whereas actually the fellow upper lid is retracted (*Figs 12.12, 12.13*).

In the case of ptosis that becomes worse in the afternoon, myasthenia gravis should be suspected. A history of chemosis or lid swelling upon rising in the morning associated with

photophobia, lacrimation, and burning should increase suspicion of thyroid disease (*Fig. 12.14*).

Painful exophthalmos may indicate an inflammatory origin, such as Graves' ophthalmopathy or inflammatory pseudotumor. Painful ophthalmoplegia may indicate Tolosa–Hunt syndrome or an anterior cavernous sinus involvement. Third nerve paralysis with pupilloplegia and headache may implicate an intracerebral artery aneurysm. Lacrimal gland carcinoma with or without bony involvement is commonly associated with pain and a history of short duration (6–12 months). Benign tumors of the lacrimal gland are usually painless, of longer than 12 months' duration, and without bony involvement.

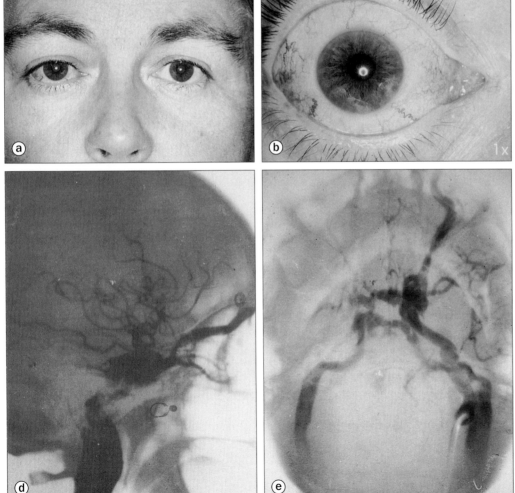

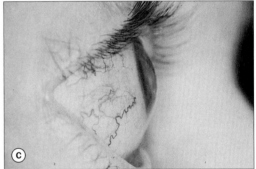

Fig. 12.10 (a) Photograph of a 54-year-old woman with right exophthalmos, pulse-synchronous swishing noises in her head, and open angle glaucoma. (b) Close-up view of the right eye of the same patient. Note corkscrew type vessels in episcleral area stopping in perilimbal area but *not* extending to limbus. (c) Lateral close-up view of the right eye. Note that corkscrew vessels stop before reaching the limbus leaving a clear perilimbal area. There was *no* pulsation of the right eye but auscultation over this eye demonstrated a systolic bruit. Intra-ocular pressure was elevated. Gonioscopy demonstrated an open anterior chamber angle with blood filling Schlemm's canal. (d) Lateral view of arterial phase of a cerebral arteriogram of the patient. Note that the right superior ophthalmic vein fills in the arterial phase as does the cavernous sinus. (e) Basal skull view of arterial phase of a cerebral arteriogram. Note that the right superior ophthalmic vein fills in the arterial phase as does the cavernous sinus.

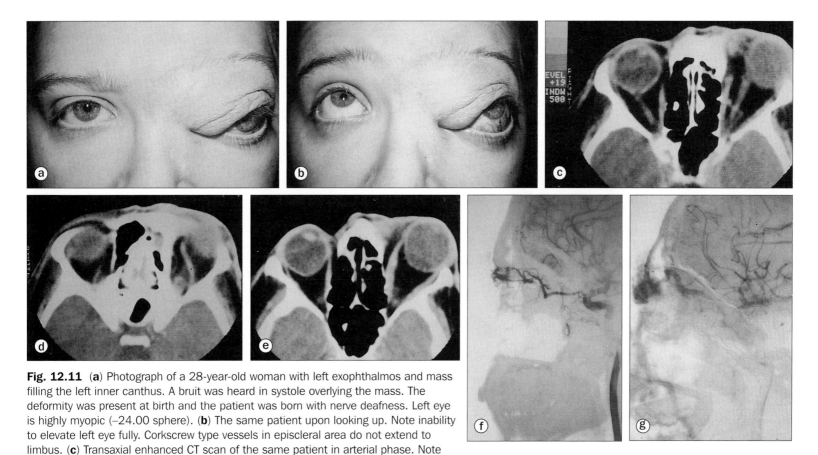

Fig. 12.11 (**a**) Photograph of a 28-year-old woman with left exophthalmos and mass filling the left inner canthus. A bruit was heard in systole overlying the mass. The deformity was present at birth and the patient was born with nerve deafness. Left eye is highly myopic (−24.00 sphere). (**b**) The same patient upon looking up. Note inability to elevate left eye fully. Corkscrew type vessels in episcleral area do not extend to limbus. (**c**) Transaxial enhanced CT scan of the same patient in arterial phase. Note that ophthalmic artery feeds the arteriovenous mass at the left inner canthus via the posterior and anterior ethmoid arteries. (**d**) Transaxial CT scan enhanced by contrast in venous phase. Note that superior ophthalmic vein remains engorged with arterial blood. (**e**) Transaxial CT scan of same patient. Note that the globe is highly myopic and is oval-shaped. The horizontal extra-ocular muscles are enlarged, a characteristic of arteriovenous malformations. (**f**) Cerebral arteriogram in arterial phase. Note that the ophthalmic artery takes origin from the internal carotid artery and feeds the mass at the left inner canthus. (**g**) Cerebral arteriogram in venous phase. Note that the superior ophthalmic vein is engorged with arterial blood.

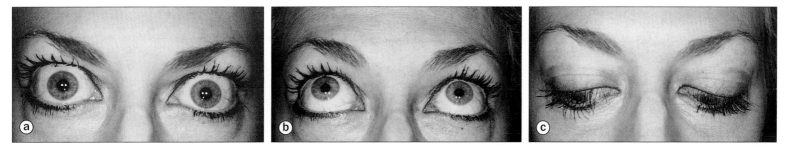

Fig. 12.12 (**a**) Full face photograph of a 32-year-old woman with hyperthyroidism. Note retraction of each upper eyelid causing an apparent exophthalmos. Baring of sclera above the upper limbus is noted. Hertel exophthalmometry was within normal limits. Diagnosis was early Graves' disease. (**b**) Up-gaze is unrestricted. (**c**) Down-gaze results in slight retraction of each upper lid with bare sclera noted above each limbus.

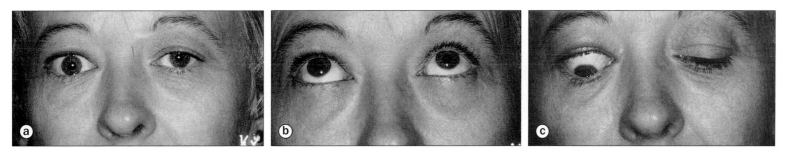

Fig. 12.13 (**a**) Full face view of a 54-year-old woman with right monocular exophthalmos and treated (I-131) hyperthyroidism. Note shortening of distance between right upper eyelashes and lid fold in primary gaze. (**b**) Note that up-gaze is unrestricted. (**c**) There is marked right upper lid retraction with tethering of the right superior levator muscle. Note bare sclera above right upper limbus, and the 'real' exophthalmos of right eye. Graves' disease usually affects both eyes (see Fig. 12.12a) but in this case only the right eye is affected. Patients often call attention to the appearance of the normal fellow eye. Note shortening of the distance from right upper eyelid fold to eyelash line when compared to the fellow left eye.

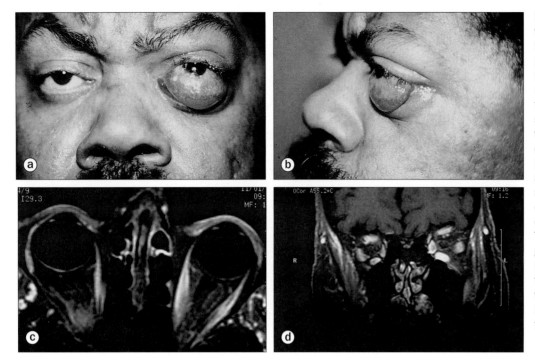

Fig. 12.14 (a) Photograph of a 42-year-old man with marked chemosis of left eye. Hyperthyroidism had been present and treated by I-131. The patient was now hypothyroid under treatment by replacement therapy. Chemosis appeared 4 months after radiotherapy. Vision was normal and there was minimal vertical diplopia. Chemosis subsided after corticosteroid therapy. (b) Lateral view. (c) T-1 weighted MR transaxial image enhanced by gadolinium – DTPA after chemosis had subsided demonstrates enlarged left medial and lateral rectus muscles in this fat suppressed section. Note normal appearing muscle tendons, a characteristic MR and CT finding in Graves' disease. There is very little 'real' exophthalmos. (d) T-1 weighted coronal MR image enhanced by gadolinium–DTPA. Medial, lateral, and inferior rectus muscles of left eye are larger than those of the right eye. This MR image is fat suppressed and was made after chemosis had subsided. Enhancement of nasal mucosa is a normal finding.

PHYSICAL EXAMINATION AND MENSURATION

After a careful history has been taken, the next step in diagnosis is the physical examination. The routine examination must include:
- Visual acuity and visual fields.
- Color vision with particular attention to red saturation.
- Position of the globe.
- Measurements of the eyelid fissures for symmetry.
- Measurements of the distance between the upper eyelid fold and eyelash line.
- Observation of injection of the globe and/or eyelids.
- Auscultation over the globe.

VISUAL ACUITY AND VISUAL FIELDS

In a patient with unilateral exophthalmos, if there is a loss of vision and a field defect in only one eye unexplained by ophthalmoscopy, there is a high likelihood that there is a disease process in only the orbit of the proptopic eye. If loss of vision is present in only the affected eye and the visual field is defective in both, the possibility of an intracranial lesion must be considered.

COLOR VISION

Every patient with proptosis should be tested for color vision in each eye. Comparison of red color saturation between the eyes may reveal optic nerve involvement before visual acuity is lost or a visual field defect occurs. Red saturation can be simply evaluated by directing the patient to observe a red bottle top which is readily available in every ophthalmologist's office. By giving a value from 1 to 100 to the intensity of red color, gross quantitative testing may be obtained.

POSITION OF THE GLOBE

By establishing the relative position of the eyes to each other and their position in regard to the orbital bony landmarks, a measure of disease and its progress within the orbit can be obtained. Disease processes within the orbit are usually due to involvement of the soft tissues. Bony margins usually remain constant, although some diseases of bone, such as meningioma invasion with osseous proliferation, osteomas, or fibrous dysplasia, may alter the position of the eyeball. Measurement devices relate the globe to the stable bony landmarks. Deviation of the eyeball may indicate paranasal sinus disease.

EYELID FISSURES

Measurement of the distance between the eyelids should be made in every case of proptosis. Malposition of the eyelids may give the appearance of exophthalmos even though the globes remain in normal relationship to each other and the bony margins. Upper eyelid retraction, lower lid paralytic ectropion, and cicatricial ectropion of the lower lid may all mimic actual proptosis. Enlargement of the globe by uniocular myopia or buphthalmos may also imitate proptosis.

Actual exophthalmos or proptosis may be determined by viewing the patient from above the eyebrow, or more accurately by use of a measuring device such as the Krahn or Hertel exophthalmometer. CT and MRI give the most accurate measurements and can be used to note progress of disease processes within the orbit.

MEASUREMENT OF DISTANCE FROM EYELASH LINE TO UPPER LID FOLD

All patients with proptosis should have an observation regarding position of the upper lid fold relative to the eyelash line. Shortening of this distance simulates real exophthalmos and is often diagnostic of Graves' disease. Lengthening of this distance may indicate paralytic ptosis, as is seen in third nerve paralysis or myasthenia gravis. Sometimes, disinsertion of the levator aponeurosis causes lengthening of this distance and is associated with thinning of the upper lid structure (see Fig. 12.13).

INJECTION OF THE GLOBE AND/OR EYELIDS

Injection of the eyelids and globe occurs in many intraorbital inflammatory diseases from orbital cellulitis (*Fig. 12.15*) to Graves' disease and inflammatory orbital pseudotumor (*Fig. 12.16*). In Graves' disease, the lids may be swollen and vessels enlarged overlying the extraocular muscle heads (*Fig. 12.17*). In orbital cellulitis, conjunctival injection extends to the limbus. In vascular anomalies or caroticocavernous fistulas, the enlarged (engorged) blood vessels stop before reaching the limbus leaving a clear zone in the perilimbal region (see Fig. 12.10).

AUSCULTATION

All proptotic eyes should be examined by the stethoscope and the patient should be queried as to noises in the head. A bruit synchronous with the heart beat is diagnostic of a caroticocavernous fistula especially if there is a high volume flow (see Figs 12.10, 12.11). In the event of a low volume flow, the patient still hears noises in the head even if the observer fails to hear a bruit.

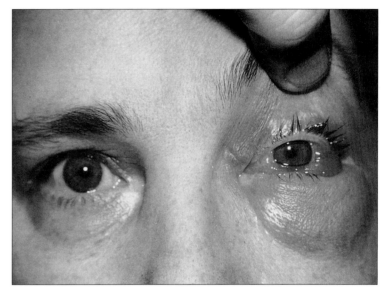

Fig. 12.15 A 34-year-old woman who developed a rupture of left ethmoid sinusitis in the left orbit. Left orbital cellulitis and proptosis developed. Note red swollen eyelids and marked chemosis of the left eye. Chemosis with distended vessels extended from the upper and lower cul-de-sacs to the limbus. (Compare to Fig. 12.14a.)

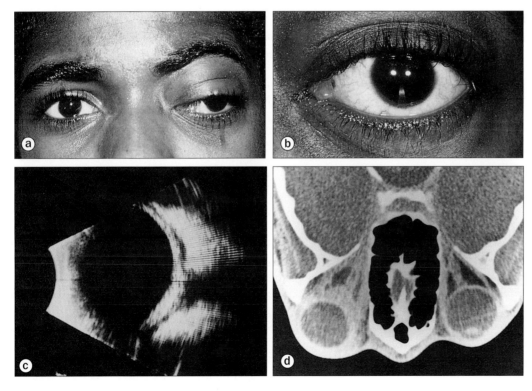

Fig. 12.16 (**a**) A 32-year-old man with painful left exophthalmos. Note lengthening of distance from left upper eyelash line to lid fold and fullness from lid fold to orbital rim. There was impaired extra-ocular motility with pain on attempted movement. Vision was diminished to 20/200, red color perception was decreased, but visual field was full. Inflammatory orbital pseudotumor was diagnosed. (**b**) Close up photograph of left eye. Note that dilated vessels extend to the limbus. (**c**) Ultrasonogram, B mode. Note anechoic area behind the sclera forming a 'T'-like sign with the optic nerve. Coleman has described this 'T' sign as characteristic of inflammatory disease. The authors have observed it in cases of lymphoma. (**d**) Transaxial CT scan. Note periocular inflammatory enhancement, beneath eyelids of the left eye. There is also retrobulbar episcleral enhancement, the so-called 'scleral rim' sign closely related to the 'T'-sign seen by ultrasonography. Feathery enhancement extends along the optic nerve and into orbital fat. The left medial and lateral rectus muscles are enlarged and their tendinous insertions are enhanced and indistinct.

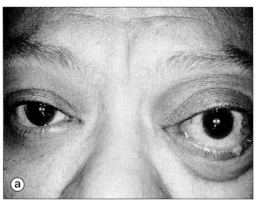
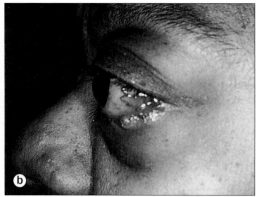
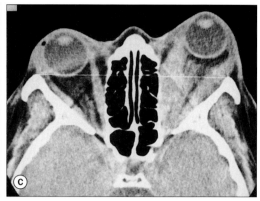

Fig. 12.17 (**a**) A 64-year-old woman with left exophthalmos and Graves' disease following I-131 treatment for hyperthyroidism. The patient was hypothyroid under treatment with thyroid replacement and corticosteroid therapy. Note engorgement of episcleral vessels in left eye. Fullness of upper and lower lids was present. Retraction of left lower eyelid showing bare sclera between lower limbus and lower eyelid was present. The distance between left upper lid fold and eyelash line was lengthened.

(**b**) Lateral view of same patient demonstrated engorgement of episcleral vessels overlying the left lateral rectus muscle. Chemosis was also present. (**c**) Transaxial CT scan. Note massive enlargement of medial and lateral rectus muscles. The tendon of the left lateral rectus muscle is normal. An imaginary line drawn from one lateral anterior orbital rim to the other noted by a cursor demonstrates the marked degree of left proptosis. Note absence of 'scleral rim' sign (compare Figs 14.17a–c to Figs 14.16a–d).

DIFFERENTIAL DIAGNOSIS

Benedict devised a simplified classification of clinical clues for differential diagnosis of orbital disease. Even in this era of sophisticated medical imaging, this author has used it to good advantage. The diagnostic clues may be divided as follows (*Fig. 12.18*):

• Neoplasms or cysts
• Inflammatory causes
• Vascular causes
• Graves' ophthalmopathy
• Associated syndromes
   Glaucoma
   Cavernous sinus syndrome
   Spencer–Hoyt syndrome

Certain associated syndromes, with or without exophthalmos, may be the first presenting physical sign of orbital disease. Elevated intraocular pressure (IOP) may be a presenting sign of Graves' disease. This is actually a pseudoglaucoma, in which the increased IOP occurs in a gaze-evoked fashion.

In 1953, Braley pointed out that elevated IOP in Graves' ophthalmopathy may appear normal in down-gaze and elevated upon up-gaze. This is thought to be due to tethering of the inferior rectus muscle, which causes an increase in IOP by compressing the globe when the patient gazes in an opposite field of action to the tethered muscle. The same phenomenon may be observed in lateral gaze when the medial rectus muscle is tethered. Recently, Gamblin and co-workers emphasized that this variation in pressure may be the first hint that Graves' ophthalmopathy is present.

Gaze-evoked pseudoglaucoma may also be seen in cases of longstanding extraocular muscle paralysis because of muscle contracture. It may occasionally be seen in Duane's syndrome.

Elevated episcleral venous pressure noted in Graves' ophthalmopathy may account for another form of glaucoma seen in Graves' disease. In this situation, Schlemm's canal is filled with blood upon gonioscopic examination. The author has had a patient with Graves' disease develop spontaneous hyphema and elevated IOP. Presumably, the blood in Schlemm's canal was under such elevated episcleral venous pressure that it ruptured into the anterior chamber, causing this unusual presentation.

In caroticocavernous fistulas and arteriovenous malformations, episcleral venous pressure becomes elevated causing pseudoglaucoma. Increased IOP may be the presenting sign in these anomalies. Neovascular glaucoma may be seen in both of these conditions after both surgical and spontaneous cures.

In a study by the author, neovascular glaucoma was seen as the presenting sign of optic nerve meningioma. This has also been reported by Waller and associates in a patient treated for optic nerve meningioma at the Mayo Clinic. Hoyt *et al.* have reported a similar complication in cases of malignant glioma of the optic nerve.

Cavernous sinus invasion by tumors that cause paresis of the third nerve may simulate orbital disease. Exophthalmos may occur with extraocular muscle paralysis. In other instances unilateral paralysis of up-gaze may result in lid retraction upon attempted up-gaze; this retraction occurs because comparable innervation is sent to the levator muscle and to the superior rectus muscle so that the eyelid moves up with the upward movement of the globe. When the branch of the third nerve innervating the superior rectus muscle is interrupted, more attempts to elevate the affected globe result in excess innervation of the ipsilateral superior levator muscle, causing an overshoot of the upper lid. This simulates Graves' upper eyelid retraction in primary gaze and upward gaze. Upon downgaze, however, the upper eyelid assumes a more normal position, confirming the diagnosis. Often the first division of the fifth nerve is paralyzed together with the third nerve, with resultant corneal anesthesia. This constellation of signs is called the 'cavernous sinus syndrome' (*Fig. 12.29*).

The Spencer–Hoyt syndrome is often the presenting sign of optic nerve meningioma, as well as meningiomas of the cranio-orbital junction. This syndrome consists of progressive visual loss, pale disc swellings and optic disc shunt vessels (*Figs 12.30, 12.31*).

Clinical diagnostic clues of orbital disease	
(1) Neoplasms or cysts (*12.19, 12.20*; see also Figs 12.1–12.5, 12.8,) 1. Distance between upper eyelid and lash line is symmetrical. 2. Axial proptosis of globe in involved orbit. 3. Baring of sclera between limbus and lower lid of involved orbit. 4. Deviation of global axis may indicate paranasal sinus disease. 5. Boggy swelling of one lower lid associated with temporal fossa fullness indicate meningioma en plaque of sphenoid ridge. **(2) Inflammatory causes (see Figs 12.15, 12.16)** 1. Axial proptosis. 2. Swelling of eyelids and chemosis with injection. 3. Distance between lash line and upper lid crease varies with degree of eyelid swelling. 4. Conjunctival injection extends to limbus. 5. Motility may be affected. **(3) Vascular causes (*12.21, 12.22*; see also Figs 12.10, 12.11)** 1. Axial proptosis in usual case – deviation of globe if vascular mass lies in anterior third of orbit. 2. Eyelid fissure symmetry varies with position of vascular anomaly. 3. Symmetry of distance between upper lid fold and eyelash line varies. 4. Conjunctival injection extends from fornix midway to limbus. 5. Systolic bruit in A/V fistulas. 6. Spontaneous hemorrhage in lymphangiomas.	**(4) Graves' Ophthalmopathy (*12.23–12.28*; see also Figs 12.12–12.14,12.17,)** 1. Unilateral or bilateral proptosis. 2. Retraction of one or both upper lids with associated widening of palpebral fissure – frequently asymmetrical. 3. Distance between upper lid crease and eyelash line shortened – frequently asymmetrical. 4. Limitation of motility is frequent. Most commonly affected is tethering of the inferior rectus muscle which limits up-gaze and simulates paralysis of the superior rectus muscle. Tethering of the medial rectus muscle simulates paralysis of the lateral rectus. Tethering of the superior rectus muscle simulates paralysis of the inferior rectus muscle. Collier's sign or retraction of the upper eyelid is often associated with a tethered inferior rectus muscle and simulates lid retraction. 5. In association with lid retraction, tethering of the superior levator muscle is often found, demonstrated by a positive upper lid forced duction test. 6. Engorged vessels are frequently seen overlying the lateral rectus muscle. 7. Chemosis is common. 8. Elevated intraocular pressure on attempted up-gaze.

Fig. 12.18 Clinical diagnostic clues of orbital disease.

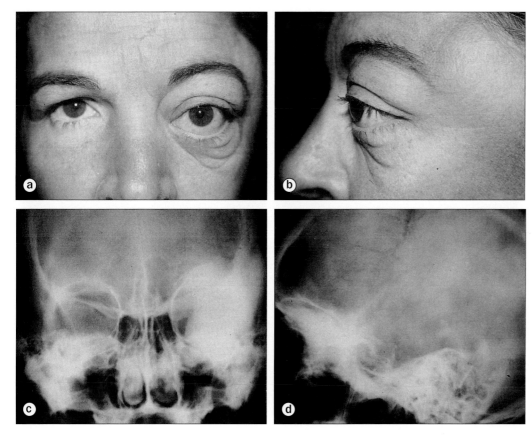

Fig. 12.19 (a) A 46-year-old woman with long-standing left monocular proptosis. Note boggy swelling of left lower lid and bare sclera between limbus and border of the lid. There was a marked widening of the left lid fissure and lengthening of the left upper lid. Axial left proptosis was present. Vision was normal and there was no visual field loss or diplopia. Note fullness in left temporal fossa. (b) Lateral view. Note the fullness in the left temporal fossa, a physical sign of meningioma en plaque. Craniotomy revealed meningioma en plaque. (c) Plain radiograph of head of patient. This is an anteroposterior view and shows a dense hyperostosis of the left sphenoid bone involving primarily the greater wing of the sphenoid with extension into the left temporal fossa. The lesser sphenoid wing is essentially undisturbed and is the reason for normal optic nerve function.

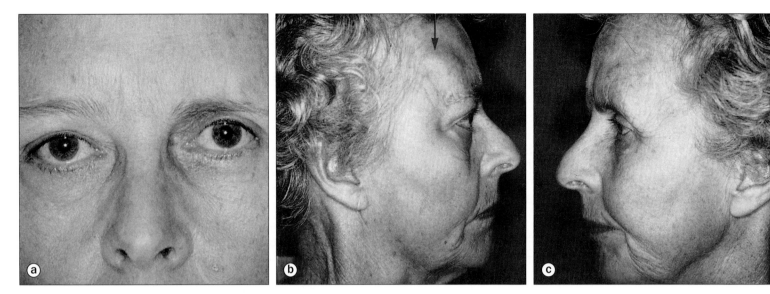

Fig. 12.20 (a) Full face photograph of a 72-year-old woman who had undergone right blepharoplasty because of a similar appearance to patient described in Fig. 12.19a. Note the right proptosis and fullness in the right supra-orbital area. The preoperative diagnosis had been blepharochalasis. (b) Right lateral view. Note fullness in right supra-orbital area extending into the temporal fossa. Diagnosis was meningioma en plaque. The plastic surgeon had failed to obtain any imaging studies to make proper diagnosis although treatment would have been the same for cosmetic reasons. (c) Left lateral view. Compare to (b).

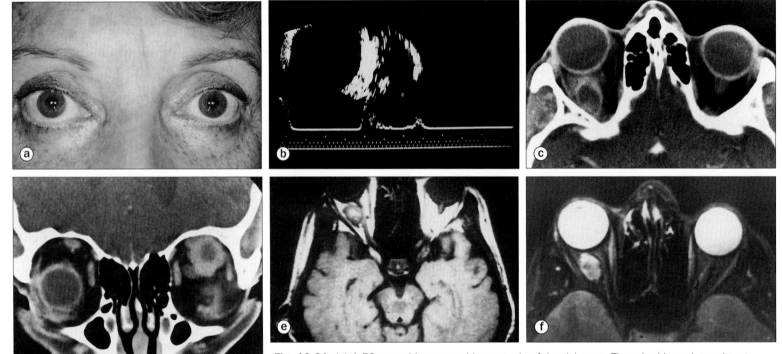
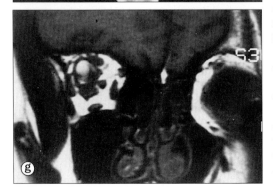

Fig. 12.21 (a) A 52-year-old woman with proptosis of the right eye. There had been intermittent subconjunctival hemorrhages and occasional ecchymosis of upper and lower eyelids. Hemorrhages resolved spontaneously. There was no loss of visual acuity or visual field, and no diplopia. Suspected diagnosis was lymphangioma. (b) Ultrasonogram, B-mode, demonstrates a well-encapsulated anechoic mass within the central surgical space. (c) Transaxial CT scan with contrast. Note enhancing mass within the central surgical space. The capsule of the mass enhances while the center is hypointense compared to the fat and to other orbital structures. Working diagnosis: lymphangioma. (d) Coronal CT scan of the same patient demonstrates the mass in central surgical space. It is well encapsulated and enhances. The center of the mass is hypointense to the capsule and orbital fat. Note that the optic nerve is displaced downward and medially. (e) Transaxial T-1 weighted MR image demonstrates a well-encapsulated mass with a central area surrounded by a low intense capsule. Note that the optic nerve in this section is displaced medially. (f) Transaxial T-2 weighted MR image demonstrates a hyperintense mass with hypointense central areas lying in the muscle cone. Note that the optic nerve is displaced medially. Axial proptosis is noted. (g) Coronal T-1 weighted MR image demonstrates a mass in the central surgical space with an area of high intensity lying in its central area. The optic nerve is pushed down and medially.

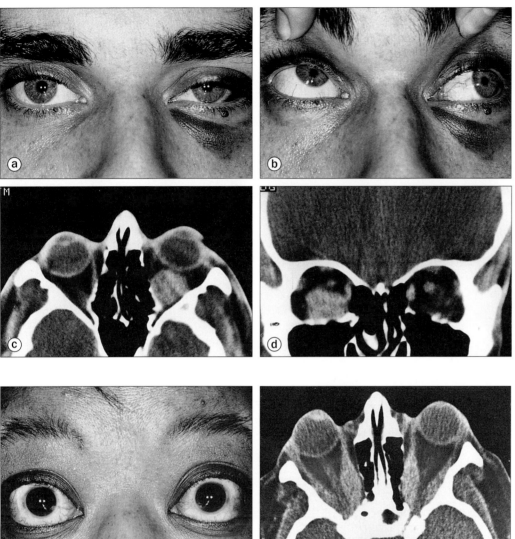

Fig. 12.22 (**a**) A 29-year-old male who had sudden spontaneous subconjunctival ecchymosis of the left upper and lower eyelids. Presumptive diagnosis was lymphangioma of left orbit. (**b**) He could not elevate the left eye and diplopia developed in this direction of gaze. The hemorrhage resolved spontaneously and vision returned to normal. (**c**) Transaxial CT scan shows a globular enhancing mass in the central surgical space of the left orbit with low density areas within the mass. (**d**) Coronal CT scan of same patient demonstrates the mass in the central and peripheral surgical space underneath the left optic nerve. The tumor enhances and shows many hypointense areas within its substance. It encompasses the inferior rectus muscle.

Fig. 12.23 (**a**) A 38-year-old woman with Graves' ophthalmopathy following treatment of hyperthyroidism with I-131 three months previously. There was bilateral visual acuity and field loss. Hertel exophthalmometry was right eye, 32 mm, left eye, 34 mm. Note widened palpebral fissures with minimal upper eyelid retraction. The lower lids are retracted exposing the sclera below the lower limbus, a sign of 'true' proptosis (compare to Figs 14.12a–c). Three bony walls were removed from each orbit, and this decompression restored acuity and visual fields to normal. (**b**) Transaxial CT scan demonstrates enlarged, swollen extra-ocular muscles with normal tendons. An imaginary line drawn from one anterior orbital rim to the other demonstrates the degree of exophthalmos. The orbital apex shows crowding with impingement on the optic nerves by swollen muscle bellies. This results in optic nerve compression and visual loss. Note inward bowing of ethmoid bone from encroachment by swollen medial rectus muscles.

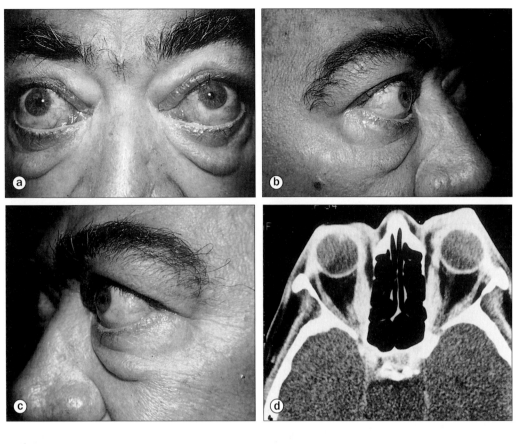

Fig. 12.24 (**a**) A 54-year-old man with Graves' ophthalmopathy 1 year after thyroidectomy for hyperthyroidism associated with diffuse goiter. Note bilateral exophthalmos, edema of lower lids, widened palpebral fissures, retraction of upper lids with herniation of retrobulbar fat through orbital septum, and edema of caruncles. Conjunctival hyperemia and chemosis were present. Note bare sclera above lower lids and that up-gaze is uninhibited, suggesting that there is no contracture of the inferior recti. (**b**) Right lateral view of same patient demonstrates retraction of upper lid, herniation of retrobulbar fat through upper and lower orbital septum and engorged episcleral vessels. (**c**) Left lateral view of same patient shows similar features. Note edema of lower lid extending onto cheek. (**d**) Transaxial CT scan demonstrates enlarged extra-ocular muscles with normal tendons and exophthalmos. Note enlarged lacrimal glands, a common finding in Graves' disease.

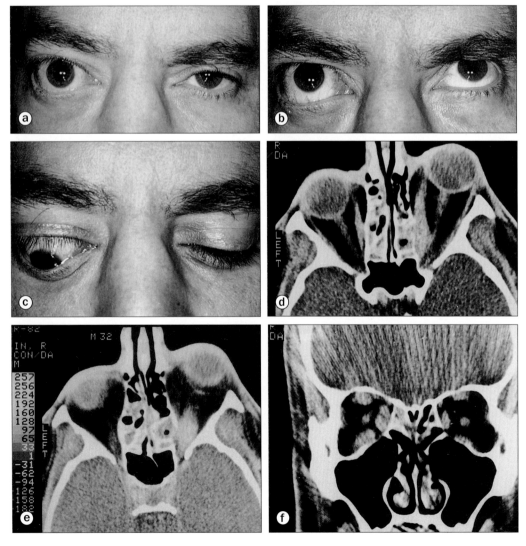

Fig. 12.25 (**a**) A right proptosis with vertical diplopia developed in this 32-year-old man 1 year after treatment for hyperthyroidism with I-131. Right monocular exophthalmos developed with vertical diplopia. Note retraction of right upper lid and baring of sclera above the right lower eyelid. (**b**) Note inability of right eye to elevate on attempted up-gaze indicating tethering of right inferior rectus muscle. (**c**) Note retraction of right upper eyelid with shortening of the distance between right upper fold and eyelash line. There was tethering of the right levator muscle. (**d**) Transaxial CT scan of right orbit. Note enlarged right medial rectus muscle encroaching on right ethmoid sinus. (**e**) Transaxial CT scan demonstrates enlarged right inferior rectus muscle, which caused right hypotropia on up-gaze (see (**b**)). (**f**) Coronal CT scan of right mid-orbit of the patient demonstrates enlargement of all extra-ocular muscles. In this section the optic nerve lies free without obvious compression. However, a scan through the apex is important to determine whether or not there is compression.

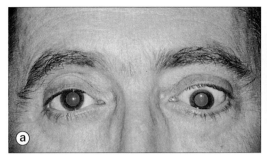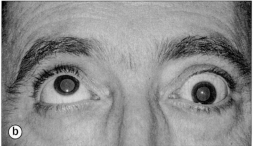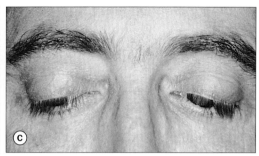

Fig. 12.26 (**a**) A 48-year-old man with Graves' disease. Note left behypotropia and retracted left upper eyelid. (**b**) The same man demonstrates marked left upper lid retraction on attempted up-gaze. This is due to tethering of the left inferior rectus muscle which prevented the left eye from moving up. When looking upward, the superior rectus muscle cannot overcome the tethered inferior rectus muscle. This effort leads to excessive neural stimulation by the left third cranial nerve. Because the levator and superior rectus muscles are innervated by the same branch of the third nerve, overstimulation affects the left upper eyelid as noted in this patient. This is *not* due to a tethered left superior levator muscle so commonly seen in Graves' disease. (**c**) Upon down-gaze there is no lid retraction confirming the fact that the left superior levator muscle is not tethered. The motility defect in this patient was corrected by surgical recession of the left inferior rectus muscle.

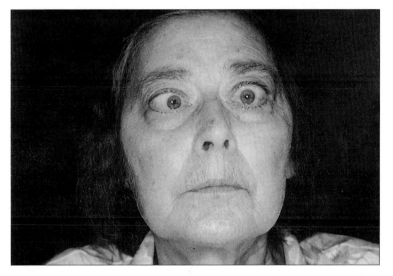

Fig. 12.27 A 68-year-old woman with longstanding Graves' disease after treatment for hyperthyroidism. Tethering of both medial and inferior rectus muscles as well as superior levator muscles in each side was present. The inferior rectus muscle is most commonly tethered simulating superior rectus palsy. The medial rectus muscle tethering simulates lateral rectus muscle palsy while tethering of the levator muscle causes lid retraction which must be distinguished from that caused by a tethered inferior rectus muscle.

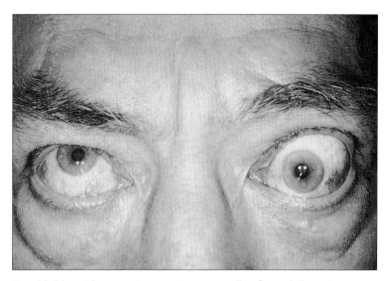

Fig. 12.28 A 73-year-old man with longstanding Graves' disease demonstrates the marked left upper eyelid retraction upon attempted up-gaze that can develop in the presence of tethering of the left inferior rectus muscle.

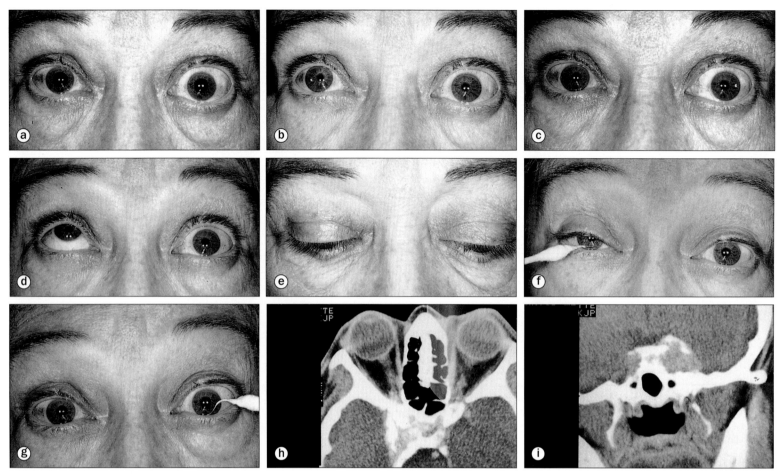

Fig. 12.29 (**a**) Full face photograph of a 60-year-old woman referred for evaluation with a presumptive diagnosis of Graves' ophthalmopathy. Evaluation demonstrated diminished visual acuity in the left eye to 20/40 (6/12). Note left proptosis and retracted left upper lid. Thyroid function studies were normal. There was a left afferent pupillary defect.
(**b**) More light reaction with the light in the right eye. (**c**) Less light reaction when the light was shining in the left eye. (**d**) Upon attempted up-gaze the left eye fails to move upward in concert with the right eye and the left upper lid retracts further than it was in primary gaze. This sign is consistent with tethering of the inferior rectus muscle seen in Graves' disease. (**e**) Upon down-gaze, the left eye moves downward without difficulty. In Graves'
disease, the left upper lid would have descended with the globe. Compare to Figs14.13a–c. (**f**) Testing the corneal sensation of the right eye as noted in this photograph is normal indicating an intact fifth cranial nerve. (**g**) Upon testing the corneal sensation of the left eye, an anesthetic left cornea was noted. This complex of symptoms and signs noted in (**a**) to (**g**) is called the 'cavernous sinus syndrome'. (**h**) Transaxial CT scan through the base of the skull at the cavernous sinus area notes an enhancing mass involving the lateral wall of the left cavernous sinus and the lesser wing of the left sphenoid bone. Presumptive diagnosis was meningioma. (**i**) Coronal CT scan through area seen in (**h**) demonstrates involvement of the left cavernous sinus and lesser sphenoid wing.

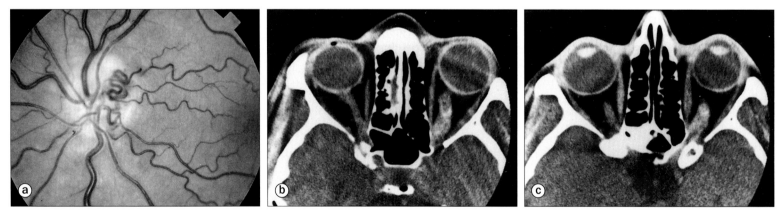

Fig. 12.30 (**a**) Fundus photograph demonstrates pale optic nerve swelling with shunt vessels on its surface (Spencer–Hoyt syndrome) in a 45-year-old woman with loss of vision in her left eye. Examination demonstrated left visual acuity of 20/50 (6/15). There was a large afferent pupil defect in the left eye. The presumptive diagnosis was perioptic nerve meningioma. (**b**) Transaxial enhanced CT scan demonstrates tubular enlargement of the left optic nerve. Calcium deposits are noted in the nerve sheath. The
enlargement extends from the globe to the orbital apex at the optic canal entrance. (**c**) Another transaxial CT view of the orbits in the same patient whose optic nerve photograph is seen in (**a**). Note that the tubular swelling of the left optic nerve extends through the optic canal. Calcium is seen in the nerve in mid-orbit. Railroad tracking or 'tram-tracking' sign is visible as a slight central lucency in the tumor at the apex of the orbit. This represents the optic nerve itself surrounded by the enhancing tumor.

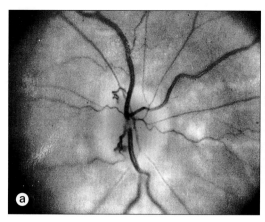
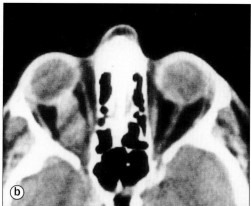

Fig. 12.31 (**a**) Fundus photograph of a 52-year-old woman with longstanding visual loss in her right eye. Note the pale swollen optic nerve and the shunt vessels on its surface (Spencer–Hoyt syndrome). (**b**) Transaxial CT scan demonstrated fusiform swelling of the optic nerve. The sheath enhances and the nerve itself is not seen. A diagonal shadow that crosses the nerve is the superior ophthalmic vein. The perioptic meningioma extends from the globe to the orbital apex.

DIAGNOSTIC EVALUATION OF EXOPHTHALMOS

With so many clinical clues pointing to diverse disease processes within the orbit, a routine logical approach to investigation is important in the diagnostic evaluation. A team approach to such a study must be developed. Such investigative studies should separate primary orbital from intracranial and paranasal sinus lesions that involve the orbit secondarily. Furthermore, these studies should select the surgical approach and the surgical team.

Working with experienced neuroradiologists, neurosurgeons, and endocrinologists, the following steps have been devised to study unilateral exophthalmos:
- Establish presence of exophthalmos.
- Rule out thyroid disease.
- Medical imaging.

ESTABLISH PRESENCE OF EXOPHTHALMOS

The techniques to establish presence of exophthalmos have been dealt with above. In a clinical setting, use of Hertel's exophthalmometer has been the most reliable method in the author's experience. Ultrasound studies rule out exophthalmos from high myopia or buphthalmos. CT scanning and MR imaging are expensive techniques but also evaluate the degree of proptosis and study orbital tissues for a cause.

RULE OUT THYROID DISEASE (GRAVES' OPHTHALMOPATHY)

Since Graves' ophthalmopathy is the most common cause for proptosis (both unilateral and bilateral), this condition must always be uppermost in the differential diagnosis. Discussion for evaluation of this disease complex is beyond the scope of this chapter. The reader is referred to standard texts on thyroid disease for further information. Cooperation with an endocrinologist is important and this specialist should be included in the 'orbital team'.

MEDICAL IMAGING

Medical imaging is the most important step in diagnostic evaluation of orbital disease and proptosis once the history and physical examination have been performed. Medical imaging evaluates the bone, soft tissue, and vasculature of the orbit. These studies separate orbital from periorbital and intracranial lesions; proceed in a logical sequence with little or no risk to the patient; and finally, select the surgical team and surgical approach.

Because of the importance of this examination, the neuroradiologist should be consulted prior to sending the patient for evaluation. The referring physician must point out the provisional diagnosis and the area to be examined. Failure to communicate with the radiologist has led to mistakes in diagnosis in the author's experience.

Of those medical imaging techniques available to us, the most useful for studying the orbit are ultrasonography, conventional and pleuridirectional X-rays, CT, and MRI. Each of these modalities performs a different function in diagnostic evaluation of orbital disease. It is beyond the scope of this chapter to describe each of these in detail.

Ultrasonography
Ultrasonography is a nonionizing technique which creates an image by utilizing low megaHertz (MHz) frequency transducers to measure reflectivity of sound in a preselected area of soft tissue. The optimal frequencies for examination of the orbit are 8 MHz (A-scan) and 10 MHz (B-scan).

Various tissues differ in sound velocity. The areas between the borders of these tissues are called acoustic interfaces. The ultrasonic beams are modified at these interfaces and are either reflected or scattered upon return to the ultrasonic probe. Evaluation of these reflected sound echoes forms the basis of ultrasonic diagnosis.

Ultrasonography has certain advantages and disadvantages. It provides a rapid inexpensive technique for examining the orbit in an office setting. There is no need for outside referral. However, it is useful only in the anterior or mid-orbit. It can measure the anterior–posterior diameter of the globe and is indispensable in determining the power of intraocular lenses to be implanted during cataract surgery. It can demonstrate such ocular changes as retinal detachments, intraocular tumors, and vitreous hemorrhages. In the orbit it can demonstrate enlarged extraocular muscles of Graves' ophthalmopathy and identify orbital inflammation (see Fig. 12.16c). Its dynamic nature makes it useful in the diagnosis of such conditions as varices, cysts, and lymphangiomas. By testing their compressibility with pressure exerted by the probe, information about the consistency of the lesion can be obtained. Lesions can be characterized according to their anechoic or echoic nature, which is useful in guiding a needle into a mass in the anterior or mid-orbit during fine needle aspiration biopsy (*Fig. 12.32b*).

However, ultrasonography is incapable of studying periorbital lesions, the bony walls, and the orbital apex. It cannot give information of adnexal or intracranial extension of orbital lesions nor orbital extension of intracranial or adnexal lesions.

Radiography

Conventional and pleuridirectional X-rays project radiation to form an image of radio-opaque structures. The techniques used are little changed from those first demonstrated by Conrad Roentgen in 1895. These techniques are excellent for demonstrating bony details but soft tissues are not seen. By use of intravenous contrast media, the blood vessels become visible. Orbital phlebography (venography) is rarely used nowadays, but may show orbital varices and arteriovenous malformations. Arteriography is still routinely used for intracranial mass lesions, caroticocavernous fistulas, and orbital arteriovenous malformations (see Figs 12.10, 12.11). Retrobulbar injection of water-soluble contrast media to demonstrate mass lesions in contrast orbitography has been abandoned as too dangerous.

Computed tomography

CT utilizes computer reconstruction techniques to calculate the absorption of radiation in a preselected slice of body tissue. The orbit is ideally constructed for evaluation by CT. It is, in effect, a bony box filled with structures of various density. Retrobulbar fat – a tissue of low density – surrounds the globe, optic nerve ,and extraocular muscles – structures of greater density. Because of this difference in tissue density, more dense structures become very well defined. With the use of intravenous contrast material, the orbital vessels can be seen. The bony walls of the orbit and apex at the orbitocranial junction become exquisitely defined with appropriate window settings upon CT scanning of these structures.

Expanding orbital masses are characterized by CT scanning as to density, size, shape, and location. Density, size, and shape suggest the etiologic possibilities, but localization in three dimensions is the most important tissue characteristic for the orbital surgeon. CT scanning determines whether a mass arises in the orbit and is confined to it, extends from the orbit into adjacent structures, or involves the orbit secondarily from an intracranial, paranasal, or adnexal site of origin. Furthermore, it relates the mass to the surgical spaces, the apex, and bony walls and the optic nerve and globe. The choice of the surgical approach and surgical team depends upon CT localization of the expanding mass. When

performing fine needle aspiration biopsy in the posterior one-third of the orbit, CT scanning is absolutely necessary in accurately placing the needle into the mass (*Fig. 12.32*).

Although CT scanning has been generally available for only 20 years, it has revolutionized orbital surgery. Fourth generation scanners give exquisite definition in characterizing the bone and soft tissue of the orbit. With the use of intravenous contrast material, the orbital and intracranial blood vessels are seen but are less well defined than the images achieved by arteriography.

Modern scanners are safe, accurate, fast, and cost effective. Successful use, however, demands close consultation between the referring physician and neuroradiologists. It is imperative that the correct anatomic site to be examined and the diagnostic possibilities be communicated. In the experience of the author, most of the mistakes in diagnosis have arisen because of a failure to make these facts known. Another source of error results from placing the patient in a wrong position for an orbital scan. The proper orbital scan should be made at either 0° to (–)25° to Read's canthomeatal line. To insure against these inbuilt errors the referring ophthalmologist should personally review the scans with the neuroradiologist before surgery.

Because certain lesions have a propensity to develop in different surgical spaces, the ophthalmologist should be familiar with these anatomic landmarks. There are four surgical spaces recognizable in proper CT scans of the orbit. They are described as follows:

- Subperiosteal space – that space between the bony orbit walls and periorbita.
- Peripheral surgical space – that area between the periorbita and extraocular muscles.
- Central surgical space – that area within the muscle cone.
- Tenon's space – that area surrounding the posterior aspect of the globe.

The former two spaces are referred to as 'extraconal' and the latter two as 'intraconal' (*Fig. 12.33*).

In the subperiosteal space, dermoids, bony tumors, plasmacytomas, and orbital extension of intracranial meningiomas have been encountered by the author. This space is continuous intracranially with the epidural space. Hematomas have been found in this area within the orbit continuous with epidural hematomas after head trauma. In the peripheral surgical space, the author has most commonly encountered cavernous hemangiomas, dermoids, fibrous histiocytomas, and lacrimal gland tumors.

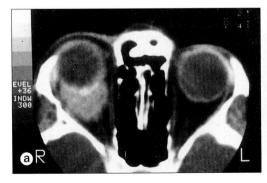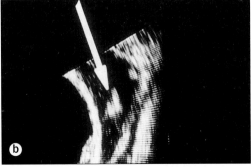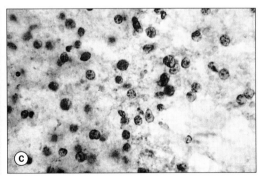

Fig. 12.32 (a) Enhanced transaxial CT scan of a 50-year-old woman who presented with clinical signs of right inflammatory orbital pseudotumor. There was right monocular proptosis of 3 mm and inflammatory signs analogous to those seen in Fig. 12.16a. This scan demonstrates a 'rim' sign in the right eye and an enhancing mass that moulds to the posterior aspect of the right globe. Presumptive diagnosis was 'inflammatory pseudotumor'. A fine needle aspiration biopsy was planned. (b) Ultrasonogram -B mode with needle in anechoic retrobulbar space demonstrates the technique of fine needle aspiration biopsy under guidance by ultrasound. Arrow points to needle in retrobulbar mass. (c) Aspirate from fine needle aspiration demonstrates large lymphomatous cells. Diagnosis was orbital lymphoma.

In the central surgical space, the author has noted optic nerve tumors (most commonly meningiomas of the optic nerve sheath and less commonly gliomas), schwannomas, cavernous hemangiomas, fibrous histiocytomas, and dermoids. Lymphangiomas have been found in all surgical planes except the subperiosteal space.

Extraocular extension of intraocular melanomas has been seen in Tenon's space. Inflammatory lesions and lymphomas have also been encountered in this space (*Figs 12.34, 12.35; see also 12.16, 12.32*).

CT scanning demonstrates various findings in certain orbital lesions, which characterize them in general and suggest the possible etiology. Tissue characterization has been described by many authors. The reader is referred to the literature for further discussion. A summary of some of these distinguishing features seen on CT scans is described below. However, it must be stressed that final diagnosis of any of these lesions requires histopathologic evaluation.

Magnetic resonance imaging

MRI is a nonionizing technique that provides images based on the distribution of hydrogen nuclei in the body. Instead of measuring density of tissue as in X-rays, this method measures the MR of protons as they occur predominantly in fatty acids and tissue water. Of the various proton nuclei that can be caused to resonate, hydrogen is the most abundant in tissue. It produces the strongest signal when stimulated by an external static magnetic field and applied radiofrequency (RF) stimulus.

In clinical practice, a patient is placed inside a large magnet, which generates a strong magnetic field up to 25 000 times that of the earth's magnetic force. Some of the hydrogen nuclei in the body tissue to be examined line up with the induced magnetic field. RF stimulus is then applied to the protons. This causes the hydrogen nuclei to 'wobble' about their axis or process. When the radiowaves are removed, the nuclei return to their original axis of rotation. In doing so they give back the energy from the radiowaves they have received. The manner in which they do this is characteristic of their chemical environment. The radiowaves given off by the hydrogen nuclei are received by a radio antenna near the patient. The signals are then processed by a computer and transformed into an image, which can be obtained from any desired angle without moving the patient. All of the orbital structures can be differentiated by MRI. The tissue examined is characterized as to proton density, spin lattice relaxation time (T-1), spin–spin relaxation time (T-2), and linear motion.

Proton density is a measure of the concentration of nuclei of elements with an odd number of charged particles. Hydrogen is the proton of choice to be analyzed because of its abundance in tissue.

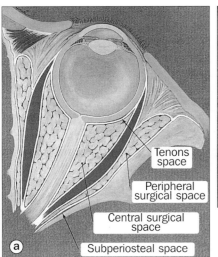
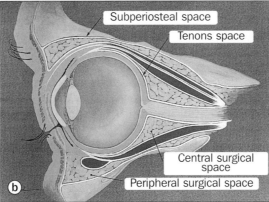

Fig. 12.33 (a) Artist's conception of transaxial view of the surgical spaces within the orbit. (b) Artist's conception of a sagittal view of the surgical spaces within the orbit.

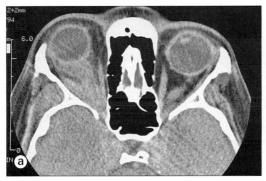
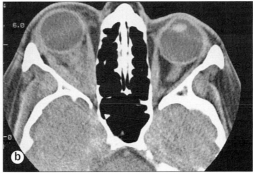
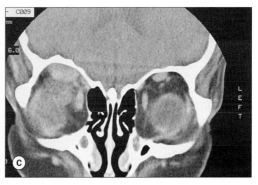

Fig. 12.34 (a) Transaxial CT scan of a 32-year-old woman with recurrence of a dormant lymphoma that had been treated by irradiation and chemotherapy in the past. In this section right monocular proptosis is seen. There is disorganization by an enhancing mass of normal retrobulbar orbital architecture. The right temporal fossa shows loss of intramuscular spaces as compared to the left temporalis muscle. A fine needle aspiration of this area revealed large cell lymphoma. (b) Another transaxial CT scan of the same patient through the right orbit demonstrates enlarged right medial and lateral rectus muscles probably due to lymphomatous invasion by large cell lymphoma. (c) Coronal CT scan demonstrates enhancing mass in orbit and enlarged extra-ocular muscles in the right orbit. Note that right temporalis muscle enhances in this section and demonstrates loss of normal architecture when compared to the left side.

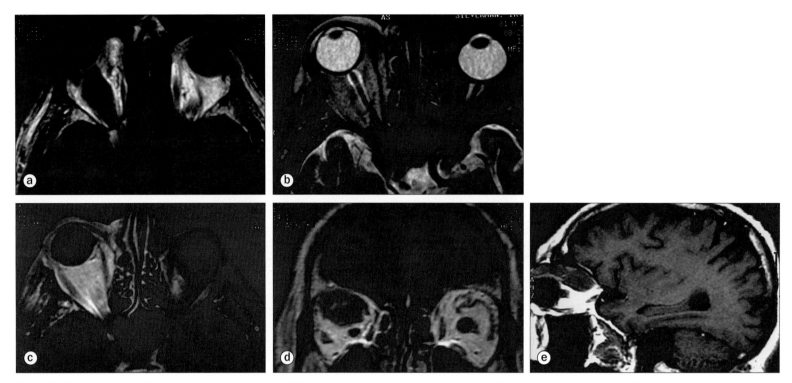

Fig. 12.35 (**a**) Transaxial T-1 weighted MR image of a 72-year-old man with known large cell lymphoma in right orbit (to viewer's left). Note mass hypointense to orbital fat fills central surgical space. (**b**) Transaxial T-2 weighted MR image of same patient demonstrates that mass fills central surgical space. It is hypointense to orbital fat. (**c**) Transaxial T-1 weighted MR image enhanced by gadolinium–DTPA. The enhanced mass is hyperintense and fills central surgical space. (**d**) Coronal view. In this T-1 weighted MR image, a hypointense mass is noted filling the superior orbit. (**e**) A sagittal view of a T-1 weighted MR image of the large cell lymphoma filling the superior orbit. Note that the mass is hypointense compared to orbital fat.

Spin lattice relaxation time (T-1) is related to the physical state of the nuclei of the proton in its environment. Spin–spin relaxation time (T-2) is a measure of the local interactions of the nuclei with one another.

Motion is a measure of volume flow of nuclei through the resonance region. By utilizing MRI with fat saturation after administering a contrast medium, gadolinium diethylenetriamine pentacetic acid (Gd–DTPA), meningiomas of the optic nerve sheath are exquisitely demonstrated. Furthermore any lesion that breaks the brain–vascular barrier is also better demonstrated by use of this contrast medium than any other technique. All lesions in the orbit are enhanced by gadolinium and fat suppression, including extraocular muscles in Graves' disease, tumors, and cysts, as well as inflammatory masses.

In a clinical setting, the practicing physician is often faced with the question of when to utilize CT or MRI in evaluating orbital pathology of an individual patient. Both CT and MRI visualize soft tissue changes. In the orbit, accuracy of diagnosis approaches 95% with both techniques.

Assuming that both modalities are available, the schema in *Figure 12.41* should be considered when referring a patient for medical imaging.

With the use of contrast media (iodinated media in CT and gadolinium diethylenetriamine pentacetic acid [Gd–DTPA] in MRI) the capabilities of both techniques are enhanced. Fat suppression and use of surface coils for orbital imaging further improve the quality of images obtained by MR.

As noted in Figure 14.41, patients with cardiac pacemaker and/or intracranial or intraorbital ferromagnetic material *must* be *excluded* from MRI. Sensitivity to iodinated contrast media is very common and every patient should be queried for this allergy before evaluating with CT since there is always a remote possibility of anaphylactic shock and death. In the event of such allergy, MRI with Gd–DTPA would be the examination of choice. There are no reports of such reactions to Gd–DTPA.

Except for evaluation of bony pathology and detection of calcium, both techniques reveal orbital pathology in 97% of cases. However, MRI with Gd–DTPA and fat suppression is the examination of choice for optic sheath meningiomas; CT is the examination of choice for intraocular calcium and bony pathology. MRI with Gd–DTPA is the test of choice for evaluation of intracranial extension of orbital tumors or orbital extension of intracranial tumors. MRI is also the examination of choice for evaluation of the sellar and perisellar region.

Patulous optic nerve sheaths mimic enlarged optic nerves and are commonly seen as a normal variant or in cases of intracranial pressure. MRI can differentiate these by its ability to distinguish between the signal intensity of the optic nerve and surrounding spinal fluid.

Invasive studies, such as venography and arteriography, are of limited value in the study of intraorbital disease. Venography may be indicated in rare instances to evaluate varices and in cases of Tolosa–Hunt syndrome if MRI is unavailable. Cerebral arteriography continues to be used by most neurosurgeons prior to surgery, especially in cases of intracranial aneurysms and arteriovenous malformation.

Distinguishing features of CT scans	
Graves' ophthalmopathy (see Figs 12.12–12.14, 12.24, 12.25)	**Cavernous hemangiomas (see Figs 12.2–12.4)**
(1) Exophthalmos. (2) Enlarged extraocular muscles with normal tendons. (3) Distortion of the ethmoids by the medial rectus muscles. (4) Orbital fat may be increased and is frequently prolapsed through the septum. (5) Bilateral involvement.	(1) Intra- or extraconal mass. (2) Spherical or elliptical in shape. (3) Smooth wall. (4) Modest enhancement with contrast media. (5) Usually located lateral to optic nerve displacing it medially. (6) No erosion of bone.
Inflammatory orbital pseudotumor (see Fig. 12.16)	**Optic nerve tumors**
(1) Exophthalmos. (2) Swollen extraocular muscles with abnormal tendons. (3) Anterior orbit is most often affected. (4) Normal CT landmarks may be obliterated. (5) Dense sclero uveal rim ('rim sign'). (6) Usually, unilateral involvement.	**A. Gliomas (Fig. 12.38)** (1) Fusiform swelling optic nerve. (2) Optic nerve may be kinked. (3) Cyst formation within nerve. (4) Areas of varying density. (5) Modest enhancement with contrast media. (6) Optic canal enlarged but may be normal.
Dermoid cyst (*Fig. 14.37*)	**B. Optic nerve sheath meningiomas** **(*12.39*; see Figs 12.30, 12.34)**
(1) Well-encapsulated mass, usually located in the anterior or mid-orbit. (2) May occur in any surgical space – frequently involves the subperiosteal or peripheral surgical space. (3) Variable coefficients of attenuation occur within the mass, some of which have low Hounsfield numbers consistent with fat. (4) Pressure erosion of surrounding bone.	(1) Tubular swelling of optic nerve from apex to sclera. (2) Bulbous or fusiform swelling of optic nerve at apex. (3) Optic canal may be normal or enlarged – may show hyperstosis late. (4) Perineural sheath enhances with contrast media. (5) Low density center noted on coronal cuts and 'railroad tract sign' on transaxial section. (6) Perineural structures may be invaded late in course. (7) Intracranial invasion late in course.
Lacrimal gland tumors	**Fibrous histiocytoma (see Fig. 12.40)**
A. Inflammatory or lymphoid origin (1) Oblong enlargement. (2) May be compressed or diffuse. (3) Molds to surrounding structures. (4) Contour usually sharply angulated. (5) Enhances with contrast media. (6) Bone is normal. (7) Located in anterior orbit.	(1) Intra- or extraconal mass. (2) Elliptical or spherical shape. (3) Marked enhancement with contrast media. (4) No erosion of bone.
B. Neoplasia (see Fig. 12.8) (1) Rounded or globular mass. (2) If benign – smooth margins. (3) If malignant – serrated margins. (4) Bony erosion. (5) Globe may be flattened. (6) Extends posteriorly.	**Lymphoid tumor of orbit (see Figs 12.32, 12.34, 12.35)** (1) Retrobulbar mass usually in superior compartment. (2) Mass molds to adjacent structures. (3) Contours usually sharply demarcated. (4) Streaky profiles in orbital fat. (5) Bone is normal. (6) Benignancy and malignancy similar.

Fig. 12.36 Distinguishing features of CT scans.

SUMMARY

A method for evaluation of orbital disease has been presented. Whenever the physician is presented by a patient with proptosis, careful examination is demanded in order to make a diagnosis. The techniques outlined in this chapter have proved of benefit to the author during the past 40 years of practice.

A team approach to evaluate orbital disease is emphasized and should include the ophthalmologist, endocrinologist, ear nose and throat surgeon, neurosurgeon, neuroradiologist, and pathologist. Although discussion of treatment is beyond the scope of this chapter, frequent consultation in this group should lead to better treatment and a happier outcome for the patient.

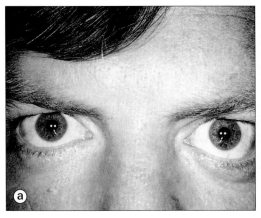
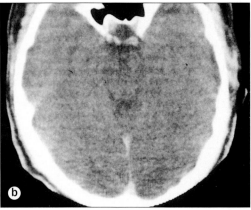
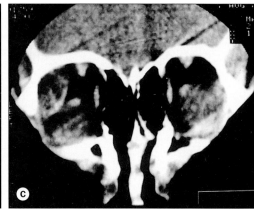

Fig. 12.37 (**a**) Photograph of a 45-year-old man with long-standing proptosis of his left eye (left monocular proptosis). Note the widened left palpebral fissure and baring of sclera above left lower eyelid. Visual acuity was normal. Vertical diplopia developed on left gaze. (**b**) Transaxial CT scan. Note the elongated mass in the peripheral surgical space of left orbit. There was a low density center iso-intense to orbital fat. The mass moulded to the bone and globe. Differential diagnosis included lacrimal gland tumor and dermoid cyst. Pathologic diagnosis was dermoid cyst. (**c**) Coronal CT scan. This scan in left mid-orbit shows that the tumor lies in the peripheral surgical space. Note low intensity center of tumor iso-intense to orbital fat. The tumor encroaches on the central surgical space in this view but does not affect the optic nerve.

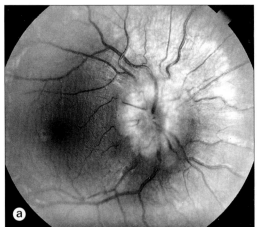
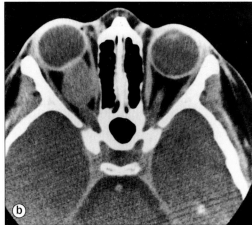

Fig. 12.38 (**a**) Optic nerve photograph of a 5-year-old girl who displayed 2 mm of right monocular proptosis and visual loss. There was minimal right exotropia. Note the nerve head is pale and swollen. There are no shunt vessels. Compare to Fig. 12.30a. (**b**) Transaxial CT scan. The right eye is slightly exotropic and there is enhancement of the flattened optic nerve head. The retrobulbar portion of the optic nerve has a large bulbous swelling starting just behind the globe. In the orbital apex an enlarged fusiform swelling of the optic nerve extends into the optic canal which appears larger than the left optic canal.

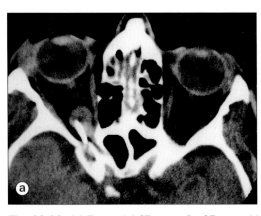
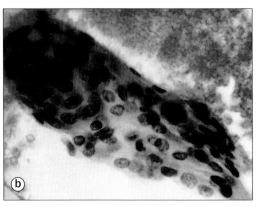

Fig. 12.39 (**a**) Transaxial CT scan of a 65-year-old man who presented with a blind, proptotic right eye. The right optic nerve was white and there were no shunt vessels on its surface. This scan demonstrates a globular-shaped optic nerve mass in the orbital apex extending into the optic canal. The linear density in the orbital apex is a fine needle placed in the optic nerve under CT guidance to obtain the aspiration biopsy shown in (**b**). These types of cells are typical of optic nerve meningioma. Because of the patient's age and the fact that he was already blind in that eye, it was elected to continue to observe him without transcranial surgery.

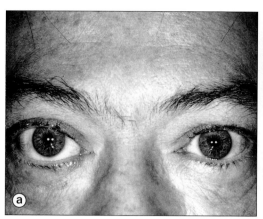
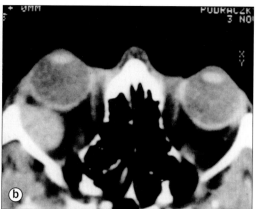

Fig. 12.40 (**a**) Photograph of a 54-year-old man with painless right proptosis. There was no visual acuity loss but horizontal diplopia developed on gazing to the right. Note slightly widened right lid fissure and exposure of the right sclera beneath the limbus and above the right lower eyelid. There was axial proptosis and no asymmetry of eyelids. (**b**) Transaxial CT scan. A large homogeneous globular mass was noted in the mid-third of the right orbit occupying both the peripheral and central surgical spaces lying against the lateral wall of the orbit. Diagnosis was fibrous histiocytoma. At operation a 20 mm tumor was removed. The diagnosis was benign fibrous histiocytoma. Ten years later the tumor became malignant with local invasion.

Comparison of CT and MRI	
Advantages of CT	**Advantages of MRI**
1. Bone visualization.	1. No ionizing radiation.
2. Calcium detection.	2. Multiplanar views.
3. Superior spatial resolution.	3. Superior soft tissue (contrast) resolution.
4. Decreased cost.	4. Low incidence of allergy to
5. Increased availability.	MI contrast media compared to
6. Ability to scan patients with intracranial	iodinated contrast media used in CT.
or orbital ferromagnetic material.	5. Better contrast sensitivity
7. Rapid data acquisition; artifact from	permitting improved visualization of subtle
eye movement.	zones of enhancement or edema; MS
	plaques; tangles of Alzheimer's disease.
	6. No bone artifact.

Fig. 12.41 Comparison of CT and MRI.

Further reading

Ahmadi J, Teal JS, Segall HD, *et al.* Computed tomography of carotid-cavernous fistula. *Am J Neuroradio.* 1983; 4:131–136.

Alper MG, David DO, Pressman BD. Use of computerized axial tomography (EMI scanners) in diagnosis of exophthalmos. *Trans Am Acad Ophthalmol Otolaryngol* 1975;**79**:150–165.

Alper MG and Davis DO. Computed tomography in diagnosis ofnon-neoplastic unilateral exophthalmos. In: DiChiro G. ed. *Book of Abstracts* (International Symposium on Computer Assisted Tomography in Non-tumoral Diseases of the Brain, Spinal Cord, and Eye.) Oct 11–15, 1976.

Alper MG. Endocrine orbital disease. In: Erger PH ed. *Orbit Roentgenology.* New York:John Wiley and Sons. pp. 70–92, 1977.

Alper MG. Computerized tomography (CT) in diagnosis of inflammatory orbital pseudotumor and Graves' disease. In: Thompson HS, ed. *Topics in Neuro-Ophthalmology.* Williams and Wilkins: Baltimore, pp. 347–68, 1979.

Alper MG. Computed tomography in planning and evaluating orbital surgery. *Ophthalmology.* 1980:**87**:418–431.

Alper MG. Management of primary optic nerve meningiomas. *J. Clin Neuro-Ophthalmol.* 1981:**1**:101–117.

Alper MG and Aitken PA. Anterior and lateral microsurgical approaches to orbital pathology. In: Schmidek HH and Sweet WH eds. *Operative Neurosurgical Techniques* Vol 1. Grune and Stratton:Inc. pp 245–277, 1982.

Alper MG, Bray M. Evolution of a primary lymphoma of the orbit. *Br J Ophthalmol.* 1984:**68**:255–260.

Alper MG, Wartofsky L. Endocrine ophthalmopathy. In: Becker KL, ed. *Principles and Practice of Endocrinology.* Philadelphia, Pennsylvania: JB Lippincott Company, In Press, Chapter 42, p. 335

Ambrose J. Computerized x-ray scanning of the brain. *J. Neurosurg.* 1974:40:679–695.

Ambrose J, Hounsfield GN. Computerized transverse axial tomography. *Br J Radio* 1973:46:148–149.

Benedict WL. Diseases of the orbit. *Trans Am Acad Ophthalmol Otolaryngeal.* 1949:54:26–36.

Benedict WL. Surgical treatment of tumors and cysts of the orbit. *Am J Ophthalmol.* 1949:**32**:763.

Bernardino ME, Zimmerman PD, Citrin CM, *et al.* Scleralthickening: A CT sign of orbital pseudotumor. *Am J Roentgenol* 1977:**129**:703–706.

Brailey W, Eyre J. Exophthalmic goitre with increased tension. *Ophthalmol Rev.* 1901:**20**:147–148.

Braley AE, Malignant exophthalmos. *Am J Ophthalmol* 1953:**36**:1286–1290.

Brant-Zawadzki M, Davis P, Crooks LE, Mills CM, Norman D, Newton TH, Sheldon P, Kaufman L. Nuclear magnetic resonance demonstration of cerebral abnormalities: Comparison with CT. *Am J Neuro-Rad* 1983:4:117–124.

Brant-Zawadzki M, Kaufman L, Crooks L. NMR of the normal and pathologic eye and orbit. *Am J Neuro-Rad* 1984:**5**:345–350.

Bull J. The changing face of neuroradiology over nearly forty years. *Neuroradiology* 1995:**9**:111–115.

Bullock J, Waller RR. Choroidal folds experimentally produced by traction on the optic nerve. Presented at first Scientific Program of the Orbital Society. Pittsburgh, PA. March 20, 1972.

Chavis RM, Garner A, Wright JE. Inflammatory orbital pseudotumor. A clinicopathologic study. *Arch Ophthalmol* 1978:**96**:1817–1822.

Coleman DJ, Jack RL, Franzen LA and Werner SC. High resolution B-scan ultrasonography of the orbit: V. Eye changes of Graves' disease. *Arch Ophthalmol* 1972:**88**:465–471.

Coleman DJ, Jack RL, Franzen LA and Werner SC. High resolution B-scan ultrasonography of the orbit: VI. Pseudotumors of the orbit. *Arch Ophthalmol* 1972:**88**:472–480.

Coleman DJ, Liyzi FL, Jack RL. Ultrasonography of the eye and orbit. Lea and Febiger, Philadelphia, 1977.

Dallow RL, Momose KJ, Weber AL, Wray SH. Comparison of ultrasonography, computerized tomography (EMI scan), and radiographic techniques in evaluation of exophthalmos. *Trans Am Acad Ophthalmol Otolaryngol* 1976:**81**:OP305–322.

Dandy WE. Results following the transcranial operative attack on orbital tumors. *Arch Ophthalmol* 1941:**25**:191–216.

Dandy WE. Orbital tumors. Results following the transcranial operative attack. New York Oskar Piest, 1941.

Davis DO, Alper MG. Computerized tomography of the orbit and orbital lesions. In: Pefer H ed. *Orbit Roentgenology.* Arger New York:John Wiley & Sons, pp 196–214, 1977.

Davis FA. Primary tumors of the optic nerve. *Arch Ophthalmol* 1940:**23**:735–957.

Dolva LO. Side-effects of thyrotropin releasing hormone. *Br Med J* 1983:**287**:532.

Dubois PJ, Kennerdell JS, Rosenbaum AE. Advantages of a fourth generation CT scanner in the management of patients with orbital mass lesions. *Comput Tomogr* 1979:**3**:279–290.

Drews LC. Exophthalmometer. *Am J Ophthalmol* 1957:**43**:37–58.

Dutton JJ. Optic Nerve sheath meningiomas. *Surv Ophthalmol* 1992:**37**:167–183.

Enzmann D, Donaldson SS, Marshall WH, Kriss JP. Computed tomography in orbital pseudotumor. *Radiology.* 1976:**120**:597–601.

Enzmann D, Marshall WH, Rosenthal QR, Kriss JP. Computed tomography in Graves' exophthalmopathy. *Radiology.* 1976:**118**:615.

Ferry AP, Font RL. Carcinoma metastatic to the eye and orbit. I. A clinicopathologic study of 227 cases. *Arch Ophthalmol* 1974:**92**:276–286.

Font RL, Hidayat AA. Fibrous histiocytoma of the orbit. *Human Pathology.* 1982:**13**:199–209.

Forbes GS, Sheedy II PF, Waller RR. Orbital tumors evaluated by computed tomography. *Radiology* 1980:**136**:101–111.

Foster J. The diagnosis and treatment of orbital tumors. *Ann R Coll Surg Engl.* 1955:**17**:114.

Frisen L, Hoyt WF, Tengroth BM. Optociliary veins, disc pallorand visual loss; a triad of signs indicating spheno-orbital meningioma. *Acta Ophthalmol* 1973:**51**:241–249.

Gamblin GT, Harper DG, Galentine P, Fuck DR, Chernow B, Ril C:

Prevalence of increased intraocular pressure in Graves' disease – evidence of frequent subclinical ophthalmopathy. *N Eng J Med.* 1983:**308**:420–424.

Gay AJ, Wolkstein MA. Topical guanethidine therapy for endocrine lid retraction. *Arch Ophthal.* 1966:**76**:364–367.

Gorman C. Editorial. Ophthalmopathy of Graves' disease. N Eng J Med 308:453-454, 1983.

Grossman RI. Neuroradiology in the brave new world. In: Cohen EJ, ed). *Year Book of Ophthalmology.* St Louis, Missouri: Mosby-Year Book Inc. p 269, 1994.

Grove AS. Evaluation of Exophthalmos. *N Eng J Med* 1975:**292**:1005–1013.

Hanafee WN. Orbital Venography. *Radio Clin North Am* 1972:**10**:63.

Hanafee WN. Section of contrast studies of the orbit. In: Symposium. Modern examination methods of orbital disease. *Trans Am Acad Ophthalmol Otolaryngol.* 1974:**78**:OP599–600.

Harris GJ, Jakobiec FA. Cavernous hemangioma of the orbit. *N Neurosurg.* 1979:**51**:219–228.

Hauer J. Additional clinical sign of "unilateral" endocrine exophthalmos. *Br J Ophthalmol.* 1969:**53**:210–211.

Heaps RS, Miller NR, Albert DM, Green WR, Vitale S. Primary adenocarcinoma of the lacrimal gland. A retrospective Study. *Ophthalmology.* 1993:**100**:1856–1860.

Henderson JH. *Orbital tumors* (second edition). Stuttgart-New York:Georg Thieme, 1980.

Hertel E. Ein einfaches exophthalmometer. *Arch V Ophthal* 1905:**60**:171–178.

Hilal SK, Trokel SL, Coleman DJ. High resolution computerized tomography and B-scan ultrasonography of the orbits. *Trans Am Acad Ophthalmol Otolaryngol* 1974:**81**:607–617.

Hilal SK, Trokel SL. Computerized tomography of the orbit using thin sections. *Semin Radiol.* 1977:**12**:137.

Hollenhorst RW Jr, Hollenhorst RW Sr, MacCarty CS. Visual prognosis of optic nerve sheath meningiomas producing shunt vessels on the optic disc. *Mayo Clin Proc.* 1978:**53**:84–92. Also: *Trans Am Ophthalmol Soc* 1977:**75**:141–163.

Hoyt WF, Meshel LG, Lessel S, *et al.* Malignant optic glioma of adulthood. *Brain* 1973:**96**:121–132.

Iliff CE. Tumors of the orbit. *Trans Am Ophthalmol Soc.* 1957:**55**:505.

Iliff WU, Green WR. Orbital lymphangiomas. Ophthalmology 1979:**86**:914–929.

Jakobiec FA, McLean I, Font RL. Clinicopathologic characteristics of orbital lymphoid hyperplasia. *Ophthalmology.* 1979:**86**:948–966.

Jakobiec FA, Henkind P. Editorial. Ophthalmic CT scanning: The quest for precision and specificity. *Ophthalmology* 1980:**87**:13A.

Jakobiec FA, Yeo JH, Trokel SL, Abbott GF, Anderson RL, Alper MG, and Citrin CM: Combined clinical and computed tomographic diagnosis of primary lacrimal fossa lesions. *Am J Ophthalmol* 1982:**94**:785–807.

Jakobiec FA, Rootman J, Jones IS: Secondary and metastatic tumors of the orbit. In: Duane TD, Jaeger EA eds. *Clinical Ophthalmology*. Philadelphia:Harper and Row. **Vol 2**, pp 1067, 1982.

Jakobiec FA, Depot MJ, Kennerdell JS, Shults WT, Anderson RL, Alper MG, Citrin CM, Hosepian EMN, Trokel SL: Combined clinical and computed tomographic diagnosis of orbital glioma and meningioma. *Ophthalmology* 1984:**91**:137–155.

Karp LA, Zimmerman LE, Borit A, Spencer WH. Primary intraorbital meningiomas. *Arch Ophthalmol* 1974:**91**:24–28.

Kennerdell JS, Dekker A, Johnson BL: Orbital fine needle aspiration biopsy: The results of its use in 50 patients. *Neuro-Ophthalmol.* 1980:**1**:117–121.

Knowles DM II, Jakobiec FA. Orbital lymphoid neoplasms. A clinico-pathologic study of 60 patients. *Cancer.* 1980:**46**:576–589.

Kronlein RU. Zur pathologie und opeerativen behandlung der Dermoidcysten. *Beits Klin Chir* 1888:**4**:149.

Lindblom B, Truwit CL, Hoyt WF: Optic nerve sheath meningioma: Definition of intraorbital, intracranial and intracranial components with magnetic resonance imaging. *Ophthalmology*, 1992:**99**:560–566.

Lloyd GAS: CT scanning in diagnosis of orbital disease. *Comput Tomogr* 1979:**3**:227.

Lombardi G: *Radiology in neuro-ophthalmology*. Baltimore:Williams and Wilkins, 1967.

Manchester PT, Bonmati J: Idopyacet (Diodrast) injection for orbital tumors. *Arch Ophthalmol* 1955:**54**:591.

Moseley IF, Sanders MD: Diseases of the orbit. In: *Computerized tomography in neuro-ophthalmology*. Philadelphia:Toronto:W.B. Saunders Company pp 209–82, 1982.

Moseley I, Brant-Zawadzki M, Mills C. Nuclear magnetic resonance imaging of the orbit. *Br J Ophthalmol* 1983:**67**:333–342.

Naffziger HC: Pathologic changes in the orbit in progressive exophthalmos. *Arch Ophthalmol* 1932:**9**:1.

Naffziger HC: Progressive exophthalmos. An R Coll Surg Engl 1954:**15**:1–24.

Newton TH, Potts DG: *Advanced imaging techniques. Modern Neuroradiology*, **Vol 2**, Clavedel Press:California. 1983.

Parsons C, Hodson N: Computed tomography of paranasal sinus tumors. *Radiology* 1979:**132**:641–645.

Partain CL, James Jr AE, Rollo FD, Price RR. *Nuclear magnetic resonance (MRI) imaging.* Philadelphia:L.W.B. Saunders Co. 1983.

Reese AB: *Tumors of the eye* (second edition). Hagerstown, MD:Harper & Row, 1963.

Reese AB: *Tumors of the eye* (third edition). Hagerstown, MD:Harper & Row, 1976.

Rose GE: Orbital meningiomas: Surgery, radiotherapy, or hormones? *Br J Ophthalmol.* 1993:**77**:313–314.

Silva D: Orbital tumors. *Am J Ophthal.* 1968:**65**:318–339.

Spencer WH: Primary neoplasms of the optic nerve and its sheaths: Clinical features and current concepts of pathogenetic mechanisms. *Trans Am Ophthalmol Soc* 1972:**70**:490–528.

Spoor TC, Kennerdell JS, Kekker A, Johnson BL, Rehkopf P. Orbital fine needle aspiration biopsy with B-scan guidance. *Am J. Ophthalmol* 1980:**89**:274–277.

Spoor TC, Kennerdell JS, Martiney AJ, Zorub D. Malignant gliomas of the optic nerve pathways. *Am J Ophthalmol.* 1980:**89**:284–292.

Trokel SL, Hilal SK: recognition and differential diagnosis of enlarged extraocular muscles in computed tomography. *Am J Ophthalmol.* 1979:**87**:503–512.

Unsold R, DeGroot J, Newton TH. Images of the optic nerve: Anatomic CT Correlation. *AJNR* 1980:**1**:317–323.

Unsold R, DeGroot J, Newton TH: Images of the optic nerve. Anatomic CT Correlation. *AJR* 1980:**135**:767–773.

Walton PG: An instrument for measuring ocular displacement; the ocular topometer. *Trans Ophthalmol Soc UK* 1967:**87**:409–430.

Werner SC: Classification of eye changes of Graves' disease. *Am J Ophthalmol.* 1969:**68**:646–648.

Werner SC: Modification of the classification of eye changes of Graves' disease; recommendations of the Ad Hoc Committee of the American Thyroid Association. *J Clin Endocrinol Metab.* 1977:**44**:203–204.

Werner SC, Ingbar SH. *The thyroid* (third edition). New York:Harper & Row Publishers. 1971.

Wright JE. The role of surgery in the management of orbital tumors. *Mod Probl Ophthalmol.* 1975:**14**:553.

Wright JE. Primary optic nerve meningiomas: Clinical presentation and management. *Tr Am Acad Ophthalmol and Otolaryngol* 1977:**83**:OP617–625.

Wright JE, Rose GE, Garner A. Primary malignant neoplasms of the lacrimal gland. *Br J Ophthalmol.* 1992:**76**:401–407.

Wright JE, Stewart WB, Krohel GB. Clinical presentation and management of lacrimal gland tumors. *Br J Ophthalmol.* 1979:**63**:600.

Wright JE, Call NB, Liaricos S: Primary optic nerve meningiomas. *Br J Ophthalmol* 1980:**64**:553–558.

Zimmerman LE: Arachnoid hyperplasia in optic nerve glioma. *Br J Ophthalmol* 1980:**64**:638–639.

Zimmerman LE: Pathology and computed tomography. *Ophthalmology* 1980:**87**:602.

CHAPTER 13

The Pupil

Randy H Kardon, H Stanley Thompson

EXAMINING THE PUPILS

THE BEDSIDE OR OFFICE EXAMINATION

Conditions and Equipment for the Pupil Exam

Good Visibility. Clinical decisions about pupillary function are based on observations, so the examiner must, of course, be able to see the pupils well. It is astonishing that this needs to be stated, but one cannot depend upon pupillary abnormalities to be immediately obvious. They must be searched for.

Comfort. Both the patient and the examiner should be comfortable. There are several important observations to make – so take your time, get comfortable, and do it correctly. Patients should be instructed to 'lean forward a little' before being asked to look at a distant point. The patient must be close enough for the details of the iris to be seen, and the examiner should not be straining forward or holding his or her breath.

Room Lights Out. Begin in darkness or in very dim light. This allows the pupils to start their constriction from a bigger size, and increases the amplitude of the pupillary movement making it easier to see. The light switch should be in easy reach, so that the room lights can be turned on and off without the examiner taking his or her eyes off the patient's pupils.

Hand Light Well Focused and Reasonably Bright. A fiberoptic transilluminator (*Fig. 13.1*) is preferred because it provides a bright,

even beam without hot spots or dim areas (for example, a Welch-Allyn Halogen 3.5v Finhoff transilluminator with a fresh bulb; see *Figures 13.2* and *13.3*).

Pupil Gauge and Neutral Density Filters. Estimating pupil diameter in millimeters is a skill that can be quickly learned by using any pupil gauge calibrated in half millimeter steps.

Estimating the amount of the pupillomotor input asymmetry (the 'relative afferent pupillary defect') can of course be done

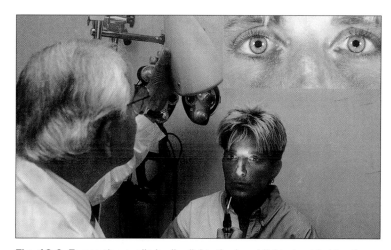

Fig. 13.2 To see the pupils in dim light, the hand light should shine from below while the patient looks up into the darkness. The room lights can then be turned on and off to see if the pupils respond to light and whether the illumination influences the pupillary inequality.

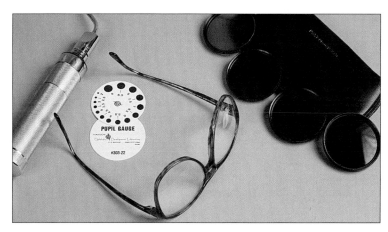

Fig. 13.1 The equipment required for the basic clinical examination of the pupils: a bright hand light with an even spread of light (in this case a halogen-bulb, fiberoptic transilluminator), a simple pupil gauge in 0.5 mm steps, and a few neutral density filters (0.3, 0.6, 0.9, and 1.2 log).

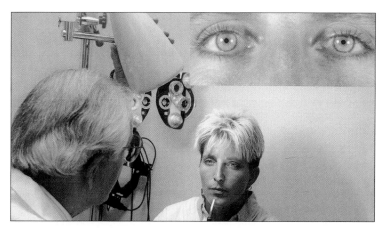

Fig. 13.3 When the room lights are turned on, look to see how the anisocoria has changed. In this normal subject there is a clinically trivial 'simple anisocoria' in darkness that goes away with light.

roughly using the alternating light test – without any neutral density filters; but when done by this method, some wild errors can occur due to age variations in pupil size and pupil mobility. Estimating the size of a relative afferent pupillary defect without using filters is very much like estimating an ocular deviation 'by Hirschberg', without doing a prism cover test. Photographic neutral density filters are recommended (49 mm, screw mount, 0.3 log, 0.6 log, and 0.9 log). These are sometimes available through local photographic supply stores.

The Examination
There are three stages to the examination of the pupils: 1) evaluation of anisocoria; 2) evaluating the input (afferent) arm of the light reflex arc; and 3) evaluation of the near response.

Evaluation of Anisocoria. Pupillary inequality – anisocoria – is usually due to an iris innervation problem, so evaluating this condition is a matter of deciding whether all four iris muscles are properly wired up. In the office, the best way to decide whether it is the sphincter muscle or the dilator muscle that is weak is to compare the amount of anisocoria in darkness and in light. This can be done without any special equipment. The examiner has to be able to change the lighting and still see the pupils, as demonstrated in *Figures 13.2* and *13.3*.

Of course, there is usually no anisocoria in darkness or in light. At this point the output (efferent) arm of the light reflex arc can be presumed to be intact, and the examiner can proceed to check for an afferent defect. But if there is an anisocoria, it should be established whether this increases in darkness or in light (*Fig. 13.4*).

Evaluating the Input (Afferent) Arm of the Light Reflex arc. Measuring the relative afferent pupillary defect (RAPD) is the most important part of the pupil examination – it is the most frequently used part of the exam, and it gives the most valuable clinical information. The alternating light test for an afferent

defect is usually based on the assumption that the subject has a matched pair of irises, each of them with both muscles in good shape and properly innervated, so that the light reactions can be compared. It is important, therefore, to decide first that there is no output (efferent) defect.

If one sphincter is weak, the examiner can, of course, still check for an afferent defect by watching the pupil that still works, and comparing its direct reaction and its consensual reaction. If there seems to be no asymmetry, this should be confirmed with the 'tilt test' (see 'Tilting' the dubious RAPD, below; *Figures. 13.5* and *13.6*).

Measuring the Relative Afferent Pupillary Defect.
- **Check for an impaired light reaction.** If one pupil has a consistently poor reaction to light ('an output defect'), then all observations should be made in the eye with the better light reaction.
- **Will an anisocoria influence the estimate of the pupillary input asymmetry?** Small pupils let in less light and large pupils let in more. If neither pupil is smaller than 3 mm in light, however, then any anisocoria of less than 2.0 mm can be disregarded, at least with respect to a false afferent defect induced by the pupillary inequality. In short, only very large anisocorias cause enough difference in retinal illumination between the two eyes to produce an apparent asymmetry of pupillomotor input.
- **Alternate the light from one eye to the other** (*Fig. 13.7*). If the light is too bright the pupils will not redilate promptly, so very little pupillary movement will be seen. There are two ways to get around this problem: 1) reduce the stimulus intensity by backing the light away to 3 or 4 inches from the eyes and then continue to alternate the light; or 2) increase the darkness interval by deliberately passing the light under the patient's nose on the way from one eye to the other; this allows for a brief further dark adaptation, and sets the starting pupil diameter of the about-to-be-illuminated eye at a higher level. The second way gives a more visible light reaction, but it reduces the slight

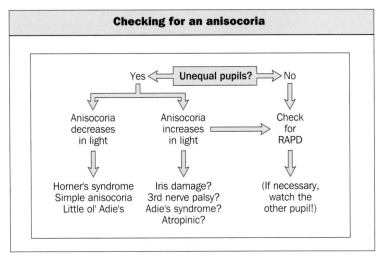

Fig. 13.4 Before checking for an input asymmetry, look for an output asymmetry (an anisocoria) that may influence the measurement. If the anisocoria decreases in light (i.e. the anisocoria is greater in darkness), then look for other signs of Horner's syndrome. If none can be seen, then it may be a 'simple anisocoria' (see below). If the bigger pupil does not constrict well in light (resulting in more anisocoria in light than in darkness) then the sphincter is weak or has poor innervation. Is the iris damaged? Has the patient had a mydriatic drop or ointment? Is there a third nerve palsy? Is it an Adie's pupil? The anisocoria should be explained first, in order to select which pupil should be watched when looking for an afferent defect.

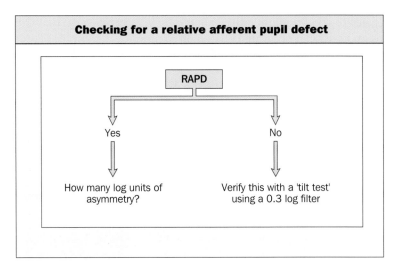

Fig. 13.5 If the pupils constrict better when the light shines in one eye than they do when it shines in the other, the degree of asymmetry of pupillomotor input should be estimated. If there seems to be no asymmetry, the 'tilt test' should be attempted.

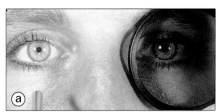

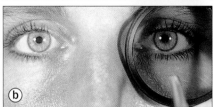

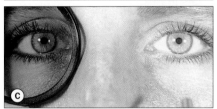

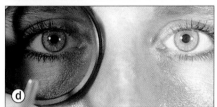

Fig. 13.6 The tilt test. In this normal subject, with no afferent defect, a pupillary input defect can be artificially induced by simply holding a 0.3 log neutral density filter over one eye and repeating the alternating light test. Since roughly the same size of relative afferent pupillary defect was induced with the filter over the left eye (**a** and **b**) as with the filter over the right eye (**c** and **d**), there is no significant asymmetry of input. If, for example, the patient had a very small input defect in the left eye (say 0.2 log units), then adding a 0.3 log filter over the suspected left eye would increase it to 0.5 log units – an easily visible asymmetry of response; whereas the same filter over the right eye would produce a negligible defect (0.1 log) in the other direction. This difference in behavior when the filter is over different eyes indicates that the RAPD is real.

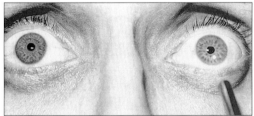

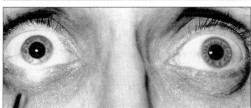

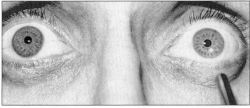

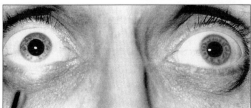

Fig. 13.7 This patient has a large afferent defect in the right eye. It is best demonstrated by alternating the light from eye to eye at a steady rate. The light should be kept just below the visual axis and one to two inches from each eye. Each eye should be illuminated for about 1 full second and then the light switched quickly to the other eye; this allows comparison of the initial direct contraction to light in each eye. If the examiner prefers to look for pupillary escape, the light should be held on each eye for 3 seconds and pupillary dilatation observed before switching to the other eye.

amplification of the difference between the two responses that comes with prompt alternation of the light.

- **Observe the illuminated eye.** If the pupils react relatively weakly when one eye is stimulated and better when the other is stimulated, an afferent defect relative to the better eye (an RAPD) has been identified.
- **Balance the responses with filters.** This should be done by holding a filter up over the good eye and repeating the alternating light test. If the input asymmetry is still visible, the density of the filter over the good eye should be increased until the amplitude of the direct light reactions of the two eyes is balanced. The balance point should be deliberately overshot and then returned to, for the measurement to be confirmed. When a dense filter is used it may be necessary to peek behind the filter just to see the pupil (*Fig. 13.8*).
- **'Tilting' the dubious RAPD.** If a very small asymmetry is suspected, e.g. a defect of less than 0.3 log in the left eye, but the examiner is unsure whether this is just noise in the system (i.e. 'hippus'), an effort can be made to confirm the asymmetry by 'tilting' the RAPD to the right and to the left with a 0.3 log filter (see Fig. 13.6).
- **Moment to moment variability.** Unfortunately, the pupillary response to a repeated light stimulus is far from constant; it changes from moment to moment. This means that, for practical purposes, every clinical measurement of an RAPD should have '+/- 0.2 log' appended to it.
- **Small children. Infants and small children may appear to have weak pupillary responses to light.** This is due to excitement and apprehension. When the light stimulus is repeated several times the light reaction usually improves. A baby's pupils can be checked from about a meter away with a direct ophthalmoscope. The brightest light with the smallest spot should be used, in a dark room, focusing on the red reflex and alternating from eye to eye. The baby is usually fascinated, and a filter can sometimes be placed in the beam to one eye.
- **Only one working pupil.** When the input defect is in an eye with an injured iris or a dilated pupil, attention should be on the pupillary responses of the uninjured eye. The direct and consensual responses of the working pupil can still be compared by alternating the light from one eye to the other. While a measurement is being made, the good eye is behind the filter and it may be hard to see the pupil. Sometimes it is necessary to use a side light on the good iris in order to see its consensual pupil reaction. This may corrupt the measurement, so, if pos-

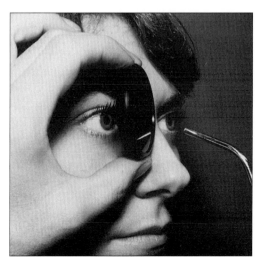

Fig. 13.8 A dark iris will, naturally, seem even darker behind the filter so that it may be hard to see the pupil; in this situation it helps to peek behind the filter to get a better view of the iris.

sible, an infrared video system should be used.
- **Kestenbaum's number.** Kestenbaum was the first to suggest, in 1946, that it might be valuable to quantify the amount of damage to the pupillomotor input fibers in one optic nerve compared to the other. He suggested comparing the direct pupil response in each eye by covering one eye and measuring the pupil diameter attained in the illuminated eye (*Fig 13.9*). The difference (in mm) between the two pupils thus measured he called a *'pseudoanisocoria'*, and this number comes surprisingly close to the RAPD measured with filters. This estimate of pupillary input asymmetry requires that both muscles in each iris be working normally; it works best in young people with mobile pupils. This technique should be used only when filters are unavailable.

Evaluation of the near response. The pupillary response to a near effort must be checked. If the light reaction seems a little weak, the examiner should look to see if the pupils constrict better to a near stimulus than they do to light. If they do, this is called a 'light–near dissociation'.
- **How to test for a pupillary near response.** The pupillary near reaction is usually weak when tested in dim light or in the dark. The patient needs to see what he or she is looking at before trying to get it into focus. A near response should not be attempted at the slit lamp unless the magnification is necessary to see segmental contractions of the iris sphincter; the room is usually dark and there is too much equipment in the patient's face.

The near response should be looked for in moderate room light so that the patient's pupils are mid-sized, and the near object is clearly visible.

The patient should be given an accommodative target to look at: something of interest or with fine detail on it (*Fig. 13.10*). Sometimes a better response is obtained if some other sensory input is added to the stimulus. Something auditory, for example, such as a ticking watch or clicking fingernails, or something proprioceptive, for example the patient's own

thumbnail, can be held up in front of him or her; perhaps, in the case of a child, with a little face drawn on it (see Fig. 13.10).

The examiner should watch for convergence to help him or her judge how hard the patient is trying. Remember that the near response, although it may be triggered by blurred or disparate imagery, has a large volitional component, and the patient may need encouragement. If, for some reason, the patient has not been making a near effort recently (for example, because stereopsis is not achieved at near), then the patient may need a few practice runs. Often on the third or fourth try the patient will produce a good response. If a good near response is not achieved, it is usually because the patient (or the examiner) has not been trying hard enough.

A patient who is completely blind and has no pupillary reaction to light will still sometimes produce a good near response if you ask him or her to 'cross your eyes like you did when you were a child'. If a patient fails to produce a near response, the 'lid closure reflex' should be attempted: the patient should be asked to look at the examiner and squeeze his or her eyes shut while the examiner tries, with both hands, to hold one of them open. This will often produce a surprisingly strong near response. This is called the *'eye-closure pupil reaction'*.
- **Recognizing a light–near dissociation.** Sometimes, in a doubtful case, it is hard to know where to draw the line. When is the near response clearly greater than the light reaction? When facing the patient, with pocket light in hand, there are usually three levels of light available to the examiner: (1) darkness, with a light shining tangentially on the pupils from below; (2) room light; (3) room light with an additional bright light in the eyes.

With the patient looking into the distance, bright light should be shone into the patient's eye three or four times, each time for only 1 or 2 seconds. This tells the examiner how small the pupils will go with just a light stimulus. The near response should never be judged by adding a near stimulus to a bright light stimulus; this almost always produces an apparent light–near dissociation because the near stimulus inevitably adds something to the light stimulus. A real light–near dissociation is present only if the near response (tested in moderate light) exceeds the best constriction that bright light can produce.

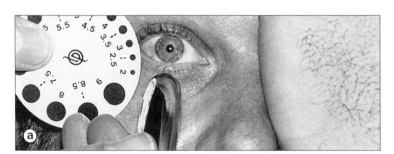
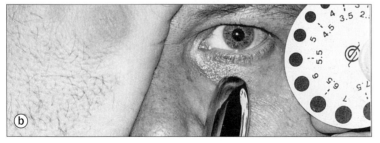

Fig. 13.9 (a) Measuring Kestenbaum's number. The patient should cover one eye firmly; a bright light should be shone in the exposed eye from a distance of about 1 inch and a pupil gauge used to estimate the average pupil diameter attained. (b) This should be repeated for the other eye. The difference (in mm) between the two pupils is Kestenbaum's number. This patient appears to have had a large relative afferent pupillary defect – about 2.0 log units (5 mm OS *minus* 3 mm OD).

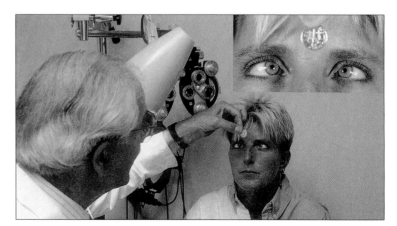

Fig. 13.10 The near response of the pupils is best checked in moderate light, using an accommodative target.

A MAGNIFIED VIEW

Neurologists who do not have a slit lamp at hand may achieve adequate results with the magnification provided by an otoscope or ophthalmoscope; ophthalmologists, however, will insist on a slit lamp because they are comfortable with it and know that it provides an excellent view of the iris. This magnification is necessary to make sure that there is no local iris cause for pupil distortion or immobility. Segmental palsy of the iris sphincter can be immediately recognized; this is a clear indication of denervation of the sphincter due to neuropathy or injury. In addition, structural abnormalities of the iris can be identified (*Fig. 13.11*).

The slit beam feature of the slit lamp should not be used to examine the iris. It is not necessary, as the iris is usually all on one plane. A broad beam should be used, coming from one side, so that shadows of the stromal details bring out all the dips and bumps.

PHOTOGRAPHY OF THE PUPIL

Self-developing photographs are very helpful because the examiner knows, before the patient leaves, whether he or she has the right picture. If not, another can be taken.

The 'Polaroid CU-5 Close-Up Camera' uses type 669 color film, which is pulled out of the camera and the paper peeled off the picture. This type of camera can be used on a day to day basis to record diagnostic pupillary pharmacologic tests (*Fig. 13.12a*), droopy lids and eye movement abnormalities, and an occasional MRI for the chart. Newer Polaroid cameras (*Fig. 13.12b*) use Type 339 color film, which automatically ejects out of the camera. Other manufacturers have recently introduced digital (filmless) cameras suitable for pupillary work. A camera should be able to take a life-size picture showing both eyes at the same moment in time. As the exposure has already been

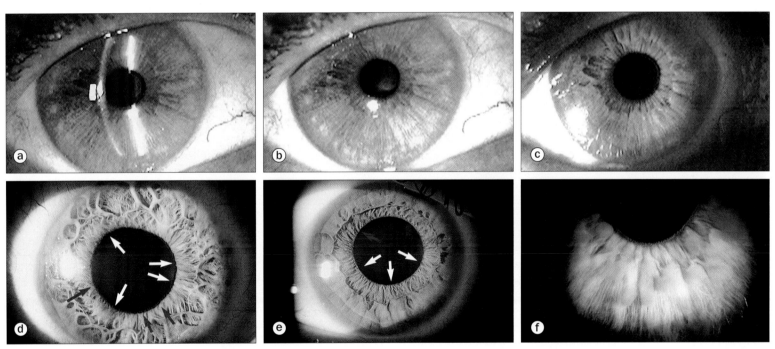

Fig. 13.11 (**a**) A normal iris, illuminated with a slit beam in the usual way. Only a small sliver of the iris is brightened by the beam and the stromal details are not well seen. (**b**) Full frontal illumination flattens the image of the iris, diminishing the iris details. (**c**) A broad beam of light shining from the side throws shadows into the stromal crypts of the same normal iris and adds depth to the view of the iris. This makes it easier to recognize the features that are characteristic of regional palsy of the iris sphincter muscle. (**d**) A 33-year-old man with Adie's tonic pupil. The white arrows are pointing to sectors of the sphincter that are contracting well, and the red arrowheads indicate areas in which the iris sphincter is weak. Notice that the curvature of the pupillary margin is usually tighter in the sections that are functional and flatter in the palsied parts. (**e**) A 50-year-old woman with Adie's tonic pupil. The lower half of the iris sphincter (white arrows) still contracts reasonably well, but the top half is weak (red arrow). The red arrow points to a weak section at 10 o'clock, over which the corrugated iris stroma can be seen to stream towards 9 o'clock, pulled by the tightened sphincter segment in that area. (**f**) A patient with neurofibromatosis (type 1). The brown Sakurai–Lisch nodules stand out when tangential light rakes across the iris stroma.

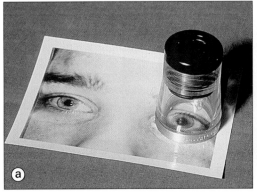
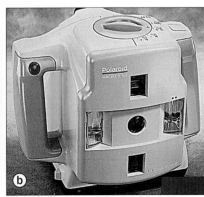

Fig. 13.12 (a) As Polaroid pictures are exactly 1:1, the pupil diameters (and the anisocoria) can be measured directly from the photographs with the help of a magnifying loupe. (**b**) The Polaroid Macro 5 SLR also has separate lenses for different magnifications and uses no-touch, laser beam focusing.

made before the pupil has had a chance to constrict, flash photography can be used to capture pupil size and anisocoria in darkness or in light, and with the patient looking in the distance or at near.

INFRARED VIDEOGRAPHY

Infrared videography (*Fig. 13.13*) allows the examiner to see the movement of both pupils at once clearly in the dark (*Fig. 13.14*). This is especially helpful for checking difficult afferent pupil defects, e.g. when one pupil is fixed, or both irises are very dark. Videography is also useful when looking for dilatation lag of a Horner's pupil, for catching the brief paradoxical constriction when the lights are turned out in patients with some retinal abnormalities, and for transilluminating the iris in pigment dispersion syndrome and in Adie's syndrome (*Fig. 13.15*).

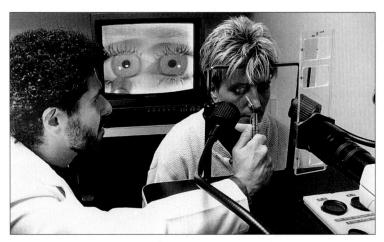

Fig. 13.13 Infrared video-pupillometer. The infrared sources (clusters of LEDs) are mounted in gooseneck lamps. The double base-out prisms bring the pupils close together on the screen.

COMPUTERIZED PUPILLOMETRY

Various computerized, infrared-sensitive pupillometers are commercially available (*Fig. 13.16a*). Most of these elegant instruments can record precisely the dynamics of pupillary movement in the light or in the dark. Once recorded, the pupillary information can be analyzed by sophisticated software (*Fig. 13.16b*).

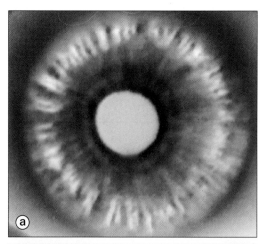

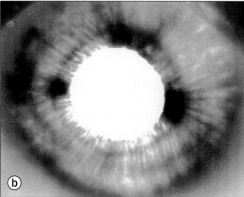

Fig. 13.15
(a) Transillumination of the iris in a patient with pigment dispersion syndrome. Glaucoma experts feel that infrared videography is a sensitive technique for detecting early iris lucencies in this condition.
(b) Transillumination of the iris in a patient with Adie's syndrome. The segmental sphincter palsies (light zones) and the areas of aberrant innervation (the dark zones of contracted sphincter) can be seen better with infrared video transillumination than with color slit lamp examination of the iris stroma.

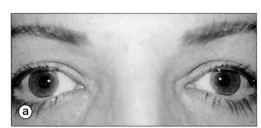

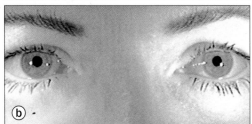

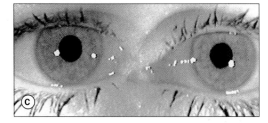

Fig. 13.14 (a) A pair of brown eyes in room light showing how difficult it often is to see the pupils. (b) The same eyes as seen in infrared illumination by the video-pupillometer. Melanin in the iris stroma reflects the infrared light, enhancing the contrast. (c) The same infrared video view, with the base-out prisms in place. Eliminating the nose makes better use of the video screen area available and allows added magnification of the pupils.

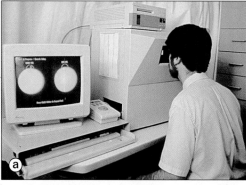

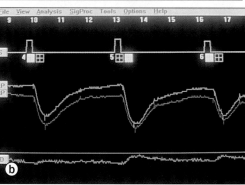

Fig. 13.16 (a) An example of a binocular infrared computerized pupillometer. (b) Tracings of the pupil diameter of both pupils in a normal subject with anisocoria, analyzed and diplayed by computer software.

PUPIL PERIMETRY

An automated perimeter can be modified to record pupillary responses. A video camera is pointed at the pupil and the amplitude of each light reaction is measured and stored in the computer. This is helpful for localizing lesions in the pupillary pathways (*Fig. 13.17*), and for demonstrating that messages are indeed going normally into the brain from parts of the visual field in which the patient claims to see nothing because of functional visual loss.

PUPILLARY ABNORMALITIES

ANISOCORIA

As mentioned above, pupillary inequality usually means that one of the four iris muscles, or its innervation, is damaged (*Figs 13.18, 13.19*). To establish which muscle is not working properly, it helps to know how the anisocoria is influenced by light. It is also worth noting that an anisocoria always increases in the direction of action of the paretic iris muscle, just as an esotropia increases when gaze is in the direction of action of a weak lateral rectus muscle.

The Patient with a Pupillary Inequality that Increases in the Dark

In such patients, the problem is distinguishing a Horner's syndrome from a 'simple anisocoria' (or 'physiologic anisocoria'), in which the inequality is also greater in dim light compared to bright light. A simple anisocoria may vary from day to day, or even from hour to hour, and is visible in about one-fifth of the normal population; it is not related to refractive error. Clinically, Horner's syndrome is recognized by looking for the associated signs, such as ptosis, 'upside down ptosis' of the lower lid, and, in a fresh case, conjunctival injection and lowered intraocular pressure.

Simple anisocoria is common (about 10% of normal subjects, examined in room light, will have an anisocoria of 0.4mm or more), is not associated with disease, and may change from day to day. Simple anisocoria also, like Horner' syndrome, decreases slightly in light, but it does not show a dilatation lag of the smaller pupil (*Fig. 13.20*), as would be seen in Horner's syndrome.

Is the smaller pupil slow to dilate?

The characteristic 'dilatation lag' of the Horner's pupil can be easily seen in the office with a hand light shining from below. The room lights should be switched off and the smaller pupil examined to see if it appears reluctant to dilate. Pupillary dilatation is normally a combination of sphincter relaxation and dilator contraction. This combination produces a prompt dilatation. The patient with Horner's syndrome has a weak dilator muscle in one iris and, as a result, that pupil dilates more slowly than the normal pupil. If the sympathetic lesion is complete, the affected pupil will dilate only by sphincter relaxation. This asymmetry of pupillary dilatation produces an anisocoria which is most prominent 4 to 5s after the lights are turned out. This is a much slower process than most people imagine. Ten to 20s after the lights are out, the anisocoria lessens as the sympathectomized pupil gradually catches up (*Fig. 13.21*).

This test is a quick and simple way of distinguishing Horner's syndrome from simple anisocoria, and it is a test that does not require pupillary drug testing. It works well most of the time, especially in young people with mobile pupils, but if the dilatation asymmetry is inconclusive, cocaine eye drops may be used to confirm the diagnosis of Horner's syndrome.

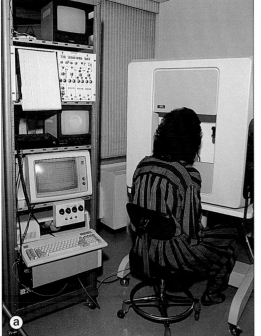
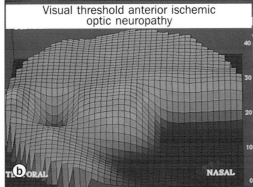
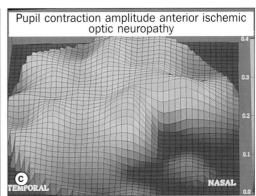

Fig. 13.17 (a) Pupil perimetry. An automated perimeter has been modified to record pupil responses to the same light stimuli, in the same locations that are used for conventional perimetry. **(b)** A visual field in a patient with anterior ischemic optic neuropathy, showing inferior nasal and arcuate defects in the left eye. This was done with a Humphrey perimeter (30-2) and the threshold was plotted to give the illusion of a three-dimensional 'island of vision'. **(c)** A 'pupil field' of the same eye, plotted in the same way, showing the amplitude of the pupillary responses obtained from the same 76 locations as the 30-2 field (but using a size V stimulus). Note that there is a pupil defect inferonasally, in the same region as the visual field defect. The obvious advantage of this technique is that the data jump into the computer automatically – with the help of a brainstem reflex arc. The patient has only to keep his eyes open and maintain fixation.

The innervation of the iris muscles

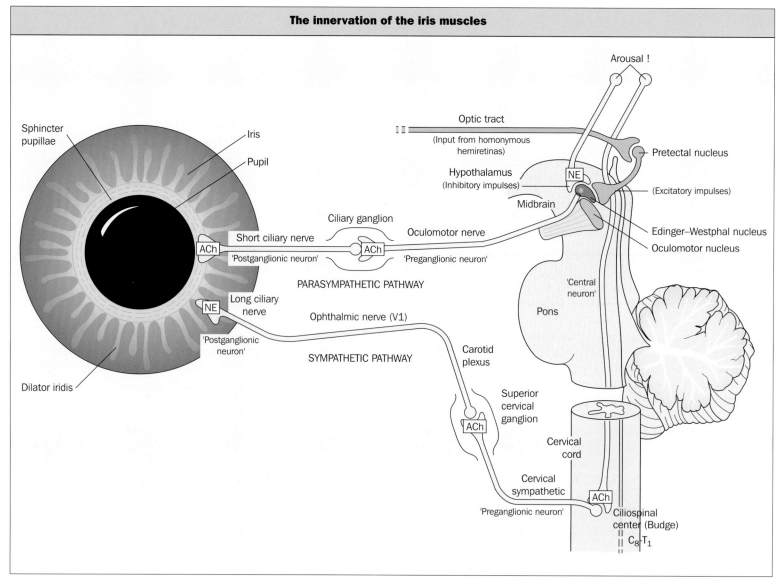

Fig. 13.18 The parasympathetic and sympathetic innervation of the iris muscles. From the CNS to the effector muscle there are always two neurons (pre- and postganglionic). This is also true for the ciliary muscle that controls accommodation. Both ganglia (ciliary and superior cervical) are cholinergic, but the sympathetic neuro-effector junction is adrenergic. Notice that the inhibitory fibers to the sphincter nucleus (Edinger–Westphal) are also adrenergic, so that both centrally and peripherally norepinephrine acts to dilate the pupil.

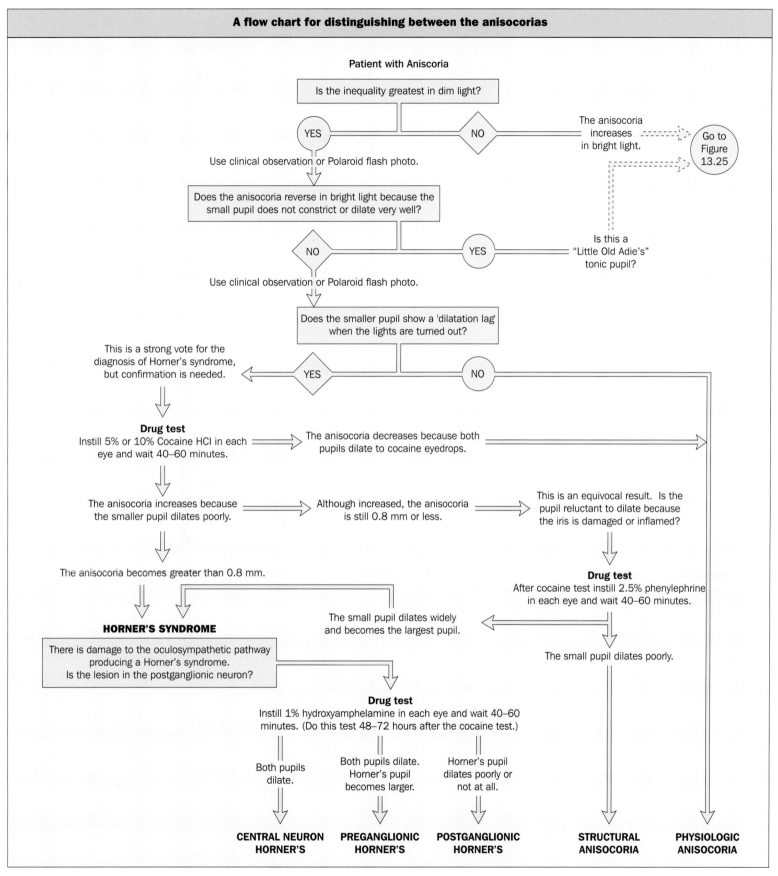

A flow chart for distinguishing between the anisocorias

Patient with Aniscoria

Is the inequality greatest in dim light?

YES — NO

The anisocoria increases in bright light. → Go to Figure 13.25

Use clinical observation or Polaroid flash photo.

Does the anisocoria reverse in bright light because the small pupil does not constrict or dilate very well?

NO — YES

Is this a "Little Old Adie's" tonic pupil?

Use clinical observation or Polaroid flash photo.

Does the smaller pupil show a 'dilatation lag' when the lights are turned out?

This is a strong vote for the diagnosis of Horner's syndrome, but confirmation is needed. ← YES — NO

Drug test
Instill 5% or 10% Cocaine HCl in each eye and wait 40–60 minutes.

The anisocoria decreases because both pupils dilate to cocaine eyedrops.

The anisocoria increases because the smaller pupil dilates poorly.

Although increased, the anisocoria is still 0.8 mm or less.

This is an equivocal result. Is the pupil reluctant to dilate because the iris is damaged or inflamed?

The anisocoria becomes greater than 0.8 mm.

HORNER'S SYNDROME

There is damage to the oculosympathetic pathway producing a Horner's syndrome. Is the lesion in the postganglionic neuron?

The small pupil dilates widely and becomes the largest pupil.

Drug test
After cocaine test instill 2.5% phenylephrine in each eye and wait 40–60 minutes.

The small pupil dilates poorly.

Drug test
Instill 1% hydroxyamphelamine in each eye and wait 40–60 minutes. (Do this test 48–72 hours after the cocaine test.)

Both pupils dilate.

Both pupils dilate. Horner's pupil becomes larger.

Horner's pupil dilates poorly or not at all.

CENTRAL NEURON HORNER'S | **PREGANGLIONIC HORNER'S** | **POSTGANGLIONIC HORNER'S** | **STRUCTURAL ANISOCORIA** | **PHYSIOLOGIC ANISOCORIA**

Fig. 13.19 If the anisocoria is greatest in dim light and diminishes in bright light, then the pupillary inequality is either physiologic (a 'simple anisocoria') or due to loss of sympathetic innervation to the dilator muscle (Horner's syndrome). There are a few other conditions to consider, but this chart is concerned only with acute damage to a single intraocular muscle or its innervation. (Reproduced with permission of the American Academy of Ophthalmology)

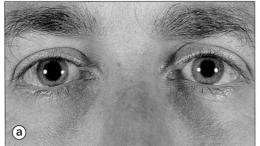
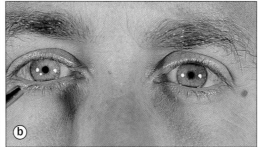
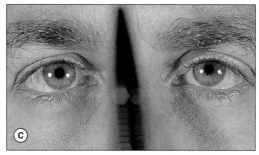

Pupillogram of simple anisocoria

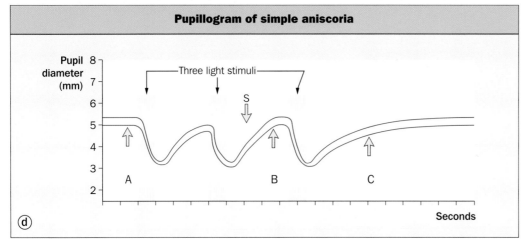

Pupil diameter (mm) — Three light stimuli — S — A — B — C — Seconds

Fig. 13.20 (a) Simple anisocoria – patient in dim light. The right pupil is definitely larger than the left pupil. (**b**) Simple anisocoria – patient in bright light. The pupils are now about equal in size. (**c**) Simple anisocoria – a near response. Anything that makes the pupils smaller will diminish a simple anisocoria. (**d**) Pupillogram of a patient with simple anisocoria: A, there is more anisocoria in darkness – just as in Horner's syndrome; B, unlike Horner's syndrome, a sudden noise (S) causes both pupils to dilate; C, there is no dilatation lag of the smaller pupil, and thus no transient decrease in anisocoria during the ensuing 10–15s.

Pupillogram of oculosympathetic defect

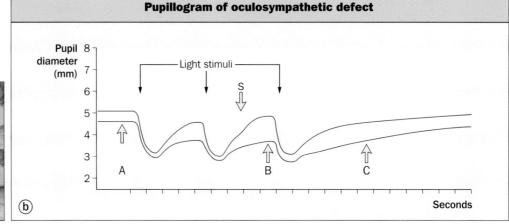

Pupil diameter (mm) — Light stimuli — S — A — B — C — Seconds

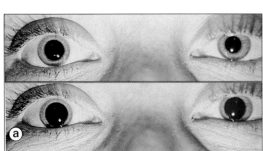

Fig. 13.21 (a) Left Horner's Syndrome – Dilatation lag in a patient with Horner's syndrome. The top photograph was taken 5 s after the lights went out: the right pupil has already dilated but the left pupil has fallen behind because the radial dilator muscle is not pulling the pupil open. The bottom picture was taken 15 s after lights-out: both pupils have now dilated fully. This delay of dilatation as the iris sphincter relaxes in darkness is characteristic of Horner's syndrome. (**b**) Pupillogram of patient with Horner's syndrome. Note the characteristic fluctuations in anisocoria: A, more anisocoria in darkness than in light; B, an abrupt increase in anisocoria after a sudden noise (S) – due to a sympathetic discharge to the innervated dilator muscle; C, a temporary increase in anisocoria after the lights have gone out, then a decrease, due to 'dilatation lag' of the Horner's pupil.

Is it really a Horner's syndrome?

Cocaine acts by blocking the re-uptake of the norepinephrine that is normally released from the nerve endings. If norepinephrine is not being released, because of an interruption in the sympathetic pathway, cocaine has no adrenergic effect (*Fig. 13.22a*). A Horner's pupil will dilate less to cocaine than the normal pupil, regardless of the location of the lesion. Forty-five minutes after putting cocaine drops in both eyes the anisocoria should have increased markedly because the normal pupil has dilated more than the Horner's pupil (*Fig. 13.22b–d*).

We recommend 10% cocaine HCl (never more than 2 drops) in both eyes to ensure that even the darkest iris receives a full mydriatic dose, without producing a corneal epithelial defect.

(Note that 2%, 4%, and 5% cocaine have also been used successfully as a diagnostic test for Horner's syndrome.) Forty to sixty minutes should be allowed to elapse before the anisocoria is measured.

What is an abnormal cocaine test ?

The likelihood of a diagnosis of Horner's syndrome increases steadily with increasing degrees of pupillary inequality (measured after the instillation of cocaine). Unlike the hydroxyamphetamine test, calculation of the change in the anisocoria from before to after cocaine application is unnecessary. If there is at least 0.8 mm of pupillary inequality after cocaine, the presence of a Horner's syndrome is confirmed (*Fig. 13.22e, f*).

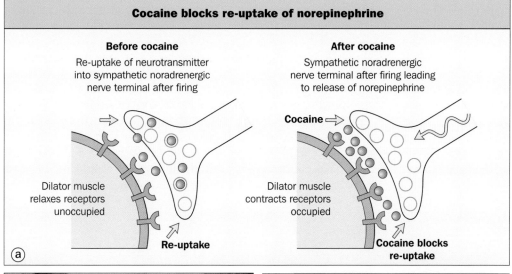

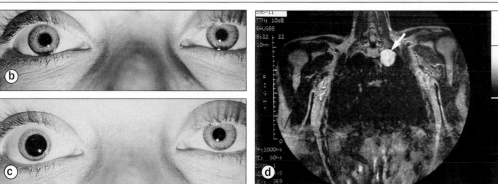

Fig. 13.22 (**a**) The normal re-uptake of norepinephrine into the adrenergic nerve ending contributes to the prompt termination of its action. Cocaine's action is to block this re-uptake, and the norepinephrine still being released from the nerve now piles up at the receptors of the dilator muscle, pulling the pupil wide open. (**b**) Same patient as in Fig. 13.21a, taken in room light before cocaine drops in each eye (**c**) 45 minutes after cocaine HCl 10% had been placed in both eyes. Notice that in the right eye the pupil has dilated and the palpebral fissure has widened, but that the left eye is unaffected by the cocaine. (**d**) Same patient's MRI showing a benign ganglioneuroma in the left pulmonary apex (arrow) damaging the preganglionic sympathetic pathway. (**e**) Frequency distribution for anisocoria measured 60 minutes after cocaine HCl 10% was administered in 50 normal subjects (green bars) and 119 patients with Horner's syndrome (purple bars). (**f**) The odds ratio that a given patient has Horner's syndrome, based on the anisocoria after cocaine eye drops.

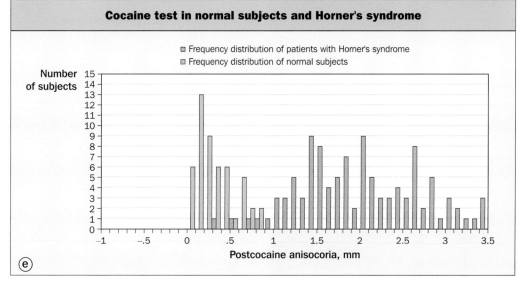

Postcocaine anisocoria		
Anisocoria, mm	Mean odds	Lower 95% confidence
0.0	1:1	1:1
0.1	2:1	2:1
0.2	6:1	2:1
0.3	14:1	4:1
0.4	32:1	6:1
0.5	77:1	10:1
0.6	185:1	15:1
0.7	441:1	24:1
0.8	1050:1	37:1
0.9	2510:1	58:1
1.0	5990:1	92:1

Is the damage to the sympathetic pathway in the postganglionic neuron?

This is a question of considerable clinical importance, as many postganglionic defects are caused by benign vascular headache syndromes, or a carotid dissection and a preganglionic lesion is sometimes due to the spread of a malignant neoplasm.

Hydroxyamphetamine eyedrops help to localize the lesion in Horner's syndrome. The clinician needs to know where the lesion is in order to direct the radiographic work-up, e.g. to the internal carotid artery rather than to the pulmonary apex. Horner's syndrome sometimes presents itself in such a characteristic setting that further efforts at localizing the lesion are not necessary. This is true of patients with 'cluster headaches'.

Hydroxyamphetamine acts by releasing norepinephrine from storage in the sympathetic nerve endings (*Fig. 13.23a*). (Hydroxyamphetamine hydrobromide 1% is now available in the USA from certain independent, licensed, compounding pharmacists. In Europe, 'Pholedrin' is a good substitute; tyramine HCl 5% has the same action, and has been used.) When the lesion is postganglionic, the nerve is dead and no norepinephrine stores are available for release. When the lesion is complete, a pupil like this will not dilate at all. Horner's pupils that are due to preganglionic or central lesions will dilate *at least* normally, because the postganglionic neuron, with its stores of norepinephrine, although disconnected, is still intact (*Fig. 13.23a–c*). In fact, when the lesion is in the preganglionic neuron, the Horner's pupil often becomes larger than the normal pupil, due apparently to 'decentralization supersensitivity'.

Interpreting the hydroxyamphetamine test

The test is simple (*Figs. 13.23b,c*): the pupils are measured *before* and 40–60 minutes *after* hydroxyamphetamine drops have been put into both eyes, and the change in anisocoria in room light is noted. If the Horner's pupil – the smaller one – dilates less than the normal pupil, increasing the anisocoria, the lesion is in the postganglionic neuron. If the smaller pupil dilates well so that it becomes the larger pupil, then the lesion is preganglionic and has left the postganglionic neuron intact. The examiner should wait at least 2 days, preferably 3, after using cocaine before using hydroxyamphetamine; cocaine seems to block its effectiveness.

It is the authors' experience that in about half of ambulatory Horner's syndrome patients, the location of the lesion can be satisfactorily identified by the nature and location of the injury or disease. The other half of Horner's patients offer no clues as to the location of the damage, and a pharmacologic localization of the lesion in these patients would be most helpful.

The authors have attempted to apply what has been learned about hydroxyamphetamine mydriasis in those patients with a known lesion location to those where the lesion location is unknown. (*Fig. 11.23e*). It appears that postganglionic lesions (along the carotid artery) can be separated from the non-postganglionic lesions (in the brainstem, spinal cord, upper lung, and lower neck) with a degree of certainty that varies with the amount of anisocoria induced when the drops are put in both eyes. (*Fig. 13.23f*) shows the chances of the lesion being postganglionic, based on the change in anisocoria.

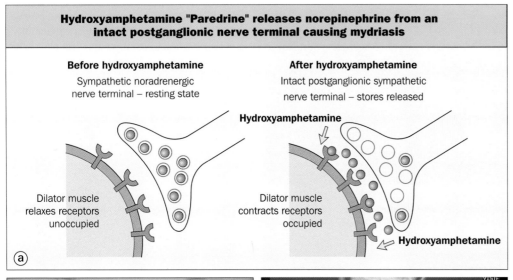

Hydroxyamphetamine "Paredrine" releases norepinephrine from an intact postganglionic nerve terminal causing mydriasis

Before hydroxyamphetamine
Sympathetic noradrenergic nerve terminal – resting state

Dilator muscle relaxes receptors unoccupied

After hydroxyamphetamine
Intact postganglionic sympathetic nerve terminal – stores released

Hydroxyamphetamine

Dilator muscle contracts receptors occupied

Hydroxyamphetamine

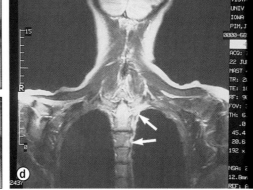

Fig. 13.23 (**a**) Hydroxyamphetamine acts to release norepinephrine from the stores in the adrenergic nerve terminal. If the postganglionic adrenergic nerve fibers no longer exist, there will be no stores of norepinephrine to be released and the hydroxyamphetamine drop will have no mydriatic effect. If, however, it is the central or preganglionic neuron that is interrupted, there will still be stores of norepinephrine in the postganglionic neuron, ready for release. (**b**) Patient with Horner's syndrome before hydroxyamphetamine drops in both eyes. (**c**) Same patient 1 hour after hydroxyamphetamine drops. Notice that there is very little change in the anisocoria; both pupils have dilated. (**d**) MRI of the same patient showing metastatic breast carcinoma along the pleura of the pulmonary apex, presumably damaging the stellate ganglion (arrows).

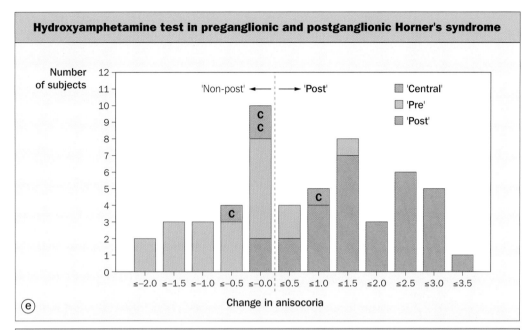

Hydroxyamphetamine test in preganglionic and postganglionic Horner's syndrome

(e)

Fig. 13.23 (**e**) This histogram shows the difference in dilatation induced by instilling hydroxyamphetamine drops in both eyes of 54 patients with Horner's syndrome. The apparent location of the damage to the sympathetic pathway, as judged clinically before the test, is indicated by the color of the bars. Usually, in postganglionic lesions, the affected pupil failed to dilate and the anisocoria increased ('positive' change), whereas in the non-postganglionic lesions both pupils dilated so that there was little change in anisocoria, or the smaller pupil actually became the larger pupil ('negative' change). The four patients believed to have central lesions are marked with a 'C'; the vertical dashed line roughly divides the preganglionic from the post-ganglionic cases based on the change in anisocoria. (**f**) This distribution shows the chances that a lesion is postganglionic for any measured change in anisocoria (from –1.5 to +2.5 mm) with hydroxyamphetamine drops in both eyes.

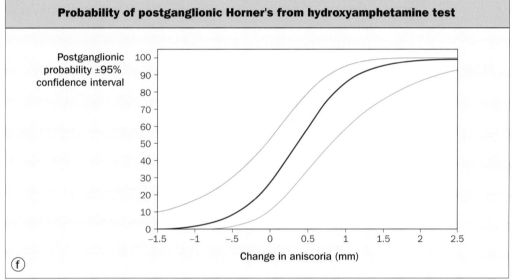

Probability of postganglionic Horner's from hydroxyamphetamine test

(f)

Congenital Horner's syndrome

When a child with a unilateral ptosis and miosis is seen, the first question is whether it is really a Horner's syndrome. The ptosis of Horner's syndrome is moderate, never complete. Sometimes the elevation of the lower lid is persuasive (*Fig.13.24a*). A child with a congenital Horner's and naturally curly hair will, on the affected side of his or her head, have hair that seems limp and lank. The shape of the hair follicles apparently depends on intact sympathetic innervation, as does the iris pigment. A child with blonde, straight hair and very pale blue eyes will not have any visible hair straightness or iris heterochromia.

Cocaine eye drops may be of some diagnostic help. The authors have often used 10% drops with no ill effect, but recommend a weaker solution (two drops of 2% in each eye). The most telling symptom is the hemifacial flush/blanch that occurs with nursing or crying. It is generally the affected side that is pale. In an

air conditioned office it may be hard to decide whether there is an asymmetry of sweating.

A cycloplegic refraction can sometimes produce an atropinic flush everywhere except on the affected face and forehead, and thus unexpectedly solve the diagnostic problem (*Fig. 13.24b*).

In infants, hydroxyamphetamine drops are not helpful in localizing the lesion because orthograde transynaptic dysgenesis takes place at the superior cervical ganglion after an early interruption of the preganglionic oculosympathetic neuron. This results in fewer postganglionic neurons, even though there was no postganglionic injury; this, in turn, produces weak mydriasis and ambiguous answers from the hydroxyamphetamine test.

A Horner's syndrome that has been clearly acquired in infancy should be evaluated for neuroblastoma, a treatable tumor (*Figs 13.24c–f*).

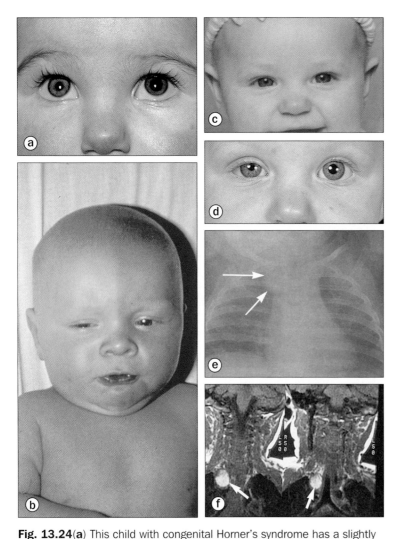

Fig. 13.24 (**a**) This child with congenital Horner's syndrome has a slightly paler iris on the side of the smaller pupil, but there was very little ptosis of the right upper lid. The palpebral fissure was narrower on the right, mainly because the right lower lid was elevated. This 'upside-down ptosis' is a characteristic feature of Horner's syndrome – it may masquerade as 'increased scleral show' in the normal eye. (**b**) This baby, with a right ptosis and miosis, developed a flush during cycloplegia that made the vasomotor abnormality very clear; the Horner's side remained pale. (**c**) This photo from the family album showed that this infant had no signs of Horner's syndrome during her first 8 months. (**d**) The same infant, aged 16 months, with an obvious Horner's syndrome. Note the ptosis, miosis, and up-side-down ptosis. (**e**) Because the syndrome was acquired, a chest x-ray was ordered; this showed a mass in the pulmonary apex (arrows). (**f**) MRI confirmed the lesion (arrows) in two adjacent slices through the neck and surgery showed it to be a neuroblastoma.

If the Patient has a Pupillary Inequality that Increases in the Light
In this situation, there are several questions to be asked (*Fig 11.25*):

Is the iris normal to slit lamp examination?
Trauma to the globe will usually result in a torn sphincter and an iris that transilluminates at the slit lamp. The pupil is often not round and there may be other evidence of ocular injury. Naturally, such a pupil will not constrict well to light. The residual reaction is often segmental in a traumatic iridoplegia. If, however, the iris looks normal, the following questions should be asked:

Is there any residual light reaction at all?
If not, the possibility of atropinic mydriasis arises. However, a completely blocked light reaction can sometimes be seen when the sphincter is denervated by either a preganglionic lesion (third nerve palsy) or a postganglionic lesion (fresh tonic pupil), in acute angle closure (iris ischemia), or in the presence of an intraocular iron foreign body (iron mydriasis). If the dilated pupil still has some response to light, the dilatation could be due to partial denervation of the sphincter, to incomplete atropinization or to adrenergic mydriasis. When the light reaction is poor, because the dilator muscle is in spasm (due to adrenergic mydriatics like phenylephrine), the pupil will be very big, the conjunctiva blanched, and the lid retracted. In such a case, if the amplitude of accommodation is decreased, it will be due to spherical aberration and to a shallow depth of field – both purely optical results of the dilated pupil.

When there is some residual light reaction, the next step is to look with the slit lamp for sector palsy of the iris sphincter.

Is there a segmental paralysis of the iris sphincter?
When the dilator is in a drug-induced adrenergic spasm, or when the cholinergic receptors in the iris sphincter are blocked by an atropine-like drug, the entire sphincter muscle (all 360° of it) is less effective. This is not the case when nerve fibers have been interrupted; all Adie's pupils with a residual light reaction (about 90% of them) have segmental contractions of the sphincter, and many preganglionic partial third nerve palsies also have regional sphincter palsies, but these can usually be attributed to an associated diabetic autonomic neuropathy. This means that when a pupil with a weak light reaction and no segmental palsy is seen, the examiner should think about a drug-induced mydriasis and then perhaps look again for lid and motility signs of a third nerve paresis.

Is the pupil supersensitive to cholinergic drugs?
If weak pilocarpine (0.0625%, 0.1%, 0.125%), or weak methacholine (2.5%), is applied to both eyes (both corneas being healthy and untouched, tear function normal, and the eyelids working properly in both eyes) and the affected (dilated) pupil constricts more than the normal pupil so that it actually becomes the smaller pupil, then the iris sphincter has probably lost some of its innervation. It seems likely that with a postganglionic denervation (ciliary ganglion to the eye) the sphincter will show slightly higher supersensitivity than in the preganglionic case (third nerve palsy). It appears, however, that the differences are not great. For all of these reasons, cholinergic supersensitivity of the iris sphincter is now considered only a weak sign of Adie's syndrome.

Ptosis or diplopia should be looked for once more, as it is very rare for an ambulatory patient to have an isolated sphincter palsy as a result of damage to the intracranial third nerve.

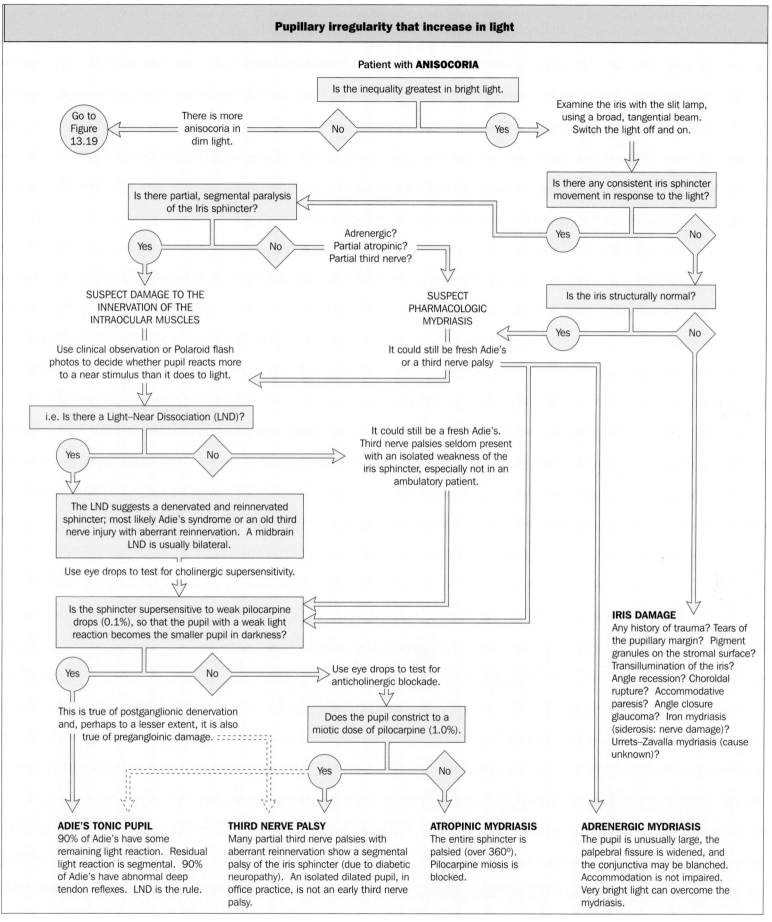

Pupillary irregularity that increase in light

Patient with **ANISOCORIA**

Is the inequality greatest in bright light.

No — There is more anisocoria in dim light. — Go to Figure 13.19

Yes — Examine the iris with the slit lamp, using a broad, tangential beam. Switch the light off and on.

Is there any consistent iris sphincter movement in response to the light?

Yes — Is there partial, segmental paralysis of the Iris sphincter?

No — Is the iris structurally normal?

Is there partial, segmental paralysis of the Iris sphincter?

Yes / No — Adrenergic? Partial atropinic? Partial third nerve?

Yes → **SUSPECT DAMAGE TO THE INNERVATION OF THE INTRAOCULAR MUSCLES**

SUSPECT PHARMACOLOGIC MYDRIASIS

Is the iris structurally normal?

Yes → It could still be fresh Adie's or a third nerve palsy

No → **IRIS DAMAGE**

Use clinical observation or Polaroid flash photos to decide whether pupil reacts more to a near stimulus than it does to light.

i.e. Is there a Light–Near Dissociation (LND)?

Yes / No →

It could still be a fresh Adie's. Third nerve palsies seldom present with an isolated weakness of the iris sphincter, especially not in an ambulatory patient.

The LND suggests a denervated and reinnervated sphincter; most likely Adie's syndrome or an old third nerve injury with aberrant reinnervation. A midbrain LND is usually bilateral.

Use eye drops to test for cholinergic supersensitivity.

Is the sphincter supersensitive to weak pilocarpine drops (0.1%), so that the pupil with a weak light reaction becomes the smaller pupil in darkness?

Yes / No → Use eye drops to test for anticholinergic blockade.

This is true of postganglionic denervation and, perhaps to a lesser extent, it is also true of pregangloinic damage.

Does the pupil constrict to a miotic dose of pilocarpine (1.0%).

Yes / No

IRIS DAMAGE
Any history of trauma? Tears of the pupillary margin? Pigment granules on the stromal surface? Transillumination of the iris? Angle recession? Choroldal rupture? Accommodative paresis? Angle closure glaucoma? Iron mydriasis (siderosis: nerve damage)? Urrets–Zavalla mydriasis (cause unknown)?

ADIE'S TONIC PUPIL
90% of Adie's have some remaining light reaction. Residual light reaction is segmental. 90% of Adie's have abnormal deep tendon reflexes. LND is the rule.

THIRD NERVE PALSY
Many partial third nerve palsies with aberrant reinnervation show a segmental palsy of the iris sphincter (due to diabetic neuropathy). An isolated dilated pupil, in office practice, is not an early third nerve palsy.

ATROPINIC MYDRIASIS
The entire sphincter is palsied (over 360º). Pilocarpine miosis is blocked.

ADRENERGIC MYDRIASIS
The pupil is unusually large, the palpebral fissure is widened, and the conjunctiva may be blanched. Accommodation is not impaired. Very bright light can overcome the mydriasis.

Fig. 13.25 If, at the start, the pupillary inequality is greatest in *bright light* rather than in the dark, this indicates that the sphincter of the larger pupil is weak, or that there is a parasympathetic lesion on that side. Is the iris normal to slit lamp examination? Is there any residual light reaction at all? Is there a segmental paralysis of the iris sphincter? Is the pupil supersensitive to cholinergic drugs? Does the pupil constrict to a miotic dose of pilocarpine (e.g. 1%)?

If the normal pupil constricts a little and the dilated pupil not at all, the mydriasis may be due to a local dose of an anticholinergic drug like atropine. A stronger concentration of pilocarpine is needed to settle this point.

Does the pupil constrict to a miotic dose of pilocarpine (e.g. 1%)?
If, on application of 1% pilocarpine in each eye, the affected pupil does little or nothing, and the unaffected pupil constricts normally, the pupil was dilated because of:
- Anti-cholinergic mydriasis. (e.g. scopolamine, cyclopentolate, atropine, hyoscine)
- Traumatic iridoplegia. (look for sphincter rupture, pigment dispersion, angle recession)
- Angle closure glaucoma (ischemia of the iris sphincter)
- Fixed pupil following anterior segment surgery

The cause for this complete loss of function of the iris muscles is unknown. Is does not appear to be ischemic, or toxic. Is it an auto-immune process? Is it the same as the Urrets–Zavalia syndrome, the dilated fixed pupil that occasionally follows a penetrating keratoplasty?

Adie's tonic pupil
Young adults (more women than men) may suddenly find that one pupil is large or that they cannot focus one eye up close. Slit lamp examination usually shows segmental denervation of the iris sphincter. Within the first week, supersensitivity to cholinergic substances can be demonstrated. After about 2 months, nerve regrowth has been active and fibers originally bound for the ciliary muscle (they outnumber the sphincter fibers by 30:1) start arriving (aberrantly) at the iris sphincter at about 8 weeks. This produces the characteristic 'light–near dissociation' of Adie's syndrome. Eventually the affected pupil becomes the smaller of the two pupils, especially in dim light (*Fig. 13.26*).

The segmental palsy of the iris sphincter can be seen particularly well by infrared video recording of transillumination of the iris (see Fig. 13.15b)

The fixed, dilated pupil
When a pupil is dilated by some atropinic medication (*Figs 13.27a–c*), it can be distinguished with some confidence from an innervational palsy by its tendency to resist the miotic effects of cholinergic drops such as pilocarpine or arecoline.

A 1% solution of pilocarpine is a firmly miotic dose for any eye, but a sphincter with all its cholinergic receptors blocked with atropine or tropicamide will not constrict to 1% pilocarpine. If the anticholinergic drug is wearing off, so that a small light reaction is beginning to return, 1% pilocarpine may cause a minimal constriction (*Fig. 13.27d*).

Third nerve palsy
There is an old clinical rule of thumb that says that if the pupillary light reaction is spared, then the third nerve palsy is probably not due to compression or trauma, but more likely to small vessel disease, such as might be seen in diabetes (*Figs 13.28, 13.29*). This is still a fairly good rule, provided it is borne in mind that the small but definite number of pupil-sparing third nerve palsies are due to midbrain infarcts, which should have neuroimaging studies (*Fig. 13.30*).

Aberrant regeneration in the third nerve
The third cranial nerve carries instructions to several different muscles, so when the nerve is injured and the fibers re-grow, they often end up in the wrong place. For example, the eye may inappropriately turn in when the patient is trying to look down, or the pupil may inappropriately constrict with depression of the globe (*Fig. 13.31*).

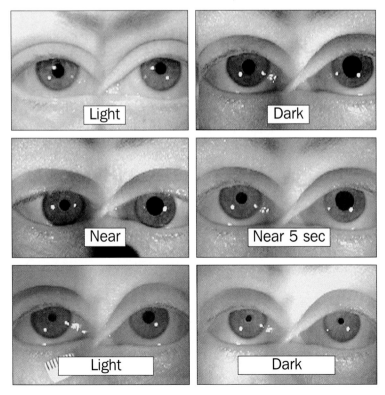

Fig. 13.26 A patient with Adie's pupil OD. Notice that the right pupil constricts imperfectly – in light it is slightly larger than the left pupil. However, in the darkness it dilates poorly, and has definitely become the smaller pupil. It does not constrict well because some of the sphincter's original innervation has been lost; it does not dilate well because the sphincter now has inappropriate tone due to aberrant innervation by fibers originally destined for the ciliary muscle. This is also the cause of the evident light–near dissociation. Notice that the right pupil is 'tonic', in that it stays small after a strong near effort when, 5 s after looking back into the distance, the pupil of the unaffected left eye has already begun to let go. In addition, cholinergic supersensitivity is demonstrated by the fact that, while looking in the distance, in the dark, the right pupil becomes the smaller one after weak pilocarpine has been put in both eyes. However, after 1% pilocarpine, both pupils became equal and miotic.

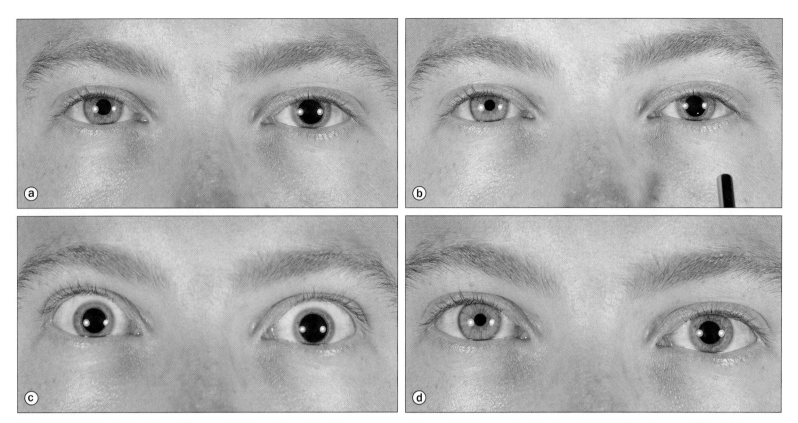

Fig. 13.27 (a) A patient with a left eye anticholinergic mydriasis in room light. (b) Same patient in bright light, showing that the light reaction is not entirely lost. No segmental palsy of the iris sphincter was seen with a slit lamp. (c) Same patient in the dark (d) still in darkness 30 minutes after pilocarpine 1% had been placed in both eyes. Note that the left pupil constricted a little, but not nearly as much as the unmedicated eye.

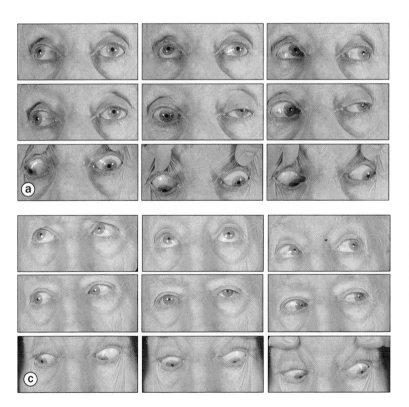

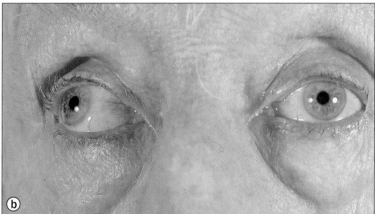

Fig. 13.28 (a) Patient with an ischemic left third nerve palsy. (b) Same patient, in room light, showing that both pupils constricted equally to light.(c) 3 months later, the patient showed full recovery of eye movements, without aberrant regeneration.

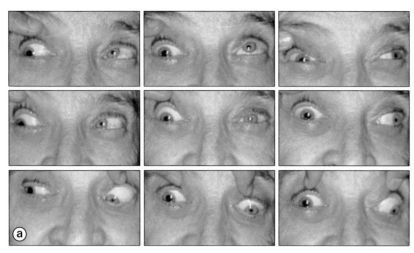

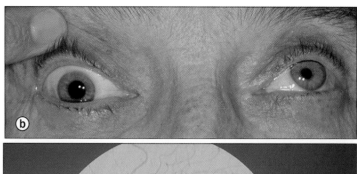

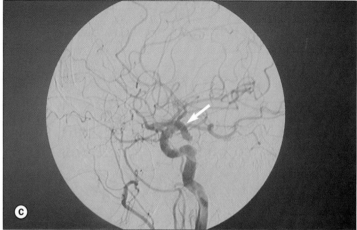

Fig. 13.29 (**a**) Patient with a right compressive third nerve palsy. (**b**) Same patient, in room light, showing that the right pupil constricted poorly to light. (**c**) The patient's carotid angiogram showing a Circle of Willis aneurysm (arrow).

Pupil involvement in third nerve palsies			
	Extraocular muscles		
	Total impairment of the extraocular muscles (90%)	Partial impairment of the extraocular muscles	No impairment of the extraocular muscles (10% or less)
Total impairment of the parasympath. Intraocular muscles (i.e. no pupil light reaction) or accommodation.	highest risk of aneurysm (Send promptly to neurology or neurosurgery for evaluation and possible carotid angiography to rule out aneurysm – even if age, gender, and pain do not strongly support the diagnosis)	Highest risk of aneurysm (Send promptly to neurology or neurosurgery for evaluation and possible carotid angiography)	Little or no risk of aneurysm. In an ambulatory patient, this is almost certainly a peripheral problem (i.e. orbital or ocular), and not a third nerve paresis. Atropinic? (1.0% pilo?) Adie's? (Slit lamp exam) Trauma? Iron? Angle closure glaucoma?
Partial impairment of the parasympath. Intraocular muscles (i.e. the pupillary light reaction is weak)	Uncertain risk of aneurysm This could be an ischemic third on top of pre-existing diabetic autonomic neuropathy of the Iris sphincter. Examine both Irises at the slit lamp and view recent face pictures. (Would probably send for studies anyway – especially if age, gender, and pain suggest an aneurysm)	High risk of aneurysm. This is a partial third nerve palsy without any relative sparing of the pupil. (Send promptly to neurology or neurosurgery for evaluation and possible carotid angiography)	Little or no risk aneurysm. In an ambulatory patient, this is almost certainly a peripheral problem (i.e. orbital or ocular) and not a third nerve paresis. Atropinic? (1.0% pilo?) Adie's? (0.1% pilo) Trauma? Iron? Angle closure glaucoma?
No impairment of the parasympath. Intraocular muscles (i.e. the pupillary light reaction is normal).	Low risk of aneurysm. Almost certainly an ischemic mononeuropathy. Does patient have diabetes? (Would postpone the studies)	Low risk of aneurysm. Almost certainly an ischemic mononeuropathy. Does the patient have diabetes? (Would postpone the carotid angiography)	Not applicable (normal).

Left axis label: Intraocular muscles (pupil and accommodation)

Fig. 13.30 Third nerve palsies, indicating, according to the proportion of intraocular and extraocular muscle involvement, the relative risk that the third nerve may be damaged in its sub-arachnoid course by an aneurysm of the Circle of Willis.

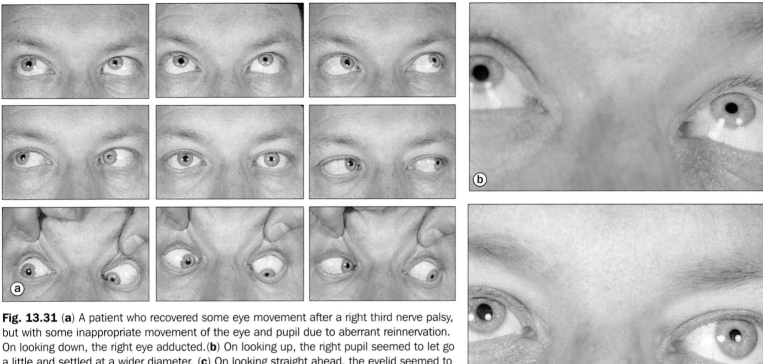

Fig. 13.31 (**a**) A patient who recovered some eye movement after a right third nerve palsy, but with some inappropriate movement of the eye and pupil due to aberrant reinnervation. On looking down, the right eye adducted.(**b**) On looking up, the right pupil seemed to let go a little and settled at a wider diameter. (**c**) On looking straight ahead, the eyelid seemed to be working well. (**d**) On looking down the right pupil constricted.

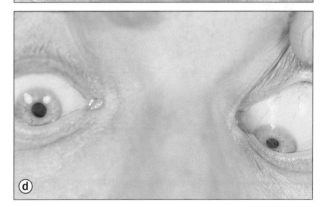

CHAPTER 14

The Visual Pathway from Optic Chiasm to Striate Cortex

Jason JS Barton

INTRODUCTION

The optic chiasm is formed from the partial decussation of axons from retinal ganglion cells. The effect of this is to sort visual information by right and left hemifields instead of right and left eyes. Lesions at or after the chiasm have characteristic visual field defects that reflect this reorganization, with binocular involvement and restriction of visual loss to the right or left field with unilateral lesions; furthermore, the presence of an abrupt step along the vertical meridian almost always means a lesion at or after the chiasm. This step is an important clue of bilateral disease affecting postchiasmal pathways; perimetrists should always search for it in patients with binocular visual loss of unknown cause.

The section of the visual relay formed by the axons of the retinal ganglion cells (i.e. optic nerve, chiasm, and tract) is also called the anterior visual pathway, whereas that formed by geniculostriate axons (i.e. optic radiations and striate cortex) is the posterior pathway. This distinction is useful in patients with hemifield visual defects because a chiasmal or tract lesion is more likely than a lesion of the posterior pathway to be a compressive mass. Two signs point to anterior disease: optic atrophy and a relative afferent pupillary defect (RAPD). However, it must be stressed that their absence does not exclude anterior pathway compression.

The clinical signs and pattern of visual field defect offer mainly localization clues. They also offer etiologic clues in that certain pathologies are more likely at certain sites. More etiologic information will be gained from clinical features such as the temporal course of symptoms and signs, including serial changes in visual fields.

OPTIC CHIASM

GROSS ANATOMY

The optic chiasm is formed anteriorly by the convergence of the optic nerves and divides posteriorly into the optic tracts. It inclines downwards anteriorly and is readily seen on MR sagittal images (*Fig. 14.1a*). Laterally, the internal carotid arteries emerge from the cavernous sinus. The third ventricle and the hypothalamus, including the infundibulum and mamillary bodies, lie posteriorly and superiorly. The interpeduncular cistern is below, just anterior to the midbrain. Above the chiasm are the anterior cerebral and anterior communicating arteries, and above these the medial aspects of the frontal lobes.

The most important relation is the inferiorly placed pituitary gland, resting in the sella turcica and separated from the chiasm by the diaphragma sella and the suprasellar cistern (*Fig. 14.1b*). The relation of the chiasm to the sella varies. The chiasm's anterior margin may lie as much as 2 mm anterior (pre-fixed) or 9 mm posterior (post-fixed) to the tuberculum sellae. A pituitary tumor in a patient with a pre-fixed chiasm may compress the optic tracts instead of the chiasm; similarly, it may compress the optic nerves in a patient with a post-fixed chiasm.

The dorsal chiasm is supplied by several branches from the A1 segment of the anterior cerebral arteries and also from the anterior communicating and internal carotid arteries (*Fig. 14.2*). The ventral chiasm has branches from the internal carotids, with perhaps some contribution from the posterior communicating, posterior cerebral, or basilar arteries. The extensive collateral supply explains why ischemic lesions of the chiasm are rare.

FUNCTIONAL ANATOMY

As the optic nerves approach the chiasm, the macular fibers that entered the nerve temporally assume a more central location. The location of peripheral axons mirrors their retinal origins (i.e. inferior retina inferiorly, nasal retina medially). The axons of the temporal retina cross in the lateral part of the intracranial optic nerve and pass uncrossed through the lateral edge of the chiasm. The axons of the nasal retina cross, with superior nasal fibers crossing in the superior (dorsal) aspect of the chiasm and inferior nasal fibers in the inferior (ventral) chiasm (*Fig. 14.3*). As the ventral fibers from the inferior nasal retina cross, they loop slightly anteriorly into the opposite optic nerve, forming Wilbrand's knee. Macular axons cross diffusely in the chiasm, although they are concentrated in the central and posterior aspects.

CLINICAL SYNDROMES

The hallmark of chiasmal lesions is damage to the crossing nasal fibers, causing bitemporal hemianopia. This can vary from complete loss of temporal fields, with respect of the vertical meridian and macular splitting (*Fig. 14.4*), to subtle deficits of central or peripheral vision. Lesions that compress the chiasm from below, such as pituitary tumors, affect the superior temporal fields first (*Fig. 14.5*). Lesions that impinge on the posterior chiasm may cause bitemporal central scotomata. However, most compressive masses are large and the radiology seldom delineates compression this precisely. The variations on bitemporal loss are important to recognize: any kind of bitemporal visual loss suggests a chiasmal lesion, usually a mass requiring surgical intervention and

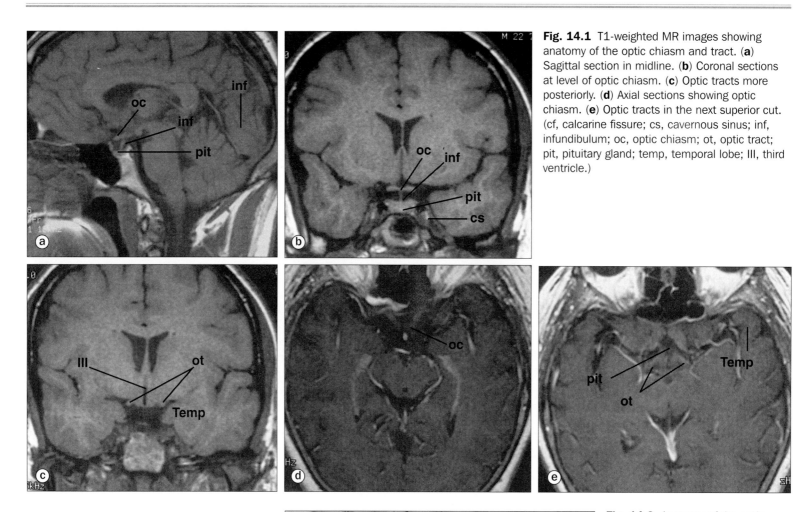

Fig. 14.1 T1-weighted MR images showing anatomy of the optic chiasm and tract. (**a**) Sagittal section in midline. (**b**) Coronal sections at level of optic chiasm. (**c**) Optic tracts more posteriorly. (**d**) Axial sections showing optic chiasm. (**e**) Optic tracts in the next superior cut. (cf, calcarine fissure; cs, cavernous sinus; inf, infundibulum; oc, optic chiasm; ot, optic tract; pit, pituitary gland; temp, temporal lobe; III, third ventricle.)

Fig. 14.2 Anatomy of the optic chiasm and tract. Inferior surface of brain with midbrain transected and left temporal lobe partly removed. (ica, internal carotid artery; inf, infundibulum; lgb, lateral geniculate body; m, mamillary bodies; pulv, pulvinar; pcomm, posterior communicating artery; oc, optic chiasm; olf, olfactory nerve; on, optic nerves; ot, optic tract; unc, uncus of temporal lobe.)

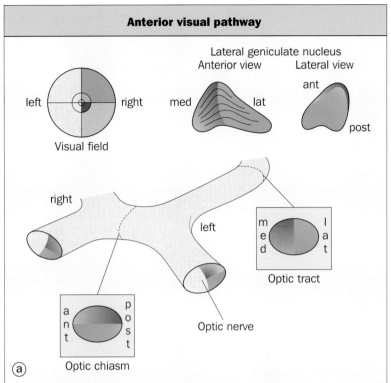

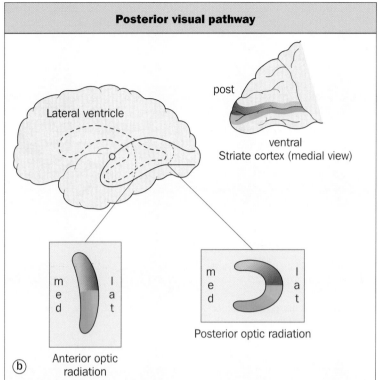

Fig. 14.3 Approximate retinotopic representations within the anterior (**a**) and posterior (**b**) visual pathways from the optic chiasm to the striate cortex.

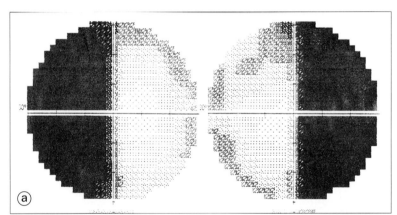

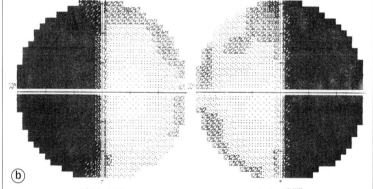

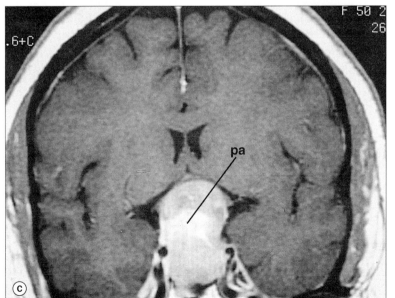

Fig. 14.4 Complete bitemporal hemianopia on Humphrey 30-2 perimetry. (**a**) In a 51-year-old woman who presented with complaints of diplopia and 'jumbled reading'. The examination showed normal optic discs. (**b**) Repeat perimetry 6 weeks after resection of a pituitary adenoma seen on MR imaging (**c**) was much improved. pa, pituitary adenoma

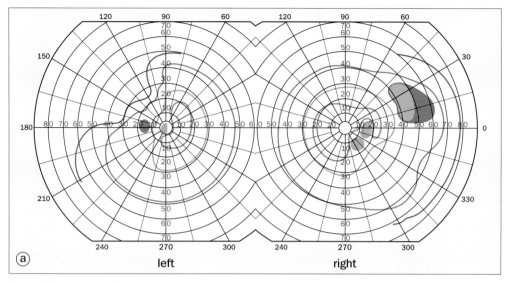
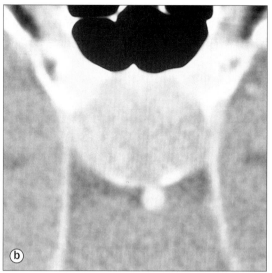

Fig. 14.5 (**a**) Partial bitemporal hemianopia on Goldmann perimetry. (**b**) In a 76-year-old man with a large pituitary adenoma seen on axial non-contrast CT. Note that visual loss affects primarily superior visual fields.

Lesions of the optic chiasm or tract	
Major causes	Pituitary adenomas:
	Prolactinoma
	Nonsecreting
	Growth-hormone
	ACTH
	Meningioma
	Craniopharyngioma
	Giant aneurysm
Minor causes	Other tumors
	Glioma (optic nerve/hypothalamus)
	Dysgerminoma
	Chordoma
	Metastases
	Inflammation
	Sarcoidosis
	Multiple sclerosis
	Arachnoiditis
	Basilar meningitis (bacterial, TB, cryptococcus)
	Arachnoid cyst
	Sphenoid mucocele
	Empty sella syndrome
	Hydrocephalus
	Trauma
	Radiation necrosis

Fig. 14.6 Lesions of the optic chiasm and tract.

a potentially treatable cause of visual loss (*Fig. 14.6*).

As a result of the variable relation of the chiasm to the sella turcica, tumors here can compress the optic nerve or tract as well. One clue to a parasellar compressive optic neuropathy is the junctional scotoma. Visual loss in one eye may be accompanied by an asymptomatic defect in the superior temporal quadrant of the other eye. This means the optic nerve has been affected at its junction with the chiasm, with dysfunction of the fibers in Wilbrand's knee. The differential diagnosis is that of chiasmal syndromes rather than optic neuropathy. Other combinations of optic nerve and chiasmal patterns of visual loss can also occur (*Fig. 14.7*).

Complete bitemporal hemianopia occasionally causes an unusual diplopia. Most people have small phorias but the eyes are

aligned by keeping overlapping regions of the visual field in registration. However, no portion of the visual field is seen simultaneously by both eyes after complete bitemporal loss. Without overlapping regions, phoric deviation may emerge. With vertical phorias, this 'hemifield slide' may cause a vertical step in the midline when both eyes are viewing. With exodeviations objects in the midline are doubled and with esodeviations, there is a midline scotoma. Intermittent diplopia alternating with the disappearance of objects is a pathognomonic story for bitemporal hemianopia (as in the patient illustrated in *Fig. 14.24*).

Chiasmal lesions may or may not be accompanied by optic atrophy. Visual recovery is more likely if atrophy is absent at the time of surgical decompression (see Fig. 14.24). Atrophy is usually diffuse but can have a bow-tie pattern. Fibers from nasal fovea enter the disc temporally, wheras fibers from the nasal peripheral retina enter the disc nasally; fibers from the temporal peripheral retina arch around the papillomacular bundle to enter the disc superiorly and inferiorly. Disc atrophy in temporal hemianopia spares these superior and inferior wedges, forming the bow-tie appearance.

Relative afferent pupillary defects do not accompany complete bitemporal hemianopia because the visual loss in both eyes is the same but they can occur with partial asymmetric lesions or with combined optic nerve and chiasm lesions.

OPTIC TRACTS

GROSS ANATOMY

After the optic chiasm, axons subserving the contralateral hemifields travel in the optic tracts. Each tract initially points posterolaterally after branching from the chiasm, then sweeps around the lateral aspect of the cerebral peduncle towards its ending in the lateral geniculate nucleus (LGN) (see Fig. 14.1e). Anteriorly it forms part of the roof of the interpeduncular cistern. Between the paired tracts lie the third ventricle and hypothalamic structures such as the mamillary bodies and infundibulum. The optic tract abuts diencephalic structures superiorly, wheras inferolaterally it faces the uncus and amygdala of the temporal lobe across

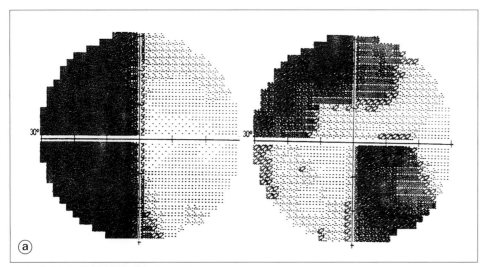

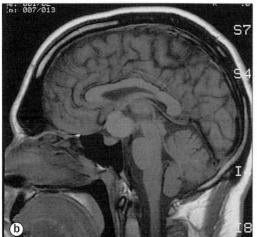
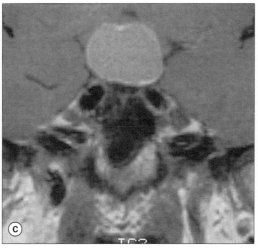
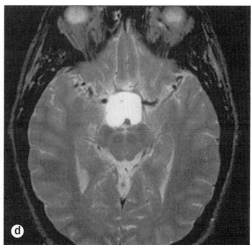

Fig. 14.7 Visual loss in a 26-year-old man with craniopharyngioma seen on MR (**b**) to (**d**). Visual fields (**a**) suggest a combination of incomplete bitemporal hemianopia from optic chiasm compression and a superonasal field defect (respecting horizontal meridian) from optic nerve compression.

the choroidal fissure (Fig. 14.1c). Important inferior relations are the posterior communicating artery anteriorly and the posterior cerebral artery posteriorly (see Fig. 14.2). The anterior choroidal artery is the main blood supply, although small branches from carotid and posterior communicating arteries have been described.

FUNCTIONAL ANATOMY

Two transformations to the retinotopic organization of the retinal axons occur during passage through the tract. First, there is a gradual rearrangement of fibers so that those of one location in a retina are associated spatially with those of the corresponding location in the other retina. Retinal correspondence is only approximately achieved by the termination of the tract, however. Second, the retinotopic map is tilted, so that macular fibers come to lie dorsally, inferior retinal axons laterally, and superior retinal axons medially (see *Fig. 14.3*). This arrangement is also reflected in the LGN.

Not all retinal axons end in the LGN. Just before this point, axons that subserve the pupillary light reflex leave the optic tract and pass inferior to the medial geniculate body, through the brachium of the superior colliculus, and end in the pretectal nuclei of the rostral midbrain. Some axons also leave the dorsal optic chiasm to enter the suprachiasmatic and supraoptic nuclei, where they play a role in hormonal circadian rhythms.

CLINICAL SYNDROMES

Lesions of the optic tract cause a contralateral homonymous hemianopia. There are three distinct features that distinguish this retinogeniculate hemianopia from the more common hemianopias of the geniculostriate pathway.

First, there may be marked incongruity with partial tract lesions (*Fig. 14.8*), because of imprecise correspondence of points in the visual field of the right and left eyes. Mild incongruity also occurs with lesions of the optic radiation, but marked incongruity always suggests a tract lesion. A complete tract lesion will cause complete hemianopia similar to that from lesions elsewhere.

The fact that tract lesions affect axons of retinal ganglion cells leads to the next two points. An RAPD is often seen with tract lesions because axons involved in the pupillary light reflex also travel in the optic tract. Only rarely does a lesion affect the short segment of optic tract after the exit of these fibers. The RAPD may correlate with the incongruity of the hemianopia, being present in the eye with more visual loss. However, complete hemianopias are also associated with an RAPD in the eye with temporal field loss, reflecting both the greater size of the temporal field and the 53:47 ratio of crossed (nasal) to uncrossed (temporal) retinal fibers in the optic tract.

Degeneration of retinal ganglion axons causes optic disc atrophy and loss of the retinal nerve-fiber layer. These findings are not seen with geniculostriate lesions, except for rare perinatal or

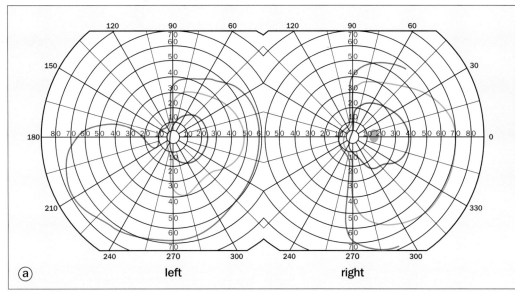
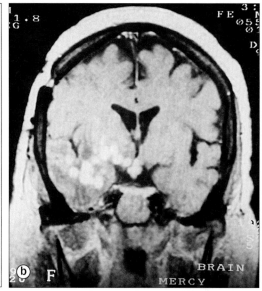

Fig. 14.8 (**a**) Incongruous left homonymous hemianopia in a 53-year-old woman with 7 years of complex partial seizures and biopsy-proven neurosarcoidosis. (**b**) Coronal MR with gadolinium showed multiple foci of enhancement in the temporal lobe, which also involved the right optic tract.

longstanding lesions with presumed retrograde trans-synaptic degeneration. The pattern of atrophy can be distinctive. The eye with temporal hemianopia can exhibit bow-tie atrophy, as discussed in chiasmal syndromes, whereas the eye with nasal hemianopia has a diffuse pallor involving temporal, superior, and inferior aspects.

The optic tract, like the chiasm, is most often affected by masses. An unusual fundoscopic picture is 'twin-peaks papilledema', in which bow-tie atrophy in the nasal and retinal quadrants of the optic disc is combined with papilledema in the superior and inferior quadrants (*Fig. 14.9*).

LATERAL GENICULATE NUCLEUS

GROSS ANATOMY

The LGN is a subnucleus of the thalamus, lying in its ventro-postero-lateral corner. It is lateral to the medial geniculate nucleus, ventral and lateral to the ventral posterior nucleus, and ventral and anterior to the pulvinar. The optic radiations emerge from its dorsolateral aspect, whereas the acoustic radiations from the medial geniculate body to auditory cortex traverse its dorsomedial aspect. The ventral surface of the LGN abuts the ambient cistern and, more laterally, the inferior horn of the lateral ventricle; directly opposite lies the hippocampus and parahippocampal gyrus. The lateral choroidal artery branches from the posterior cerebral artery and supplies the hilu and the middle zone of the LGN. The anterior choroidal artery branches from the internal carotid and supplies the lateral and medial aspects of the LGN, in addition to the optic tract.

FUNCTIONAL ANATOMY

The retinogeniculate neurons synapse in the LGN with cells whose axons project to striate cortex. The LGN has six layers: the ipsilateral eye projects to layers 2, 3, and 5 and the contralateral eye to layers 1, 4, and 6. The ventral two layers contain large cells (magnocellular) and the dorsal four layers contain small cells (parvo-

cellular). The retinal ganglion M cells that project to magnocellular layers have large receptive fields and transient responses to the onset or offset of a light; it is likely that the M cells are responsible for high temporal resolution and low-contrast sensitivity. P cells that project to parvocellular layers have small receptive fields and, therefore, finer spatial resolution; in addition, P cells but not M cells are sensitive to color. The bulk of foveal fibers are from P cells.

The retinotopic arrangement in the LGN is an approximate continuation of the rotation seen in the optic tract (see Fig. 14.3). Macular fibers terminate in a dorsal wedge that includes the hilum and is angled posteriorly. Superior retinal fibers, subserving the opposite lower quadrant, end in the medial horn and inferior retinal fibers end in the lateral horn. The more peripheral fibers of either quadrant are located towards the ventral surface.

CLINICAL SYNDROMES

Lesions of the LGN are rare. As the LGN is small it is often difficult to know radiologically whether a visual field defect associated with a posterior thalamic lesion represents damage to the LGN or to the optic tract or radiations. Nevertheless, three types of visual loss have been attributed to LGN lesions. The first is an incongruous homonymous hemianopia, reflecting the segregation of the inputs of the two eyes in different layers. The second occurs with ischemia of the middle wedge supplied by the lateral choroidal artery, causing a congruous sectoral hemianopia that straddles the horizontal meridian (*Fig. 14.10*). Ischemia of the territory of the anterior choroidal artery leads to the third type, which is the converse of the second. Upper and lower sectors of the hemifield are affected with sparing of the sector straddling the horizontal meridian.

Atrophy of the optic disc and nerve-fiber layer accompanies both tract and LGN lesions but LGN lesions causing incongruous hemianopias can be distinguished from optic tract lesions by the absence of an RAPD.

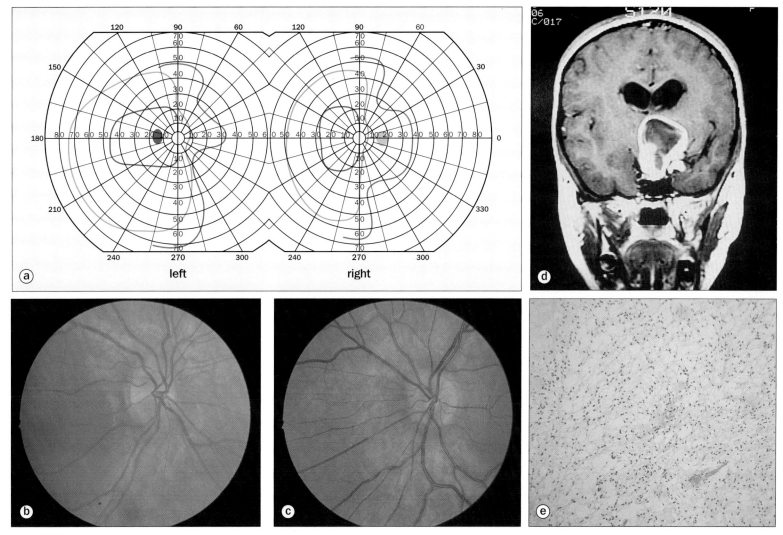

Fig. 14.9 Mildly incongruous right homonymous hemianopia (**a**) in a 7-year-old girl with 'twin-peaks' papilledema in the right eye (**b**) and disc swelling in the left eye (**c**), suggesting a mass compressing the left optic tract. Coronal MR with gadolinium showed hydrocephalus and a large off-midline enhancing tumor with cysts (**d**) that proved to be an astrocytoma (**e**).

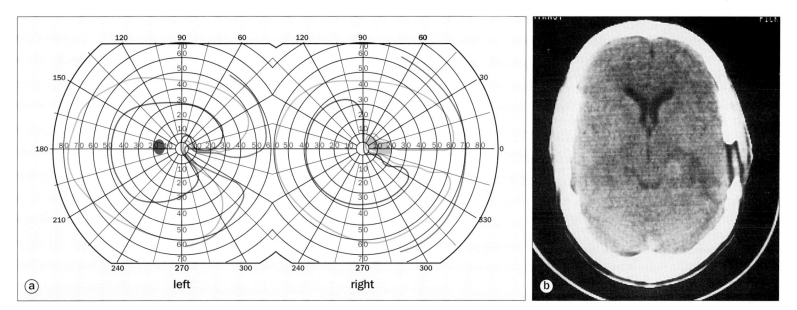

Fig. 14.10 Right sectoral homonymous hemianopia (**a**) in a 60-year-old man with hemorrhage in the region of the left lateral geniculate nucleus on noncontrast axial CT (**b**). Involvement of the optic radiation cannot be excluded.

OPTIC RADIATIONS

GROSS ANATOMY

After leaving the dorsal aspect of the LGN, the geniculostriate fibers form a bundle crossing the retrolenticular region of the posterior limb of the internal capsule. The fibers spread out laterally over the dorsal (superior) aspect of the inferior horn of the lateral ventricle. The ventral half of the radiation is directed anteriorly and curves over the tip of the inferior horn of the ventricle as Meyer's loop; these anterior-most fibers do not approach within 4–5 cm of the tip of the temporal lobe. The remaining dorsal half of the radiation projects posteriorly and passes over the main body of the inferior horn. Both halves course through the external sagittal stratum together and pass lateral to the trigone and occipital horn, before turning medially to end in the striate cortex. The dorsal fibers, underlying the parietal cortex, receive branches from the middle cerebral artery; the ventral fibers in Meyer's loop receive branches from the posterior cerebral artery.

FUNCTIONAL ANATOMY

The ventral optic radiation contains fibers representing the contralateral superior quadrant of the visual field. The most anterior of these fibers in Meyer's loop are from the wedge abutting the vertical meridian; as they turn to pass lateral to the temporal horn of the ventricle these meridional fibers lie in the inferior radiation. Macular fibers travel on the lateral surface of the middle of the radiation in its posterior course (see Fig. 14.3).

CLINICAL SYNDROMES

Lesions of the internal capsule that affect the radiations are usually ischemic or hemorrhagic. As the radiations are a compact bundle here, complete hemianopia usually results.

Lesions of the anterior temporal lobe damage fibers from the lower retina and so cause a superior quadrantanopia. This is usually a wedge of field loss bordering the vertical meridian and sparing the macula but can be a complete quadrantanopia extending to the horizontal meridian because the ventral (upper quadrant) fibers in Meyer's loop are well separated from the dorsal fibers (*Fig. 14.11*). The defect is sometimes incongruous but mildly so compared with tract lesions. Lesions more posterior than 8 cm from the tip of the lobe almost always affect the fibers from the inferior quadrant as well. Associated signs can include uncinate fits, complex partial seizures, auditory or visual hallucinations, and aphasia if the dominant hemisphere is involved.

In the parietal lobe, a superior lesion may cause a homonymous inferior quadrantanopia, usually congruous (*Fig. 14.12*). This seldom aligns with the horizontal meridian because the ventral and dorsal fibers run together at this point. More extensive lesions cause a homonymous hemianopia, sometimes splitting the macula. A parietal hemianopia occasionally is distinguished from occipital hemianopias by impaired optokinetic nystagmus or smooth pursuit towards the side of the lesion. Other signs include cortical sensory disturbances and aphasia and Gerstmann's syndrome in the dominant hemisphere.

Sectoral hemianopias can result from acute lesions of the optic radiations but these differ from LGN lesions by the absence of optic atrophy (*Fig. 14.13*).

STRIATE CORTEX

GROSS ANATOMY

The primary visual cortex is located on the superior and inferior banks of the calcarine fissure, which is in the medial occipital cortex and runs parallel to its ventral surface (see Fig. 14 1a). The visual cortex extends from immediately posterior to the splenium of the corpus callosum to the first 1–2 cm of the posterior surface of the occipital lobe. The falx cerebri and the interhemispheric fissure separate the right and left occipital lobes. The primary visual cortex possesses a unique histologic feature, the line of Gennari. This thin white lamina is easily seen running parallel to the cortical surface within gray matter. The bulk of the blood supply of the striate cortex derives from the posterior cerebral artery. A parieto-occipital branch supplies the superior bank whereas a posterior temporal branch supplies the inferior bank. A calcarine branch also supplies the central region. The occipital pole is a watershed zone between the posterior and middle cerebral arteries, with significant individual variation in the supply of the foveal representation.

FUNCTIONAL ANATOMY

The superior bank of the calcarine fissure contains cortex corresponding to the superior retina (inferior visual field), whereas the inferior bank contains the representation of the superior visual field. The foveal region is concentrated in the occipital pole, with the more peripheral field lying anterior (see Fig. 14.3). Most anterior is the representation of the monocular temporal crescent, the region of temporal field in the contralateral eye that lies beyond the limits of the nasal field (60°) of the ipsilateral eye.

Throughout the visual system the macular region is more heavily represented than peripheral vision. This remains true in the occipital cortex; over half of the striate cortex is devoted to the central 10° of vision ('cortical magnification'). The occipital cortex contains a mixture of monocular and binocular cells, arranged in ocular dominance columns; however, there is no gross separation of ocular inputs.

CLINICAL SYNDROMES

Highly congruous homonymous hemianopias are the rule with lesions of the striate cortex. The most severe visual loss after a unilateral lesion is complete homonymous hemianopia with macula splitting. This often represents a posterior cerebral artery infarction in a patient whose entire calcarine cortex lies within the territory of that artery. In a patient whose macular pole is supplied by or has abundant collateral circulation from the middle cerebral artery, the hemianopia may be macula sparing (*Fig. 14.14*). Macula sparing in some patients may also be a result of bilateral representation of the central 3° of foveal vision in the cortex.

Lesions of all types can affect portions of the striate cortex while sparing other regions. Involvement of either the upper or

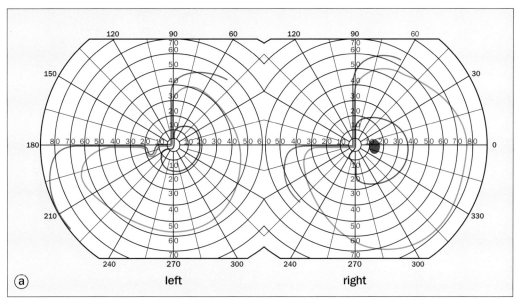
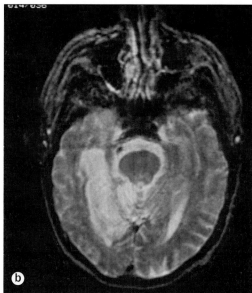

Fig. 14.11 An unusually congruous left superior homonymous quadrantanopia respecting the horizontal meridian (**a**) in a 54-year-old man with infarction of the right medial temporal lobe, sparing the occipital lobe, on axial MR (**b**). The lesion presumably affects the ventral optic radiation in Meyer's loop.

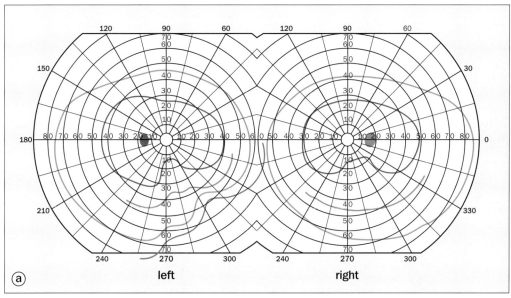
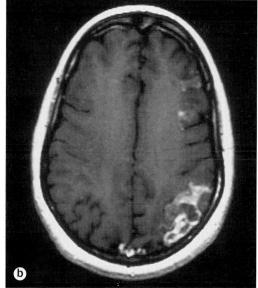

Fig. 14.12 (**a**) Subtle and mildly incongruous partial right inferior homonymous quadrantanopia in a 35-year-old woman with a 7-month history of intermittent numbness of the right hand and left-sided headache. (**b**) Axial MR with gadolinium showed a parietal arterio-venous malformation.

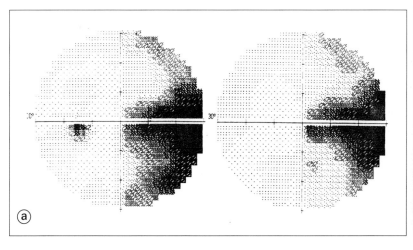
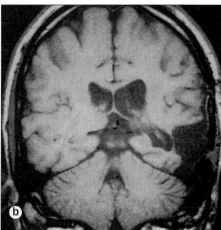

Fig. 14.13 Right sectoral homonymous hemianopia (**a**) in a 27-year-old man with infarction of the left lateral temporal lobe affecting the optic radiations, as shown on coronal MR (**b**). No lesion was seen in the region of the lateral geniculate nucleus.

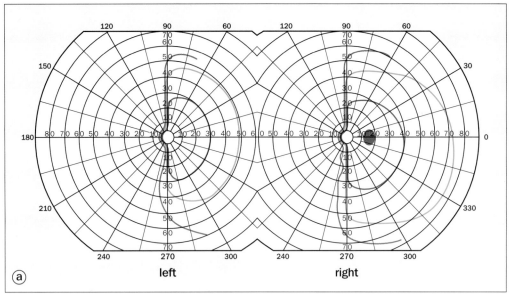

Fig. 14.14 Macula sparing left homonymous hemianopia (**a**) in a 49-year-old woman with a right medial occipital infarct not involving the occipital pole on MR (**b**).

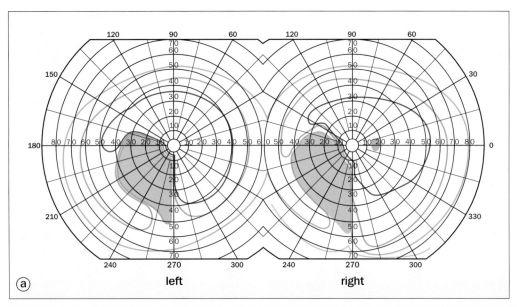

Fig. 14.15 (**a**) Right inferior homonymous quadrantanopia sparing the macula but not respecting the horizontal meridian in a 50-year-old woman with an infarct of the striate cortex. (**b**) Axial MR showed sparing of the occipital pole. (**c**) Sagittal MR showed that the infarct involved mainly the superior bank of the calcarine fissure .

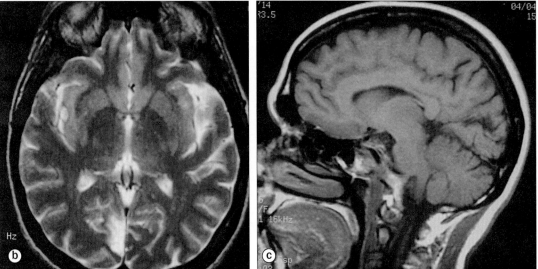

14.16). Such defects may not respect the horizontal meridian (see Fig. 14.15) because the representation of the upper and lower fields is continuous across the meridian in the depths of the sulcus. In fact, Horton and Hoyt argue that a quadrant defect respecting the horizontal meridian implies a lesion of the (extra-striate) V2 cortex. Occasionally, though, there are patients for whom the horizontal meridian is respected by a striate lesion (see Fig. 14.16).

Partial involvement can also occur along the anteroposterior extent of the striate cortex. A lesion of the occipital pole alone will cause a macular hemianopic scotoma (*Fig. 14.17*). This sometimes results from watershed infarcts during systemic hypoperfusion. Lesions that spare the pole spare the macula (see Fig. 14.14). Lesions that affect a midzone of the striate cortex may

spare both the macula and the far periphery (*Fig. 14.18*).

One type of peripheral sparing results in a defect that is the sole exception to the highly congruous nature of striate hemianopias. Lesions that do not extend to the anterior cortex representing the temporal crescent create an incongruous hemianopia that involves the whole hemifield of the ipsilateral eye but spares this crescent in the contralateral eye (see Fig. 14.16). This pattern may be mistakenly attributed to an optic tract lesion. However, the absence of both optic atrophy and RAPD, along with the location of the crescent outside 60° and the high congruity of the defect inside 60°, indicates a striate lesion. The opposite picture, a monocular field defect affecting only the temporal crescent, is rarely seen, reflecting infrequent occurrence, infrequent symptomology, and the improbability of detection.

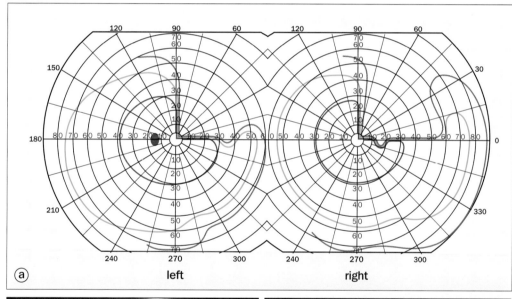

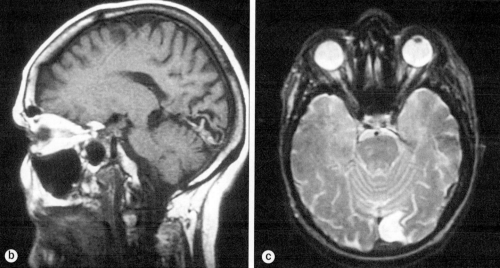

Fig. 14.16 (**a**) Right superior homonymous quadrantanopia extending to the macula, respecting the horizontal meridian, and with sparing of the monocular temporal crescent (beyond 60°) in the right eye. This 77-year-old woman had a medial occipital infarction limited to the striate cortex. The infarct involved the inferior bank of the calcarine fissure and did not extend to the splenium on sagittal MR (**b**) and also involved the occipital pole on sagittal and axial MR (**c**).

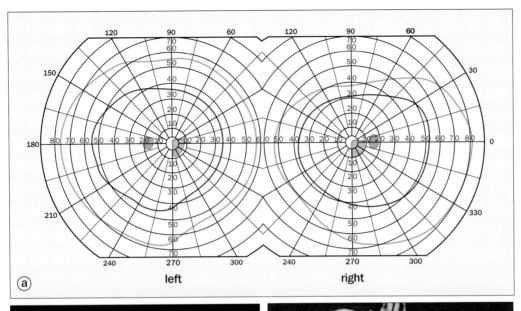

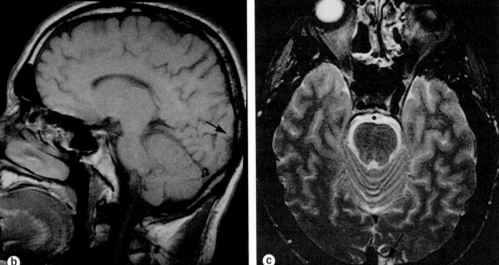

Fig. 14.17 Homonymous right inferior central scotomata (**a**) in a 38-year-old man who suddenly complained of difficulty in reading. MR showed a very subtle lesion of the occipital pole (**b**) and (**c**), most likely an infarct (arrow).

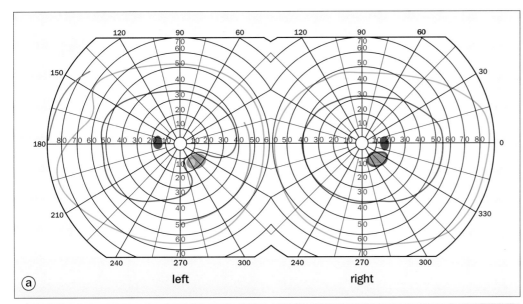

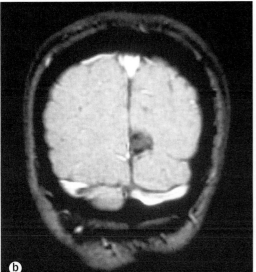
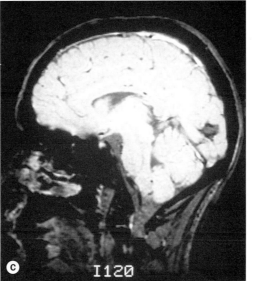

Fig. 14.18 (**a**) Homonymous right inferior paracentral scotomata in a 14-year-old girl with perinatal occipital infarction. (**b**) Coronal MR showed an infarct of the superior bank of the calcarine fissure. (**c**) Sagittal MR showed a midstriate lesion sparing both the occipital pole, corresponding to macular vision, and the more anterior striate cortex, corresponding to a more peripheral visual field.

Further reading

Bell RA, Thompson HS. Relative afferent pupillary defect in optic tract hemianopia. *Am J Ophthalmol.* 1978;**85**:538–540.

Bunt AH, Minckler DS. Foveal sparing. *Arch Ophthalmol.* 1977;**95**:1445–1447.

Carter JE, O'Connor P, Shacklett D, Rosenberg M. Lesions of the optic radiations mimicking lateral geniculate nucleus visual field defects. *J Neurol Neurosurg Psychiatry.* 1985;**48**:982–988.

Czarnecki JSC, Weingeist TA, Burton TC, Thompson HS. 'Twin peaks' papilledema. The appearance of papilledema with optic atrophy. *Can J Ophthalmol.* 1976;**11**:279–281.

Gunderson CH, Hoyt WF. Geniculate hemianopia: incongruous homonymous field defects in two patients with partial lesions of the lateral geniculate nucleus. *J Neurol Neurosurg Psychiatry.* 1971;**34**:1–6.

Hollenhorst RW, Younge BR. Ocular manifestations produced by adenomas of the pituitary gland: analysis of 1000 cases. In: Kohler PO, Ross GT, eds *Diagnosis and Treatment of Pituitary Tumors.* New York: Elsevier. 1973 pp.53–64.

Horton JC, Hoyt WF. Quadrantic visual field defects. A hallmark of lesions in extrastriate (V2/V3) cortex. *Brain.* 1991;**114**:1703–1718.

Horton JC, Hoyt WF. The representation of the visual field in human striate cortex: a revision of the classic Holmes map. *Arch Ophthalmol.* 1991;**109**:816–824.

Kirkham TH. The ocular symptomology of pituitary tumours. *Proc R Soc Med.* 1972;**65**:517–518.

CHAPTER 15

Infranuclear and Nuclear Ocular Motor Palsies

Jason JS Barton

INTRODUCTION

The three ocular motor cranial nerves, the oculomotor (III), trochlear (IV), and abducens (VI), innervate all extraocular muscles that rotate the globe, as well as the main lid elevator and the intraocular muscles for accommodation and pupil constriction. Dysfunction of these nerves is the most common cause of diplopia. Other symptoms include lid droop, blurred near vision, and photophobia from a dilated pupil.

Each nerve can be divided into three anatomic segments. The nuclei contain the cell bodies of the neurons and are located near the midline in the dorsal brainstem tegmentum, just ventral to either the Sylvian aqueduct or the fourth ventricle. Axons from these nuclei travel a variable distance through the medial brainstem as fascicles, then exit the brainstem to form peripheral nerves. This peripheral portion also has three sections: one traversing the subarachnoid space, another passing through the cavernous sinus and superior orbital fissure, and a final intraorbital section.

The first question with ocular motor palsies is whether the cause lies in the CNS or in the peripheral nerve. Anatomic localization is useful in narrowing the etiologic differential diagnosis (*Fig. 15.1*). Although lesions of the nuclei of these nerves often create distinctive ocular motor defects, the eye movements resulting from fascicular lesions may be indistinguishable from those of peripheral nerve lesions. It is important, therefore, to seek signs and symptoms arising from involvement of adjacent neurologic structures. A knowledge of the anatomic relations of the ocular motor nerves is essential to understand the clinical ocular motor syndromes.

OCULOMOTOR NERVE (THIRD CRANIAL NERVE)

FUNCTION AND ANATOMY

In contrast to the other two ocular motor nerves, the third nerve innervates several extraocular muscles. These are the inferior oblique and the superior, inferior, and medial recti. It also innervates the levator palpebrae superioris, the iris sphincter, and the ciliary muscle.

The third nerve nuclear complex extends in the midbrain from the trochlear nucleus at the pontomesencephalic junction up to the posterior commissure rostrally (*Fig. 15.2*). The Sylvian aqueduct lies dorsal to the complex, and the medial longditudinal fasciculus (MLF) runs rostrocaudally just ventral to the oculomotor complex. Also ventral to its rostral part are the interstitial nucleus of Cajal and the rostral interstitial nucleus of

Differential diagnosis of lesions of the ocular motor nerves by anatomic site
Nuclear and fascicular lesions:
Ischemia (small perforating branches of basilar artery)   Hemorrhage (hypertension, lymphoma)   Compression by extra-axial masses   Infiltration (cerebrospinal fluid)   Trauma   Inflammation (multiple sclerosis)
Peripheral nerve lesions:

Subarachnoid space
 	
 Meningitis (basilar)
 Meningeal carcinoma or lymphoma
 Increased intracranial pressure
 Ischemia (microvascular: diabetes, hypertension)
 Compressive saccular aneurysms
 Compressive extra-axial neoplasms
 Trauma
 	
 Cavernous sinus
 	
 Compression
   Metastatic
   Nasopharyngeal carcinoma
   Carcinoma (breast, lung)
   Lymphoma
   Myeloma
   Meningioma
   Pituitary adenoma
   Chordoma
   Giant carotid aneurysm
 Inflammation
   Tolosa–Hunt
   Granulomatous (Wegener's)
 Infection
   Mucormycosis
   Carotid: cavernous fistula

Fig. 15.1 Differential diagnosis of lesions of the ocular motor nerves by anatomic site.

the MLF, pre-nuclear structures for vertical gaze. The oculomotor nuclear complex contains subnuclei for the individual muscles, arranged as rostrocaudal columns (*Fig. 15.3*). The inferior rectus subnucleus is most dorsal and the superior rectus subnucleus most medial. The superior rectus subnucleus differs from the rest in that it innervates the contralateral eye, its axons crossing in the nucleus to join the opposite fascicle. Dorsal to the caudal end of the complex is the central caudal nucleus, a single midline structure that supplies the levators of both eyes. The fibers to the iris sphincter and ciliary muscles arise primarily from the Edinger–Westphal nuclei, located dorsal to the rostral end of the subnuclei.

The fascicle of the oculomotor nerve projects anteriorly with a caudal tilt, fans slightly laterally in the tegmentum, and emerges from the medial face of the cerebral peduncle (see Fig. 15.2b). This course associates it with the reticular formation, red nucleus, substantia nigra, and pyramidal tract in succession.

The subarachnoid nerve is sandwiched between the superior cerebellar artery below and the posterior cerebral and posterior communicating arteries above (*Figs 15.4, 15.5*). The free edge of the tentorium approaches laterally as the nerve nears the clivus and enters the cavernous sinus adjacent to the posterior clinoid. The nerve continues forward in the wall of this sinus, superior to the trochlear nerve. Near the end of the sinus the oculomotor nerve divides into an inferior and superior division, which pass through the superior orbital fissure and the annulus of Zinn into the orbit, where both shortly divide into terminal branches.

VASCULAR SUPPLY

The nucleus and fascicle are supplied by median perforating branches from the junction of the basilar, superior cerebellar, and posterior cerebral arteries. Branches of the latter two arteries also supply the proximal part of the subarachnoid nerve. Branches of the meningohypophyseal trunk supply the remaining distal subarachnoid nerve as well as the proximal part of the intracavernous segment. Branches of the ophthalmic artery supply the remainder of the intracavernous nerve.

CLINICAL SYNDROMES OF THE THIRD NERVE

A third nerve palsy causes symptoms of diplopia, ptosis, and blurred near vision. With severe ptosis the patient will of course have no diplopia. Diplopia varies between horizontal, vertical, and oblique forms according to the direction of gaze. A complete unilateral palsy has absent elevation and adduction of the eye, with some residual depression that is accompanied by intorsion

---

Brainstem anatomy of the ocular motor nerves

Fig. 15.2 Brainstem anatomy of the ocular motor nerves. (**a**) Midline sagittal section. (**b**) Axial sections from the midbrain (top), rostral pons (center), and caudal pons (bottom). Nuclei of cranial nerves III, IV, V, VI, and VII are indicated. (BC, brachium conjunctivum; CCN, central caudal nucleus; CP, cerebral peduncle; CS, corticospinal fibers; IC, inferior colliculus; inC, interstitial nucleus of Cajal; MGN, medial geniculate nucleus; ML, medial lemniscus; MLF, medial longitudinal fasciculus; riMLF, rostral interstitial nucleus of the MLF; RN, red nucleus; SN, substantia nigra.)

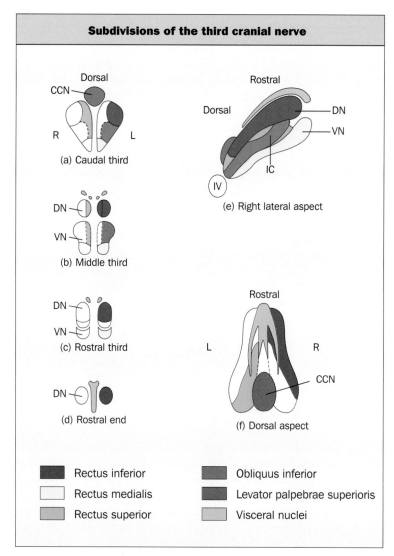

Subdivisions of the third cranial nerve

■ Rectus inferior	■ Obliquus inferior
□ Rectus medialis	■ Levator palpebrae superioris
▨ Rectus superior	▨ Visceral nuclei

Fig. 15.3 Subdivisions of the third cranial nerve, viewed from its dorsal aspect. (CCN, central caudal nucleus; EW, Edinger–Westphal nucleus. Extraocular muscle subnuclei are: IO, inferior oblique; IR, inferior rectus; MR, medial rectus; SR, superior rectus [crossed innervation].)

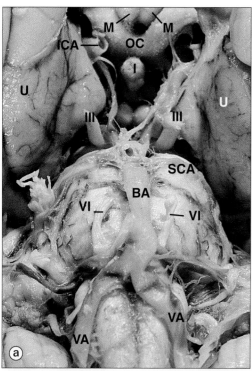

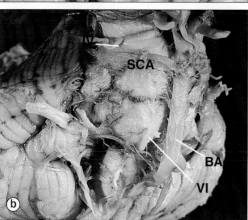

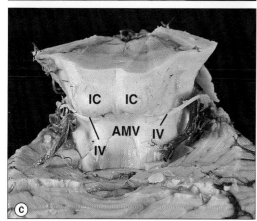

Fig. 15.4 Anatomy of the ocular motor nerves. (**a**) Ventral view of brainstem, showing the emergence of the sixth nerve from the pontomedullary junction medially, and the third nerve from the interpeduncular fossa just inferior to the uncus and the posterior cerebral and posterior communicating arteries. (**b**) Oblique view, also showing the fourth nerve wrapping around the midbrain between the posterior cerebral and superior cerebellar arteries. (**c**) Dorsal view with portion of cerebellum removed to show the emergence of the fourth nerve after decussation in the anterior medullary velum.
(AMV, anterior medullary velum; BA, basilar artery; I, infundibulum; IC, inferior colliculus; ICA, internal carotid artery; M, mamillary bodies; OC, optic chiasm; PCA, posterior cerebral artery; PCommA, posterior communicating artery; SCA, superior cerebellar artery; U, uncus of temporal lobe; VA, vertebral artery.)

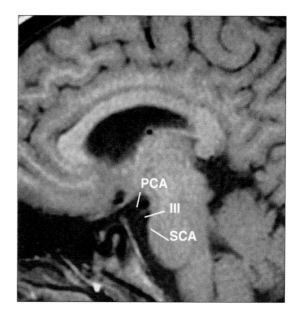

Fig. 15.5 Sagittal section just lateral to the midline, showing the subarachnoid third nerve as it passes between the posterior cerebral and superior cerebellar arteries. (BA, basilar artery; PCA, posterior cerebral artery; SCA, superior cerebellar artery.)

(indicating fourth nerve action) but normal abduction (*Fig. 15.6*). As a result, the eye in primary gaze is depressed and abducted ('down and out'). There is a pronounced ptosis and a large unreactive pupil, with impaired accommodation. Partial syndromes sparing various of these features are common.

Nuclear Lesions

The anatomy of the third nucleus leads to certain patterns of ocular palsy that are distinct from palsies of the fascicle or nerve (*Fig. 15.7*). Furthermore, some fascicular or nerve patterns are not consistent with nuclear damage. For example, a complete third nerve palsy with normal elevation of the other eye cannot be due to a nuclear lesion because of the crossed innervation of the superior rectus. Other patterns and explanations are given in *Figure 15.8*.

Fascicular Lesions

Partial or complete palsies occur with fascicular lesions. Several eponymous syndromes exist to describe their association with other signs. Involvement of the brachium conjunctivum is responsible for ipsilateral limb ataxia (Nothnagel's syndrome), the red nucleus for contralateral resting hemitremor, hemichorea, or hemiballismus (Benedikt's syndrome), and the cerebral peduncle for contralateral paresis of the limbs or face (Weber's syndrome, which may also be caused by an extra-axial mass within the interpeduncular fossa). These syndromes can exist in combination.

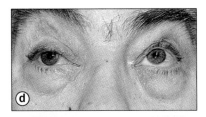
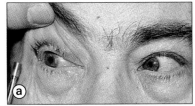
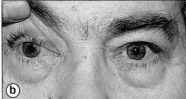
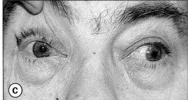
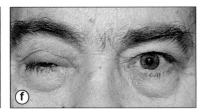
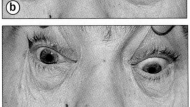

Fig. 15.6 Complete right third nerve palsy with pupil-sparing, in a 66-year-old man with an 18-year history of diabetes. The palsy resolved spontaneously 10 weeks later.

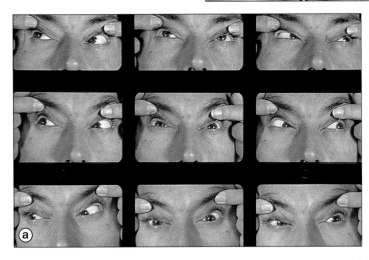

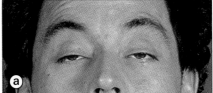

Fig. 15.7 (**a**) Bilateral ptosis and impaired down-gaze in a 39-year-old man with AIDS. (**b**) Axial MRI showed an enhancing periaqueductal lesion, probably affecting the dorsal aspect of the third nucleus. Autopsy showed HIV encephalitis.

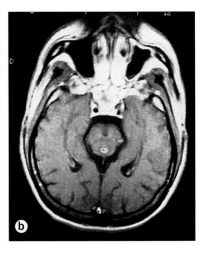

Fig. 15.8 Nuclear syndromes of the third nerve. (CCN, central caudal nucleus; EW, Edinger–Westphal nucleus; SR, superior rectus subnucleus.)

Nuclear syndromes of the third nerve	
Clinical involvement	**Explanation**
Obligate nuclear syndromes	

Unilateral third nerve palsy, with
  Contralateral palsy of superior rectus
  Bilateral ptosis
	Crossed innervation of SR
	Single unpaired CCN

Bilateral third nerve palsy with spared lid function	Ventral lesion sparing CCN
Possible (but not exclusively) nuclear syndromes	

Isolated bilateral
  Ptosis
  Internal ophthalmoplegia
  Superior rectus palsy
	Dorsal lesion affecting CCN
	Dorsal lesion affecting EW
	Midline lesion affecting decussating SR

Isolated unilateral palsy of single muscle Medial rectus, inferior rectus, or inferior oblique	Small subnuclear lesion
Complete bilateral third nerve palsies	Large midline lesion
Fascicular or nerve syndromes that cannot be nuclear	
Unilateral dilated pupil Unilateral ptosis Complete unilateral third nerve palsies with spared contralateral superior rectus Isolated superior rectus palsy	The 2 EW nuclei are fused at midline CCN supplies both lids Crossed innervation of SR SR fibers decussate in nucleus

Nerve Lesions

Although cavernous sinus lesions often affect several nerves simultaneously, mononeuropathies can also occur. In the anterior portion of the sinus the superior or inferior subdivisions of the third nerve may be affected separately (*Figs 15.9, 15.10*). A superior or inferior division palsy should be investigated for a mass in this area, although they may also be caused by partial lesions of the nerve or fascicle elsewhere.

ETIOLOGY

In children, congenital palsies account for nearly half of the third nerve palsies. When acquired, however, the proportion of identified causes is similar to adults, with trauma and inflammatory conditions accounting for one-third (*Fig. 15.11*). Unusual congenital syndromes include adduction palsy with synergistic divergence, vertical retraction syndrome, and cyclic oculomotor paresis, in which the eye alternates between underaction and overaction of the third nerve over several minutes. Compressive vascular or neoplastic lesions account for a significant number of adult palsies (*Fig. 15.12*). Distinguishing these from benign ischemic palsies, which recover over several months, can be difficult. Two useful signs are pupil involvement and aberrant regeneration.

The 'Pupil Rule'

Life-threatening aneurysms of the posterior communicating artery commonly present with third nerve palsies. These first compress the superomedial periphery of the subarachnoid nerve, where pupillary axons travel. Clinical studies estimate that more than 86% of aneurysmal third nerve palsies have pupillary involvement. In contrast, 73% of ischemic third nerve palsies spare the pupil. The blood supply of the nerve is from the periphery in, so that ischemia affects the center more than the periphery where pupil fibers lie.

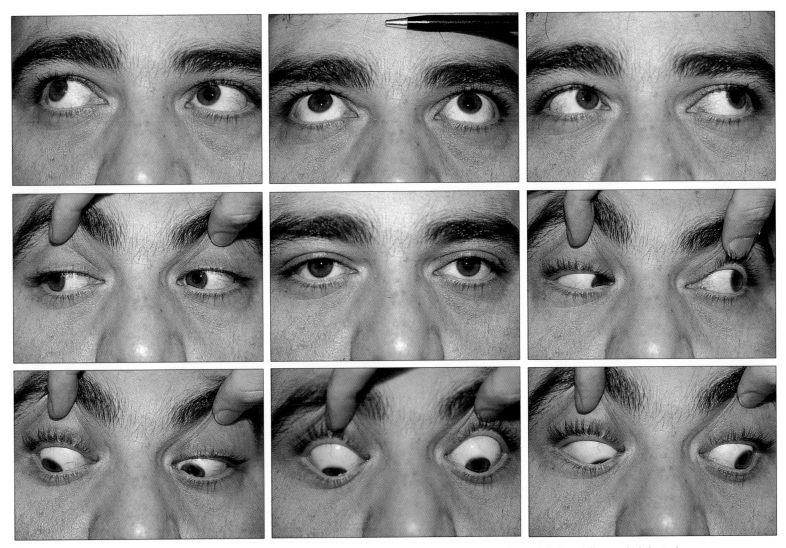

Fig. 15.9 Lesion of left inferior division of the third nerve, with impaired adduction and depression (especially in midline and abducted positions) of the left eye, and a dilated pupil, in a 28-year-old man with periorbital pain and presumed Tolosa–Hunt syndrome.

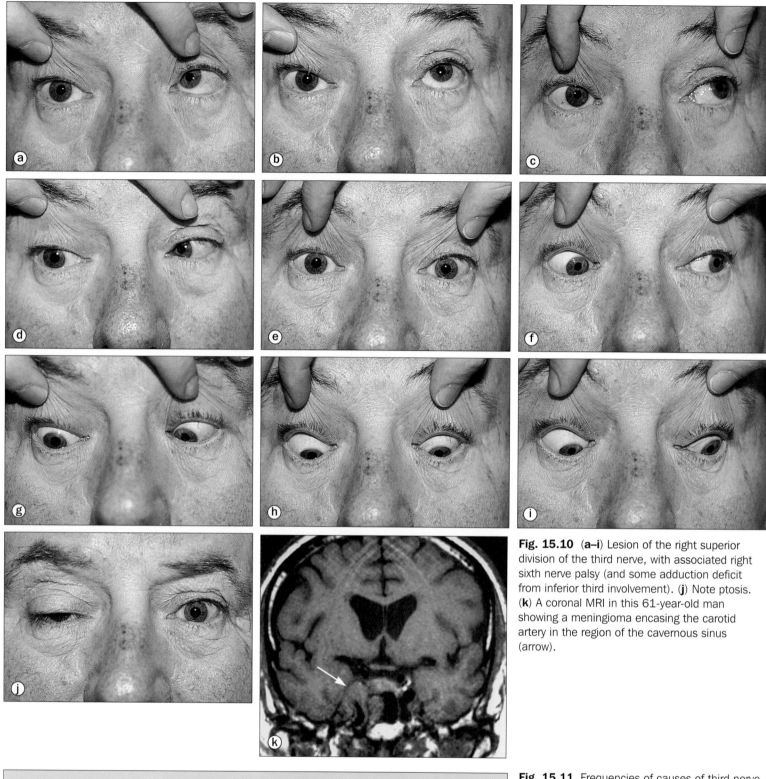

Fig. 15.10 (**a–i**) Lesion of the right superior division of the third nerve, with associated right sixth nerve palsy (and some adduction deficit from inferior third involvement). (**j**) Note ptosis. (**k**) A coronal MRI in this 61-year-old man showing a meningioma encasing the carotid artery in the region of the cavernous sinus (arrow).

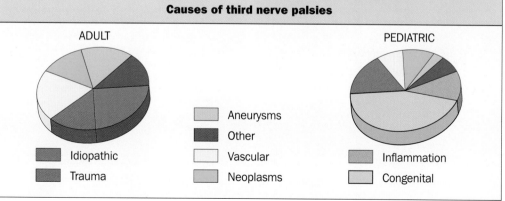

Fig. 15.11 Frequencies of causes of third nerve palsies in adults and children. (Data derived from Harley 1980 and Richards *et al.* 1992.)

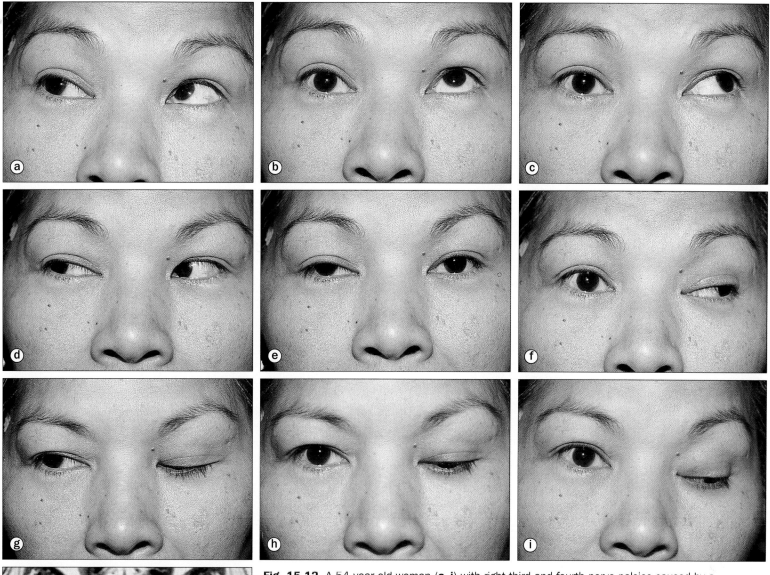

Fig. 15.12 A 54-year-old woman (**a–i**) with right third and fourth nerve palsies caused by a cavernous sinus meningioma seen in axial MRI (**j**) that had been partially resected 4 years earlier. Note the elevation of the ptotic right lid in down-gaze and left gaze, signs of aberrant regeneration.

Complete pupil-sparing in an otherwise complete third nerve palsy is virtually never due to an aneurysm (*Fig. 15.6*). Partial pupil-sparing does not count. 'Apparent pupil-sparing' from a co-existent Horner's syndrome should be excluded because this combination means a cavernous sinus mass. Complete pupil-sparing with a partial third nerve palsy can occur with aneurysms. In such cases, the pupil is usually affected within a few days. Some of these pupil-sparing palsies occur with basilar aneurysms, which compress the nerve from a different angle than posterior communicating aneurysms.

As ischemic palsies recover over 1 to 3 months and provided imaging shows no alternative diagnosis the patient can be reassured of this time span.

Aberrant Regeneration
Regeneration after some third nerve insults can be misdirected, leading to abnormal synkinetic movements. The pupil may be innervated by fibers initially destined for the inferior or medial recti, causing pupillary constriction on down-gaze or adduction. Lid elevation with similar movements is caused by the misdirection of these fibers to the levator (*Fig. 15.12*). Fibers from one extraocular muscle may also be re-routed anomalously to another; unwanted adduction during down-gaze is one example. As ischemic or idiopathic third nerve palsies rarely, if ever, cause aberrant regeneration, compressive lesions should be suspected. Occasionally these signs occur in a patient with no history of third nerve palsy. This 'primary aberrant regeneration' also implies a compressive lesion. Aberrant regeneration is not as ominous in children because it occurs frequently with congenital palsies.

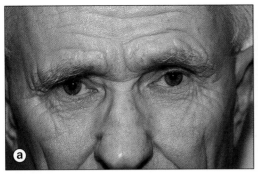 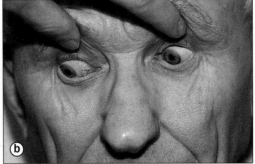 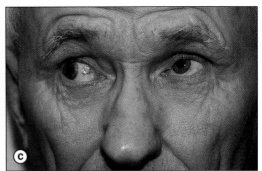

Fig. 15.13 Left fourth nerve palsy in a 70-year-old man. Note (**a**) head tilt away from the lesion, (**b**) poor depression in adducted position, and (**c**) inferior oblique overaction in gaze away from the side of the lesion.

TROCHLEAR NERVE (FOURTH CRANIAL NERVE)

FUNCTION AND ANATOMY

The fourth cranial nerve innervates the superior oblique muscle, whose primary function is intorsion of the eye, most prominently when the eye is abducted. It also depresses the eye, mainly during adduction, and has a minor contribution to abduction.

The fourth nuclei are paired medial structures in the periaqueductal gray matter, lying ventral to the Sylvian aqueduct at the pontomesencephalic junction. The oculomotor nuclear complex is rostral, whereas immediately ventral is the MLF. Like the superior rectus subnuclei of the third nerve, the fourth nerve nuclei innervate the superior oblique of the contralateral eye.

The fascicle of the fourth nerve follows an unusual course. It heads posteriorly, curving around the aqueduct in the periaqueductal gray matter, decussates in the anterior medullary velum, and emerges caudal to the inferior colliculi (see Figs 15.2, 15.4c). As it starts dorsal and remains dorsal, the fascicle does not lie close to major structures within the brainstem.

The long subarachnoid course of the fourth nerve carries it around the midbrain between the superior cerebellar and posterior cerebral arteries (see Fig. 15.4b) to the cavernous sinus, where it lies inferior to the oculomotor nerve but superior to the ophthalmic nerve (V^1). It then traverses the superior orbital fissure, passes outside the annulus of Zinn laterally, and crosses above the superior rectus to reach the superior oblique muscle.

CLINICAL SYNDROMES OF THE FOURTH NERVE

The patient with a unilateral palsy has diplopia, primarily vertical but often oblique, with the images tilted with respect to each other. On examination, there is decreased depression of the adducted eye and relative excyclotorsion of the eyes. The patient may have an obvious head tilt away from the side of the lesion, which minimizes the diplopia (Fig. 15.13). On occasion, patients tilt the head towards the lesion, if they find a wide separation of the images less confusing than a narrow separation. The Bielschowsky three-step test shows ipsilateral hypertropia which increases on contralateral gaze and on ipsilateral head tilt. Inferior oblique overaction can occur on contralateral gaze (see Fig. 15.13c). A bilateral palsy usually shows a small hypertropia looking straight ahead which increases with gaze to the side opposite the hypertropia but reverses direction with gaze to the same side. Head tilt also produces an alternating hypertropia.

Nuclear Lesions
There is no specific ocular motor pattern of fourth nerve nuclear damage. Associated damage to brainstem tegmental structures is the only clue. The proximity of the MLF to the nuclei (see Fig. 15.2) may lead to a combination of internuclear ophthalmoplegia (INO) and hypertropia due to fourth nerve palsy. The palsy will be missed unless a three-step test is done because hypertropias with INO are common and often attributed to skew deviation.

Fascicular Lesions
The fascicle is usually affected as it decussates in the superior medullary velum, often causing bilateral fourth nerve palsies (*Fig. 15.14*). Such lesions may be associated with other signs of dorsal midbrain compression, such as the pretectal syndrome. Rarely, the fascicle is interrupted in the lateral periaqueductal gray matter, with associated signs of a Horner's syndrome contralateral to the palsy (but ipsilateral to the lesion), contralateral limb ataxia from superior cerebellar peduncle involvement, or diminished sensation in the ipsilateral body and face from involvement of the sensory lemniscus.

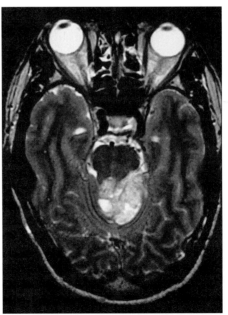

Fig. 15.14 An axial MRI of a 43-year-old man who presented with bilateral fourth nerve palsies. Note the large germinoma compressing the dorsal brainstem at the level of the anterior medullary velum.

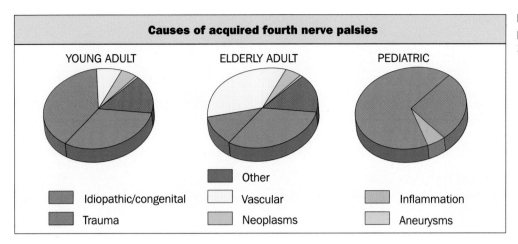

Fig. 15.15 Frequencies of causes of fourth nerve palsies in adults and children. (Data from Harley 1980 and Richards *et al.* 1992.)

Nerve Lesions

There are no characteristic signs pointing to trochlear nerve involvement in the subarachnoid space. Associated involvement of third, fifth (V₁ or V₂), or sixth nerves or the oculo-sympathetic fibers points to the cavernous sinus.

ETIOLOGY

Most fourth nerve palsies are not due to ominous lesions. Aneurysms and neoplasms account for less than 6% of isolated fourth nerve palsies (*Fig. 15.15*). Lesions dorsal to the midbrain as well as anterior and in the cavernous sinus may compress the fourth nerve (see Fig. 15.14). Trauma is the most common identified cause, responsible for almost one-third of these palsies. Congenital palsies account for another quarter. In children these two are responsible for the vast majority of fourth nerve palsies.

As many as four-fifths of congenital ocular motor nerve palsies are IV nerve palsies. These are often unilateral but can be bilateral. They appear similar to acquired palsies but the presence of large vertical fusional amplitudes is characteristic. Some palsies after minor head trauma represent decompensation of congenital palsies, evident when previous photographs of the patient show a head tilt.

ABDUCENS NERVE (SIXTH CRANIAL NERVE)

FUNCTION AND ANATOMY

The sixth nerve innervates the lateral rectus, which abducts the eye. The sixth nerve nucleus, however, contains two intermingled populations of neurons, one which projects through the sixth fascicle and nerve to the lateral rectus and another whose axons cross immediately to join the contralateral MLF and project to the contralateral medial rectus subnucleus of the third nerve. The sixth nerve nucleus thus controls conjugate ipsilateral horizontal eye movements.

The abducens nuclei lie in the medial dorsal pontine tegmentum, close to the floor of the fourth ventricle (see Fig. 15.2). The fascicle of the facial nerve (VII) curls around each nucleus dorsally, forming the facial colliculi on the floor of the ventricle. The MLF, which carries fibers from the contralateral sixth nerve nucleus to the ipsilateral medial rectus subnucleus, lies ventromedially.

The sixth nerve fascicle, like the third nerve fascicle, projects anteriorly with a caudal tilt, passing through the medial brainstem to emerge at the pontomedullary junction between the basis

pontis and the pyramids. Through this course it is associated with the parapontine reticular formation, the facial (VII) nucleus and fascicle, the central tegmental tract, the superior olivary nucleus, and the corticospinal tract.

The two sixth nerves ascend through the subarachnoid space closely parallel, dorsal to the clivus and the anterior inferior cerebellar artery. Each nerve penetrates the dura below the petrous crest, travels under the petroclinoid ligament, and enters the cavernous sinus, where it lies lateral to the internal carotid artery. For a brief period the sympathetic fibers may attach to it before passing to the first branch of the fifth nerve. The sixth nerve enters the superior orbital fissure, passes through the annulus of Zinn laterally, and quickly penetrates the lateral rectus.

CLINICAL SYNDROMES OF THE ABDUCENS NERVE

A unilateral sixth nerve palsy causes horizontal diplopia, with images that grow wider apart in far gaze and with gaze to the side of the palsy. On examination there is impaired abduction of the eye, although this may be minimal with partial lesions. Usually there is esotropia in the primary position which increases on ipsilateral gaze, although a subtler lesion may cause esotropia only on ipsilateral gaze. Esotropia is more prominent when a far target is used and may be absent with a near target. Abducting saccades are often slowed and there may be a dissociated nystagmus of the other eye during adduction (*Fig. 15.16*). This presumably represents the effects of central adaptation, analogous to the situation with INO. A bilateral sixth nerve palsy usually presents with esotropia in the primary position which increases on gaze to either side, with or without an obvious limitation of abduction.

Nuclear Lesions

As the sixth nerve nucleus contains a mix of sixth nerve neurons and interneurons projecting to the contralateral medial rectus, lesions of the nucleus do not create an abduction palsy. Instead, they cause an ipsilateral gaze palsy that affects all types of eye movements (*Fig. 15.17*). This distinguishes it from a lesion of the parapontine reticular formation, in which the vestibulo-ocular reflex eye movements are spared.

If the lesion involves the adjacent MLF, the ipsilateral gaze palsy will be accompanied by contralateral INO, a 'one-and-a-half' syndrome. Involvement of both sixth nerve nuclei will cause bilateral horizontal gaze palsy. The fascicle of the facial nerve is often affected by these lesions, causing an ipsilateral lower-motorneuron type of facial palsy (see Fig. 15.17).

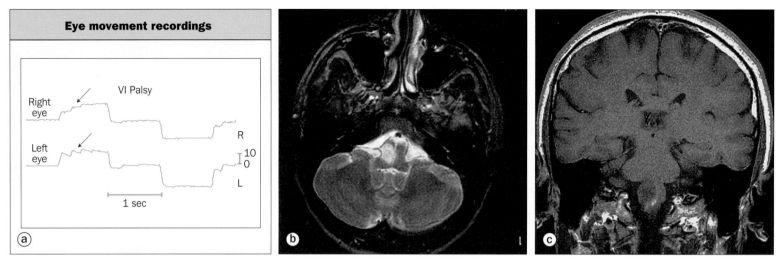

Fig. 15.16 A 32-year-old man with a right sixth nerve fascicular palsy. (**a**) Eye movement recordings, showing hypometric abducting movements in the right eye and adduction nystagmus in the left eye (arrows). Axial (**b**) and coronal (**c**) MRIs showing the presumed demyelinating lesion in the right ventral pontomedullary junction.

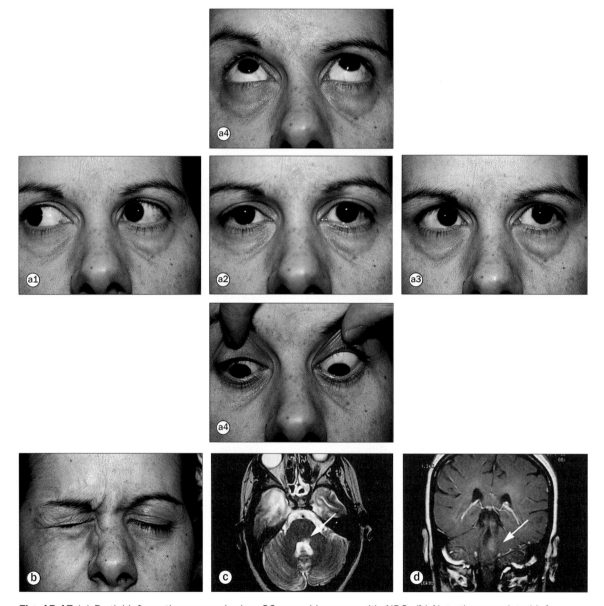

Fig. 15.17 (**a**) Partial left pontine gaze palsy in a 36-year-old woman with AIDS. (**b**) Note the associated left facial palsy. An axial (**c**) and coronal (**d**) MRI showing the lesion in region of the sixth nucleus (arrows).

Fascicular Lesions

There are three eponymous fascicular syndromes. Foville's syndrome arises from occlusion of the anterior inferior cerebellar artery, with infarction of the lateral pontine tegmentum. Extension medially will include either the fascicle or the nucleus. Associated signs are all ipsilateral: facial analgesia (V^1), flaccid facial palsy and loss of taste in the anterior tongue (VII), deafness (VIII), and Horner's syndrome. More ventral lesions of the medial basis pontis cause a contralateral hemiparesis (Raymond), sometimes also with ipsilateral facial palsy (Millard–Gubler).

Nerve Lesions

Cerebellopontine tumors that impair seventh and eighth nerve function may progress to a unilateral sixth nerve palsy too. In its subarachnoid course the two sixth nerves are close to each other; compressive tumors here often cause bilateral sixth nerve palsies. Other pathologies that affect the subarachnoid nerve, such as increased intracranial pressure and meningitis, may likewise cause unilateral or bilateral palsies (*Fig. 15.18*). Petrous apex lesions can lead to sixth and seventh nerve palsies, with involvement of the trigeminal ganglion as well. Cavernous sinus lesions can affect the VI nerve alone or in combination with the other nerves of the sinus, particularly the sympathetic fibers, giving a sixth nerve palsy with Horner's syndrome.

Etiology

Of the known causes of isolated sixth nerve palsy in adults, neoplasms and ischemia account for about one-quarter each

(*Fig. 15.19*). Neoplasm and trauma are more common causes of sixth nerve palsy in children. Hypertension and diabetes are particularly common causes of microvascular ischemic palsies in the elderly. Childhood tumors are usually brainstem gliomas or posterior fossa tumors, such as medulloblastoma or cerebellar astrocytoma. Ischemia and aneurysms are rare. Congenital syndromes include conjugate horizontal gaze palsy in children, Möbius syndrome (sixth and seventh nerve palsies), and Duane's retraction syndrome (*Fig. 15.20*). Duane's syndrome is relatively common. Three types exist, all distinguished from other VI palsies by co-contraction phenomena caused by anomalous innervation. In type 1 there is limited abduction but during adduction the eye retracts because both medial and lateral recti contract. Aplasia of the oculomotor cranial nerves is the common feature of all these syndromes.

MULTIPLE OCULAR PALSIES

Idiopathic and ischemic lesions are less common and compressive lesions are more common among multiple ocular motor nerve palsies (*Fig. 15.21*). Almost 40% of combined third, fourth, and sixth palsies are due to neoplasms, usually in the cavernous sinus. Combinations of third and fourth alone, or third and sixth alone, are due to neoplasms about 20% of the time. Aneurysms are unusual except for combined third and fourth nerve palsies, because only these two nerves are closely situated in their subarachnoid course. The combination of fourth and sixth nerve palsies alone is extremely rare and likely to arise only from a lesion in the cavernous sinus. If torsion is visible in a patient with III cranial nerve palsy and the eye is fully abducted then the IV nerve is intact.

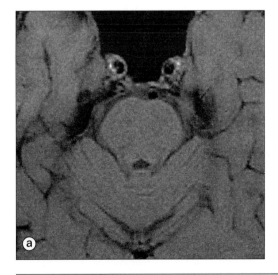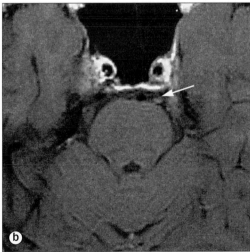

Fig. 15.18 Axial MRI without (**a**) and with (**b**) gadolinium in a 41-year-old man with ulcerative colitis, who presented with bilateral hearing loss and left sixth nerve palsy. The left subarachnoid sixth nerve enhances (arrow). Spinal fluid showed meningeal carcinomatosis from a previously unknown adenocarcinoma of the colon.

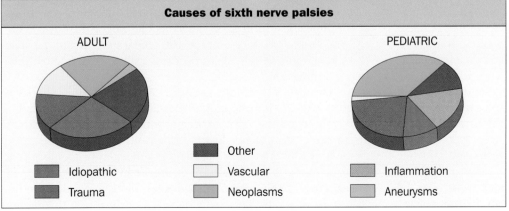

Fig. 15.19 Frequencies of causes of sixth nerve palsies in adults and children. (Data from Harley 1980 and Richards *et al.* 1992.)

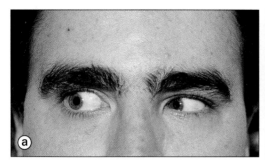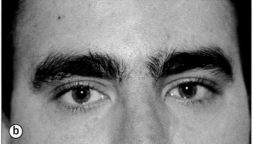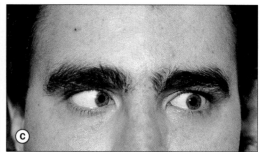

Fig. 15.20 Left Duane's retraction syndrome in a 29-year-old man. (**a**) The eyelids narrow in the left eye on right gaze. (**b**) Central gaze. (**c**) The left eye does not abduct well.

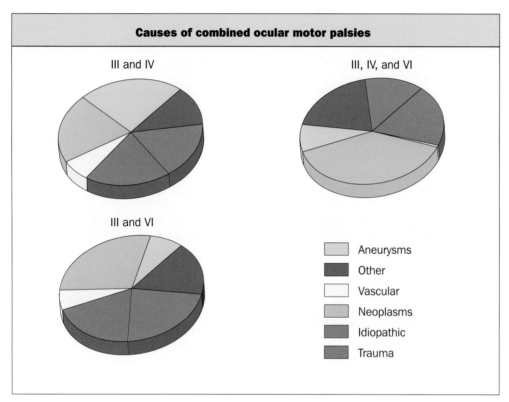

Causes of combined ocular motor palsies

III and IV

III, IV, and VI

III and VI

- Aneurysms
- Other
- Vascular
- Neoplasms
- Idiopathic
- Trauma

Fig. 15.21 Frequencies of causes of multiple ocular motor palsies. (Data from Harley, 1980 and Richards *et al.* 1992.)

CAVERNOUS SINUS

Anatomy, Clinical Features, and Lesions

The cavernous sinus is the venous confluence of the superior ophthalmic vein and the inferior petrosal sinus. The two sinuses flank the pituitary sella, extending from the clivus posteriorly to the superior orbital fissure anteriorly. Laterally lie the temporal lobes, whereas medially is the sella and the sphenoid sinus. Above the sinus is the suprasellar cistern, with structures of the optic pathway and circle of Willis.

The internal carotid artery enters the sinus, bends anteriorly as the siphon, gives off the ophthalmic artery, and exits the sinus. The sympathetic fibers to the eye leave the carotid within the sinus to join V$_1$. The sixth nerve also lies within the sinus, whereas cranial nerves third, fourth, V^1, and variably V^2 (proceeding from superior to inferior) lie within the sinus wall.

Lesions within the cavernous sinus can affect all or some of these nerves (see Fig. 15.10). Superior or inferior division palsies of the third nerve suggest a lesion here. The combination of a sixth nerve palsy with a Horner's syndrome also suggests a lesion within the sinus. Pain accompanying ophthalmoplegia may result from V^1 or V^2 involvement, which commonly occurs. More anteriorly, at the superior orbital fissure, lesions may affect the optic nerve, causing visual loss. Interference with the drainage from the superior ophthalmic vein leads to proptosis, lid edema, and conjunctival chemosis (*Fig. 15.22*).

Neoplasms account for as many as 70% of cavernous sinus syndromes, with about one-half of these being metastatic (see Fig. 15.1). Up to another 25% are due to intracavernous giant carotid aneurysms. Thus, mass lesions cause 90% or so of these syndromes. In the immunosuppressed population, pyogenic thrombosis or fungal infections such as mucormycosis require urgent treatment. It must be stressed that benign conditions like Tolosa–Hunt syndrome are diagnoses of exclusion in this region.

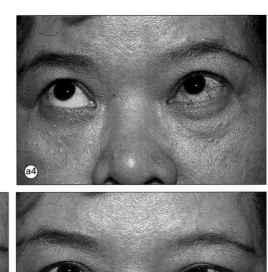

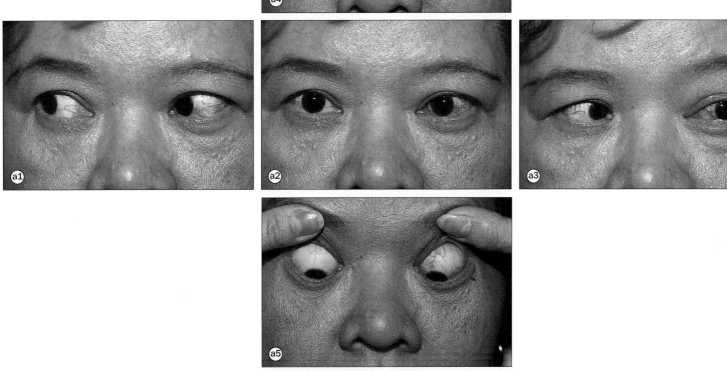

Fig. 15.22 A 53-year-old woman with a left carotid–cavernous sinus fistula causing (**a**) left sixth nerve palsy, mild proptosis, and (**b**) injection of conjunctival and scleral vessels. A left carotid angiogram (**c**), lateral view, shows abnormal filling of cavernous sinus (CVS) and superior ophthalmic vein (SOV).

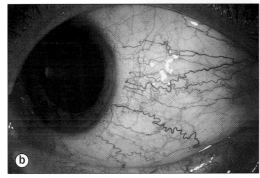

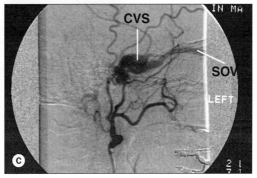

Further reading

Harley RD. Paralytic strabismus in children. Etiologic incidence and management of the third, fourth and sixth nerve palsies. *Ophthalmology.* 1980;**87**:24–43.

Linskey ME, Sekhar LN, Hirsch WL, Yonas H, Horton JA. Aneurysms of the intracavernous carotid artery: clinical presentation, radiographic features, and pathogenesis. *Neurosurgery.* 1990;**26**:71–79.

Nadeau SE, Trobe JD. Pupil sparing in oculomotor palsy: a brief review. *Ann Neurol.* 1983;**13**:143–148.

Richards BW, Jones FR, Younge BR. Causes and prognosis in 4,278 cases of paralysis of the oculomotor, trochlear, and abducens nerves. *Am J Ophthalmol.* 1992;**113**:489–496.

Thomas JE, Yoss RE. The parasellar syndrome: problems in determining etiology. *Mayo Clin Proc.* 1970;**45**:617–623.

Trobe JD. Third nerve palsy and the pupil. *Arch Ophthalmol.* 1988;**106**:601–602.

Trobe JD, Glaser JS, Post JD. Meningiomas and aneurysms of the cavernous sinus. Neuro-ophthalmologic features. *Arch Ophthalmol.* 1978;**96**:457–467.

CHAPTER 16

Cerebral and Brainstem Ocular Motor Disorders

James A Sharpe

Eye movements serve vision by placing the image of an object on the fovea of each retina, and by preventing slippage of images on the retina. Stability of retinal images is necessary, since slippage of images on the retina over 2–3 degrees/second blurs visual acuity. The brain employs two modes of ocular motor control: fast eye movements (saccades) and smooth (slow) eye movements. Fast eye movements bring the fovea to a target, and smooth eye movements prevent retinal image slip. Six distinct ocular motor systems are utilized to achieve clear vision (*Fig. 16.1*):

- The saccadic system.
- The smooth pursuit system.
- The optokinetic system.
- The vergence system.
- The vestibulo-ocular system.
- The fixation system.

Four of these systems generate conjugate gaze (or version) which is the subject of this chapter. Fixation maintenance and disjunctive horizontal movements, (or 'vergence'), are not considered here.

CONTROL SIGNALS

Recordings from ocular motor neurons in alert monkeys demonstrate that the innervational change during all types of eye movements consist of an eye velocity command (a phasic discharge) and an eye position command (a tonic discharge). During saccades, the phasic discharge consists of a high-frequency pulse of innervation that moves the eyes rapidly against orbital viscous forces (*Fig. 16.2*). When a new eye position is attained, the position command, called a step change in innervation, is required to sustain eye position against elastic restoring forces of the eye muscles. This is the pulse–step change of innervation for saccades (see Fig. 16.2). The pulse and step must be appropriately matched to prevent slow drift of the eyes after saccades.

The pulse is generated by burst neurons. For horizontal saccades, the burst neurons are located in the paramedian pontine reticular formation (PPRF). Burst neurons for vertical saccades reside in the rostral interstitial nucleus of the medial longitudinal fasciculus (riMLF) located within the medial longitudinal fasciculus (MLF) rostral to the third nerve nucleus. Between saccades, the burst neurons are kept silent by pause neurons located in the midline of the caudal pons (*Fig. 16.3*). When a saccade is dispatched, a trigger signal inhibits the pause neurons, thereby releasing the burst neurons to create the pulse. The step discharge (a position command) is generated from the pulse (a velocity command) by a neural integrator that 'integrates', in the mathematical sense, the pulse. This neural integrator for horizontal gaze is located in the medial vestibular nucleus and the nucleus prepositus hypoglossi, which lies just medial to the vestibular nuclei. The velocity-to-position integrator for vertical eye motion resides principally in the interstitial nucleus of Cajal, located within the MLF and just caudal to the riMLF in the rostral

Ocular motor control systems
Two goals
Binocular foveation
Prevent retinal slip
Two modes
Fast eye movements (saccades, quick phases)
Smooth eye movements
Six systems
Saccadic
Smooth pursuit
Vergence
Vestibulo-ocular
Optokinetic
Fixation

Fig. 16.1 Ocular motor control systems.

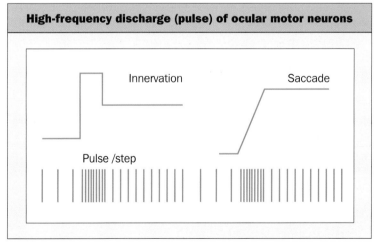

Fig. 16.2 Schema of high-frequency discharge (pulse) of ocular motor neurons that dispatch saccades and nystagmus quick phases and the level of tonic firing (step) of motor neurons required to sustain any desired eye position in the orbit. This innervation is represented as a histogram of the motor neuron firing rate.

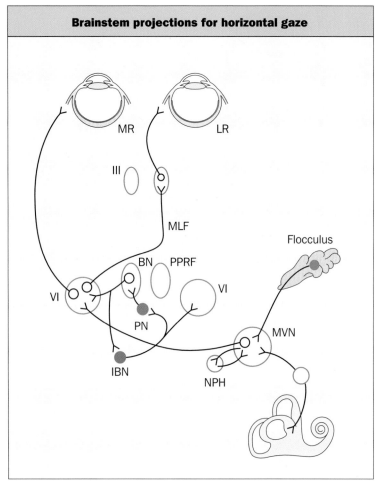

Brainstem projections for horizontal gaze

Fig. 16.3 Schema of some brainstem projections for horizontal gaze. Saccades are dispatched when a trigger signal turns off pause neurons, which inhibit burst neurons. Reciprocal inhibition of antagonist muscles is achieved by excitation of inhibitory burst neurons. (MR, medial rectus; LR, lateral rectus; III, oculomotor nucleus; MLF, medial longitudinal fasciculus; PPRF, pontine paramedian reticular formation; PN, pause neurons; BN, excitatory burst neurons; IBN, inhibitory burst neurons; NPH, nucleus prepositus hypoglossi; MVN, medial vestibular nucleus; VI, abducens nucleus.)

midbrain. The cerebellar flocculus also regulates the step of discharge via its connections with the neural integrator. Lesions of the integrator or its cerebellar connections cause gaze-evoked (gaze paretic) nystagmus.

Similarly, eye velocity commands for smooth pursuit, vestibular, and optokinetic smooth eye movements are transmitted directly to ocular motor neurons and also integrated by the neural integrator to yield appropriate position commands. The position commands are transmitted to ocular motor neurons from tonic cells of the neural integrator. All eye movement systems utilize the same velocity-to-position integrator.

OCULAR MOTOR SYSTEMS

SACCADIC SYSTEM

Saccades achieve rapid refixation of targets that fall on the extrafoveal retina by moving the eyes at peak velocities that can exceed 700 degrees/s. Their high speed minimizes the time of visual blurring created by the eye movement. The rapid eye movements that comprise the quick phases of optokinetic or vestibular nystagmus are also saccades. Refixation saccades and nystagmus quick phases have identical dynamic qualities, measured by the relationship by which their peak velocity increases as their amplitude increases. They are generated by the same burst neurons in the midbrain or pons.

Abnormalities of saccadic trajectory can by interpreted as disorders of triggering saccades, or as disorders of generating either the pulse or the step (*Fig. 16.4*). Horizontal saccades are initiated in the PPRF by supranuclear trigger signals from the frontal lobe eye fields, and from the superior colliculi (*Fig. 16.5*). The amplitude of saccades is established by a signal of desired eye position, usually the error between the fovea and the target position on the retina. This retinal error signal is derived from the striate cortex and processed by the parietal and frontal lobes before it is delivered to the PPRF. Similarly, vertical saccades are initiated by burst neurons in the riMLF in response to supranuclear trigger and retinal error signals. The frontal eye field in the posterior part of the middle frontal gyrus and the precentral sulcus and gyrus participates in dispatching saccades to predictable visual target locations and to remembered targets. The supplementary eye fields in the dorsomedial frontal lobe are important in planning sequences of saccades with or without visual cues. The dorsolateral prefrontal cortex plays a role in preparing saccades to memorized positions or imagined targets.

Saccades should be tested for their accuracy and speed by having the patient refixate between two targets, such as the examiner's fingers. Normal refixation movements are accomplished by one or two saccades. Inaccurate saccades are called dysmetric. Refixation movements of three or more saccades are termed hypometric saccades, which are abnormal if they predominate in one direction or comprise most large amplitude refixations. Saccades that consistently overshoot the target constitute overshoot dysmetria. Each dysmetric saccade is corrected by a return saccade after an interval of about 200 ms, the visual reaction time. If the examiner can see the eye move throughout the trajectory of a saccade, it is abnormally slow.

Saccadic Paralysis
Massive acute cerebral hemispheric lesions cause inability to trigger contralateral saccades. This cerebral saccadic palsy is transient, lasting hours or days. It may be explained by withdrawal of corticofugal innervation to the superior colliculus, in effect collicular shock. The horizontal vestibulo-ocular reflex is spared.

Acute unilateral frontal or parietal lobe hemispheric lesions cause transient ipsilateral deviation of the eyes and inability to make contralateral saccades beyond the orbital midposition (*Fig. 16.6*). An exception to the ipsilateral deviation after acute cerebral hemispheric lesions is the contralateral, 'wrong side' deviation (*Fig. 16.7*) for several hours to days that can follow hemorrhage in one thalamus (*Fig. 16.8*). In contrast to cerebral lesions, unilateral lesions of the PPRF (*Fig. 16.9*) cause contralateral deviation of the eyes and paralysis of ipsilateral saccades (*Fig. 16.10*). If the dorsal part of the caudal pontine tegmentum is damaged, the ipsilateral vestibulo-ocular reflex (VOR) is abolished; however, the VOR is spared if involvement is confined to the rostral or caudal pons, damaging the PPRF which lies ventral to the projections from the vestibular nuclei to the ocular motor nuclei (see Fig. 16.9).

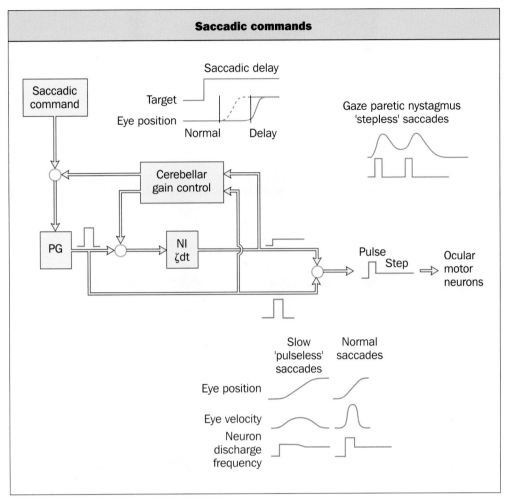

Fig. 16.4 A saccadic command from the cerebral hemisphere is delivered to the pulse generator (PG), consisting of burst neurons in the pontine paramedian reticular formation, for horizontal saccades, and the rostral interstitial nucleus of the medial longitudinal fasciculus, for vertical saccades. The saccadic command consists of both a trigger signal and a retinal error signal to the PG. The pulse (an eye velocity command) is transformed to step (eye position command) by the neural integrator (NI). The pulse and step are added and delivered to motor neurons. Different parts of the cerebellum separately control the output of the saccadic command and the step. The insets depict saccadic delay, gaze-evoked nystagmus, and slow versus normal saccades.

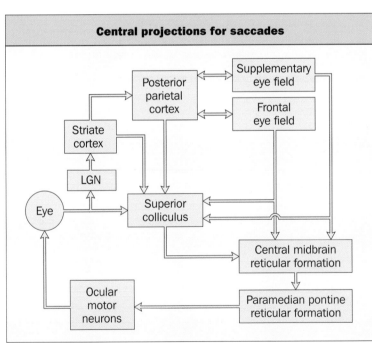

Fig. 16.5 Projections from the retina via the lateral geniculate nucleus (LGN) to the striate and extrastriate parietal lobe cortex, and to the frontal eye field and supplementary eye field in the supplementary motor area. These two frontal lobe areas project to the central midbrain reticular formation directly, and indirectly through a parallel pathway to the superior colliculus. Commands for horizontal saccades are delivered to the saccade generator in the paramedian pontine reticular formation. A direct retinocollicular projection to brainstem saccade generators is another parallel pathway.

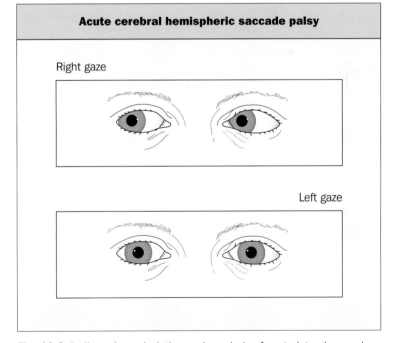

Fig. 16.6 Ipsilateral eye deviation and paralysis of contralateral saccades, beyond the midposition, after acute right cerebral hemispheric lesion.

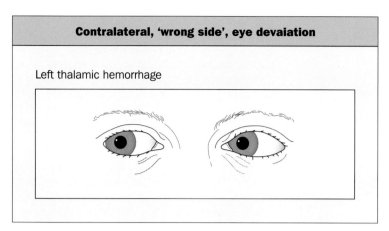

Fig. 16.7 Contralateral ('wrong side') eye deviation after left thalamic hemorrhage.

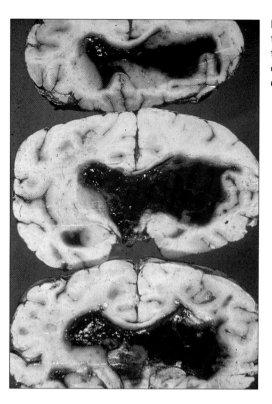

Fig. 16.8 Left thalamic hemorrhage that caused contralateral eye deviation.

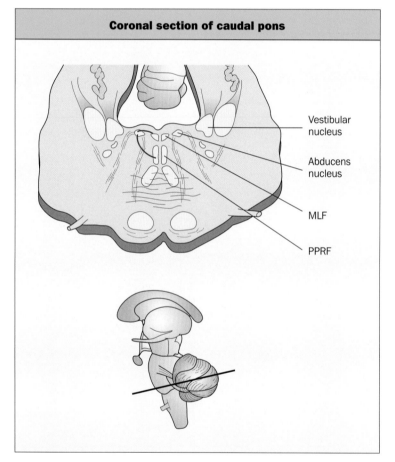

Fig. 16.9 Coronal section of caudal pons showing projections from paramedian pontine reticular formation (PPRF) to the abducens nucleus motor neurons and to interneurons which ascend in the contralateral medial longitudinal fasciculus (MLF). (Modified with permission from Sharpe JA, Rosenberg MA, Hoyt WF, Daroff RB. Paralytic pontine exotropia. *Neurology.* 1974;**24**:1076–1081.)

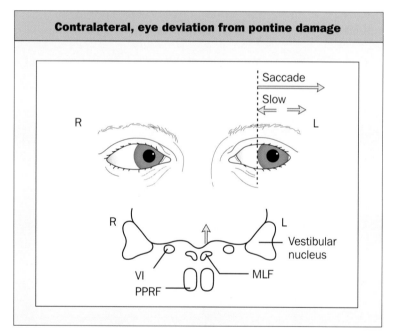

Fig. 16.10 Contralateral eye deviation after unilateral lesion in pontine tegmentum that involves paramedian pontine reticular formation (PPRF) and probably vestibular projections to abducens nucleus (VI). Ipsilateral saccades are paralyzed or slow. Slow (smooth) eye movements are possible in both directions in the contralateral hemifield of gaze.

Unilateral lesions of the midbrain reticular formation (MRF) cause paresis of contralateral saccades (and of ipsilateral smooth pursuit). Such lesions are usually associated with unilateral involvement of the oculomotor nucleus (*Fig. 16.11*). Unilateral nuclear third nerve palsy is evidenced by limited depression and adduction in the ipsilateral eye, limited elevation of both eyes (*Fig. 16.12*), and bilateral ptosis (*Fig. 16.13*). One oculomotor nucleus transmits axons to the opposite superior rectus muscles and axons from one oculomotor nucleus pass through the one opposite. Corticofugal projections that initiate contralateral saccades traverse the MRF to the caudal midbrain tegmentum where they decussate *en route* to the contralateral PPRF. Lesions rostral to this decussation of the saccadic pathway explain the paresis of contralateral saccades. Involvement below the decussation would cause paresis of ipsilateral saccades. Saccadic paresis is manifested by hypometria and slowing.

Exploded view of the oculomotor subnuclei

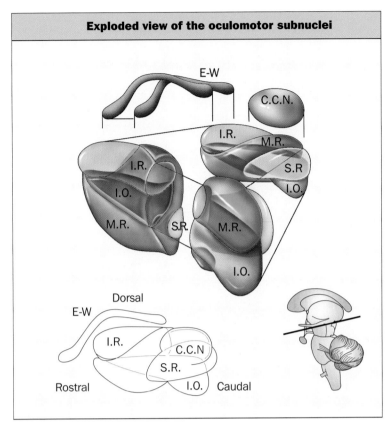

Fig. 16.11 A diagram of oculomotor nuclei, which are paired midline structures in the ventral periaqueductal gray matter. The right superior rectus subnucleus (SR) innervates the left superior rectus muscle and vice versa. The caudal central nucleus (CCN) is a midline unpaired structure that innervates both levator palpebrae muscles. All other subnuclei innervate the ipsilateral eye. (E–W, Edinger–Westphal nucleus to the sphincter pupillae and intraocular ciliary muscles; IR, inferior rectus; MR, medial rectus; IO, inferior oblique subnuclei.) (Adapted with permission from Sharpe JA. Analysis of diplopia. *Medicine North America.* 1986;**35**:5002–5026.)

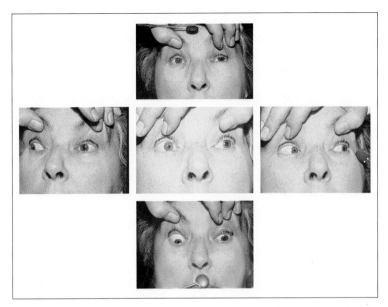

Fig. 16.12 Patient with left nuclear third nerve palsy form metastatic carcinoma in left midbrain tegmentum shows left exotropia in primary position, limited depression of left eye, and elevation palsy of both eyes.

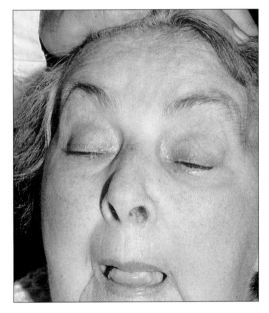

Fig. 16.13 Bilateral ptosis from unilateral metastatic carcinoma in left midbrain tegmentum, involving the caudal central nucleus (see Fig. 16.11) of ocular motor nucleus, in the same patient shown in Figure 16.12.

Slow Saccades

Slow saccades are caused by damage to excitatory burst neurons, inhibitory burst neurons, or pause neurons (see Fig. 16.3), or burst cell projections to the third, fourth, and sixth ocular motor nuclei. Lesions of the pontine tegmentum cause marked reduction of saccadic peak velocity (see Fig. 16.4). Slow saccades are a feature of focal lesions in the pontine tegmentum (see Fig. 16.9), such as infarcts and tumors, and of degenerations such as progressive supranuclear palsy (PSP), Huntington's disease, and variants of olivopontocerebellar degeneration (*Fig. 16.14*). Multiple sclerosis (MS), lipid storage diseases, or infections (e.g. acquired immunodeficiency syndrome [AIDS], Whipple disease) involving the tegmentum also cause slow saccades. The fast phases of optokinetic nystagmus (OKN) are also saccadic eye movements; they are also slowed when voluntary and reflex saccades to targets are slowed.

Another cause of slow saccades is peripheral neuromuscular disease (ocular myopathy, myasthenia gravis, and nerve palsies). Involvement of cerebral corticotegmental projections by strokes, and degenerations in the cerebral hemispheres, such as Parkinson's disease and Alzheimer's disease, cause mild, clinically imperceptible, slowing. Mental fatigue, reduced vigilance, and ingestion of sedative drugs also cause slight slowing of saccades.

Saccadic delay

Saccades are dispatched about 200 ms after a visual stimulus (see Fig. 16.4). Saccadic delay in all directions can be an enduring sign of cerebral cortical or basal ganglia involvement, as in Alzheimer's disease and Parkinson's disease. Saccadic latency measures neural conduction in the visual afferent and central ocular motor pathways. Although often clinically undetected in those conditions, prolonged saccadic latency is an obvious and fundamental defect in congenital ocular motor apraxia. Patients use head motion to dispatch coincident saccades. Combined motor programs for triggering eye and head movements serve to trigger saccades in ocular motor apraxia. This congenital disorder improves with maturation into adulthood. CT scanning is mandatory in ocular motor apraxia, since structural lesions of the posterior fossa or cerebral hemispheres may mimic congenital ocular motor apraxia.

Slow saccades
Paramedian pontine lesions
Demyelination
Infarct, hematoma
Neoplasm
Degeneration
Olivopontocerebellar
Progresive supranuclear palsy
Huntington's disease
Ataxia telangiectasia
Alzheimer's disease*
Parkinson's disease*
Anticonvulasant drugs
Midbrain lesions*
Cerebral hemispheric damage
Lipidosis
Tay Sachs
Gaucher: horizontal
Niemann–Pick: vertical
Infections
Acquired immunodeficiency syndrome (AIDS)
Whipple disease
Peripheral neuromuscular disease
Nerve palsy
Dysthyroid myopathy
Progressive external ophthalmoplegia
Myasthenia gravis
* Cerebral hemispheric or midbrain lesions, drugs, or mental fatigue cause mild slowing not evident clinically

Fig. 16.14 Slow saccades.

Hypometric Saccades

Saccadic refixations usually consist of one or two steps. Refixations of three or more saccadic steps are called multiple-step hypometric saccades (*Fig. 16.15*). They occur in some normal subjects after fatigue. They are conclusively abnormal if they predominate in one direction. Hypometric saccades reflect low gain in the saccadic system. The ratio of output (saccadic amplitude) to input (saccadic command) is subnormal.

Hypometric saccades occur contralateral to cerebral hemispheric damage and ipsilateral to cerebellar cortical lesions. Omnidirectional hypometric saccades accompany bilateral cerebral, basal ganglia, or cerebellar disease.

The occurrence of delayed and innacurate saccades in Parkinson's disease and Huntington's disease indicates that the basal ganglia participate in saccadic eye movements. The pars reticulata of the substantia nigra (SNr) and globus pallidus are major outflow pathways of the basal ganglia (*Fig. 16.16*). In monkeys, neurons of the SNr decrease their tonic discharge rate before saccades to visual, auditory, or remembered targets. The frontal

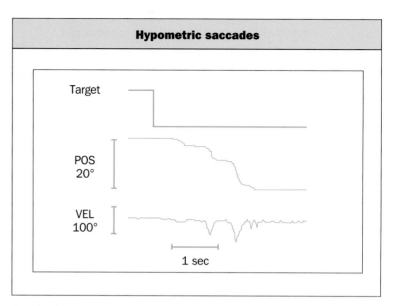

Fig. 16.15 Hypometric saccades consisting of three or more saccadic steps between two foveal target positions. Each hypometric saccade is slow. (POS, eye position; VEL, velocity)

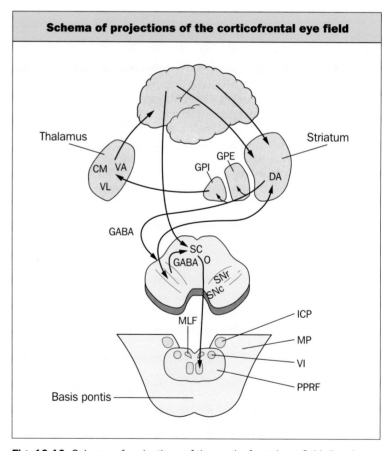

Fig. 16.16 Schema of projections of the corticofrontal eye field directly to the superior colliculus (SC) and indirectly via the caudate nucleus (striatum) to globus pallidus (GP) and substantia nigra pars reticulata (SNr). Inhibitory projections from SNr to SC and from the striatum to SNr are GABA-ergic. After crossing the midbrain in the dorsal tegmental decussation, projections from the superior colliculus and midbrain reticular formation reach the paramedian pontine reticular formation (PPRF). (VI, abducens nucleus; MLF, medial longitudinal fasciculus; ICP, inferior cerebellar peduncle; MP, middle cerebellar peduncle; VA, ventroanterior; VL, ventrolateral; CM, centromedian nulclei of thalamus; SNc, substantia nigra pars compacta.) (With permission from Sharpe JA. Supranuclear disorders of horizontal eye motion. *Semin Neurol.* 1986;**6**:155–166.)

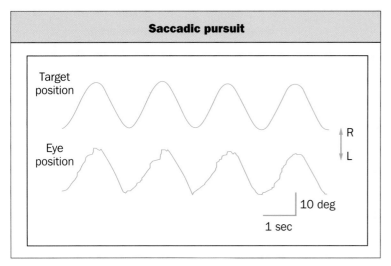

Fig. 16.17 Saccadic pursuit in one direction, ipsilateral to the side of a right parietotemporal hematoma, and smooth contralateral pursuit. Right is upward, left downward.

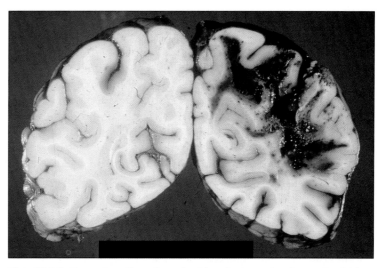

Fig. 16.18 Coronal section of cerebral hemisphere showing parietal lobe hemorrhage that caused saccadic pursuit toward the side of the lesion.

eye field projects to the caudate nucleus which in turn projects to the SNr. The SNr projects to the superior colliculus and inhibits it. Saccades are triggered when SNr inhibition of the superior colliculus is removed by suppression of the tonic activity of SNr neurons. During steady fixation, SNr sustains tonic inhibition of the superior colliculus, preventing extraneous saccades. Release of fixation allows the SNr to decrease its inhibitory drive upon the superior colliculus. The caudate nucleus is thought to mediate inhibition of SNr by γ-aminobutyric acid (GABA) and inhibition of the superior colliculus by SNr is also GABA-ergic (see Fig. 16.16). The striatal–SNr–superior colliculus circuit is thought to gate the release of voluntary and reflexive saccades. Inhibition of the superior colliculus by the SNr would help prevent unwanted reflexive saccades that occur in Huntington's disease in response to suddenly-appearing visual stimuli.

SMOOTH PURSUIT

Smooth pursuit maintains fixation of a slowly moving target. The pursuit system responds to slippage of an image near the fovea in order to accelerate the eyes to a velocity that matches that of the target. When smooth eye movement velocity fails to match target velocity, catch-up saccades are used to compensate for limited smooth pursuit velocities (*Fig. 16.17*). The examiner should move the target slowly (under 30–40 degrees/s) before the patient. If saccades are seen to track the target, the smooth pursuit system is inadequate. Low smooth pursuit velocity causes clinically evident saccadic tracking of a slowly moving target.

Unidirectional Pursuit Paresis
Clinical estimates of increased frequency and amplitude of saccades during tracking are used to diagnose smooth pursuit paresis. The disorder can be quantified by measurement of smooth pursuit gain, the ratio of smooth eye movement velocity to target velocity. Saccadic pursuit occurs toward the side of parietal lobe lesions (*Fig. 16.18*) and is usually associated with contralateral hemianopia, but the smooth eye movement disorder is independent of the visual defect. It does not accompany pregeniculate

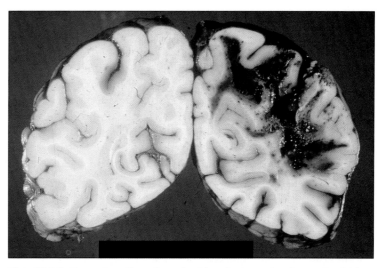

Fig. 16.19 Reconstruction of zones of lesions that overlapped in eight patients with asymmetric smooth pursuit; all had lower smooth pursuit velocities toward the side of the lesion. The area of common damage was contiguous on serial axial slices and involved Brodmann cortical areas 19 and 39, subcortical white matter, and the posterior limb of the internal capsule.

or striate cortical hemianopia. Asymmetric pursuit velocities in patients with hemianopia signify prestriate cortical damage or disruption of commissural connections that transmit retinal information from the normal cerebral hemisphere towards the visually deprived (hemianopic) hemisphere.

Unidirectional saccadic pursuit occurs towards the side of parietal lobe lesions (see Fig. 16.17), particularly involving the angular gyrus and prestriate cortical areas 19, 37, and 39 at the temporal–occipital–parietal junction (*Fig. 16.19*). These areas are the homologues of the MT (middle temporal) and MST (middle superior temporal) areas in the monkey brain. Pursuit defects similar to those seen after lesions to areas MT and MST in monkeys have been identified in humans. One type is defective smooth pursuit for targets moving towards the side of the lesion in response to stimuli presented in either visual hemifield – a directional defect. A second category is bidirectional impairment of horizontal pursuit to targets in the visual hemifield contralateral to the side of the lesion. Saccades to moving targets are also inaccurate in the contralateral hemifield. This pursuit defect is called a retinotopic defect; it is typical of lesions of the striate cortex, but it does not specify damage to the visual radiation or striate cortex, since patietotemporal lesions without hemianopia can have the same effect.

Cerebral hemispheric control of smooth pursuit is not entirely ipsilateral, since unilateral lesions can cause bidirectional impairment of pursuit. Cerebral hemidecortication in humans lowers ipsilateral gain, but does not abolish ipsilateral smooth pursuit. Partial sparing of ipsilateral pursuit may be attributed to pathways in the opposite cerebral hemisphere that contribute to contralateral smooth pursuit. Gain for contralateral low-velocity targets may exceed 1.0. When smooth eye movement velocity exceeds target velocity, back-up saccades opposite to the direction of smooth eye motion are utilized to refoveate the target. Above-normal pursuit gains in patients with large hemispheric lesions can be associated with ipsilaterally beating nystagmus; the slow phase velocities of this pursuit paretic nystagmus are too low (1–3 degrees/s) to account for the measured pursuit asymmetry. This nystagmus may be explained by imbalanced drive of smooth eye tracking systems, either pursuit or optokinetic.

Retinotopic pursuit defects can be identified in the laboratory, but not by bedside or clinic examination. A target that jumps away from the fovea into one hemifield and then moves at constant speed either towards or away from the fovea is called a step-ramp target; it enables the examination of the initiation of smooth tracking towards a pursuit stimulus from any desired location on the retina close to, or remote from, the fovea. In contrast, pursuit of a continuous to-and-fro target elicits steady-state pursuit (pursuit maintenance) with the fovea at or near the target.

Visual inattention to contralateral space does not produce a unidirectional smooth pursuit deficit, just as hemianopia does not. Inattention to contralateral space with reference to head position (craniotopic space) does not cause unidirectional pursuit defects either. Inattention to contralateral craniotopic space causes a bidirectional pursuit defect within the contralateral zone of target motion. Some patients with acute frontal or parietal lobe damage do not track targets past the midline into the contralateral craniotopic field of gaze. Cerebral hemispheric pursuit defects can be grouped into four categories (*Fig. 16.20*):

- Unidirectional saccadic pursuit towards the side of the lesions. Contralateral smooth pursuit velocities may be normal, high, or low (but above ipsilateral smooth eye movement velocities).
- Bidirectional saccadic pursuit in both hemifields without asymmetry.
- Retinotopic impairment of pursuit in all directions in the contralateral visual hemifield.
- Paralysis of pursuit contralateral to the craniotopic midline after acute hemisphere lesions.

Frontal lobe lesions may also cause asymmetric pursuit paresis that appears to be symmetric on clinical examination. Quantitative eye movement recording demonstrates lower smooth pursuit gain toward the side of damage in some patients. Reduced ipsilateral pursuit gain with frontal lobe lesions may result from

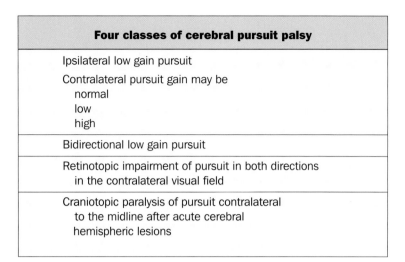

Four classes of cerebral pursuit palsy

Ipsilateral low gain pursuit
Contralateral pursuit gain may be
normal
low
high
Bidirectional low gain pursuit
Retinotopic impairment of pursuit in both directions in the contralateral visual field
Craniotopic paralysis of pursuit contralateral to the midline after acute cerebral hemispheric lesions

Fig. 16.20 Four classes of cerebral pursuit palsy.

involvement of the human homologue of the simian frontal eye fields. The ipsidirectional pursuit defects caused by damage to either of two distinct cerebral regions, angular gyrus or dorsolateral frontal lobe, imply two parallel routes through which cortical pursuit commands are conveyed to the brainstem. Lesions within the posterior limb of the internal capsule cause asymmetric pursuit. Ipsilateral pursuit impairment that accompanies posterior thalamic hemorrhage may be explained by involvement of the posterior limb of the capsule (see Fig. 16.19). A descending pathway in monkeys from the MST to the pons traverses the posterior limb of the internal capsule and adjacent pulvinar. A putative pursuit pathway is depicted in *Figure 16.21*.

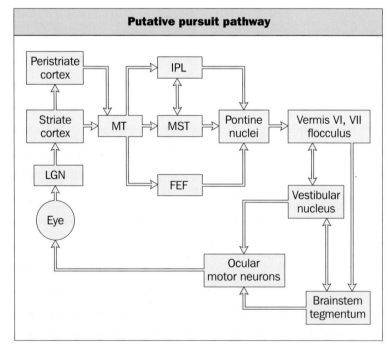

Putative pursuit pathway

Fig. 16.21 Schematic organization of circuit used for generating smooth pursuit, based on data from monkeys. Homologues of area of MT and MST in the human brain are Brodmann areas 19 and 39. (LGN, lateral geniculate nucleus; MT, middle temporal area; MST, middle superior temporal area; IPL, inferior parietal lobule; FEF, frontal eye field; VI, VII, lobules VI and VII of the cerebellar vermis.)

Smooth pursuit paresis
Ipsilateral
Parieto–temporo–occipital (areas 37, 39, 19)
Posterior lateral frontal lobe
Midbrain tegmentum
Basis pontis
Cerebellum (flocculus)
Contralateral
Caudal pontine tegmentum
Lateral medulla
Fastigial nucleus of cerebellum

Fig. 16.22 Smooth pursuit paresis.

Unilateral lesions of the MRF may impair smooth pursuit toward the side of damage. Ipsilateral saccadic pursuit also occurs towards the side of lesions that involve the cerebellar flocculus (*Fig. 16.22*).

The routes through which pursuit motor commands are transmitted to motor neurons in the brainstem are uncertain; it is probable that pontine nuclei, particularly the dorsolateral pontine nuclei (DLPN), relay excitatory mossy fiber efferents to the cerebellum. Projection from the pontine nuclei to the flocculus are scanty, and contralateral. The smooth pursuit

pathway undergoes double decussation (*Fig. 16.23*), the first decussation occurring in the projection from the brainstem to the cerebellum, and the second decussation occurring between the vestibular nucleus and the contralateral abducens nucleus. Experimental chemical lesions confined to neurons in the PPRF leave smooth pursuit intact. Selective infarction of the midline and medial part of both PPRFs paralyzes saccades and nystagmus quick phases in all directions, while sparing smooth pursuit and the VOR.

In contrast to unilateral lesions in the cerebral hemisphere, vestibulocerebellum, or rostral pons, unilateral tegmental damage in the caudal pons and rostral medulla impairs contralateral smooth pursuit (see Fig. 16.22). Damage to the fastigial nucleus of the cerebellum impairs contradirectional pursuit. Greater paresis of contralateral pursuit with pontomedullary damage may signify disruption of projections from the vestibular nucleus to the abducens nucleus (see Fig. 16.23).

Omnidirectional Pursuit Paresis
Saccadic pursuit in all directions results from diffuse cerebral, cerebellar, or brainstem disease. For example, MS, Parkinson's disease, Alzheimer's disease, and cerebellar degenerations all cause saccadic tracking of slowly moving targets (*Fig. 16.24*). Advanced age (over 65 years), sedative drugs, fatigue, and inattention also lower smooth pursuit velocities and thereby cause saccadic tracking. When qualified by these influences, omnidirectional saccadic pursuit is the most sensitive ocular motor sign of brain dysfunction.

Fig. 16.23 Putative brainstem pursuit pathway showing double decussation. The first decussation is from pontine nuclei (mainly the dorsolateral pontine nucleus) to the cerebellar flocculus. Mossy fibers excite basket and stellate cells which inhibit Purkinje cells. Purkinje cells, in turn, inhibit neurons in the medial vestibular nucleus (MVN). Excitatory projections from the MVN to the contralateral abducens nucleus (VI) constitute a second decussation. (With permission from Johnston JL, Sharpe JA, Morrow MJ. Paresis of contralateral smooth pursuit and normal vestibular smooth eye movements after unilateral brainstem lesions. *Ann Neurol.* 1992;**31**:495–502.)

Causes of omnidirectional pursuit impairment
Degenerative diseases
Acquired immunodeficiency syndrome
Alzheimer's disease
Parkinson's disease
Progressive supranuclear palsy
Cerebellar ataxias
Schizophrenia
Drugs
Ethanol
Barbiturates
Benzodiazepines
Carbamazepine
Chloral hydrate
Lithium
Methadone
Phenytoin
Other causes
Senescence
Inattention

Fig. 16.24 Causes of omnidirectional pursuit impairment.

VESTIBULO-OCULAR SYSTEM

The VOR subserves vision by generating conjugate eye movements that are equal and opposite to head movements. In that way, images of the stable world remain stationary on the retina. The reflex keeps gaze (the sum of eye position and head position) stable relative to the world. The ratio of eye velocity to head velocity – the VOR gain – must approximate 1.0 as the eyes and head move in opposite directions. If the gain is too high or too low, the target image is off the fovea. Head motion stimulates the semicircular canals to activate the VOR. Oscillopsia is an illusionary to-and-fro movement of the environment. It is provoked by head movement in many patients with abnormalities of VOR gain. For example, patients with bilateral labyrinthine disease or brainstem lesions who have low gain often experience oscillopsia during rapid head movements (*Fig. 16.25*). Oscillopsia is sometimes noted when the eyes and head are not perfectly out of phase (by 180 degrees) as they move in opposite directions. Imbalance of the VOR causes nystagmus when the head is still, which can cause oscillopsia. Abnormalities of VOR gain and balance can be assessed in the clinic and at the bedside (*Fig. 16.26*). High frequency active head motion causes nystagmus if the reflex gain is hyperactive or hypoactive. If the VOR gain is hyperactive (gain > 1), nystagmus fast phases are in the same direction as head motion. If the VOR is hypoactive (gain < 1), nystagmus is directed opposite to head motion. The patient may perceive movement of images in the direction of the fast phase (see Fig. 16.25), which is actually a corrective foveating saccade.

The VOR can also be tested in the clinic by having the patient make active head movements at a high frequency (2–3 Hz) while viewing Snellen test letters. Acuity should remain the same as that recorded with the head immobile. If visual acuity falls during active to-and-fro head oscillation, then the VOR is overactive or underactive. It is also possible to assess the VOR during ophthalmoscopy with the pupil dilated. The patient is instructed to shake his/her head from side to side at about 2–3 Hz. The nonvisualized eye is covered. If the VOR is functioning normally, the optic disc

Bedside tests of the VOR
Head shaking over 1.0 Hz
Test visual acuity
Look for nystagmus
Examine the optic disc
Oculocephalic maneuvers
Caloric tests

Fig. 16.26 Bedside tests of the VOR.

(or other fundus landmark) does not move during head rotation. If VOR gain is hyperactive, the disc oscillates in the same direction as the head. If the reflex is hypoactive, the head and optic disc oscillate in opposite directions. It is important that head motion be sustained at well over 1 Hz, since smooth pursuit and optokinetic following reflexes can compensate for VOR deficits during head motion below that frequency. Care must be taken that the head does not shift from side to side, since translation of the head causes movement of the optic disc even when the VOR is normal. The patient should wear his/her regular spectacles, since VOR gain is adapted to the power of corrective lenses.

Oculocephalic Maneuvers

In unconscious patients, oculocephalic maneuvers assess the VOR in the absence of visual following reflexes. In unconscious patients, nystagmus fast phases are absent and the eyes deviate in the direction of stimulation. Failure of deviation indicates structural interruption or severe metabolic depression of brainstem VOR pathways. Drug intoxication can paralyze the VOR in the early stages of coma. Discrete involvement of brainstem VOR connections by structural lesions sometimes causes perverted vestibular responses in directions different from the VOR stimulus vector. Sedative drug intoxication may mimic structural lesions by causing monocular paresis of adduction (internuclear ophthalmoplegia – INO) or delayed downward deviation in response to unilateral caloric stimulation.

In alert patients, however, full ocular excursion does not necessarily indicate that the VOR is normal. If the head is moved at low accelerations, intact smooth pursuit and optokinetic following reflexes may compensate for a defective VOR and elicit full excursion despite a subnormal VOR. Nonetheless, oculocephalic responses are useful in detecting the range of VOR excursion; in patients with paralysis of saccades and pursuit, the presence of active oculocephalic reflexes indicates sparing of the VOR and signifies that the ophthalmoplegia is caused by supranuclear damage to saccadic and pursuit pathways.

OPTOKINETIC SYSTEM

Optokinetic smooth eye movements aid vestibular eye movements by stabilizing images on the retina during constant velocity or very low-frequency head movement, when the VOR does not function optimally. The optokinetic system is the helpmate of the vestibulo-ocular system; they act in concert to keep the eyes still as the head moves. During constant velocity head rotation in darkness, the vestibular nystagmus response fades away as a cupula returns

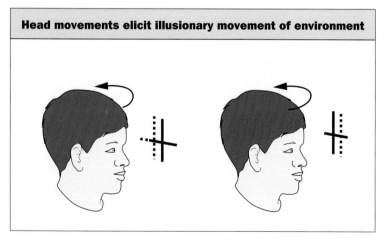

Head movements elicit illusionary movement of environment

Fig. 16.25 Head movements elicit illusionary movement of environment, when vestibulo-ocular reflex gain is abnormal. If the gain is too high, the image moves in the same direction as head movement (left). If the vestibulo-ocular reflex is too low, the images seem to move opposite to the direction of head movement (right). (With permission from Bender MB, Feldman M. *Arch Neurol.* 1967;**17**:354–364.)

to its initial position. During rotation in the light, however, optokinetic smooth eye movements compensate for the deficient VOR. The retinal slip generates eye movements to stabilize images on the retina. The optokinetic system requires a full-field stimulus for an optimal response.

Small hand-held striped tapes or drums (*Fig. 16.27*) that are used in the clinic to test optokinetic nystagmus (OKN) activate both smooth pursuit and optokinetic smooth eye movements, but they do not appreciably activate the optokinetic system. The slow phases of nystagmus stimulated by small targets are probably generated largely by the pursuit system. The recording of optokinetic-after nystagmus (OKAN) in darkness is a means of detecting function of the optokinetic system without the influence of the smooth pursuit system. The pursuit system is concerned with foveal tracking of small objects, while the optokinetic system is responsible for panretinal tracking of large objects. Genuine optokinetic nystagmus elicited by a full-field stimulus (unlike those in Fig. 16.27) is accompanied by illusionary self rotation (circularvection) and followed by OKAN in darkness. This does not negate the value of small OKN stimuli in the clinical setting, since paretic pursuit typically accompanies impaired OKN. Like smooth pursuit, OKN evoked by hand-held targets is defective when stimuli move towards the side of cerebral and cerebellar lesions. The amplitude and frequency of the nystagmus response is reduced, but the primary deficit is reduction in the slow phase velocity.

BRAINSTEM GAZE CONTROL

HORIZONTAL GAZE

Horizontal Vestibulo-Ocular Reflex

The horizontal VOR is served by an excitatory projection composed of a three-neuron pathway from the horizontal semicircular canal to the medial vestibular nucleus, through the ascending tract of Deiters, which lies just lateral to the MLF (*Fig. 16.28*), then to the ipsilateral medial rectus subnucleus of the oculomotor nucleus. Another excitatory pathway projects from the vestibular nucleus to the contralateral abducens nucleus and then through internuclear neurons in the abducens nucleus to the ipsilateral MLF and medial rectus subnucleus (see Fig.16.11). These three or four neuron reflex arcs carry the head (eye) velocity command. The integrated vestibular eye position command is generated from the head velocity command by connections to the nucleus prepositus and back to the medial vestibular nucleus. The integrated (eye position) command is transmitted to the medial rectus and lateral rectus motor neurons through the same vestibular neurons that transmit the eye velocity command.

The abducens nucleus contains both motor neurons to the lateral rectus muscle and internuclear neurons that project in the contralateral MLF to medial rectus motor neurons (Figs 16.2, 16.28). These internuclear neurons may be the most important horizontal VOR pathway to the medial rectus and they also transmit the saccadic and pursuit signals to the medial rectus. Thus, a lesion of the abducens nucleus causes ipsilateral conjugate palsy of saccades, pursuit, and vestibular movements, not isolated sixth nerve (lateral rectus) palsy. Burst neurons in the PPRF that generate horizontal saccades also project to ipsilateral abducens nucleus motor neurons and internuclear neurons.

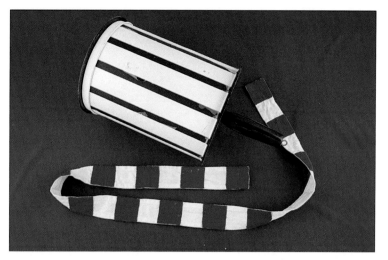

Fig. 16.27 Hand-held optokinetic tape and drum used to elicit sequential saccades and smooth tracking.

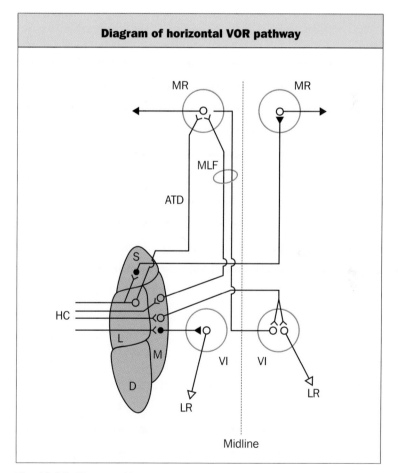

Fig. 16.28 Diagram of horizontal VOR pathway that carries eye velocity commands from the semicircular canal (HC) to medial rectus (MR) subnucleus of the oculomotor nucleus and to the abducens nucleus (VI). Excitatory second-order vestibular neurons project to the MR through the medial longitudinal fasciculus (MLF) and the ascending tract of Deiters (ATD). The abducens nucleus contains motor neurons of the lateral rectus muscle and interneurons that project through the opposite MLF to the MR. Open symbols indicate excitatory neurons and filled symbols indicate inhibitory neurons. Inhibition of internuclear neurons in the ipsilateral abducens nucleus is not illustrated. (S, superior; L, lateral; M, medial; and D, descending vestibular nuclei; LR, lateral rectus muscles.) (With permission from Sharpe JA and Johnston JL. The vestibulo-ocular reflex: clinical, anatomic and physiologic correlates. In: Sharpe JA, Barber HO, eds. *The Vestibulo-Ocular Reflex and Vertigo*. [New York: Raven Press; 1993] 15–39.)

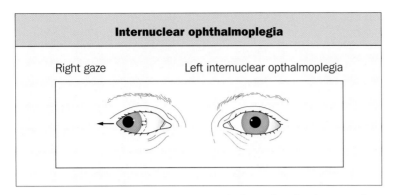

Internuclear ophthalmoplegia

Right gaze   Left internuclear opthalmoplegia

Fig. 16.29 Internuclear ophthalmoplegia of left eye from involvement of the left medial longitudinal fasciculus. During leftward gaze, adduction of the left eye is paralyzed and there is abducting jerk nystagmus of the right eye.

Lesions of the PPRF burst neurons cause conjugate paralysis or slowing of ipsilateral saccades.

Internuclear ophthalmoplegia consists of impaired adduction on the side of the lesion in the MLF and abducting jerk nystagmus of the opposite eye (*Fig. 16.29*). In total INO, adduction is paralyzed to saccadic, pursuit, and vestibular stimulation. Slow adducting saccades are the only manifestation of incomplete or chronic lesions. Subtle INO is made obvious by dissociated OKN, when targets move in the direction of the paretic eye; that is, towards the side of MLF damage. The intensity of nystagmus is reduced on the side of the INO, when contrasted with active OKN in the fellow eye. Lesions of the MLF disrupt vertical vestibular and pursuit commands that ascend from the vestibular nuclei through the MLF (see below). In INO vertical pursuit and vertical VOR, movements are slowed but vertical saccades are normal. Gaze-evoked nystagmus occurs during upward, and sometimes downward, fixation.

The combination of unilateral pontine gaze palsy and INO causes the one-and-a-half syndrome. Damage to the PPRF or abducens nucleus and the MLF on one side (*Fig. 16.30*) is manifested by paralysis of horizontal movements of the ipsilateral eye in both directions and paralysis of adduction in the opposite eye. In the acute phase the opposite eye is exotropic (*Fig. 16.31*). This 'paralytic pontine exotropia' is distinguished from other types of exotropia by slowed adducting saccades in the laterally deviated eye and the horizontal immobility of the eye on the side of pontine damage.

VERTICAL GAZE

As a general principle, vertical gaze is mediated by bilateral circuits and vertical gaze palsies signify bilateral or paramedian lesions.

Vertical Saccades
Commands from the caudal PPRF are carried rostrally in the brainstem tegmentum to the riMLF. Burst neurons in the riMLF that generate upward saccades project across the posterior commissure (*Fig. 16.32*) and then to motor neurons in the third nerve nucleus (*Fig. 16.33*). Burst neurons in the riMLF that generate downward saccades project, predominately ipsilaterally, to the third and fourth nerve nuclei (see Fig. 16.33). Projections from the riMLF to the interstitial nucleus of Cajal (INC) are also important in mediating vertical gaze.

Vertical Vestibulo-Ocular Reflex
Each semicircular canal activates two extraocular muscles that

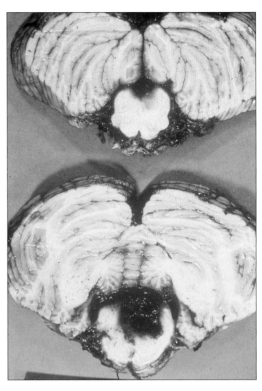

Fig. 16.30 Hemorrhage in right side of the tegmentum at the junction of the pons and the medulla caused a one-and-a-half syndrome (right internuclear ophthalmoplegia, and rightward gaze palsy) in a child with a brainstem arteriovenous malformation.

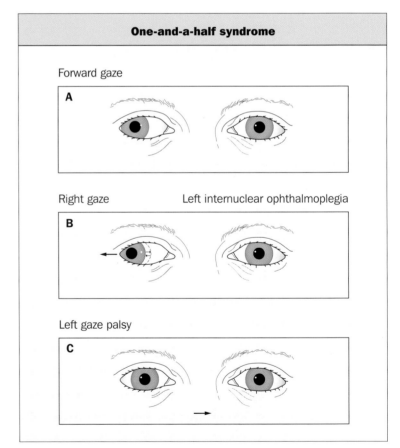

One-and-a-half syndrome

Forward gaze

A

Right gaze   Left internuclear ophthalmoplegia

B

Left gaze palsy

C

Fig. 16.31 One-and-a-half syndrome from lesion in the left caudal pontine tegmentum involving the left medial longitudinal fasciculus and abducens nucleus (or paramedian pontine reticular formation). There is exotropia of the right eye (**a**). During rightward gaze (**b**) a left internuclear ophthalmoplegia is evident. Attempted leftward gaze (**c**) shows a leftward saccadic palsy. (With permission from Sharpe JA, Rosenberg MA, Hoyt WF, Daroff RB. Paralytic pontine exotropia. *Neurology.* 1974;**24**:1076–1081.)

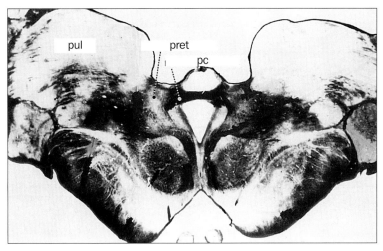

Fig. 16.32 Transverse section of the caudal diencephalon and rostral midbrain showing the posterior commissure dorsal to the third ventricle, and the adjacent pretectum. Lesions with the posterior commissure, and unilateral or bilateral lesions of the immediately adjacent pretectum, interrupt fibers from the rostral interstitial nucleus of the medial longitudinal fasciculus (mediating upward and torsional saccades), and fibers from the interstitial nucleus of Cajal (mediating upward smooth eye movements).Pul, pulvinar; pret, pretectum; pc, post commissure.

rotate each eye in the same plane as the semicircular canal is oriented. One anterior canal excites the ipsilateral superior rectus and the contralateral inferior oblique muscles (*Fig. 16.34*), resulting in elevation and contralateral torsion of both eyes. Each posterior semicircular canal excites the ipsilateral superior oblique and contralateral inferior rectus muscles (*Fig. 16.35*). One posterior canal activates depression and contralateral torsion of both eyes. Both anterior canals activate the upward VOR during downward head acceleration and both posterior canals activate the downward VOR during upward head acceleration.

Axons from the vertical canals on one side synapse in the vestibular nucleus. Their excitatory projections cross the midline to innervate the contralateral inferior oblique and inferior rectus muscles and the ipsilateral superior rectus and superior oblique muscles (see Figs 16.34, 16.35). The motor neurons innervating those four muscles are all located on the same side of the brainstem. Excitation from the anterior canals ascends in the brachium conjunctivum (see Fig. 16.34) and a ventral tegmental pathway beneath the MLF. Excitatory projections from the posterior canal ascend in the contralateral MLF (see Fig. 16.35). Thus, lesions of the MLF cause INO (see above), and also impair

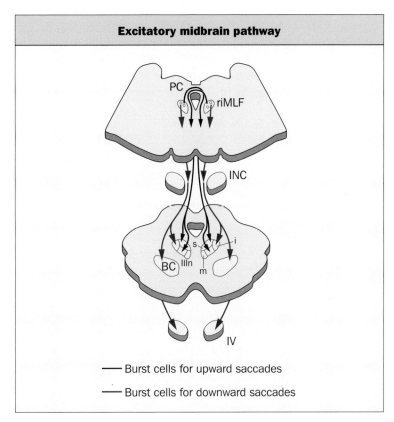

Fig. 16.33 Excitatory midbrain pathway that generated vertical saccades showing projections from the riMLF across the posterior commissure (PC) to the superior rectus (s) and inferior oblique subnuclei of the oculomotor nucleus (III). Projections from the rostral interstitial nucleus of the medial longitudinal fasciculus (riMLF) to the inferior rectus subnucleus (i) and the trochlear nucleus (IV) mediate downward (and torsional) saccades. Lesions in the ventral pretectum, interrupting fibers from the interstitial nucleus of Cajal (INC) and riMLF ventral to the aquaduct of Silvius, as they project to the oculomotor and trochlear nuclei, cause selective paralysis of downward gaze. (BC, brachium conjunctivum.) (With permission from Ranalli PJ, Sharpe JA, Fletcher WA. Palsy of upward and downward saccadic, pursuit and vestibular movements with unilateral midbrain lesion: pathophysiologic correlations. *Neurology.* 1988;**38**:114–122.)

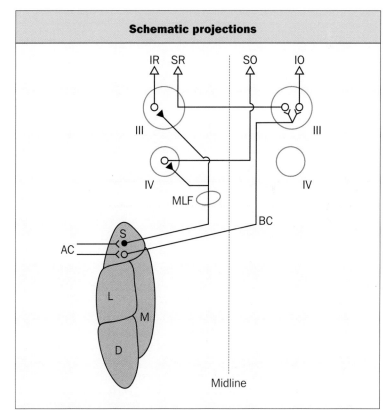

Fig. 16.34 Schematic projections from the anterior semicircular canal to the oculomotor (III) and trochlear (IV) nuclei. Excitatory anterior canal (AC) signals traverse the brachium conjunctivum (BC) and inhibitory AC signals go through the medial longitudinal fasciculus (MLF). Open symbols indicate excitatory neurons and filled symbols indicate inhibitory neurons. (S, superior; L, lateral; M, medial; and D, descending vestibular nuclei; IR, inferior rectus; SR, superior rectus; SO, superior oblique; IO, inferior oblique muscles.) (With permission from Sharpe JA, Johnston JL. The Vestibulo-ocular reflex: clinical, anatomic, and physiological correlations. In: Sharpe JA, Barber HO, eds. *The Vestibulo-Ocular Reflex and Vertigo.* [New York: Raven Press, 1993] 15–39.)

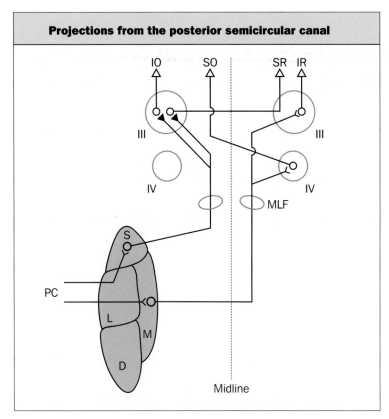

Projections from the posterior semicircular canal

IO   SO   SR IR

III   III

IV   MLF   IV

PC

Midline

Fig. 16.35 Projections from the posterior semicircular canal (PC) to the ocular motor (III) and trochlear (IV) nuclei. Second order vestibular neurons carry PC information through the medial longitudinal fasciculus (MLF). Open symbols indicate excitatory neurons, and filled symbols indicate inhibitory neurons. (S, superior; L, lateral; M, medial; and D, descending vestibular nuclei; IR, inferior rectus; SR, superior rectus; SO, superior oblique; IO, inferior oblique muscles.) (With permission from Sharpe JA, Johnston JL. The vestibulo-ocular reflex: clinical, anatomic, and physiologic correlations. In: Sharpe JA, Barber HO, eds. *The Vestibulo-Ocular Reflex and Vertigo*. [New York: Raven Press, 1993] 15–39.)

Pretectal syndrome
Upward gaze palsy
Upward saccade palsy
Upward pursuit and saccade palsy
Upward vestibulo-ocular reflex palsy
Retraction saccades
Lid retraction
Light–near dissociated pupils

Fig. 16.36 The pretectal syndrome.

the vertical VOR. The eye velocity-to-position integrator for vertical movements includes the INC.

Vertical smooth pursuit pathways include the cerebellar flocculus and posterior vermis, and the superior vestibular nucleus. Pursuit signals project rostrally through the MLF and brachium conjunctivum to the third and fourth nerve nuclei. The posterior commissure probably conveys upward VOR and smooth pursuit signals to the oculomotor nucleus.

Pretectal Syndrome

Paralysis of upward saccades, with variable sparing, or loss, of upward smooth pursuit or the VOR or both, is associated with bursts of binocular adduction and retraction (convergent–retraction saccadic pulses, not true 'nystagmus') that are elicited by attempted upward saccades, and with light–near dissociation of the pupils (*Fig. 16.36*). The upper eyelids are often retracted – a phenonemon known as Collier's sign or the posterior fossa stare. Destruction of the posterior commissure is sufficient to cause pretectal syndrome, but bilateral or unilateral extracommissural pretectal lesions that interrupt its fibers have the same effect. Limitation of vertical gaze is also an effect of senescence. Upward saccades are most vulnerable, with vertical pursuit and vestibular smooth eye movements being preserved in many cases. This pretectal syndrome is associated with a variety of ocular signs that encompass the eponyms sylvian aqueduct and dorsal midbrain syndromes. The eponym Parinaud syndrome is not appropriate for this constellation of neuro-ophthalmic signs, since Parinaud neither described it nor reported that dorsal pretectal damage was responsible for palsy of upward gaze.

Retraction saccades are evoked by attempted upward saccades. Anomalous coinnervation of extraocular muscles causes the retraction. Nearly synchronous pulses of innervation in horizontally and vertically acting ocular muscles cause saccadic bursts of retraction. Such lack of reciprocal inhibition of antagonist motor neurons is also a feature of horizontal gaze palsies. Although convergent saccadic jerks are often prominent in retraction saccades, which is sometimes called nystagmus, it is not an oscillation of the vergence system. Downward-moving optokinetic targets provide a convenient means of demonstrating the disorder; each upward fast phase of OKN elicits a burst of retraction.

Bell's phenomenon refers to upward, often oblique, ocular deviation during forced eyelid closure against manual restraint. When upward saccadic and smooth pursuit eye movements are paralyzed, preservation of Bell's phenomenon indicates a supranuclear cause of ophthalmoplegia. Preservation of Bell's phenomenon often correlates with preservation of upward doll's eye reflexes, but these two reflex stimuli for ocular elevation may be dissociated by supranuclear brainstem disease. The upward VOR may be absent with preservation of Bell's phenomenon and vice versa.

Ventral Pretectal Lesions

Lesions in the midbrain tegmentum, rostral to the third nerve nucleus, and ventral to the aqueduct of sylvius, cause selective paralysis of downward saccades, presumably by disrupting projections from the riMLF to the oculomotor and trochlear nuclei (see Fig. 16.33). The responsible lesions are usually bilateral, but unilateral paramedian lesions can also paralyze downward gaze or both upward and downward gaze; the pupils are usually of medium size and poorly reactive to both light and accommodation. The author terms these distinct ocular motor defects the ventral pretectal syndrome (*Fig. 16.37*).

In both the dorsal and ventral syndromes, the vertical VOR and smooth pursuit may appear to be spared. However, reduced gain, limited amplitude, and abnormal phase lead of the vertical VOR can accompany involvment of the INC and the riMLF, which spares the ocular motor nuclei. This indicates that supranuclear lesions of the rostral midbrain can impair the vertical VOR, thus varying from the prevailing concept that supranuclear lesions spare the vertical VOR. This misconception results from the usual method of testing the vertical VOR at the bedside, the oculocephalic

Ventral pretectal syndrome
Paralysis of downward saccades
Paralysis of downward pursuit
Paralysis of downward VOR
Paralysis may be upward and downward
Pupils medium size
Poor light and near pupillary reactions
Lesion ventral to aqueduct involving INC and rostral interstitial nucleus of the medial longitudinal fasciculus

Fig. 16.37 The ventral pretectal syndrome.

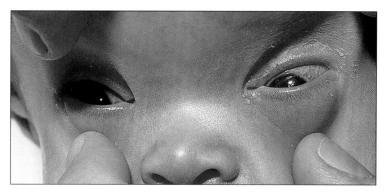

Fig. 16.38 Tonic downward deviation of the eyes in a child with hydrocephalus from congenital aqueductal stenosis, causing 'sunset eyes' appearance.

maneuver, in which the patient's head is passively flexed and extended while fixating on a target in a well-lit room. As noted above, the eye movements that result represent not only the vertical VOR, but also visual enhancement of this reflex by smooth pursuit and optokinetic smooth eye movements. Moreover, although the examiner may judge the amplitude of oculocephalic eye movements to be normal, the gain and phase of the vertical VOR cannot be measured at the bedside. Complete assessment of vertical VOR dysfunction requires oculographic recording and quantification of vertical VOR eye movements performed in darkness.

Tonic Vertical Deviation

Sustained downward deviation of the eyes can be a manifestation of caudal thalamic hemorrhage, presumably with compression of the rostral midbrain. Metabolic encephalopathy, usually hepatic, can cause downward deviation and up-gaze palsy. Aqueductal distension in patients with hydrocephalus has the same effect (*Fig. 16.38*). Otherwise healthy infants may have unexplained downward deviation during the first few weeks of life.

Sustained upward deviation of the eyes is an infrequent feature of severe hypoxic encephalopathy. The pretectum and midbrain are structurally intact and the deviation has been attributed to damage to cerebellar pathways. Paroxysms of upward deviation are a feature of epileptic seizures and oculogyric crises. Postencephalitic parkinsonism, phenothiazine drugs, and carbamazepine intoxication cause oculogyric crises.

Skew Deviation

Skew deviation refers to vertical strabismus caused by supranuclear lesions (*Fig. 16.39*). Skew is attributed to disruption of projections from the utricles to the INC, which maintains tonic innervation of motor neurons that supply extraocular muscles acting in vertical and torsional vectors. Unilateral lesions in the midbrain and rostral pons cause ipsilateral hypertropia, and lesions of caudal pons and medulla cause contralateral hypertropia. Unilateral utricular nerve stimulation elicits vertical divergence of the eyes, with the higher eye on the side of stimulation, and unilateral labyrinthine damage may transiently induce skew deviation with ipsilateral hypotropia. Myasthenia gravis and orbital disease such as thyroid ophthalmopathy, pseudotumor, and orbital blow-out fracture must be excluded. The deviation may be either comitant in different positions of gaze or incomitant, and may even simulate paralysis of a single vertically acting muscle. For example, a left hypertropia on down-

ward gaze to the left and a right hypertropia on downward gaze to the right mimic inferior rectus palsies but can result from involvement of the pontine and medullary tegmentum.

The ocular tilt reaction is a distinctive triad of skew deviation, conjugate ocular torsion, and head tilt (see Fig. 16.39). The eyes tort toward the lower skewed eye and the head is inclined laterally in the same direction. Acute unilateral labyrinthine damage may produce this synkinesis transiently; the lower eye is on the side of the peripheral vestibular lesion. This pattern of head tilt often accompanies skew deviation, and torsion of one or both eyes is typical of skew deviation; the eyes undergo cyclotorsion, with the upper poles of the cornea towards the lower eye. This torsion can be documented by fundus photography with the head erect (*Fig. 16.40*).

Monocular elevation paresis is an infrequent manifestation of unilateral damage in the rostral midbrain. The eyes are straight in the primary position. Elevation of one eye is equally limited with the eye abducted or adducted, signifying impaired innervation of contralateral superior rectus motor neurons and ipsilateral inferior oblique motor neurons. In most cases, a unilateral pretectal lesion, contralateral to the paretic eye, has been responsible for this supranuclear double elevator palsy.

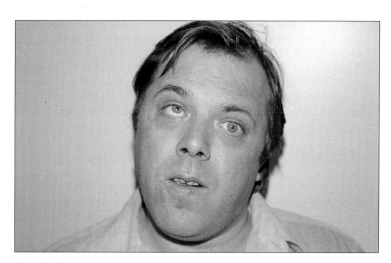

Fig. 16.39 Skew deviation showing right hypertropia while patient fixates with left eye. There is also a leftward head tilt. The eyes were torted clockwise, with the upper poles of the globes toward the left shoulder. The skew, head tilt, and torsion comprise the ocular tilt reaction. (With perrmission from Zackon DH, Sharpe JA. The ocular tilt reaction and skew deviation. In: Sharpe JA, Barber HO, eds. *The Vestibulo-Ocular Reflex and Vertigo* [New York: Raven Press, 1993] 129–140.)

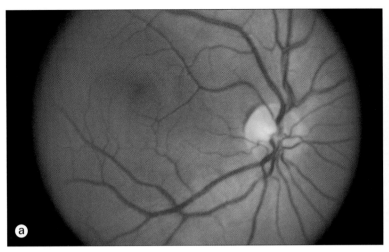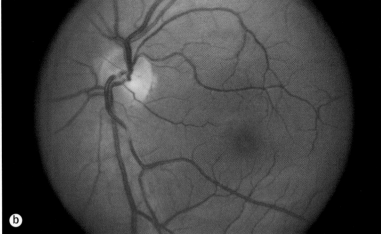

Fig. 16.40 Torsion of the eyes associated with skew deviation. Fundus photographs show intorsion of the right eye with downward displacement of the optic disc relative to the macula (**a**) and extorsion of the left eye with upward displacement of the optic disc relative to the macula (**b**).

Further reading

Bogousslavsky J, Regli F. Pursuit gaze defects in acute and chronic unilateral parieto-occipital lesions. *Eur Neurol.* 1986;**25**:10–18.

Brandt T, Dietrich, M. Skew deviation with ocular torsion: A vestibular brainstem sign of topographic diagnostic value. *Ann Neurol.* 1993;**33**:528–34.

Buttner-Ennever JA, Buttner U, Cohen B, *et al.* Vertical gaze paralysis and the rostral interstitial nucleus of the medial longitudinal fasciculus. *Brain.* 1982;**105**:125–49.

Cannon SC, Robinson DA. Loss of the neural integrator of the oculomotor system from brainstem lesions in monkey. *J Neurophysiol.* 1987;**57**:1383–409.

Dehaene I, Lammen M. Paralysis of saccades and pursuit: clinicopathological study. *Neurology.* 1991;**41**:414–5.

Ford CS, Schwartze GW. Weaver RG, Troost BT. Monocular elevation paresis caused by an ipsilateral lesion. *Neurology.* 1984;**34**:1264–7.

Hanson MR, Hamid MA, Tomsak RL, Chou SS, Leigh RJ. Selective saccadic palsy caused by pontine lesions: clinical, physiological and pathological correlations. *Ann Neurol.* 1986;**20**:209–17.

Henn V, Lang W, Hepp K, *et al.* Experimental gaze palsies in monkeys and their relation to human pathology. *Brain.* 1984;**107**:619–36.

Johnston JL, Sharpe JA, Morrow MJ. Paresis of contralateral smooth pursuit and normal vestibular smooth eye movements after unilateral brainstem lesions. *Ann Neurol.* 1992;**31**:495–502.

Johnston JL, Sharpe JA. Sparing of the horizontal vestibulo-ocular reflex with lesions of the paramedian pontine reticular formation. *Neurology.* 1989;**39**:876.

Keane JR. Sustained up gaze in coma. *Ann Neurol.* 1981;**9**:409–12.

Keane J.R. Views and reviews. Pretectal syndrome: 206 patients. *Neurology.* 1990;**40**:684–90.

Leigh RJ, Zee DS. *The neurology of eye movements.* (Philadelphia: FA Davis Co; 1991.)

Morrow MJ, Sharpe JA. Cerebral hemispheric localization of smooth pursuit asymmetry. *Neurology.* 1990;40:284–92.

Morrow MJ, Sharpe JA. Retinotopic and directional deficits of smooth pursuit initiation after posterior cerebral hemispheric lesions. *Neurology.* 1993;**43**:595–603.

Morrow MJ, Sharpe JA. Smooth pursuit eye movements. In: Sharpe JA, Barber HO, eds. *The vestibulo-ocular reflex and vertigo.* (New York: Raven Press; 1993) 141–62.

Pierrot-Deseilligny CH, Chain F, Serdaru M, *et al.* The one and a half syndrome. *Brain.* 1981;**104**:665–99.

Ranalli PJ, Sharpe JA, Fletcher WA. Palsy of upward and downward saccadic, pursuit and vestibular movements with a unilateral midbrain lesion: pathophysiological correlations. *Neurology.* 1988;**38**:114–22.

Ranalli PJ, Sharpe JA. Vertical vestibulo-ocular reflex, smooth pursuit and eye-head tracking dysfunction in internuclear ophthalmoplegia. *Brain.* 1988;**111**:1277–95.

Robinson DA. Control of eye movements. In: Brooks VB, ed. *Handbook of physiology.* (Bethesda: American Physiological Society; 1981) 1275–320.

Sharpe JA, Lo AW, Rabinovitch HE. Control of the saccadic and smooth pursuit systems after cerebral hemidecortication. *Brain.* 1979;**102**:387–403.

Sharpe JA. Supranuclear disorders of horizontal eye motion. *Semin Neurol (New York).* 1986;**6**:155–66.

Sharpe JA, Morrow MJ. Cerebral hemispheric smooth pursuit disorders. *Neuro-ophthalmology.* 1991;**11**:87–98.

Sharpe JA, Ranalli PJ. Vertical vestibulo-ocular reflex control after supranuclear midbrain damage. *Acta Otolarngol.* 1991;**481**(suppl):194–8.

Sharpe JA, Johnston JL. The vestibulo-ocular reflex: clinical, anatomic and physiologic correlates. In: Sharpe JA, Barber HO, eds. *The vestibulo-ocular reflex and vertigo.* (New York: Raven Press; 1993) 15–39.

Thier P, Bachor A, Faiss J, Dichgans J, Koenig E. Selective impairment of smooth pursuit eye movements due to an ischemic lesion of the basal pons. *Ann Neurol.* 1991;**29**:443–8.

Tijssen CC, van Gisenbergen JAM, Schulte BPM. Conjugate eye deviation: side, site, and size of the hemispheric lesion. *Neurology.* 1991;**41**:846–50.

Troost BT, Daroff RB. The ocular motor defects in progressive supranuclear palsy. *Ann Neurol.* 1977;**2**:397–403.

White OB, Saint-Cyr JA, Tomlinson RD, Sharpe JA. Ocular motor deficits in Parkinson's disease. II. Control of the saccadic and smooth pursuit systems. *Brain.* 1983;**106**:571–87.

Zackon DH, Sharpe JA. Midbrain paresis of horizontal gaze. *Ann Neurol.* 1984;**16**:495–504.

Zackon DS, Sharpe JA. The ocular tilt reaction and skew deviation. In: Sharpe JA, Barber HO, eds. *The vestibulo-ocular reflex and vertigo.* (New York: Raven Press; 1993) 129–40.

Zee DS, Yee RD, Singer HS. Congenital ocular motor apraxia. *Brain.* 1977;**100**:581–99.

Zee DS. Ophthalmoscopy in evaluation of vestibular disorders. *Ann Neurol.* 1978;**3**:373.

CHAPTER 17

The Normal Optic Nerve Head and its Variations

Emanuel Rosen

INTRODUCTION

The observation of the optic nerve head (ONH) may provide vital clues to intracranial pathology. It is a sensitive indicator for the early onset of raised intracranial pressure and thereby the existence of space occupying as well as compressive intracranial lesions. In order to evaluate the health or abnormality of the ONH, its normal anatomy must be understood. The shape, size, color, and form of the ONH is unique to each eye, although its variations fit a general structural pattern. What may clinically be referred to as a 'normal' ONH actually embraces a spectrum of appearances, for example, from the very small ONH in hyperopic or small eyes to the seemingly large ONH in a myopic eye. Atrophy of the optic nerve and swelling of the nerve head are two gross representations of malfunction. Variations in nerve head outline distinction, central cupping, temporal pallor, circumpapillary haloes, or pigmentation, on the other hand, are responsible for just some of the confusion that makes it difficult to separate normal variation from pathologic entities. Intraocular conditions, as opposed to intracranial conditions, may influence the structure of the ONH as well as its appearance, which may be partially obscured by opacification of the intraocular light path. Magnification differences may also cause variation in ONH appearance as a consequence of the optical system in a particular eye.

The aim of this chapter is to identify the normal aspects of the ONH and its immediate surrounding tissues, as well as to illustrate some of the variations that may lead to confusion when making the decision: is this nerve head normal or pathologic? Images demonstrating so-called 'normal' optic nerve heads, showing the types of variation that occur within the norm, will be provided as a basis for comparison with the 'abnormal' optic nerve heads encountered in everyday clinical practice and discussed elsewhere in this book.

OPTIC NERVE HEAD STRUCTURES

There are specific anatomical structures that comprise the ONH but in every population there is considerable variation in its size, contour, color, elevation, depression, and vascularity. Indeed, each optic nerve is as unique as a fingerprint.

The optic nerve is an important structure in the fields of both neuro-ophthalmic and neurologic medicine. As a result of its location at a visible outpost of the brain, bathed in cerebrospinal fluid (CSF) at the head of a cranial nerve, its appearance yields valuable clues to intracranial pathology as well as to local abnormalities. Constant observation of optic nerve heads is necessary, however, to gain the experience required to derive full value from this convenient window into intracranial pathology.

The optic nerve is composed of approximately 1 million nerve fibers that conduct impulses from the retinal network of more than 100 million light receptors. The nerves are bundled into sheaths which, in turn, are surrounded by the meningeal sheaths and CSF. The internal and external sheaths are comprised of connective tissue, with fine vascular support.

In microscopic longitudinal section, a normal optic nerve reveals the intraocular (i.e. within the scleral canal) and early retrobulbar portions (*Fig. 17.1*). The intraocular portion is divided into three laminae: the inner retinal lamina anteriorly, the choroidal lamina (where myelination of the optic nerve head begins) medially, and the outer scleral lamina posteriorly. The anterior surface of the retinal lamina (i.e. the optic disc or nerve head) measures about 1.5 mm in diameter. As the optic nerve leaves the scleral canal posteriorly to form the retrobulbar portion, it measures 3–4 mm in diameter. The increased width is due mainly to the addition of the nerve fiber myelin sheaths.

The nerve fiber layer of the retina is thickest at the margin of the optic nerve, where unmyelinated nerve fibers make a sharp

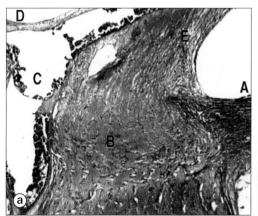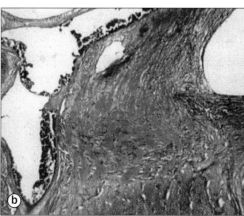

Fig. 17.1 Normal optic nerve head. (**a**) Black and white micrograph, showing A, scleral wall; B, nerve fiber bundles entering lamina cribrosa; C, physiologic optic cup plus central retinal vein; D, central retinal artery; E, right-angled turn nerve fibers thickest on nasal disc. (**b**) Color micrograph showing nerve fibers stained pink and connective tissue blue to show the astroglial support for nerve fiber bundles, optic cup surface tissue, and lamina cribrosa.

right-angled turn immediately after crossing the optic disc margin to enter the neuroglial tissue of the prelaminar optic disc (see Fig. 17.1). Here, the nerve fibers become segregated into bundles, separated from one another by columns of glial cells. Not until these glial-supported nerve fiber bundles pass through the lamina cribrosa do the nerve fibers become invested with a myelin sheath. Columns of glial cells, composed entirely of astrocytes, surround the nerve bundles in the prelaminar disc area (see Fig. 17.1). The lamina cribrosa consists of collagenous trabeculae that are contiguous with the scleral coat of the eye (see Fig. 17.1), their criss-cross pattern forming a series of outlets for the nerve fiber bundles. The central retinal artery and vein gain access to the eye via the optic nerve, which penetrate its retrobulbar portion and emerge onto the nerve as the main retinal vascular elements (see Fig. 17.1).

The scleral wall of the eye, at the level of optic nerve passage, is fenestrated by the scleral foramen but braced by the lamina cribrosa (see Fig. 17.1). The size of the scleral foramen, across which the lamina extends, varies between eyes and thereby contributes to the unique appearance of the nerve head. At the level of the choroidal vasculature, the subretinal vascular area, radial vessels penetrate the nerve head to provide an essential vascular supply from a loosely defined ring known as the 'circle of Zinn'. This vascularity, coupled with surface capillaries on and around the nerve head (the circumpapillary radial capillary plexus, which is derived from the retinal arteries), provides the ONH with its color, which in turn is influenced by the size of the ONH and the scleral foramen.

The optic nerve is embryologically and anatomically more like a tract of the brain than a true cranial nerve. It is invested by dural and arachnoidal membranes from the external scleral surface all the way to the optic canal, where the dura becomes fused with the periosteum of the sphenoid bone. The subarachnoid space of the optic nerve is contiguous with that of the intracranial contents. An elevation in intracranial pressure is directly transmitted, therefore, to the subarachnoid space surrounding the optic nerve and contained within its dural sheath. The most anterior portion of the optic nerve is that which lies across the ocular wall from the disc surface to the retrolaminar position, where myelin first becomes apparent. This portion of the nerve, approximately 2 mm in length, is a critically important location for disease. It passes through a region with a relatively high-pressure gradient and receives a complex, bipartite vascular supply at the capillary level.

A cross-section of the optic nerve (*Fig. 17.2*) shows the central parenchyma, containing axons, the central retinal artery and central retinal vein, minor blood vessels, astrocytes, oligodendrocytes, and pial septa. This is surrounded by pia mater, subarachnoid (potential) space, arachnoid mater, subdural (potential) space, and dura mater.

OPTIC NERVE HEAD TOPOGRAPHY

The topography of the ONH is shown in *Figure 17.3*. Abutting the neural components of the ONH is the retinal pigment epithelium (RPE), the subretinal layer that separates retina from choroid. The level of pigmentation of the RPE, and its occasional shortfall from the edge of the ONH, contributes to further individual variation (*Fig. 17.4*). *Figure 17.5* shows a normal ONH with a minimal optic cup, dense aggregation of nerve fibers on the 'pink' nasal aspects, and less dense nerve-fiber covering of the temporal aspect: the temporal pallor of a normal optic nerve head.

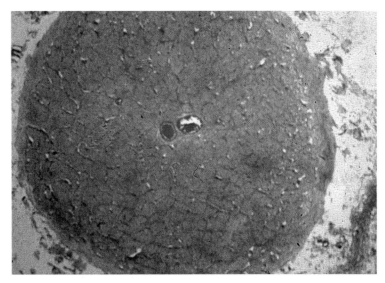

Fig. 17.2 Cross-section of the optic nerve showing the central parenchyma containing axons, the central retinal artery and central retinal vein, minor blood vessels, astrocytes, oligodendrocytes, and pial septa. This is surrounded by pia mater, sub arachnoid (potential) space, arachnoid mater, subdural (potential) space, and dura mater.

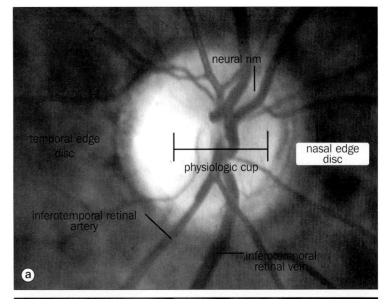
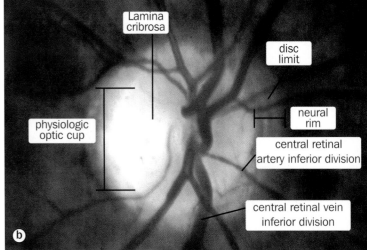

Fig. 17.3 Normal optic nerve head. (**a**) Black and white and (**b**) color retinal photographs showing the topography of the optic nerve head. In (**a**), the disc limit is clearly seen, whereas in (**b**) the vascularity of the optic nerve head blends with color of the surrounding tissue.

Large (myopic) eyes may have a diameter of up to 35 mm or more, whereas small (hyperopic) eyes may have a diameter of 20 mm or less. Such variations influence both the size of the scleral foramen and the stretching or crowding of tissues around the ONH. It is often difficult, therefore, to differentiate normal from abnormal. Myopic eyes in particular, being large in volume, have asso-ciated variations that may confuse the clinician. They are more difficult to observe, especially because the vitreous body is 'stretched' and degenerate and less clear than that of an emmetropic eye. The ONH of the highly myopic eye shown in *Figure 17.6*, is labeled to emphasize the normality of the nerve head itself while showing the stretching effects of a large eye on the circumpapillary tissues.

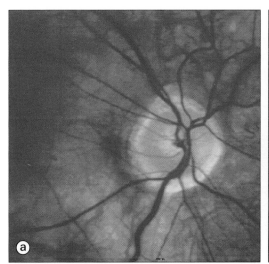
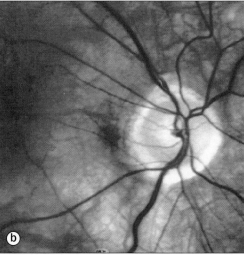
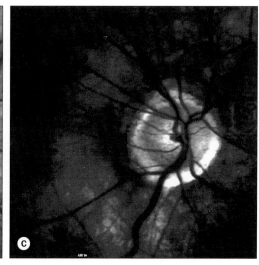

Fig. 17.4 Normal optic nerve head. (**a**) Retinal photograph of a normal optic nerve head. (**b**) Image enhancement has been used to clarify the detail. The neural tissue is seen as a 'doughnut' surrounding the central vessels. The white halo of bared scleral eye wall is revealed by the shortfall of retinal pigment epithelium through 360°. Further afield (the left side of **b**), the sparse choroidal and retinal pigment epithelial pigmentation shows choroidal larger vessels silhouetted against the scleral background contrasting with increasing density of pigmentation, especially that of the retinal pigment epithelium towards the macular area. (**c**) The contrast has been altered to emphasize the true disc margins.

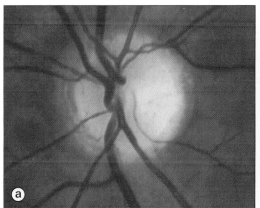
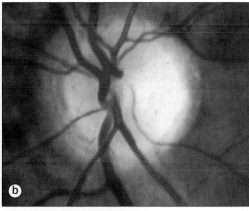

Fig. 17.5 Normal optic nerve head. (**a**) Ophthalmoscopic view. (**b**) Enhanced image of a normal optic nerve head with a minimal optic cup, dense aggregation of nerve fibers on the 'pink' nasal aspects, and less dense nerve-fiber covering of the temporal aspect. Image enhancement reveals the circumpapillary pigmentation pattern and shows the true disc margin more clearly. Vascular variations are not uncommon, as seen here in the cilioretinal artery, which emanates from the center of the disc to supply a limited area of central retina.

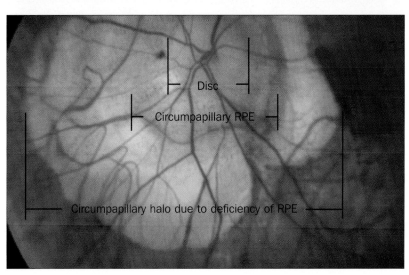

Fig. 17.6 The optic disc area of the fundus of a highly myopic eye. The ONH itself is normal but the stretching effects of a large eye are shown by the circumpapillary tissues, where the RPE has ripped through 360° and has stretched away from the residual frill of RPE surrounding the ONH.

Variations in size and form of the ONH are infinite. *Figures 17.7* and *17.8* show some of the common differences, especially in the relationship between the physiologic optic cup and the ONH as a whole: the cup to disc (C:D) ratio. This is, essentially, a result of the dimensions of the scleral optic foramen. As the central cup size increases, the nerve rim becomes more recognizable, and it is the color and form of this rim which provides clinical information on the probability of intraocular pressure damage: glaucomatous optic atrophy. The existence of one or more cilioretinal arteries adds a further element to the dissimilarity of nerve head appearances, as do the branching patterns of the main retinal vessels.

ANGIOGRAPHY OF THE OPTIC NERVE HEAD

For the past 30 years, supplementary clinical methods of evaluating the status of the ONH have been used. Fundus fluorescein angiography (FFA) provides a dynamic view of the ONH and is especially useful in showing whether the retinal and ONH capillaries are carrying blood along and whether they leak blood into adjacent tissues. Pathologic swelling of the ONH, even of a subtle degree, can be elucidated comfortably by the FFA test. As an aid to understanding the vascular supply of the optic nerve head, *Figure 17.9* illustrates FFA in use, showing a dynamic view of perfusion by fluorescein.

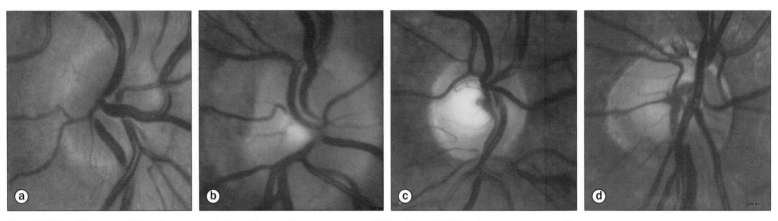

Fig. 17.7 (**a**) Right eye ONH of a hyperopic (small) eye. There is no cup. (C/D ratio = 0.) The disc is very pink with no temporal pallor. (**b**) Right eye, C/D ratio = 0.1. (**c**) Right eye, C/D ratio = 0.3. (**d**) Right eye, no cup. (C/D ratio = 0.)

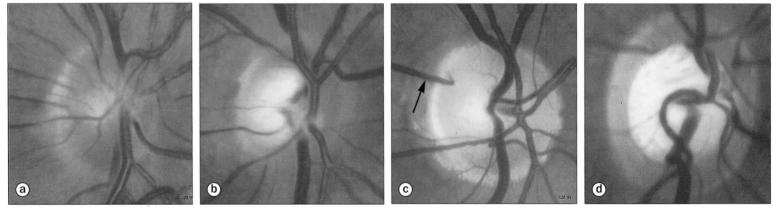

Fig. 17.8 (**a**) Right eye, C/D ratio = 0.1, showing five cilioretinal arteries. There is a crescent of RPE shortfall at temporal aspect of disc. (**b**) Right eye, C/D ratio = 0.4. The vertical element is more obvious than the horizontal element. A thick (healthy) pink neural rim is seen. (**c**) Right eye, C/D ratio = 0.2, showing cilioretinal artery (arrow), physiologic temporal disc pallor, and a slim temporal crescent of RPE deficiency.

(**d**) Right eye, C/D ratio = 0.6. This would have been regarded as glaucomatous but for the fact that the neural rim is pink, substantial, and there is no invagination of the rim in relation to the disc margin. A cilioretinal artery is present. No visual field defect would be expected with healthy neural tissue, although this type of ONH configuration is one of the risk factors in chronic open angle glaucoma.

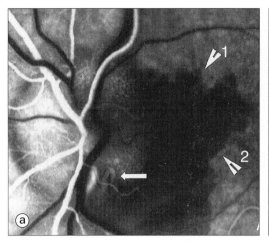
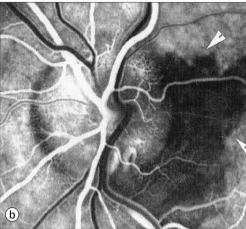
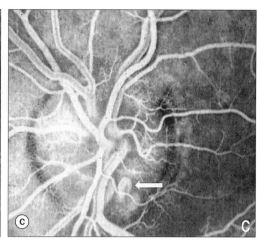

Fig. 17.9 Left eye fundus fluorescein angiogram. (**a**) The branches of the central retinal artery are filling with dye (1). The choriocapillaries in particular show the filling-flush on the nasal side (2) but not on the temporal side (arrowheads). This filling defect is the result of an aberrant ciliary artery (arrow) taking an unusually long route before appearing on the surface of the ONH. Note that at this moment, the temporal part of the anterior ONH contains little dye because capillaries fed by this slow ciliary artery supply the adjacent choroid and that portion of the disc. (**b**) 0.2 s later, dye perfusion of the filling defect is better outlined (arrows) because the adjacent choroid fluoresces more effectively. At the same time some filling of the 'defect' is seen, accompanied by an early filling-flush of the previously darkened temporal aspect of the disc. The aberrant ciliary artery is now seen clearly. (**c**) Dye filling in the temporal juxtapapillary choroid is now complete and the optic nerve head now fluoresces evenly.

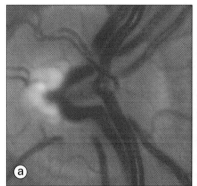
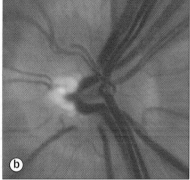
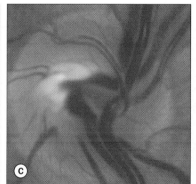
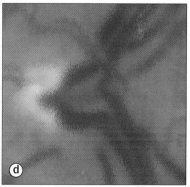

Fig. 17.10 Right eye ONH, shown via a direct ophthalmoscope. (**a**) Normal appearance. (**b**) Deliberately changed to show how it might appear in a small or hyperopic eye. (**c**) how it might be distorted in an eye with astigmatism (**d**) or blurred, in an eye with cloudy media, making its margins harder to resolve. This might be confused with early papilledema in a small or hyperopic eye.

VISUALIZATION OF THE OPTIC NERVE HEAD

A good view of the ONH is required before clinical decisions can be made. These decisions are made in spite of natural variations within the norm and an immense variety of pathologic appearances. Modern-day ophthalmologists are particularly skilled at stereoscopic viewing of the ONH and the fundus of the eye in general, even through undilated pupils, using the 78 D or 90 D aspheric lenses designed for use with the binocular slit lamp microscope. Despite the availability of such sophisticated methods, it is only through the benefit of clinical experience that normal ONH variants can be distinguished from the pathologic. Neurologists who are not equipped with slit lamp microscopes and viewing lenses rely on the direct ophthalmoscope for visualization of the ONH. Again, with practice, this is an excellent clinical tool, although it provides only a monocular view of the ONH. The direct ophthalmoscope is further handicapped by its intrinsic difficulty in providing a clear and undistorted view through cloudy ocular media, and through the media of eyes with significant refractive errors (*Fig. 17.10*). Astigmatic refractive errors may distort the appearance of the ONH and thereby lead to uncertainties in diagnosis.

In the clinical examination of the eye, once its form and reactions have been observed and its status documented, the pupil should be dilated to enable a best view of the optic nerve head. It is only in hyperopia or in older patients with small eyes that there is a remote danger of an adverse response to pupil dilation (angle closure glaucoma). A short acting mydriatic such as Tropicamide (0.5%) is appropriate. Its action is weak, rapid, brief, and easily reversed.

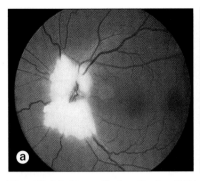 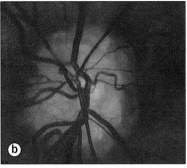 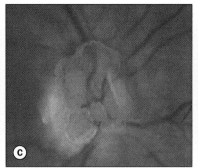 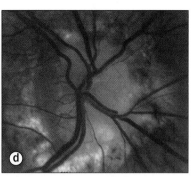

Fig. 17.11 Normally functioning ONH variants. (**a**) Myelination of prelaminar nerve fibers with extension onto the juxtapapillary retina. There is no functional variation in this left eye. (**b**) Normally functioning left eye with an unusual, evidently swollen optic nerve head, showing an irregular contour. Although the nerve is functioning normally, visual deficits may develop as the nerve head contains drusen or colloid bodies buried within its substance (see Fig. 17.12). In this case these are visible on the surface and at the margins, accounting for the irregularity of contour. (**c**) Appearance of Bergmeister's papilla. (**d**) Another variant of disc margin appearance with pigment migration and clustering (cause unknown) in a healthy right eye.

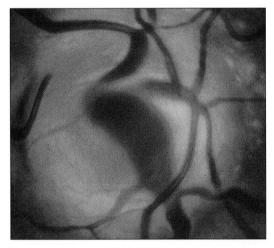

Fig. 17.12 A more obvious examples of optic disc drusen. The whole disc is pale. Buried and surface drusen in quantity suggest that visual defects will arise from these space-occupying lesions.

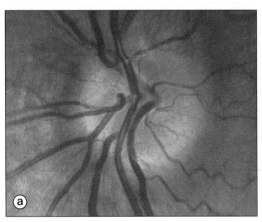 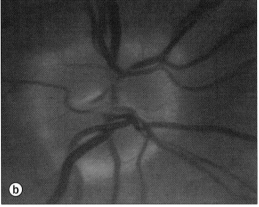

Fig. 17.13 (**a**) Absence of a physiologic cup (no space) and (**b**) a crowded (swollen) appearance with indistinct disc margins, indicates examples of pseudopapilledema.

VARIATIONS WITHIN THE NORMALLY FUNCTIONING ONH

Variations from the expected in the appearance of a normally functioning ONH are extremely common and often dramatic. *Figures 17.11* and *17.12* depict a variety of normally functioning variants, including in *Figure 17.11c* the appearance of an embryonic remnant of the central core vascular supply of the eye known as 'Bergmeister's papilla'. The remnants can obscure the disc surface and margin to give confusing signs. In this case the 'remnant' is not a Bergmeister's papilla but the remnant of a vitreal membrane forming after an intraocular hemorrhage, a sequel to a subarachnoid hemorrhage (Terson's syndrome). The membrane was removed surgically but simulates the appearance of embryonic tissue.

Small optic nerve heads can be confusing especially when a patient has symptoms that may indicate the possibility of raised intracranial pressure. *Figure 17.13* illustrates a left eye with no physiologic cup (no space) and a crowded (swollen) appearance with indistinct disc margins. In bilateral symmetry of appearance or in the monocular patient, refraction and eye globe size can be helpful in differentiating abnormal from normal.

CHAPTER 18

The Optic Nerve Head: Elevated Discs

J Corbett, M Wall

INTRODUCTION

The normal optic nerve head has a central cup diameter that is 20–30% of the diameter of the optic disc. It is slightly taller than it is wide and the vessels usually emerge on the nasal side of the nerve. It is salmon-pink to orange in color, with the temporal border normally paler than the rest of the nerve head (*Fig. 18.1*). Above and below, where the arcuate bundles from the temporal retina enter the disc, there is usually some mild obscuration of the disc margin. In some normal nerve heads, this lack of detail of the disc edge continues around the nasal border (*Fig. 18.2*). There is a wide range of normal disc size, from the small disc with no cup and a uniform red color, to the large disc with a wide cup.

ELEVATED CONGENITAL DISK ANOMALY (PSEUDOPAPILLEDEMA)

A common variant of the normal disc is the elevated congenital disc anomaly, also called pseudopapilledema (*Fig. 18.3*). This type of disc elevation is often confused with acquired optic disc edema. The congenitally elevated disc often has little or no optic cup. Vessels rise up through the center of the disc, rather than taking the usual exit route on the nasal half of the disc; the vessels may be anomalous with frequent and early branching (*Fig. 18.3c*). They are easily seen as they climb over the disc's margin (*Fig. 18.3a*), and are not obscured, as they may be in true disc edema (see 'Signs of papilledema', chapter 21). The elevated congenital disc anomaly can sometimes have drusen buried within it (see Fig. 18.3a).

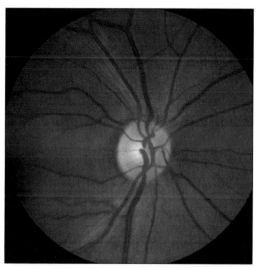

Fig. 18.1 Normal optic disc. Notice how the vessels exit from the nasal half of the nerve and that the temporal half of the disc is pale. Note also the streaming axons from retinal ganglion cells; they form the retinal nerve fiber layer, which enter the disc at its superior and inferior poles, slightly on the nasal side, following the arcades of the vessels.

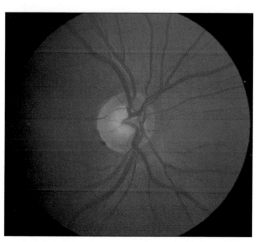

Fig. 18.2 Normal, large optic disc. Notice that the optic cup is also large.

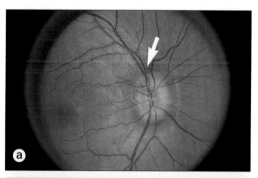

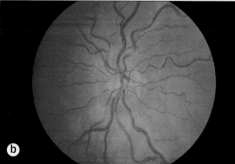

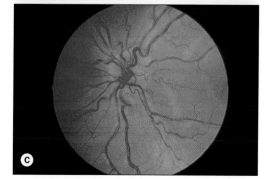

Fig. 18.3 Congenital elevated disc anomalies. (**a**) Many anomalously elevated optic nerve heads have a smooth surface that does not obscure any of the emerging vessels. Such discs often show juxtapapillary subretinal hemorrhages (arrow) that circle parts of the disc and which spontaneously absorb in weeks to months. This disc was also found to contain buried drusen (see below). (**b**) Vessels exit from the center of the nerve and appear to have more branches than usual. (**c**) This anomalous disc has many unusually tortuous blood vessels, with extra branching, emerging from the center of the disc.

LITTLE RED DISC

The English neurologist Sir William Gowers was a careful observer. He stated that 'Increased redness is of little value as a sign of hyperemia of the optic disc, on account of the great variation in the amount of structural redness'; '...abnormal redness of the disc [is] in itself of little value... unless it develops under observation.' (Gowers, 1879). He noted that small discs tend to be 'hyperemic' and large discs were 'pale' by comparison.

The size and overall appearance of the optic disc depends on the size of the scleral canal (*Fig. 18.4*), and the angle at which it penetrates the sclera. It is this canal through which the axons from the retinal ganglion cells must pass to form the optic nerve. If the scleral canal is small, there is no room for a large central cup. If the scleral canal is very small, there is no cup, the disc is crowded and red, and it is elevated more centrally than peripherally (*Fig. 18.5*). It is sometimes difficult to discern whether a small, cupless, and apparently hyperemic disc has always been that way or whether it is swollen because some other disorder is caus-

ing stasis of axoplasmic flow in the optic nerve fibers. These 'little red discs' are responsible for a lot of confusion in the clinical diagnosis of papilledema or optic disc edema. Disc anomalies, such as smallness of the disc, elevation of the disc, drusen in the disc, extra branching of the retinal vessels, may be congenitally acquired (*Figs 18.5a–c, 18.6*).

OPTIC DISC HYPOPLASIA

If the optic nerve is imperfectly formed, the disc tends to be small and pale. This developmental defect, called optic disc hypoplasia, is more common in males than in females; the optic disc is small and is usually surrounded by a yellow halo, the double ring sign (*Fig. 18.7*). The retina and retinal pigment epithelium crossing the lamina cribrosa contribute to the double ring. On histopathologic examination, there is a loss of axons with normal glial tissue and collagen indicating either a failure of differentiation of glial cells or excessive programmed cell

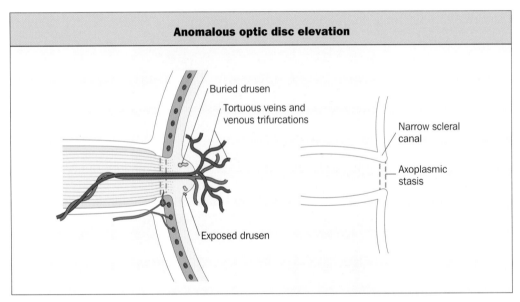

Anomalous optic disc elevation

Buried drusen
Tortuous veins and venous trifurcations
Narrow scleral canal
Axoplasmic stasis
Exposed drusen

Fig. 18.4 Anomalous disc elevation, with some buried drusen and some exposed. The origin of drusen is unknown. One hypothesis suggests that the original anomaly is a narrow scleral canal, through which over 1 million nerve fibers must pass, with axoplasmic stasis and chronic loss of axons accounting for the rest (see below).

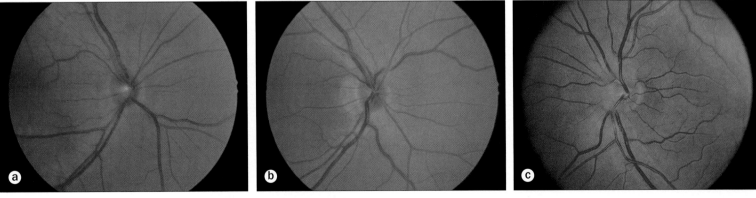

Fig. 18.5 The little red disc. (**a**) Note the small optic cup and increased redness of this patient's left optic nerve head. (**b**) The left nerve head of the twin brother of the patient in (**a**). (**c**) Another little red disc which is not so small.

death (in the fetus there are 3 million retinal ganglion cells and only about 1 million survive). However, it may also be the result of lesions at any level of the developing sensory visual system. The quality of vision in an eye with optic disc hypoplasia varies with the damage done to optic nerve axons. (*Fig. 18.7c, d*).

Optic disc hypoplasia can be linked to cranial and intracranial midline anomalies, which can be associated with life-threaten-

ing neuroendocrine deficiencies (septo-optic dysplasia of de Morsier). Optic nerve hypoplasia is also found with the fetal alcohol syndrome and may occur in association with maternal diabetes mellitus. Patients with optic nerve hypoplasia should undergo endocrine evaluation and neuroimaging to document associated anomalies so these do not cause diagnostic confusion at a later stage.

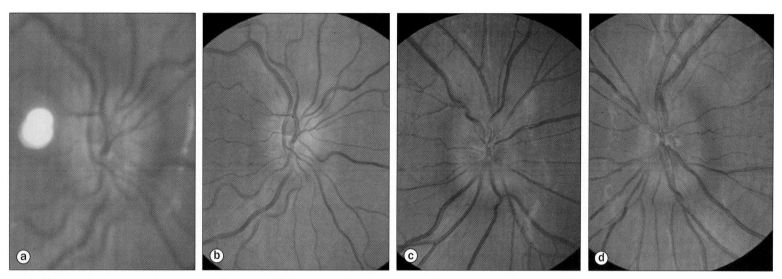

Fig. 18.6 Anomalously elevated disc. (**a**) Right optic disc in a female patient at age 12 years (in 1960). (**b**) Right optic disc at age 29 years (in 1977). If there are drusen buried in this disc they have yet to reveal themselves. (**c**) and (**d**) Both discs of the patient's 10-year-old son show anomalous elevation (in 1977).

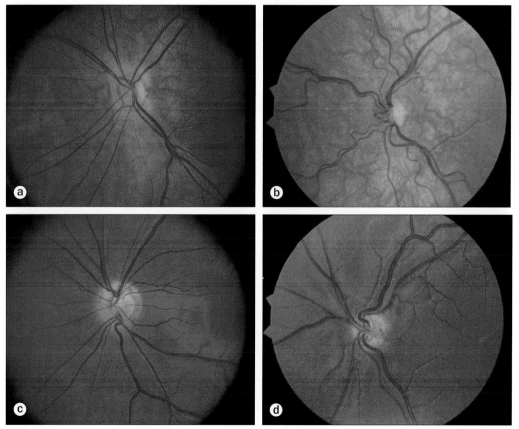

Fig. 18.7 Optic nerve hypoplasia. Hypoplastic discs are strikingly small, often pale, associated with poor vision, and usually show the double ring sign. The inside ring is the true disc margin. (**a**) Classic hypoplasia of the optic disc. (**b**) A hypoplastic disc in which the double ring is not a prominent feature. (**c**) A hypoplastic disc with a cilio-retinal artery. (**d**) A hypoplastic disc with *situs inversus* of the vessels.

COLOBOMAS, TILTED DISCS, PITS, AND OTHER CAVITARY DISC ANOMALIES

A coloboma is, generally, a congenital tissue defect of ocular development caused by abnormalities of invagination of the optic vesicle, with incomplete closure of the embryonic ocular fissure (*Fig. 18.8*) on the lower side of the developing globe. *Figure 18.9a* shows an optic disc coloboma, which is also apparent on the patient's MRI (*Fig. 18.9b*). Isolated optic nerve colobomas are rare. They are usually deeply excavated nerve head anomalies with blood vessels exiting from the margins.

The tilted disc is a non-hereditary form of bilateral optic disc anomaly which occurs sporadically in 1–2% of the population, producing a temporal elevation of the disc and a nasal excavation (*Fig. 18.10a, b*). The tilted disc anomaly is characterized by four features: (1) the disc is tilted, with the superior temporal half elevated and the inferior nasal part slightly excavated (see Fig. 18.10 a, b). The inferior pole of the disc is often rotated temporally; (2) there is an inferior crescent or conus (Fuchs' inferior coloboma) (see Fig. 18.10 a ,b); (3) the vessels emerge from the temporal half of the disc directed towards the nasal retina and then turn back towards the temporal retina; this has been termed situs inversus of the disc; (4) the posterior pigment epithelium is thin and transparent in the inferonasal quadrant of the eye, and there is often a posterior ectasia of that quadrant of the globe (an inferonasal, posterior staphyloma). Myopia with vertical astigmatism is commonly present due to this staphyloma. Associated visual loss is uncommon, but may take the form of a relative bitemporal hemianopia that does not respect the vertical meridian and can be refracted away with lenses (*Figs 18.10 c,d*).

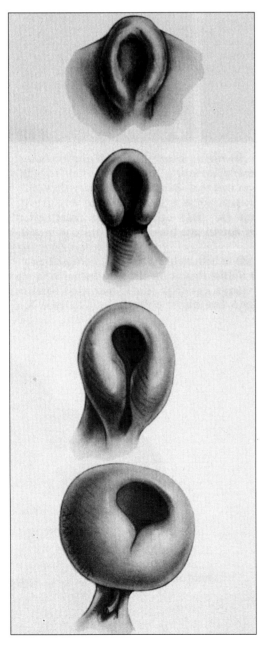

Fig. 18.8 Diagram of the normal embryologic development of the eye with invagination of the optic vesicle followed by closure of the embryonic optic fissure. Failure of closure of this fissure results in a coloboma.

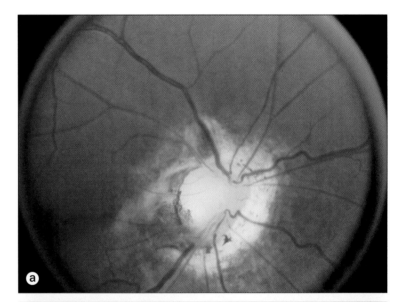

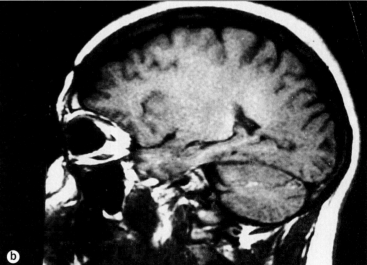

Fig. 18.9 Patient with an optic nerve coloboma. (**a**) Note the lack of tissue in the nerve head. (**b**) MRI of the same patient showing that the disc coloboma is part of an extensive posterior staphyloma of the globe. Note the conical shape of the back of the globe.

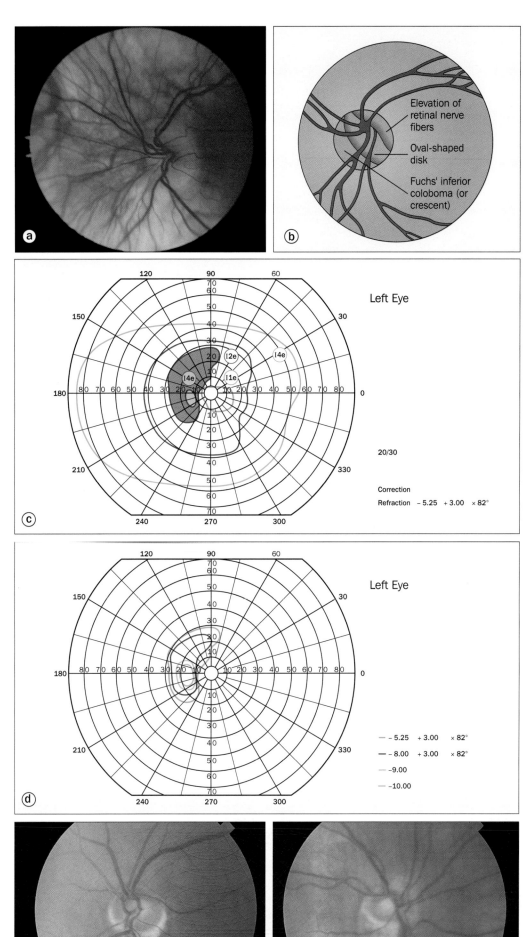

Fig. 18.10 Tilted optic discs. (**a**) The vessels emerge from the temporal rather than the nasal side of the disc. There is some extra branching of the vessels, and a white inferior crescent can be seen along the inferior rim from 3 o'clock to 7 o'clock (Fuchs' inferior coloboma). (**b**) The tilted disc is characterized by an oval shape with its inferior pole rotated towards the macula, an inferior crescent, temporal exit of the vessels (*situs inversus*), and an inferonasal posterior ectasia of the globe. (**c**) The associated visual field loss is sometimes construed as part of a bitemporal hemianopia. However, the defect does not respect the central vertical meridian. This visual field was performed using the best refraction for the fovea, but because of the ectasia of the globe this was not the best refraction for the area around the nerve head. (**d**) The pink scotoma shown in (c) above is here replotted with minus lenses of increasing strength in front of the eye. Each isopter in this visual field (d) marks the limit of an area in which the patient could not see the I2e test object. The entire superior nasal field defect can sometimes be refracted away using minus lenses because the corresponding retina is further away from the nodal point and relatively myopic. When the images in the ectatic part of the retina become sharper, the area of blurred vision becomes smaller. Two further examples of tilted optic discs (**e**) and (**f**) showing all the features described above.

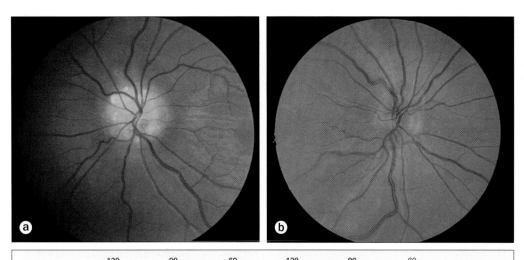

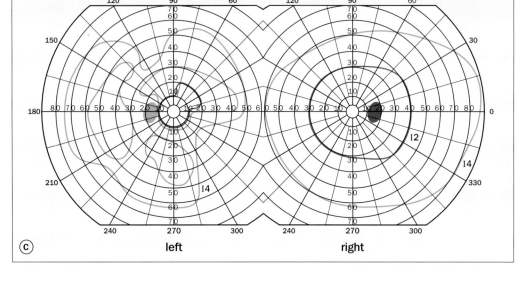

Fig. 18.11 Unilateral disc drusen. The patient's left disc (**a**) has many drusen but the right disc (**b**) has none. (**c**) The eye with the drusen shows considerable disc-related visual field loss, sparing the central 10° but the right field is normal.

MORNING GLORY DISK

The morning glory disc (*Fig. 18.12*) is caused by a defect in the closure of the optic fissure, with glial proliferation, peripapillary changes in the retinal pigment epithelium, and funnel-shaped excavation with an anomalous vascular supply and drainage. An associated retinal detachment is common and is sometimes associated with midline structural abnormalities such as shown in *Figure 18.13*. The morning glory disc is usually unilateral and in over 90% of patients the visual acuity in the affected eye is worse than 20/200.

OPTIC PITS

Optic pits (*Fig. 18.14*) are small, yellow or grayish excavations, usually found on the inferior and temporal portion of the disc. They are rare and usually unilateral. Some believe they are colobomas and this may well be the case for inferiorly located pits. However, most believe they are developmentally of unclear origin

and not colobomas because they are not associated with any of the systemic conditions seen with colobomas. Many large, temporally located optic pits allow fluid to accumulate under the retina in the region of the papillomacular bundle, leading to an area of retinal detachment with associated cystic macular changes. These detachments may be mistaken for and treated as optic neuritis.

MYELINATED NERVE FIBERS

Myelination of the optic nerve begins in the fetus, approaching the optic chiasm by about the seventh month of gestation. Myelination usually stops at the lamina cribrosa at about 1 month of age, and is complete by about the tenth month after birth. In approximately 0.5% of the population, however, myelination continues past the optic disc and into the nerve fiber layer of the retina (*Fig. 18.15*). The opaque white fibers with feathered edges can be seen as a congenital anomaly.

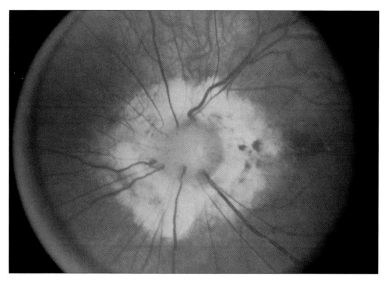

Fig. 18.12 Morning glory disc showing peripapillary retinal pigment epithelial changes, glial proliferation, and anomalous vessels.

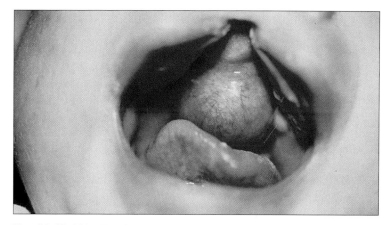

Fig. 18.13 This child had a morning glory disc anomaly and evident midline structural defects: a cleft lip and palate and a basal encephalocele that has allowed some brain and possibly the optic chiasm to push down into the child's throat. (A few generations ago this child's vision might have been at some risk had his doctor been a facile tonsillectomist 'operating with a snare and a delusion'!) (Courtesy of WF Hoyt)

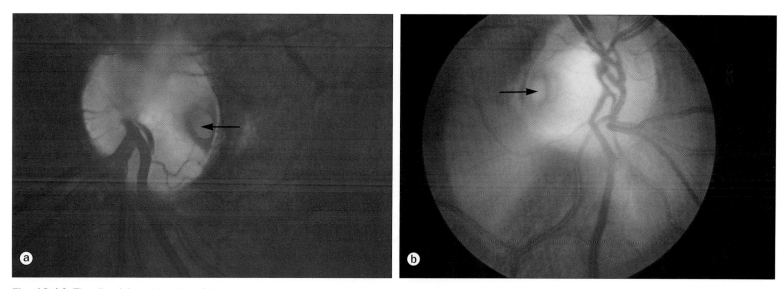

Fig. 18.14 The disc (**a**) and the disc (**b**) are both anomalous. Each shows an optic pit. A pit is a congenital disc anomaly, is a deep hole in the temporal side of the disc, often with a related loss of nerve fibers.

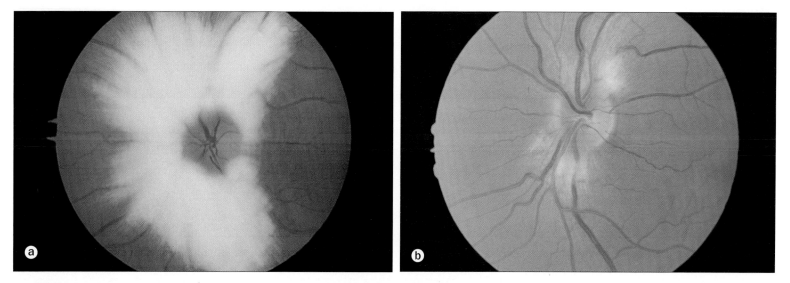

Fig. 18.15 Myelinated nerve fibers are characteristically white and feathered at the edges. These fibers may have no effect on the patient's visual field, but in this case (**a**) the blind spot was definitely enlarged. This myelin has the potential to demyelinate in multiple sclerosis. In (**b**) only a few fibers are myelinated at the upper and lower edges of the nerve head.

OPTIC DISK DRUSEN

Drusen is a German word that means 'geode' (a nodule of stone with a cavity lined with crystals or mineral matter; *Fig. 18.16*). Intrapapillary drusen are crystalloid, acellular refractile bodies that often appear in long standing anomalously elevated discs (*Fig. 18.17*). Their incidence in the general population is 0.3–2%. The anomaly seems to be most common in people of European origin. Drusen are said to 'emerge' over time. It is thought that they may develop from stagnant axoplasm dammed up by a small disc, a tight cribriform plate, or a narrow scleral canal. Perhaps as axons are gradually lost their remains are mineralized in deposits anterior to the lamina cribrosa in the optic disc.

Drusen in the nerve head can be large or small, deep or superficial, and are associated with a spoke-like arrangement of blood vessels and a tendency for disc vessels to be tortuously displaced by drusenous masses. Drusen may be 'buried' deep in the disc so that they are best seen with side lighting using the slit beam of the ophthalmoscope or slit lamp (*Fig. 18.18b*). An optic nerve head with a severe burden of intrapapillary drusen is shown in *Figure 18.19*.

Drusen may be familial in origin. Figure 18.6a, b showed the same disc photographed when the patient was aged 12 and 29 years respectively; Figure 18.6c,d showed that both discs in the patient's 10-year-old son have a similar anomalous elevation with optic nerve drusen.

Figure 18.3 showed a typical anomalous elevation of the disc, with buried drusen and a typical partial peripapillary subretinal hemorrhage at 12 o'clock. The other eye was normal. Occasionally, disc and vitreous hemorrhage may occur with prominent visual symptoms at the time of a posterior vitreous detachment.

Disc drusen often produce arcuate field loss, usually sparing the central 10° of the visual field. It is common for a patient to have more drusen in one disc than in the other but it is rare to have one disc severely involved when the other eye has no drusen at all (Figure 18.11 showed such a case with unilateral field loss).

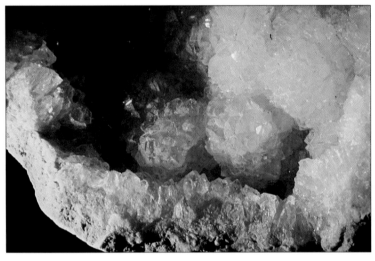

Fig. 18.16 A geode (drusen in German) is a rocky nodule lined with clusters of crystals.

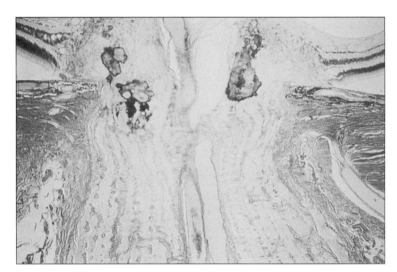

Fig. 18.17 A section through an anomalously elevated optic nerve head showing the calcific nature of buried drusen.

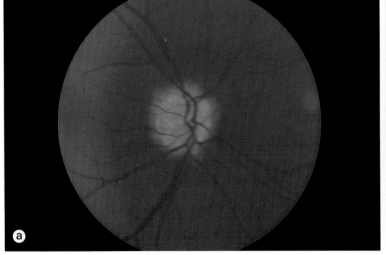

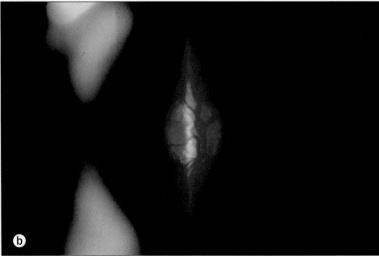

Fig. 18.18 An atrophic optic nerve head filled with drusen. (**a**) With flat frontal lighting commonly used in fundus photography, the drusen are not easy to see. (**b**) If the same disc is illuminated with a slit beam that scatters light laterally, the crystals are easily seen.

SPECIAL STUDIES TO IDENTIFY DISC DRUSEN

Fluorescein Angiography

In general, anomalously elevated discs, with or without drusen, show late staining with fluorescein, whereas in papilledema the staining disc often shows feathery 'leakage' into the adjacent nerve fiber layer.

Autofluorescence

The disc is illuminated with a 430-mm wavelength (blue) light source and photographs of the fundus are taken through a yellow filter designed to block blue light. The short (blue) wavelength light stimulates the drusen to emit a yellow light that passes through the yellow filter. This autofluorescence identifies and outlines the more superficial drusen, and is often of great help clinically (*Fig. 18.20*).

CT Scan

As they are mineralized, drusen tend to block X-rays and can be seen at the optic nerve head on CT scanning (*Fig. 18.21*).

Pseudodrusen

In patients with chronic papilledema, the appearance of many small, sharply defined exudates is associated with constriction of the visual field and loss of the nerve fiber layer. These pseudodrusen (see Figs 20.15, 20.19 and 20.20) tend to appear in the temporal margin of the disc or over the whole disc surface but they are superficial and are usually small and of a uniform size. Drusen, on the other hand, can be large or small, and may be deep or at the surface (see Figs 18.19, 18.20a).

Ocular Echography

Standardized ocular echography is a very sensitive technique for detecting disc drusen because they reflect sound waves more than the surrounding disc tissue (*Fig. 18.22*). This technique is especially useful when drusen are buried and have caused some optic disc elevation but are not visible ophthalmoscopically.

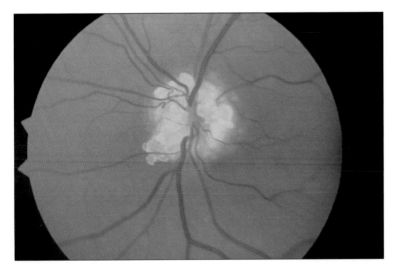

Fig. 18.19 A disc with an unusually severe burden of exposed intrapapillary drusen.

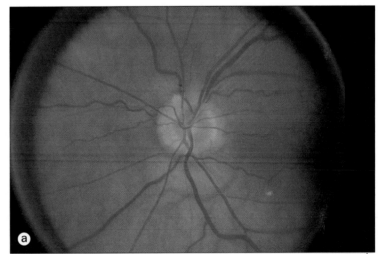

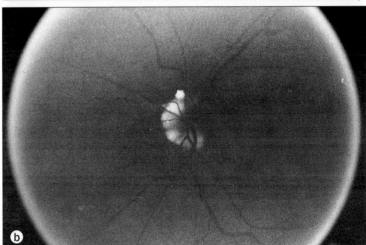

Fig. 18.20 Autofluorescence of disc drusen. (**a**) Drusen can be seen in this disc. With appropriate filters in the camera (**b**), dramatic autofluorescence of the drusen can be demonstrated.

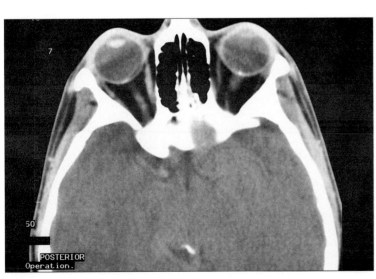

Fig. 18.21 A CT scan will sometimes confirm the presence of calcific drusen in both optic nerve heads.

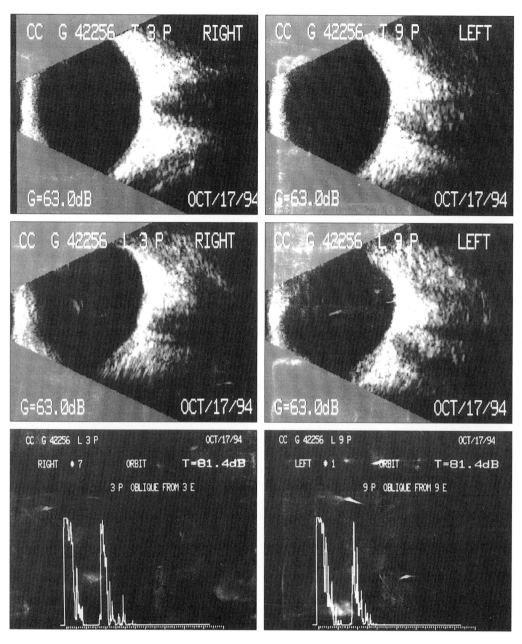

Fig. 18.22 Standardized echography of a patient with bilateral optic disc drusen (right eye more than left eye). (**Top**) Transverse B-scans (transverse to the 3 o'clock and 9 o'clock nasal meridians at the level of the optic disc), one for each eye. The drusen are indicated by bright signals underneath the disc surface and in front of the optic nerve patterns. (**Center**) Longitudinal B-scans (aligned with the nasal meridians of each eye through the optic discs and nerves). Again, the scans show bright signals from the drusen and a lack of excess spinal fluid in the sheaths of the optic nerves. (**Bottom**) A-scans (made obliquely through the ocular wall, with the probe placed nasally behind the equator of the eye), confirming the solid nature of the drusen. The high posterior echo spikes show that drusen reflect sound in the same way that a foreign body does when lodged in the coats of the eye; that is, the intensity of the drusen signal is maximal when the drusen are centered in the beam and is independent of the direction of the beam (unlike the reflections from the walls of the globe). (Courtesy of Karl Ossoinig)

Further reading

Apple DJ, Rabb MF, Walsh PM. Congenital anomalies of the optic disc. *Surv Ophthalmol.* 1982;**27**:3–41.

Brodsky MC. Congenital optic disc anomalies. *Surv Ophthalmol.* 1994;**39**:89–112.

Brodsky MC, Gladier CM, Pollock SC, *et al.* Optic nerve hypoplasia: identification by magnetic resonance imaging. *Arch Ophthalmol.* 1990;**108**:1562–1567.

Brown G, Tasman W. *Congenital Anomalies of the Optic Disc.* New York: Grune and Stratton, 1983.

Frisén L, Holmegaard L. Spectrum of optic nerve hypoplasia. *Br J Ophthalmol.* 1978;**62**:7–15.

Gowers WR. *Manual and Atlas of Medical Ophthalmology.* London: Churchill Livingstone, 1879.

Knitzinges EE, Beaumont HM. *A Color Atlas of Optic Disc Abnormalities.* Chicago: Year-Book Medical Publishers, 1987.

CHAPTER 19

Optic Atrophy

B James

INTRODUCTION

Optic atrophy indicates damage to the axons of the optic nerve, and may reflect disorders from the retina to the lateral geniculate body. The disc is pale. This reflects a reduction in the vasculature of the disc, the formation of glial tissue and, possibly, an alteration in the architecture of the remaining fibers at the nerve head, changing the reflectance of light. Careful examination of the superior and inferior arcuate regions of the retina in suspected optic atrophy may reveal dark, wedge-like defects in the nerve fiber layer. The signs of optic atrophy are seldom specific for a particular condition, however (*Fig. 19.1*).

HEREDITARY OPTIC NEUROPATHIES

Traditionally, the classification of this group has been determined by the mode of inheritance. Autosomal dominant, autosomal recessive, and mitochondrial (Leber's optic neuropathy) patterns of inheritance are described (*Fig. 19.2*).

DOMINANT OPTIC NEUROPATHY

Visual loss is of gradual onset, usually within the first 10 years of life. Those affected early in life may also have nystagmus. The degree of visual disability is very variable, even within families, and may be progressive. In the original description by Kjer, 25% of patients aged 45 years and older had vision below 20/200 but no patient had vision worse than counting fingers. Both eyes are usually affected equally. A central or centrocecal field defect is present. Blue sensitivity is particularly affected. Classically, the optic nerve shows pallor on the temporal side, and in some the disc may appear cupped. The dominant optic neuropathy gene has been located on chromosomes 18 and 3. Most patients have no associated clinical findings, but families have been described in which the condition is associated with sensorineural deafness.

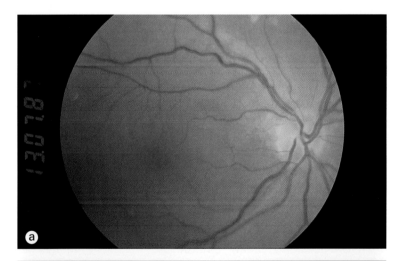

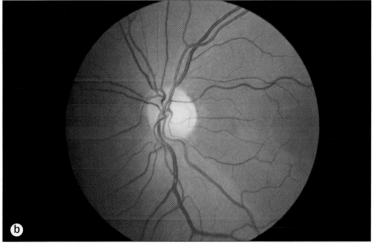

Fig. 19.1 (**a**) A normal optic disc. (**b**) Temporal pallor of the optic disc.

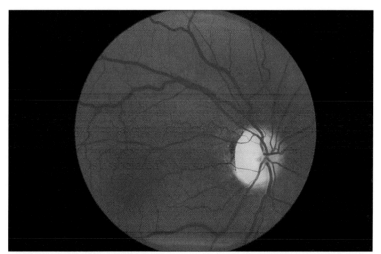

Fig. 19.2 Optic disc pallor in a patient with Leber's optic neuropathy.

RECESSIVE OPTIC NEUROPATHIES

These are very rare conditions.

In *simple* or *congenital optic atrophy*, the visual loss is worse than that seen in the dominant form and is present within the first 4 years of life. The discs are pale, and sometimes cupped, and the retinal arterioles are attenuated. There may be a history of consanguinity.

In *complicated* or *infantile optic atrophy* (also termed Behr's optic atrophy), the patient has associated neurologic problems, as well as optic atrophy. The visual loss usually appears within the first 10 years of life and may be severe. The temporal disc is pale and nystagmus and strabismus are common. Pyramidal and extrapyramidal tract signs may be present. The patient may be mentally retarded.

In *Wolfram's syndrome*, there is onset of the following combination of diseases:

• diabetes insipidus
• diabetes mellitus
• optic atrophy
• deafness

Neurologic problems, such as ataxia and epilepsy, may also be present. There may be a variety of additional ocular findings. Visual loss occurs between the ages of 5 and 21 years and is slowly progressive. The disc is pale and may be cupped. Although classified as an autosomal recessive disease, it may be that the multitudinous associations of the disease are better explained on the basis of mitochondrial dysfunction. This may result either from a nuclear or mitochondrial DNA abnormality.

LEBER'S HEREDITARY OPTIC NEUROPATHY

The disorder results from an abnormality of mitochondrial DNA, causing a defect in oxidative phosphorylation. The condition is maternally inherited and men are more commonly affected than women. There is severe, rapid visual loss (a more chronic course has also been described). Both eyes are usually affected within 1 year. Most cases present in early adulthood but later onset has also been reported. Acutely, telangiectasia may be seen around the optic disc before it becomes pale. In some patients there may be an association with multiple sclerosis. Molecular testing to determine mitochondrial DNA mutations associated with the disease is now possible. Both primary mutations (of which the 11 778 is the commonest and the 15 257 the most likely to show visual improvement) and secondary mutations, which may contribute to a reduction in oxidative phosphorylation, are recognized. Currently, no treatment is available. Individual members of families with Leber's hereditary optic neuropathy who have been found to have appropriate mitochondrial DNA mutations may benefit by abstaining from tobacco and alcohol.

TOXIC OPTIC NEUROPATHIES

TOBACCO–ALCOHOL AMBLYOPIA, NUTRITIONAL AMBLYOPIA

An inter-relationship exists between these causes of optic neuropathy. The patient presents with rapid visual loss and there is a background of poor nutrition (particularly lack of B-complex vitamins) and alcohol intake or heavy smoking, particularly pipe smoking. Cyanide is thought to be the toxin in tobacco amblyopia, while an inability to detoxify cyanide is thought to be responsible for the amblyopia seen with excess alcohol intake and poor nutrition. Clinically, visual acuity and color vision are reduced, and field testing reveals a central or centrocecal scotoma. The discs are pale. The blood film may show a macrocytic anemia. Treatment with multivitamin preparations including folic acid, and parenteral vitamin B_{12}, is effective. Long-term abstinence from alcohol and smoking and an improved diet are the ideal aims. Tropical amblyopia may also be a result of cyanide toxicity (the cyanide coming from cassava), as well as the effect of poor diet, smoking, and alcohol.

DRUG-INDUCED OPTIC NEUROPATHIES

Both isoniazid and ethambutol, used in the treatment of tuberculosis, may cause optic neuropathy. The visual loss is gradual and dose dependent. Other drugs that may cause a toxic optic neuropathy include chloramphenicol, streptomycin, amiodarone, toluene (from glue sniffing), and some drugs used in the treatment of cancer (e.g. 5-fluorouracil). Quinine toxicity causes optic atrophy by damaging the retinal ganglion cells.

Exposure to heavy metals may also result in an optic neuropathy.

GLAUCOMATOUS OPTIC ATROPHY

One of the commonest causes of optic atrophy, axonal loss results from damage at the level of the cribriform plate. This slowly progressive optic neuropathy is associated with an intraocular pressure (IOP) too high for the individual eye, although it may not be elevated beyond the statistically normal range (normal tension glaucoma). Other factors may also be important in the pathogenesis of the disease; recently the role that vascular abnormalities may play has received much attention. The optic disc cup enlarges, with an associated reduction in the volume of the neuroretinal rim, particularly in the inferior and superior quadrants. Some patients may develop notching of the optic disc cup. This may be preceded by an optic disc hemorrhage (typically seen in low-tension glaucoma) (*Fig. 19.3*).

Glaucomatous field defects are present, with paracentral scotomas or arcuate defects extending from the disc. Treatment requires the reduction of the IOP by medications, by laser, and by surgery.

VASCULAR OPTIC NERVE DISEASE

Optic atrophy results from ischemia of the retrolaminar portion of the anterior optic nerve head, termed anterior ischemic optic neuropathy. It is classified into arteritic and nonarteritic disease. The arteritic form is most commonly associated with giant cell arteritis but is also reported in other vasculitides, such as systemic lupus erythematosus (SLE) and polyarteritis nodosa. The nonarteritic form is associated with a number of systemic conditions, including hypertension, diabetes, anemia, acute systemic hypotension (e.g. in cardiac surgery), severe blood loss in middle-aged or elderly patients, migraine, and optic nerve head drusen. Abnormalities of the clotting cascade have also been reported. The condition has also been seen following cataract surgery, attributed to a rise in IOP. Ischemic optic neuropathy results in the sudden onset of variable visual loss, which is particularly severe in arteritic disease, when it may be preceded by episodes of amaurosis fugax. Classically, an altitudinal field defect is present but this is not invariable. The disc in arteritic disease is usually pale and swollen, with peripapillary cotton wool spots. In the nonarteritic form, the disc is more floridly swollen (possibly sectorially) and hemorrhagic. The discs may be small with a small cup:disc ratio (*Fig. 19.4*).

Patients with giant cell arteritis may also have anterior segment ischemia (*Fig. 19.5*). Those suspected of having giant cell arteritis require immediate treatment with systemic steroids to try and prevent second eye involvement; unfortunately these will not restore vision to the affected eye. Steroids have not been shown to have a beneficial effect in the nonarteritic disease, for which there is no treatment. A recent trial of optic nerve decompression in progressive nonarteritic ischemic optic neuropathy showed no benefit.

COMPRESSIVE OPTIC NEUROPATHY

Disc atrophy may result from compression on the optic nerve or the chiasm. The differential diagnosis is large. In the orbit, the nerve

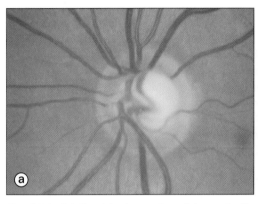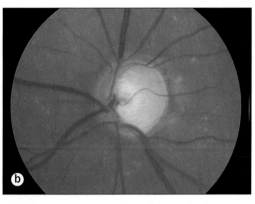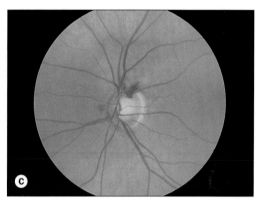

Fig. 19.3 (**a**) Physiologic cupping of the optic disc . (**b**) Glaucomatous cupping of the optic disc. (**c**) An optic disc hemorrhage in a patient without tension glaucoma.

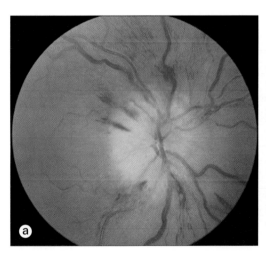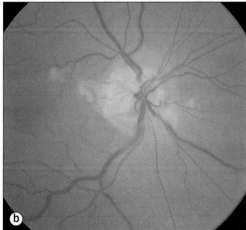

Fig. 19.4 (**a**) Non arteritic anterior ischemic optic neuropathy. (**b**) Arteritic anterior ischemic optic neuropathy demonstrating pallor compared to the fellow eye which showed a normal optic nerve head.

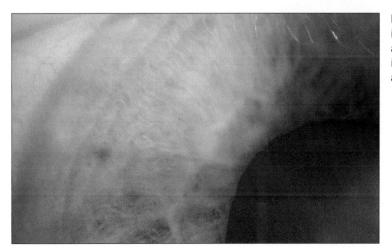

Fig. 19.5 Segmental iris atrophy following anterior segment ischemia in giant cell arteritis.

may be compressed by tumors (gliomas, meningiomas, primary and secondary orbital tumors), abnormal bone from fibrous dysplasia or Paget's disease, orbital cellulitis that has damaged the optic nerve, mucoceles from the sinuses, and by enlarged extraocular muscles, as seen in dysthyroid eye disease. The nerve may also be compressed internally by infiltrative disease, such as glioma, lymphoma, or sarcoidosis. In the cranium meningiomas, aneurysms, pituitary tumors, chiasmal gliomas, secondary metastasis, arachnoiditis around the chiasm secondary to meningitis, and craniopharyngiomas may all cause compressive optic atrophy, which is usually bilateral but not necessarily symmetric (*Fig. 19.6*).

Visual loss is usually gradual, unless the causative lesion is rapidly expanding. Color vision, particularly red sensitivity, is affected early on. Great attention must be paid to the visual field in *both* eyes; for example, looking for the bitemporal defect of a pituitary tumor or the junctional scotoma if the nerve is affected just prior to its entry into the chiasm. The discs are pale. The pallor may be localized to the nasal and temporal aspects of the disc in optic tract lesions, resulting in 'bow-tie' atrophy. Treatment is dictated by the cause of the compression.

TRAUMATIC OPTIC ATROPHY

Damage to the optic nerve may result from trauma to the orbit or head. The nerve may be injured directly, by bony injury in the region of the optic canal, through ischemic damage from disruption of the supplying blood vessels, or by compression of the nerve fibers from a hemorrhage within the optic nerve sheaf. A CT scan is helpful in diagnosis. An anteriorly placed hemorrhage within the optic nerve sheath may respond to optic nerve sheath decompression. If the site of compression lies in the optic canal, surgical decompression may be indicated. High-dose steroids, initially intravenously, have also been found to be of benefit in some patients. Treatment is often complicated by the existence of other serious injuries.

Rapid deceleration injuries, where the movement of the front of the head is suddenly stopped, may cause damage to the chiasm. Damage to this region is best demonstrated with an MRI scan. Chiasmal trauma is particularly associated with frontal bone fracture.

INFLAMMATORY OPTIC NEUROPATHIES

Optic neuritis may be associated with a variety of diseases. The incidence of demyelination is difficult to determine as it depends on the length of follow-up. In a study from Moorfields Hospital, London, UK, 57% of patients followed for 12 years developed the condition. A variety of viral infections, including upper respiratory tract infections and herpes zoster, may also cause optic neuritis, as may inflammation of the meninges, orbit, and sinuses. Granulomatous infections (syphilis, tuberculosis) and, rarely, other infections (*Toxocara*, *Toxoplasma*) may also be responsible. Classic optic neuritis has also been described in autoimmune disease, particularly SLE. There may be some overlap with ischemic optic neuropathy, however. Certainly, the histology of CNS lesions in SLE is of occlusion of small blood vessels.

The patient presents with a profound, usually uniocular, reduction in vision over a few hours or days. A characteristic finding is pain on ocular movement. A central or centrocecal scotoma is present. The disc usually appears normal in retrobulbar neuritis. If the anterior part of the nerve is involved (papillitis), the disc may become swollen and hemorrhagic; this is seen more commonly in children (*Fig. 19.7*). Vision begins to improve after 2 or 3 weeks, although it may not completely recover, leaving some evidence of optic atrophy. Some patients report a worsening of the vision with exercise or when bathing (Uhthoff's symptom), which may persist after recovery of vision. In children there is often a history of recent viral disease, and they are more likely to suffer bilateral visual loss. Devic's disease (neuromyelitis optica), seen in young adults and children, may turn out to be a juvenile form of multiple sclerosis. The optic neuropathy is bilateral and there is an associated transverse myelitis.

Peripheral retinal venous sheathing may be seen in patients

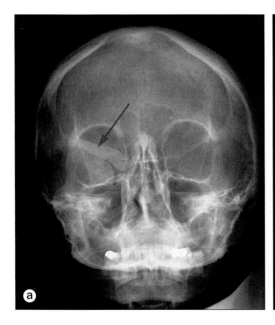
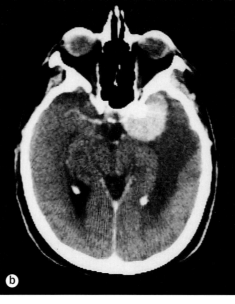

Fig. 19.6 (**a**) Hyperostosis indicates the presence of a sphenoid ridge meningioma. (**b**) CT scan showing a meningioma

with optic neuritis and demyelination. MRI scanning may also locate additional plaques of demyelination, but the patient must be appropriately counseled before performing a scan for this reason. It is not a routine investigation for a typical case of optic neuritis (*Fig. 19.8* and see chapter 20).

There is usually no indication to treat optic neuritis associated with demyelination or presumed viral infection unless both eyes are affected or it is desired to speed the recovery process. Steroids have no effect on the eventual visual outcome. A recent study suggests that treatment with oral steroids will increase the likelihood of further episodes of demyelination. Treatment, if any, should thus be with intravenous steroids because they speed the recovery of vision. Systemic steroids have also been reported as beneficial in patients with autoimmune disease.

OPTIC ATROPHY FOLLOWING RAISED INTRACRANIAL PRESSURE

Chronic papilledema secondary to raised intracranial pressure, for whatever cause, may result in axonal atrophy and contraction of the visual field. The disc loses some of the changes noted in acute papilledema, with resorption of some of the peripapillary retinal edema and loss of the acute hemorrhage and exudative changes; it is said to resemble a champagne cork (*Fig. 19.9*). Pallor of the disc slowly increases as the disc swelling subsides.

OPTIC ATROPHY ASSOCIATED WITH RETINAL DISEASE

Retinal disease and associated ganglion cell death results in axonal death and optic atrophy. The associated ophthalmoscopic picture normally makes the diagnosis. Optic disc atrophy is a feature of conditions such as retinitis pigmentosa and central retinal artery occlusion (*Fig. 19.10*). Cone dystrophies may cause particular diagnostic problems, as abnormalities in color vision may be attributed to optic nerve disease rather than a retinal photoreceptor problem that may not be apparent ophthalmoscopically. An electroretinogram (ERG) will aid diagnosis. Retinal arterial attenuation is a common accompanying sign.

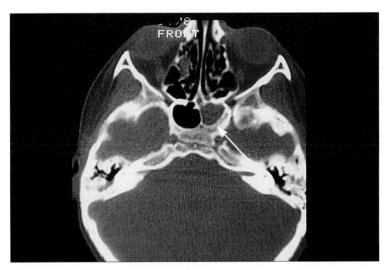

Fig. 19.7 CT scam demonstrating shenoid sinusitis in a young patient with optic

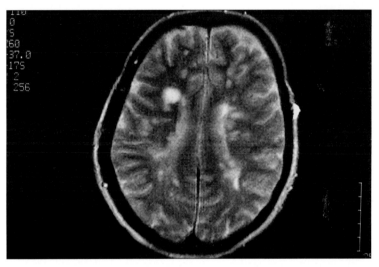

Fig 19.8 The MRI appearance of plaques of demyelination.

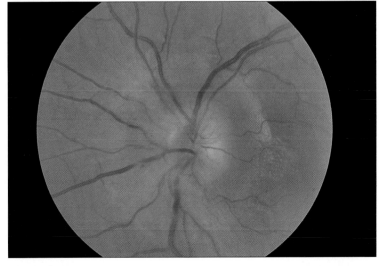

Fig. 19.9 Disc swelling in papilledema.

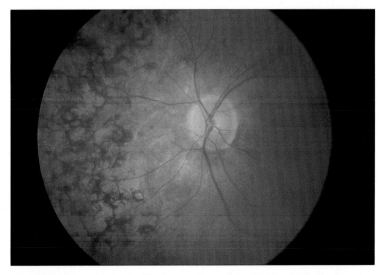

Fig. 19.10 The pale optic disc in a patient with retinitis pigmentosa.

PALE DISCS WITHOUT OPTIC ATROPHY

The disc may appear pale without atrophy of the nerve fibers. Optic nerve hypoplasia, disc colobomas or pits, optic nerve drusen, myelinated nerve fibers, and tilted optic discs may all be a cause for confusion (*Figs 19.11–19.13*) (see chapter 21).

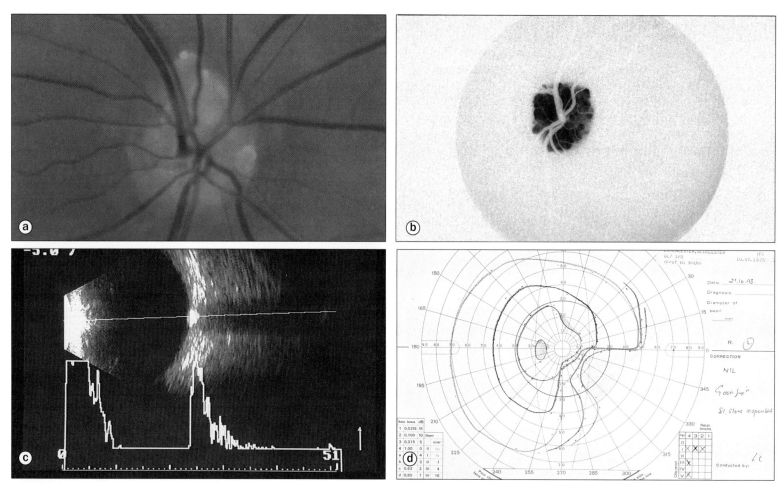

Fig. 19.11 (**a**) Optic disc drusen. (**b**) Autoflourescence of optic disc drusen. (**c**) B-mode ultrasound clearly demonstrates the optic disc drusen. (**d**) Inferonasal visual field loss due to drusen of the optic disc.

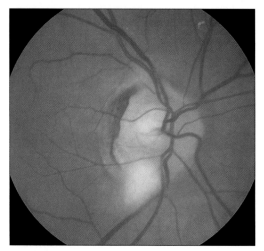

Fig. 19.12 Myelinated nerve fibers; a fuzzy white patch with edges feathered along the path of the retinal nerve fibers.

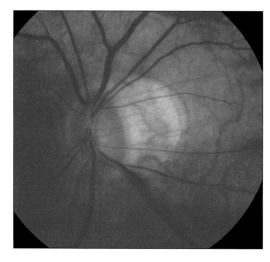

Fig. 19.13 A tilted optic disc, with a large crescent of exposed sclera.

Further reading

Katz B, Trobe JD, Beck RW. The optic neuritis treatment trial: Implications for clinicians. *Seminars in Ophthalmology*. 1995;**10**:214–220.

Kjer B. Infantile optic atrophy with dominant mode of inheritance: A clinical and genetic study of nineteen Danish families. *Acta Ophthalmol.* 1959;**54** (suppl):1–46.

Lessell S, Rossman NP. Juvenile diabetes mellitus and optic atrophy. *Arch Neurol.* 1977;**34**:759–765.

The Ischemic Optic Neuropathy Decompression Trial Research Group. Optic nerve decompression surgery for non arteritic anterior ischemic optic neuropathy is not effective and may be harmful. *JAMA.* 1995;**273**:625–632.

CHAPTER 20

Optic Neuritis: Clinical Considerations and the Relationship to Multiple Sclerosis

Roy W Beck

Optic neuritis is a term used to refer to inflammation of the optic nerve. There are a number of possible etiologies for optic neuritis but for many patients a specific cause cannot be discerned. In most patients, the etiology of the optic neuritis is related to demyelination of the optic nerve, regardless of whether multiple sclerosis (MS) has been diagnosed. In the absence of signs of MS or other systemic disease, the optic neuritis is often referred to as 'isolated'. In a small percentage of patients, primary demyelination is not the etiology and another cause, such as syphilis, sarcoidosis, a viral or postviral syndrome, systemic lupus erythematosus (SLE), or another autoimmune disease, is identified.

This chapter deals solely with demyelinative optic neuritis and the relationship of isolated optic neuritis with MS.

HISTORY AND CLINICAL PROFILE

The history of visual loss and the patient profile are critical for proper diagnosis. Patients developing optic neuritis are usually aged between 15 and 45 years. Women are affected more commonly than men.

Typically, visual loss is acute but may progress for 7–10 days. Progression for a longer period of time is possible but should make the clinician suspicious of an alternative etiology. Pain is present to some degree in more than 90% of patients. It may precede or occur concurrently with visual loss, is usually exacerbated by eye movement, and generally lasts no more than a few days. In most patients the visual loss is monocular but in a small percentage both eyes will be simultaneously affected.

CLINICAL SIGNS

Examination of the patient will show evidence of optic nerve dysfunction. Visual acuity is reduced in most patients but varies from a mild reduction to severe loss (no light perception is possible). Color vision and contrast sensitivity are impaired in almost all patients, often out of proportion to acuity. The typical visual field defect is a central scotoma; however, almost any type of field defect is possible, including altitudinal-type defects, which are most typical of anterior ischemic optic neuropathy. A relative afferent pupillary defect (RAPD) will be detectable in almost all patients with unilateral disease. If such a defect is not present, a pre-existing optic neuropathy in the fellow eye should be suspected.

The optic disc may appear normal (retrobulbar neuritis) or swollen (papillitis) (*Fig. 20.1*) in optic neuritis and clinical features are similar in both forms. Vitreous cells and retinal exudates are not generally seen. Their presence suggests an infectious or other cause for optic neuritis rather than demyelinative disease. The occurrence of macular exudates (often in a star-shaped pattern) in association with optic neuritis is termed neuroretinitis (*Fig. 20.2*). The recognition of these exudates is extremely important, as their presence virtually rules out MS as a possible etiology.

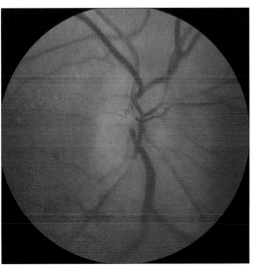

Fig. 20.1 Papillitis. Optic disc swelling due to optic neuritis typically involves the entire disc.

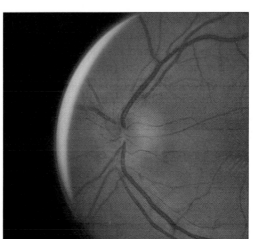

Fig. 20.2 Neuroretinitis. Note the swelling of the optic disc as well as the macular exudates in a star-shaped pattern.

PATHOLOGY

There is little known directly about the pathology of 'isolated' optic neuritis and there has not been an autopsied patient. However, optic nerve demyelination is well recognized in MS and the pathology of MS has been extensively studied. The little pathology that is available of acute optic nerve demyelinative plaques in MS has shown similar changes to the MS plaques seen in the brain, with the inflammatory response marked by perivascular cuffing, T cells, and plasma cells.

There is no evidence to suggest that the pathology of 'isolated' optic neuritis is different from the pathology of optic neuritis in MS and indeed some experimental evidence suggests that it is similar. Sergott *et al.* injected the serum from 17 patients with MS and three patients with isolated optic neuritis into the optic nerves of guinea pigs. Demyelination was found on pathological examination of the guinea pig optic nerves injected with the serum from 12 of the 17 MS patients and all three of the optic neuritis patients. There were zones of demyelination with relative sparing of axons similar to the human pathology in MS.

SPECIAL INVESTIGATIONS

The clinical profile of optic neuritis is sufficiently characteristic and specific that for most patients the diagnosis can be readily made on clinical grounds without the aid of ancillary testing. If the patient's clinical course is typical for optic neuritis, further testing is unlikely to define a cause for optic neuropathy other than demyelination (which is the presumed etiology in the absence of evidence for any other cause). The Optic Neuritis Treatment Trial (ONTT) found that blood tests, such as antinuclear antibody determination (ANA) and rapid plasma reagin (RPR), chest radiography, cerebrospinal fluid (CSF) analysis, and MRI only rarely defined a cause for optic neuritis other than MS in patients without clinical signs of a systemic disease (other than MS). Although MRI generally is not necessary to rule out causes of optic neuropathy other than optic neuritis, it is of great value in determining the patient's risk for developing other clinical signs of MS within 2 years (see details below).

NATURAL HISTORY

VISUAL

Regardless of the degree of impairment of vision, visual function for most patients with optic neuritis begins improving 1 to several weeks after the onset (without any treatment). In the ONTT, median visual acuity in the placebo group improved from about 20/60 at baseline to 20/25 by the 2-week follow-up. After 1 year, 95% of the placebo-treated patients had a visual acuity of 20/40 or better; 71% were better than 20/20.

Even with good recovery of acuity, however, there may still be significant optic nerve damage. Residual deficits in color vision, contrast sensitivity, light brightness sense, stereopsis, and other measures are frequent, and a RAPD, optic disc pallor, and prolonged visual-evoked potential latency are usually still detectable. The patient may complain of loss of vision on becoming hot, either through exercise or a hot bath (Uhthoff's syndrome).

Approximately 25% of patients will experience a recurrence of optic neuritis in the same or fellow eye. The prognosis for visual recovery decreases with each succeeding episode in an eye.

NEUROLOGIC

Previous studies reported the risk of developing MS after optic neuritis to be as low as 13% and as high as 88%. In the better designed studies, the risk appears to be in the range of 45–80% within 15 years. In one of these studies, Rizzo and Lessell reported that 58% of patients presenting with optic neuritis (69% of women and 33% of men) were diagnosed as having MS during an average follow-up of 14.9 years. Life-table analysis indicated that at 15 years' follow-up, 74% of women and 34% of men would be expected to develop MS. The average time to the development of MS was 7.8 years. The risk for MS was greater the earlier the age of onset of the optic neuritis. This study, surprisingly, did not find that recurrent attacks of optic neuritis increased the risk. Although most other studies have shown a similar risk at a younger age, not all have demonstrated such a difference in the risk of developing MS between men and women nor the lack of risk with recurrent attacks. The presence of oligoclonal banding in the CSF and of HLA haplotype DR2 have also been identified as risk factors.

The Longitudinal Optic Neuritis Study (LONS), a follow-up study of the cohort of patients entered into the ONTT, found that an abnormal brain MRI was a strong predictor of the development of other clinical signs of MS within 2 years (*Fig. 20.3*). Patients with an abnormal brain MRI had a 2-year risk of MS of about 30% (untreated), whereas patients with a normal scan had a risk of only 3%. Further follow-up will determine whether this low risk of MS with a normal scan continues in the long term.

In the LONS, a history of nons-pecific neurologic symptoms (too ill-defined to consider consistent with MS) or of optic neuritis in the fellow eye before the onset of optic neuritis at the time of entry into the ONTT was also an indicator of risk – independent of MRI – for the development of MS within 2 years. Family histo-

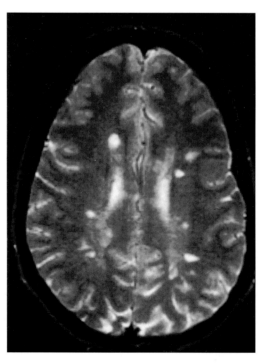

Fig. 20.3 MRI of the brain in a patient with MS. Note the multiple signal abnormalities, particularly in the periventricular areas.

ry of MS and Caucasian race were also found to be likely risk factors. Age and sex were not found to be predictors of the 2-year development of MS.

THERAPY

CORTICOSTEROIDS

Since the 1950s, corticosteroids have been frequently prescribed for optic neuritis, even though the benefit of therapy was unproven. The ONTT evaluated two corticosteroid regimens in comparison with oral placebo:
- Intravenous methylprednisolone, 250 mg, every 6 h for 3 days followed by oral prednisone, 1 mg/kg/day, for 11 days.
- Oral prednisone, 1 mg/kg/day, for 14 days.

The study found that, compared with the placebo group, the intravenous regimen provided a more rapid recovery of vision but no long-term benefit. Most of the difference in rate of recovery between groups was seen in the first 2 weeks. Thereafter, differences in visual function between groups were small. After 1 year of follow-up, there were no significant differences between the groups in visual acuity, contrast sensitivity, color vision, or visual field.

The regimen of oral prednisone alone not only provided no benefit to vision but also was associated with an increased rate of new attacks of optic neuritis in both the initially affected and fellow eyes. Within the first 2 years of follow-up, new attacks of optic neuritis in either eye occurred in 30% of the patients in the oral prednisone group, compared with 16% in the placebo group, and 14% in the intravenous group.

Unexpectedly, the study found that the group receiving the intravenous regimen had a lower rate of development of MS within the first 2 years than the placebo or prednisone groups. Among the patients in the intravenous group, definite MS developed within 2 years in only 7.5%, compared with 16.7% of the placebo group and 14.7% of the prednisone group. The 2-year adjusted rate of definite MS in the intravenous group was 0.34 (95% confidence interval [CI] 0.16–0.74) compared with the placebo group and 0.38 (95% CI 0.17–0.83) compared with the prednisone group. When the outcome was redefined to be either development of definite or probable MS, or development of definite MS or a new attack of

optic neuritis in the fellow eye, the results were similar.

Most of the treatment effect was manifested in the patients with an abnormal MRI scan at study entry. Among those patients with at least two MRI lesions, definite MS developed within 2 years in 35.9% of the 39 patients in the placebo group, 32.4% of the 37 patients in the prednisone group, and only 16.2% of the 37 patients in the intravenous group. Independent of treatment, the rate of development of definite MS in patients with a normal MRI scan was so low that therapeutic efficacy for these patients could not be judged.

OTHER TREATMENTS

No treatments, other than corticosteroids, have been shown to benefit patients with optic neuritis. However, it is reasonable to conclude that patients with optic neuritis who already show signs of MS on brain MRI may benefit from treatments such as beta interferon or copolymer A that have been shown to be beneficial in patients with well-developed MS.

MANAGEMENT RECOMMENDATIONS

In a patient with the typical clinical profile of demyelinative optic neuritis – aged between 15 and 45 years, sudden onset of visual loss with progression for less than 1 week, ocular pain worsened by eye movement, no signs of ocular inflammation (e.g. no iritis or vitritis) – a clinical diagnosis is secure without ancillary studies.

Brain MRI should be considered to establish the 2-year risk of developing new clinical signs of MS. Treatment with a course of intravenous corticosteroids is justifiable, particularly for those patients whose brain MRI scan shows signs of demyelination. However, prescribing no treatment can also be justified. To enhance the feasibility of treatment, once-a-day outpatient administration of methylprednisolone, 1 g for 3 days, could be considered in lieu of the in-hospital divided-dose schedule prescribed in the ONTT. The number of days selected for intravenous treatment is empiric and not based on scientific evidence. It is not known whether a tapering course of oral corticosteroids after the intravenous course is of any benefit.

Further reading

Beck RW, Arrington J, Murtagh FR, Cleary PA, Kaufman DI. Optic Neuritis Study Group. Brain MRI in acute optic neuritis. Experience of the Optic Neuritis Study Group. *Arch Neurol* 1993;**8**:841–846.

Beck RW, Cleary PA, Optic Neuritis Study Group. Optic Neuritis Treatment Trial: One-year follow up results. *Arch Ophthalmol.* 1993;**111**:773–775.

Beck RW, Cleary PA, Anderson MM, *et al.* A randomized, controlled trial of corticosteroids in the treatment of acute optic neuritis. *N Eng J Med.* 1992;**326**:581–588.

Beck RW, Cleary PA, Trobe JD, *et al.* The effect of corticosteroids for acute optic neuritis on the subsequent development of multiple sclerosis. *N Eng J Med.* 1993;**329**:1764–1769.

Keltner JL, Johnson, CA, Spurr JO, Beck RW. Optic Neuritis Study Group. Baseline visual field profile of optic neuritis: the experience of the Optic Neuritis Treatment Trial. *Arch Ophthalmol.* 1993;**111**:231–234.

Optic Neuritis Study Group. The clinical profile of optic neuritis: Experience of the Optic Neuritis Treatment Trial. *Arch Ophthalmol.* 1991;**109**:1673–1678.

Perkin GD, Rose FC. Visual signs at presentation. In: *Optic Neuritis and its Differential Diagnosis.* Oxford:Oxford Medical Publishers. 1979:43–73.

Rizzo JF, Lessell S. Risk of developing multiple sclerosis after uncomplicated optic neuritis. A long-term prospective study. *Neurology.* 1988;**38**:185–190.

Sergott RC, Brown MJ, Lisak RP, Miller SL. Antibody to Myelin-associated glycoprotein produces central nervous system demyelination. *Neurology* 1988,**38**:422–426.

CHAPTER 21

Raised Intracranial Pressure

W N White, J Corbett, M Wall

INTRODUCTION

Papilledema is defined as optic disc swelling due to elevated intracranial pressure. After years of speculation, the mechanism of optic disc swelling was clearly established using experimental increased intracranial pressure and decreased intraocular pressure in primate models. In these studies, intraocular injections of radioactively labeled amino acids were taken up by ganglion cells and were incorporated into the axoplasm. Normal axoplasmic flow would clear these amino acids past the lamina cribrosa within 24 h. In animals with high cerebrospinal fluid (CSF) pressure or low intraocular pressure, axoplasmic transport of these radioactive tracers is blocked at the level of the lamina cribrosa. A corollary of this observation is that where there is a major pressure differential between intraocular pressure and intracranial pressure, there is the potential for arrest of axoplasmic flow at the lamina cribrosa (*Figs 21.1, 21.2*). If axonal energy metabolism is altered, such as occurs with ischemia at the level of the lamina cribrosa or with methanol toxicity, a similar blockage of axoplasmic flow occurs. Additionally, optic disc swelling may occur transiently with indirect traumatic optic neuropathy or with retrobulbar optic neuritis as a result of transient stasis in axoplasmic transport.

PAPILLEDEMA GRADING SCHEMES AND CASE EXAMPLES

Papilledema has been characterized by a number of notations or grading schemes (*Fig. 21.3*). As it is rarely possible to date precisely the onset of optic disc swelling, temporal notations such as 'early', which suggest that one knows how long the disc swelling has been present, are not entirely suitable. 'Mild or slight' disc swelling simply denotes that the degree of swelling is not severe. However, swelling may be 'mild' in chronic papilledema due to loss of optic nerve axons. In the numerical notation devised by Lars Frisén (*Fig. 21.4*) this 'low-grade' swelling is defined as Frisén grade 1 papilledema (*Figs 21.5, 21.6*). Grade 0 represents a normal-appearing optic disc, with a radial peripapillary nerve fiber layer (NFL) without NFL thickening or tortuosity. Frisén warned that the upper and lower poles of the disc have variable NFL thickness and that these should be disregarded when staging papilledema (see Fig. 21.4). Grade 1 papilledema is characterized by mild elevation of three-quarters of the disc margin (sparing the papillomacular bundle); the nasal, superior, and inferior margins of the nerve are obscured because of peripapillary edema. This gives the appearance of a peripapillary 'C-shaped' halo.

Fully developed optic disc edema, similar to Frisén grade 2

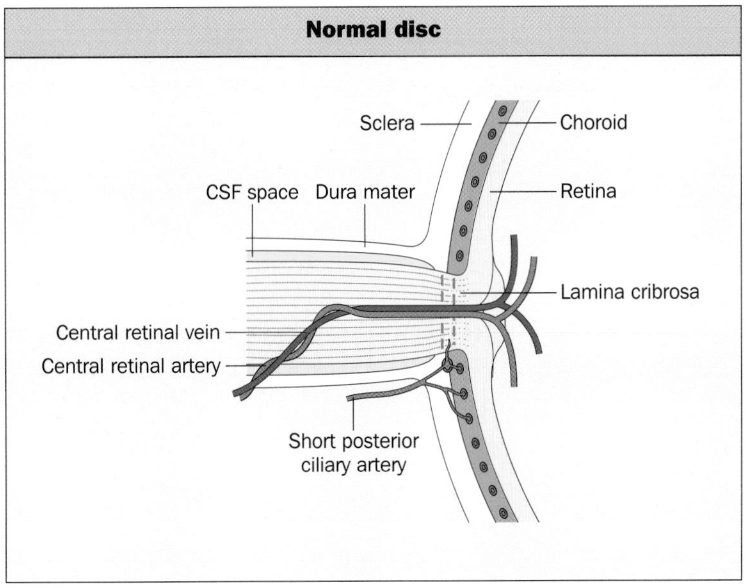

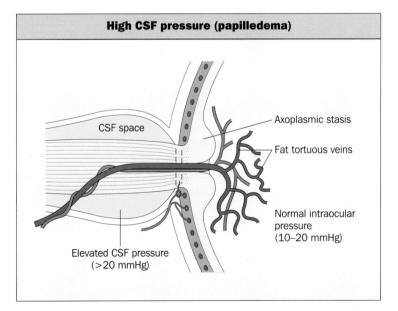

Fig. 21.1 The normal optic nerve and disc. Note the position of the lamina cribrosa, the demarcation point for axoplasmic flow spaces and optic disc edema.

Fig. 21.2 The configuration of the optic nerve subarachnoid space (CSF space) and optic nerve sheath is shown in relation to the lamina cribrosa and the elevated optic nerve head.

Fig. 21.3 Various papilledema notation schemes.

Various papilledema staging schemes						
Author	**Stage**					
Hoyt		early	fully developed	chronic		
Sanders		early	fully developed	chronic		vintage
Frisén	0	1	2	3	4	5
	normal	C-shaped halo	complete halo	vessels off disc obscured	vessels on disc obscured	mushroom disc

Papilledema grade system (Frisén scale)

Grade 0: Normal optic disc

- blurring of nasal, superior, and inferior poles in inverse proportion to disc diameter
- radial NFL without NFL tortuosity
- rare obscuration of a major vessel (usually upper pole)

Grade 1: (minimal)

- border obscuration – nasal
- elevation of borders – none (disc elevated)
- disruption of normal radial NFL arrangement with grayish opacity accentuating nerve fiber bundles
- temporal margin normal
- halo – subtle grayish with temporal gap (best seen with indirect ophthalmoscope)
- concentric or radial retinochoroidal folds

Grade 2: (mild)

- border obscuration – all (all of temporal)
- elevation – nasal border
- halo – complete

Grade 3: (moderate)

- border obscuration – all
- elevation – all borders
- increased diameter of nerve head
- obscuration of one or more segments of major blood vessels leaving disc
- halo – irregular outer fringe with finger-like extensions

Grade 4: (marked)

- elevation – whole nerve head
- border obscuration
- halo – irregular outer fringe with finger-like extensions
- total obscuration on the disc of a segment of a major blood vessel

Grade 5: (severe)

- dome-shaped protrusion (anterior expansion)
- halo – narrow and smoothly demarcated
- total obscuration of a segment of a major blood vessel may or may not be present
- obliteration of optic cup

Some findings are too variable to use; these include

- hyperemia
- vessel tortuosity
- hemorrhages
- exudates
- pallor
- cotton wool spots

Fig. 21.4 Papilledema grade system (Frisén scale).

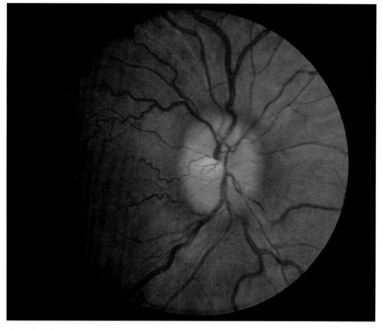

Fig. 21.5 An example of early (grade I) papilledema. Note the C-shaped halo of edema in the peripapillary region with a temporal gap.

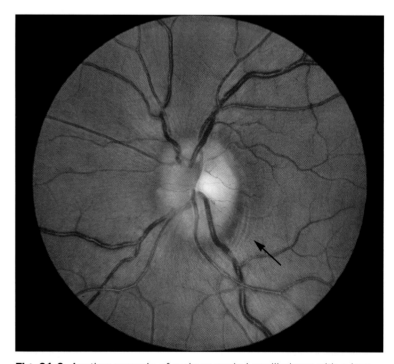

Fig. 21.6 Another example of early or grade I papilledema with a less prominent C-shaped halo. Notice also the circumferential retinochoroidal folds in the inferior-nasal quadrant ('Leslie Paton's lines')(see arrow). There is some coarsening of the nerve fiber layer seen in the inferior arcade.

papilledema, is characterized by obscuration of the vessel border 360° around the nerve, also called a full halo (of edema). It does not spare the temporal margin (*Fig. 21.7*). *Figure 21.8* is another example of Frisén grade 2 papilledema. Note how none of the major vessels is obscured by the edema. There is increased tortuosity of the retinal vasculature here; however, this is not a reliable sign of optic disc edema. The peripapillary NFL has become further opacified with grade 2 papilledema.

Figure 21.9 is an example of Frisén grade 3 papilledema. In addition to the circumferential halo, there is obscuration of major vessels as they leave the optic disc. *Figure 21.10* is another example of this grade of papilledema. Note the radial striae emanating from the disc margins.

In grade 3 papilledema, the central cup is usually obliterated (like vessel tortuosity, this is not a reliable sign of papilledema) whereas the major retinal vessels can be easily visualized on the disc. The dilated veins begin to disappear towards the periphery of the disc by undulating beneath the overlying swollen NFL

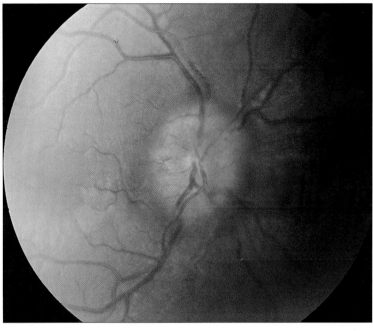

Fig. 21.7 Fully developed optic disc edema (Frisén grade 2) is present. Note the halo is now circumferential rather than C-shaped.

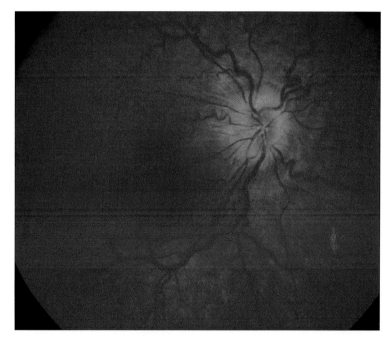

Fig. 21.8 An example of fully developed or grade 2 papilledema. Note the vessel tortuosity and the radial choroidal folds.

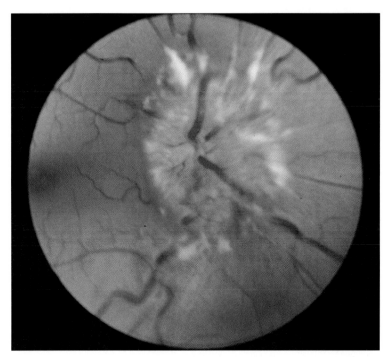

Fig. 21.9 An example of fully developed papilledema. In the Frisén classification this is grade 3 because of the major vessel obscuration as the vessels leave the disc inferiorly. Note also the fluffy white exudates (nerve-fiber layer infarcts, or cotton wool spots).

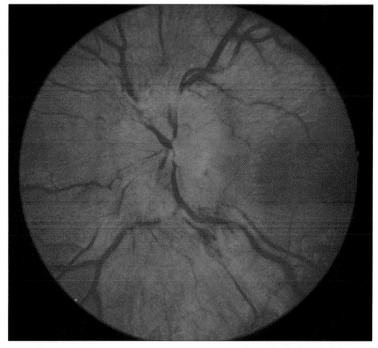

Fig. 21.10 Another example of grade 3 papilledema with a circumferential halo, coarsening of the NFL and vessel obscuration as it leaves the disc. Note the irregular outer fringe of the halo, characteristic of optic disc edema.

(Fig. 21.11). Although large nerve fiber infarctions (cotton wool spots) may obscure segments of the vasculature, this does not define the appearance of grade 3 papilledema; the NFL must be so edematous that it obscures the vessel.

In grade 4 papilledema *(Figs 21.12, 21.13)* there is total obscuration of a segment of a major branch vessel on the disc, usually with complete obliteration of the optic cup. Note the extensive dilated capillaries and microaneurysm formation involving the inferior substance of the swollen nerve in Figure 21.12. Figure 21.13 shows a less severe example of grade 4 papilledema with two peripapillary hemorrhages.

In grade 5 papilledema *(Fig. 21.14)*, anterior expansion of the optic nerve head dominates lateral expansion and the nerve head appears as a relatively smooth dome-shaped protrusion. Segments of major vessels may or may not be totally obscured by the overlying swollen tissue. Examples of findings in patients with raised intracranial pressure are given below.

Figure 21.15 shows a swollen optic nerve head (Frisén grade 2). Although the margins of the swollen nerve head are smooth and rounded in appearance, details of the optic disc rim are completely obliterated by edema. This patient was later found on neuro-imaging to have an extensive right frontal mass which on biopsy, proved to be an astrocytoma *(Fig. 21.16)*.

Papilledema is commonly due to idiopathic intracranial hypertension, also called pseudotumor cerebri. Among other causes this is a disorder of young, obese women in the child-bearing years who present with symptoms of increased intracranial pressure, often including

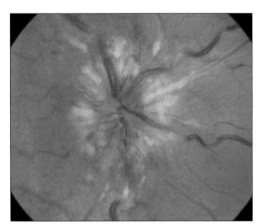

Fig. 21.11 Another example of grade 3 papilledema with vessel engorgement, tortuosity, and NFL infarcts. Note obliteration of the optic cup.

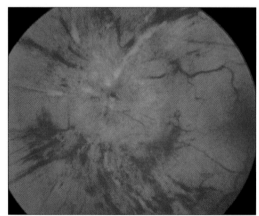

Fig. 21.12 An example of grade 4 (fully developed) papilledema. Not only are vessels obscured as they leave the disc but they are also obscured on the disc. The border of the disc is indistinct.

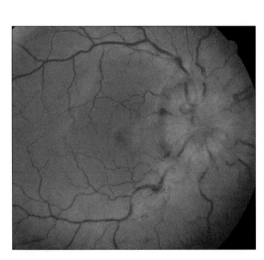

Fig. 21.13 A less severe example of grade 4 papilledema with major vessel obscuration on the disc. Note the circumferential choroidal folds and NFL thickening inferiorly and the flame-shaped hemorrhages in the peripapillary NFL.

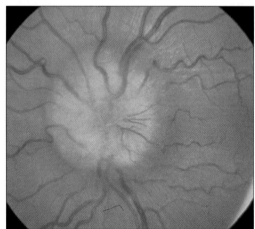

Fig. 21.14 An example of the dome-shaped protrusion of severe grade 5 papilledema.

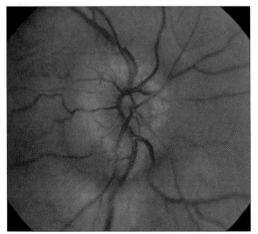

Fig. 21.15 Fully developed papilledema in a patient with a right frontal astrocytoma.

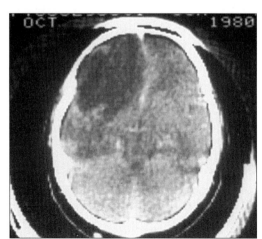

Fig. 21.16 MRI of the patient from Figure 20.15, showing the large right frontal astrocytoma.

chronic, unremitting headaches, pulse synchronous tinnitus, and transient visual obscurations. Despite the presence of papilledema, these patients show no evidence of structural pathology on neuro-imaging but typically show small slit like ventricles. *Figure 21.17* shows a patient with idiopathic intracranial hypertension who was monitored for many years. As she was treated for increased intracranial pressure (before the introduction of optic nerve sheath fenestration) her papilledema progressed from its early stages to chronic papilledema and later to optic atrophy.

In *Figure 21.17a*, the patient shows signs of early papilledema, with mild obscuration of the NFL at the optic disc margin and mild venous dilatation. Methods that have proved useful in evaluating 'early' papilledema include: ophthalmoscopy with a red-free filter, which allows better visualization of the NFL, and in addition, allows NFL hemorrhages to appear more prominent; ultrasonography, which is also useful to find buried optic disc drusen, which can create changes in the disc architecture that mimic papilledema; and fluorescein angiography, which may also be useful in evaluating leakage from dilated capillaries in acute early swelling of the disc. Baseline photographs should always be obtained in sequential examinations over time and may be necessary to distinguish papilledema from pseudo-papilledema.

In *Figure 21.17b*, the disc margin is obscured through 360° and the disc has become more elevated temporally. There is increased venous dilatation and tortuosity. In addition, there is increased prominence of the microvasculature of the disc substance, giving a hyperemic appearance to the disc. There is also a subretinal hemorrhage. This corresponds to Frisén grade 2 papilledema. Increased swelling is obliterating the optic disc cup and the previously radial NFL has become disrupted and feathery in appearance with subtle, jagged tongues of grayish NFL extending away from the disc. In *Figure 21.17c*, there is further swelling, complete obscuration, and elevation of the disc margin through 360°. A large subretinal hemorrhage is seen adjacent to the disc inferiorly.

This early papilledema (see Fig. 20.17a–c) progressed to fully developed papilledema. Four months later (*Fig. 21.17d*), at approximately the 5 o'clock position, subtle circumferential folds ('Paton's lines') can be seen

In *Figure 21.17f*, the edema has resolved after placement of a lumbar–subarachnoid peritoneal shunt. There is a circumferential ring of peripapillary atrophy and a 'high-water mark'. In addition, the area surrounding the optic nervewhere the NFL is thickest has lost the glossy sheen seen in a normal eye and has acquired a grainy, matte appearance due to loss of the NFL and optic atrophy. This gives the fundus a 'beached kelp' appearance as the arteries and veins appear to lie limply on the surface of the retina. Nine years later (*Fig. 21.17g*), frank optic atrophy is present.

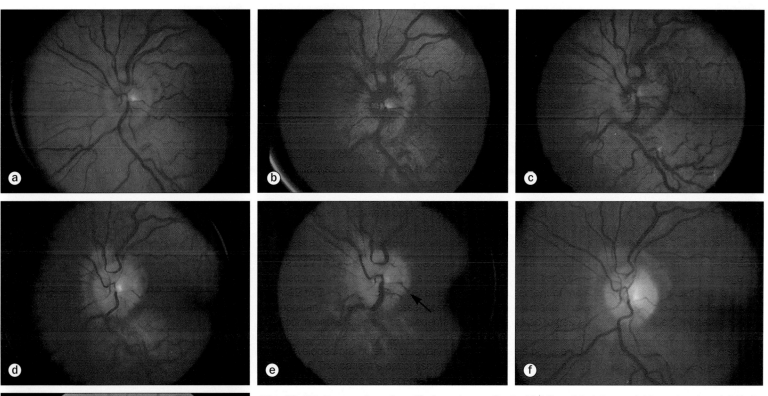

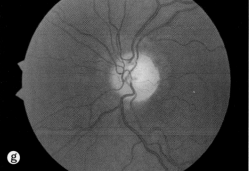

Fig. 21.17 Progression of papilledema in a patient with idiopathic intracranial hypertension. (**a**) Early papilledema. (**b**) The patient has developed grade 2 papilledema. Note the subretinal hemorrhage from 12 to 3 o'clock. (**c**) Further swelling and enlargement of the subretinal hemorrhage in the peripapillary space. Major vessel obscuration inferiorly marks this as Frisén grade 3 papilledema. (**d**) Four months later the papilledema in this patient has regressed to Frisén grade 2. Note the feathery circumferential halo and subtle retinochoroidal folds at around 5 o'clock. (**e**) The patient has now developed prominent optociliary collateral vessels between 3 and 4 o'clock on the optic disc (arrow). (**f**) The patient's optic disc after a lumbar–subarachnoid peritoneal shunt. Notice the marked defervescence of the disc edema with peripapillary pigmentation. (**g**) At a later stage with post-papilledema optic atrophy.

OPTOCILIARY COLLATERAL VESSELS

In Figure 21.17d, and more prominently in *Figure 21.17e*, another sign of chronicity, optociliary collateral vessels, has evolved. When optic discs are swollen for a long time, chronic obstruction of central retinal venous drainage causes collateral circulatory connections to open between the central retinal veins and the choroidal circulation (ciliary circulation), providing alternative drainage of venous blood via the vortex veins. These vessels are called optociliary collaterals. *Figure 21.18* shows a huge optociliary collateral in an atrophic disc that is chronically choked due to an optic nerve sheath meningioma. *Figure 21.19* shows optociliary collaterals in chronic papilledema due to an intracranial tumor.

PSEUDO-DRUSEN

With chronic optic disc swelling, superficial hard exudate residue may develop on the surface of the disc and may simulate optic disc drusen. These are termed pseudo-drusen (*Fig. 21.10;* see also Figs 20.15, 20.19). Optic nerve drusen are discussed in detail in chapter 18.

CHOROIDAL FOLDS

Various ophthalmoscopic findings can be associated with papilledema. Retinal and choroidal folds are commonly observed. *Figure 21.21* shows a complex pattern of retinal folds which, near

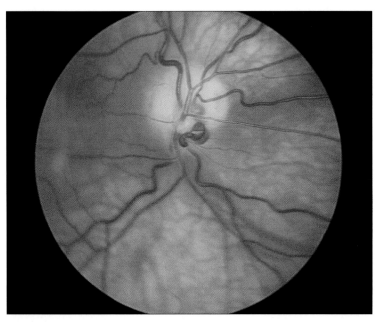

Fig. 21.18 A patient with a huge optociliary collateral vessel at 5 o'clock in a chronically edematous disc due to an optic nerve sheath meningioma.

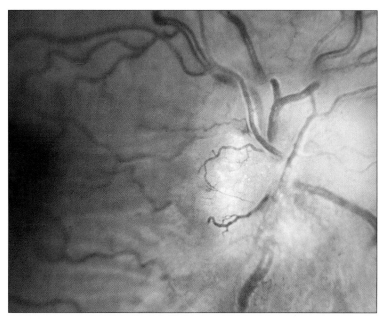

Fig. 21.19 At least three large optociliary collateral vessels in another patient with papilledema from an intracranial tumor.

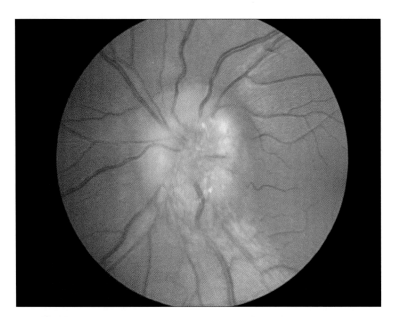

Fig. 21.20 Small 'pseudo-drusen' over the surface of the disc in a patient with chronic papilledema.

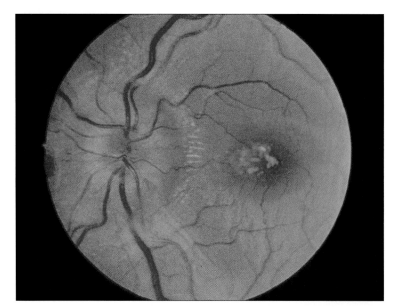

Fig. 21.21 A patient with idiopathic intracranial hypertension has radial choroidal folds and a hemimacular star with grade 2 papilledema. Circumferential folds are present superonasally.

the disc, appear circumferential but in the papillomacular bundle become radial and extend toward the fovea. Retinal pigment epithelial changes in the macula, due to the optic disc edema, are present. *Figures 21.22* (and see Fig. 21.8 – same patient) shows deeper choroidal folds, extending radially, and crossing through the center of the macula.

Circumferential folds or wrinkles called Paton's lines (see Fig. 21.6) form in the retina as it is pushed away from the optic disc. They are found in 30% of pathologically examined papilledematous discs. Horizontal or oblique linear folds in the retina can also be seen and horizontal folds in the choroid may not be visible but can be seen on fluorescein angiography. These may persist after papilledema has resolved.

EXUDATES

Different forms of exudates may be seen in association with papilledema. *Figures 21.23* (and Fig. 21.11) shows exudates that appear as white patches on the disc surface and represent infarcts in the NFL. Incomplete macular star figures with hard exudates in the macula may also be observed tracking along the course of the papillomacular bundle, as seen in *Figures 21.24a* (and Fig. 21.21). Macular stars are also seen in neuroretinitis, but visual loss is much more prominent in such patients because the retinitis produces cystic macular edema. After resolution of the papilledema, and of these exudates, retinal pigment epithelial changes involving the macula may persist, as seen in *Figure 21.24b*, and may result in visual loss.

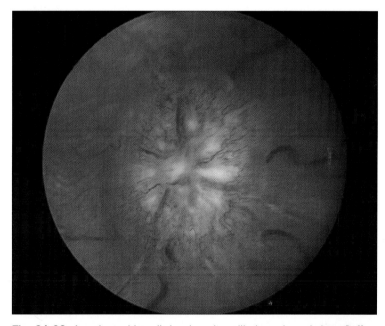

Fig. 21.22 Larger deeper chorioretinal folds extending radially across the macula in the same patient as Figure 21.19.

Fig. 21.23 A patient with well-developed papilledema has obvious fluffy white exudates on the disc.

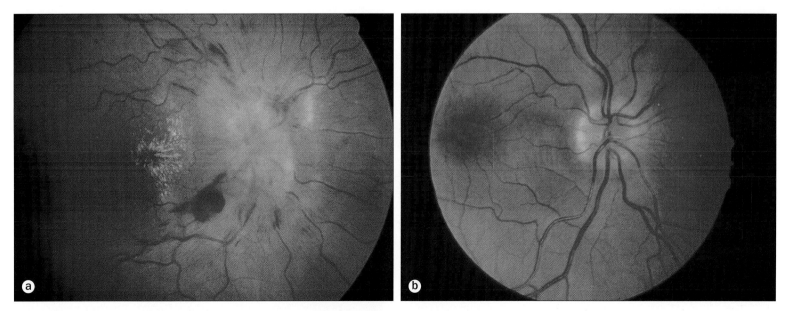

Fig. 21.24 (**a**) An incomplete macular star made up of hard exudates. (**b**) After the papilledema has resolved, macular retinal pigment epithelial changes persist. These are not the same two discs.

NEUROSENSORY RETINAL DETACHMENTS

In severe, fully developed papilledema, extensive neurosensory retinal detachments may be observed (see Fig. 21.24a). This figure also shows an incomplete macular star figure and edema of the papillomacular bundle, as well as a pre-retinal hemorrhage and numerous splinter hemorrhages.

HEMORRHAGES

Hemorrhages in almost all layers of the retina may be observed in association with papilledema. Blot-dot hemorrhages distant from the optic nerve head can be found; see *Figure 21.25*. They are thought to represent mild venous stasis retinopathy due to retinal venous congestion caused by the papilledema. The patient in

Figure 21.26 shows both an extensive subretinal peripapillary hemorrhage and a blot-dot hemorrhage distant from the disc.

Pre-retinal and vitreous hemorrhages may also be observed (*Figs 21.27, 21.28*) and are probably due to rupture of dilated capillaries on the optic disc surface. Vitreous hemorrhages in association with papilledema can also be seen in Terson's syndrome, in which a subarachnoid hemorrhage rapidly increases intracranial pressure, causing rapid onset of papilledema and extensive hemorrhage anterior to the retina and forward dissection into the vitreous.

A large peripapillary subretinal hemorrhage is seen in *Figure 21.29*; a more commonly seen smaller example is shown in *Figure 21.30*. This type of subretinal hemorrhage may be seen in congenitally elevated optic or tilted optic discs. *Figures 21.31* and *21.32* show splinter hemorrhages and peripapillary flame-shaped hemorrhages with a hemimacular star. Flame-shaped hemorrhages are also seen in *Figure 21.33*.

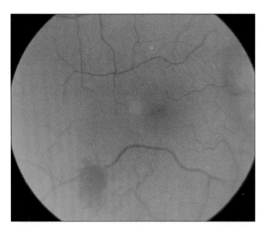

Fig. 21.25 A blot hemorrhage in a patient with papilledema due to idiopathic intracranial hypertension.

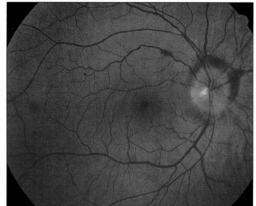

Fig. 21.26 A patient with grade 1 papilledema due to idiopathic intracranial hypertension has blot hemorrhages in the periphery along with some dot hemorrhages further out in the periphery and has a large peripapillary subretinal hemorrhage.

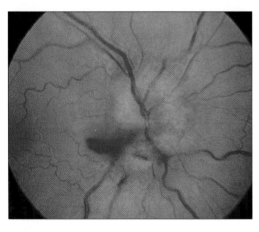

Fig. 21.27 Pre-retinal hemorrhage in a patient with high-grade papilledema.

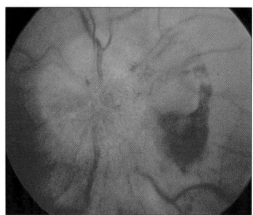

Fig. 21.28 Pre-retinal hemorrhage in a patient with chronic high-grade papilledema.

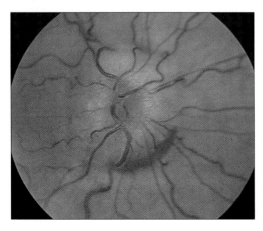

Fig. 21.29 Patient with grade 3 papilledema with a crescent-shaped inferior subretinal hemorrhage (same patient as Figure 20.33).

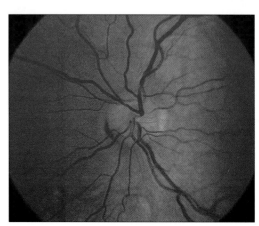

Fig. 21.30 A smaller subretinal hemorrhage is seen in this patient with early papilledema due to idiopathic intracranial hypertension. Occasionally, this type of subretinal hemorrhage is seen in patients with anomalous optic nerve heads.

Figure 21.34 shows fundus photos and fluorescein angiograms of a patient with idiopathic intracranial hypertension. There is bilateral disc swelling, complicated in both eyes by subretinal neovascular hemorrhages and peripapillary retinal detachments. Various types of hemorrhages are seen in a trumpet player with papilledema (*Fig. 21.35*).

ASYMMETRIC PAPILLEDEMA

Papilledema is usually bilateral and symmetrical; however, unilateral or highly asymmetric papilledema has been well documented (*Fig. 21.36*), occurring in about 10% of patients with papilledema. Patients may present with signs and symptoms in

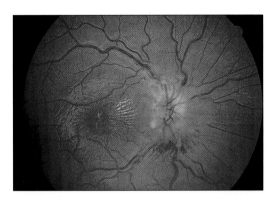

Fig. 21.31 Patient with chronic grade 2 papilledema with flame-shaped peripapillary hemorrhages and a hemimacular star.

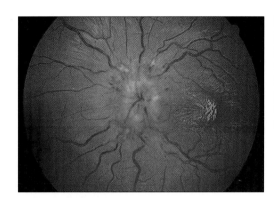

Fig. 21.32 Same patient as Figure 21.28, with macular exudates in a star formation, peripapillary flame-shaped hemorrhages, and NFL infarcts.

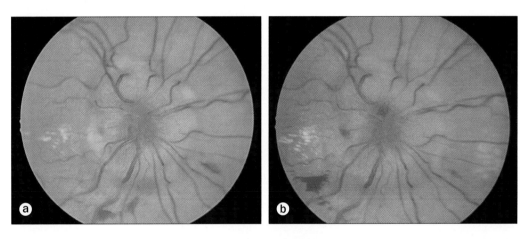

Fig. 21.33 (**a**) Chronic papilledema with marked enlargement of the optic nerve. (**b**) Findings in the same eye a year later (same patient as Figure 21.29).

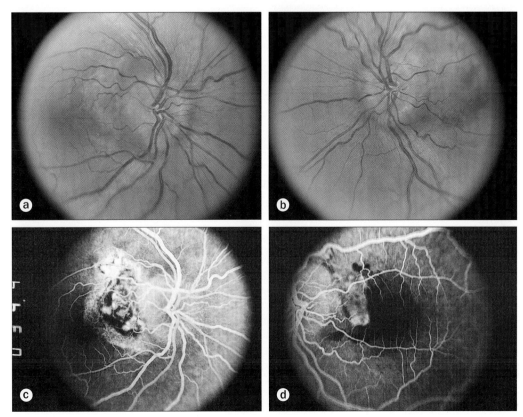

Fig. 21.34 (**a**) to (**d**) A patient with idiopathic intracranial hypertension with subretinal neovascular hemorrhages and peripapillary retinal detachments, also seen on the accompanying fluorescein angiogram. (Courtesy of WF Hoyt)

only one eye but careful observation of the asymptomatic eye usually reveals evidence of mild papilledema, as evidenced by slight elevation of the disc. This disc elevation is the first sign of papilledema, as reported by Hayreh in experimental papilledema in monkeys. However, the sign is not specific enough to be clinically useful. Nevertheless, the finding of unilateral papilledema can cause significant diagnostic confusion, committing patients to extensive, unnecessary work-ups.

ISCHEMIC DAMAGE AND OPTIC ATROPHY

Papilledema may be complicated by ischemia of the optic disc, resulting in sudden, permanent visual loss that may be complete (*Fig. 21.37a*) or segmental. *Figure 21.37b* shows the same patient's optic disc 4 months later. Unfortunately, despite treatment, some patients develop severe visual loss with post-papilledema optic atrophy (*Fig. 21.38*).

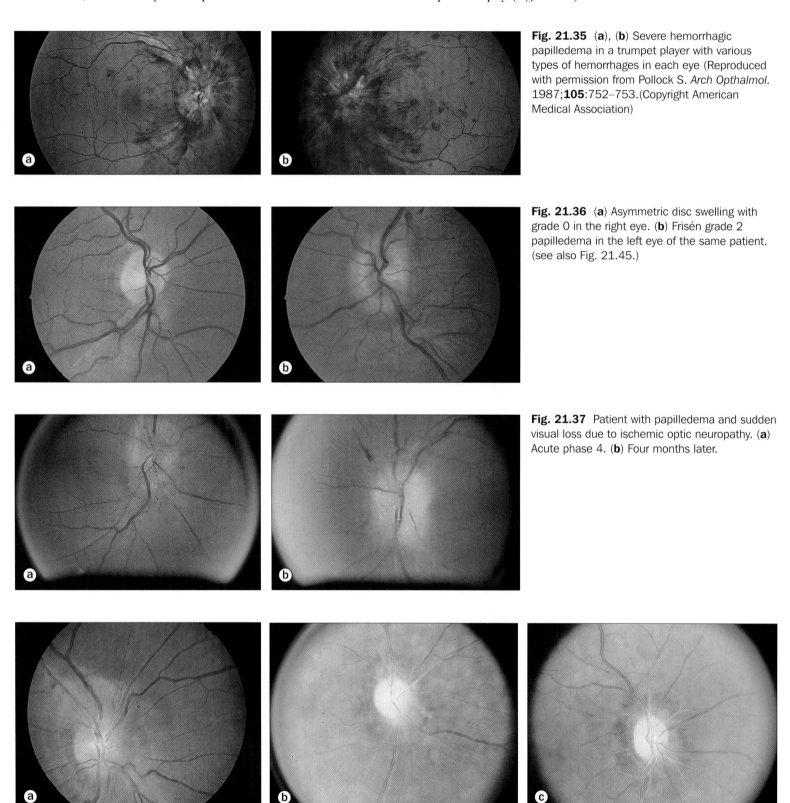

Fig. 21.35 (**a**), (**b**) Severe hemorrhagic papilledema in a trumpet player with various types of hemorrhages in each eye (Reproduced with permission from Pollock S. *Arch Opthalmol.* 1987;**105**:752–753.(Copyright American Medical Association)

Fig. 21.36 (**a**) Asymmetric disc swelling with grade 0 in the right eye. (**b**) Frisén grade 2 papilledema in the left eye of the same patient. (see also Fig. 21.45.)

Fig. 21.37 Patient with papilledema and sudden visual loss due to ischemic optic neuropathy. (**a**) Acute phase 4. (**b**) Four months later.

Fig. 21.38 Examples of post-papilledema optic atrophy. Note the series of 'high water marks' (intraretinal lipoprotein deposits) in (**a**) and the retinal pigment epithelial changes surrounding the disc in (**b**) and (**c**), along with the gliotic changes and ghosting of vessels.

OTHER CAUSES OF OPTIC DISC EDEMA

Optic disc edema that is indistinguishable from papilledema can be caused by many other conditions. Optic disc swelling due to low intraocular pressure after the removal of a cataract in the left eye is shown in *Figures 21.39* and *21.40*. Inflammation of the sclera at the back of the globe (posterior scleritis) may cause crowding of the axons as they pass through the lamina cribrosa and disc swelling. Pain on eye movement, diplopia due to swelling of muscle insertions on the globe (*Fig. 21.41*), and disc swelling (*Figs 21.42, 21.43*) are characteristic of scleritis, although all features need not be present. Optic disc swelling occurs in about 30% of patients with acute optic neuritis. *Figure 21.44a* and *b* shows the acute disc swelling and the

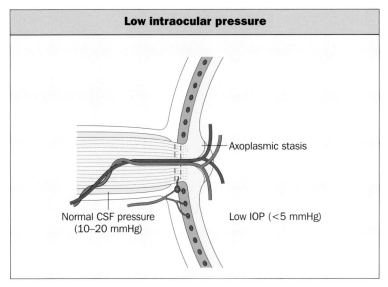

Fig. 21.39 When the intraocular pressure is low, the axoplasmic flow faces a difficult pressure gradient even when the CSF pressure is normal.

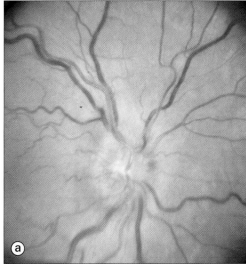

Fig. 21.40 (a) Optic disc edema secondary to hypotony after a cataract extraction. (b) The normal fellow eye of the patient.

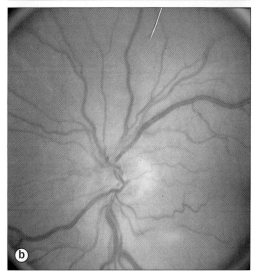

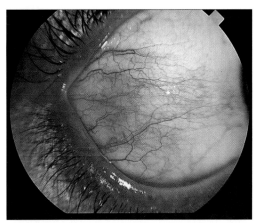

Fig. 21.41 Injection of the conjunctiva adjacent to muscle insertion and scleritis in a patient with posterior scleritis.

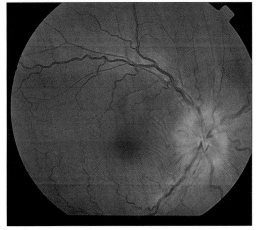

Fig. 21.42 Optic disc edema in a patient with posterior scleritis.

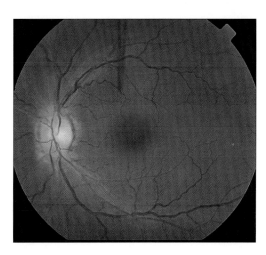

Fig. 21.43 Normal optic disc in the other eye of the patient with scleritis.

pallor of the tempopral disc after the swelling resolves, and the associated loss of the NFL. Note the clarity with which choroidal pigment and vessels are seen (see Fig. 20.44b) compared with the unaffected eye (*Fig. 21.44c*). Optic disc edema that appears pale in a blind eye is characteristic of giant cell arteritis (*Fig. 21.45*). Nonarteritic anterior ischemic optic neuropathy is another common cause of optic disc edema (*Fig. 21.37*).

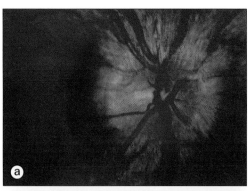

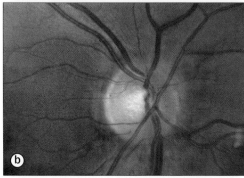

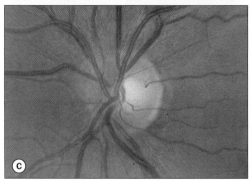

Fig. 21.44 (**a**) Optic disc edema in a patient with optic neuritis. (**b**) Resolved optic neuritis in the same patient. Note the temporal disc pallor. (**c**) The fellow (unaffected) eye for comparison.

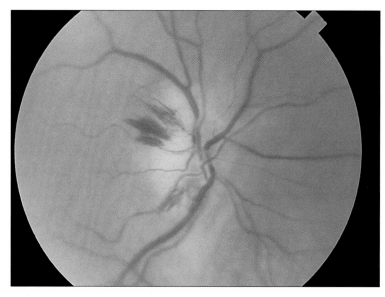

Fig. 21.45 Pale optic disc swelling with flame-shaped peripapillary hemorrhages in a patient with giant cell arteritis. The acute pale disc swelling is characteristic for this disorder.

Further reading

Akova YA, Kansu T, Yazar Z, *et al*. Macular subretinal neovascular membrane associated with pseudotumor cerebri. *J Neuro-ophthalmol.* 1994;**14**:193–195.

Bird AC, Sanders MD. Choroidal folds in association with papilloedema. *Br J Ophthalmol.* 1973;**57**:89–97.

Carter SR, Seiff SR. Macular changes in pseudotumor cerebri before and after optic nerve sheath fenestration. *Ophthalmology.* 1995;**102**:937–941.

Coppeto JR, Monteiro ML. Juxtapapillary subretinal hemorrhages in pseudotumor cerebri. *J Clin Neuro-ophthalmol.* 1985;**5**:45–53.

Frisén L. Swelling of the optic nerve head: a staging scheme. *J Neurol Neurosurg Psychiatry.* 1982;**45**:13–18.

Green GJ, Lessell S, Loewenstein JI. Ischemic optic neuropathy in chronic papilledema. *Arch Ophthalmol.* 1980;**98**:502–504.

Hayreh SS. Optic disc edema in raised intracranial pressure V. Pathogenesis. *Arch Ophthalmol.* 1977;**95**:1553–1565.

Morris AT, Sanders MD. Macular changes resulting from papilloedema. *Br J Ophthalmol.* 1980;**64**:211–216.

Tso MOM, Hayreh SS. Optic disc edema in raised intracranial pressure III. A pathologic study of experimental papilledema. *Arch Ophthalmol.* 1977;**95**:1448–1457.

Tso MOM, Hayreh SS. Optic disc edema in raised intracranial pressure IV. Axoplasmic transport in experimental papilledema. *Arch Ophthalmol.* 1977;**95**:1458–1562.

CHAPTER 22

Migraine, Tension-type Headache, and Cluster Headache

Patricia Johnston McNussen

INTRODUCTION

Headache, in its various forms, affects most of humanity. It crosses all boundaries, affecting the wealthy and the poor, the urban and the rural, male and female. Headache can strike any ethnic group, at any age. It does not respect occupation or social class. Once considered a psychologic problem by many (including the medical profession), headache has emerged as a serious health problem in recent years and is being given the attention it deserves. The tremendous cost to the individual and to society is finally being recognized. Extensive research into the pathophysiology and treatment of headache is bringing new insight and new hope to the headache sufferer and the healthcare provider (*Fig. 22.1*).

The most recent headache classification and criteria for diagnosis were published by the International Headache Society in 1988. The terminology used in this chapter is from that classification.

MIGRAINE

Descriptions of migraine date back to writings of the ancient world. The term migraine is derived from the Latin word hemicrania, which comes from the Greek hemikrania, meaning half of the skull. Many famous people throughout the ages have been afflicted. Prominent sufferers include Queen Mary Tudor of England, Friedrich Nietzsche, Immanuel Kant, Thomas Jefferson, Ulysses S Grant, Sigmund Freud, Charles Darwin, Alexander Pope, Edgar Allan Poe, Leo Tolstoi, Virginia Woolf, Frederic Chopin, Peter Ilich Tchaikovsky, John Calvin, Karl Marx, Alfred Nobel, and Mary Todd Lincoln.

Estimates of the prevalence of migraine vary widely. In adults, women are affected more than men, with 20–30% of women having migraine and 5–15% of men. In children before puberty, headache incidence is equal between the two sexes.

There does appear to be a hereditary factor in migraine, although the specific genetics and inheritance patterns are not clear. Environmental factors are also important and are discussed later.

Migraine is a complicated entity. It is true that the typical

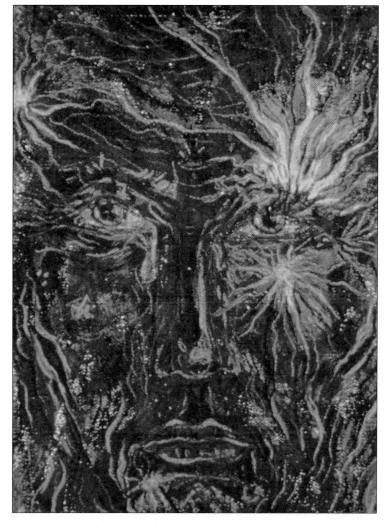

Fig. 22.1 Now that headache is being recognized as a major health problem, there is a great interest in headache art. Healthcare providers can gain tremendous insight into the suffering of their headache patients by looking at these pictures. (*Self Portrait* by Nan Quintin, from the *Through the Looking Glass* Headache Art Exhibition, courtesy of Sandoz Pharmaceuticals Corporation)

migraine headache is a unilateral throbbing pain, associated with nausea, vomiting, photophobia and, at times, other neurologic symptoms. However, that definition does not encompass the wide variety of the symptoms and signs of migraine.

MIGRAINE WITH AURA

Migraine with aura, formerly called classic migraine, refers to a migraine headache with associated neurologic symptoms. Visual disturbances are the most common type of aura and may be dramatic. Visual symptoms may be positive, negative, or a combination of the two. A fortification spectrum, or teichopsia, is a scotoma surrounded by a jagged edge that often starts as a small spot and progressively enlarges (*Fig. 22.2*). Fortification refers to the angulated, star-shaped edges that resemble a fortified city (*Figs 22.3 and 22.4*). The jagged edges often shimmer, giving rise to the term scintillating scotoma (*Fig. 22.5*). The fortified scotoma may also 'march' from the paracentral field to the temporal field. This type of disturbance is the most characteristic of the visual auras and generally lasts 20–30 min.

Many patients see flashing lights that resemble lightning bolts; some see spots or blotches (*Fig. 22.6*). Others describe wavy vision 'like heat waves off a pavement' or 'water running down a window pane'. At times the vision may just be blurry or difficult to focus. Complex visual hallucinations and palinopsia are rare but do occur. Another unusual visual disturbance is mosaic vision, where the visual image breaks up into geometric pieces (*Fig. 22.7*).

The positive visual symptoms of a migraine aura may be bright white, silver, or brilliantly multicolored. However, some patients have only negative visual symptoms, such as scotomata, homonymous hemianopsias, or quadrant defects. Diplopia may also occur (*Fig. 22.8*).

It must be remembered that, although the bizarre visual symptoms are fascinating to the physician, the distortions are often terrifying to the patient. Some people are reluctant to discuss their visual disturbances, fearful they will be considered to have a psychiatric problem. Gentle questioning and listening on the part of the examiner will often allow such patients fully to describe what they see (or do not see). Encouraging the patient to draw the aura may also be helpful (see Fig. 22.5).

RETINAL OR OCULAR MIGRAINE

Most visual auras are binocular and originate in the cerebral cortex. However, monocular visual symptoms do occur, with loss of vision more common than flashes of light. Termed retinal migraine, these events would more appropriately be called ocular migraine, because they can involve either the retinal or ciliary circulation. Permanent visual loss can occur due to central or branch retinal artery occlusion, central retinal vein occlusion, or ischemic optic neuropathy.

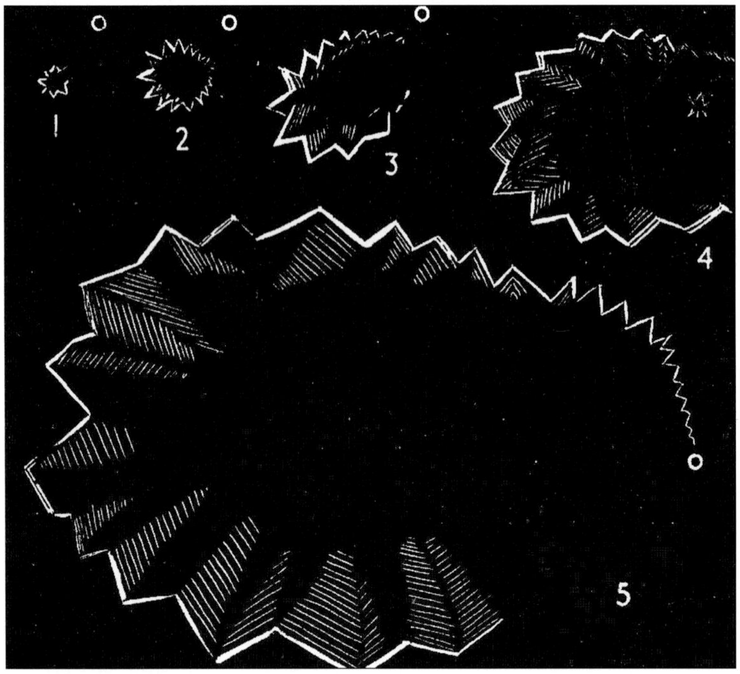

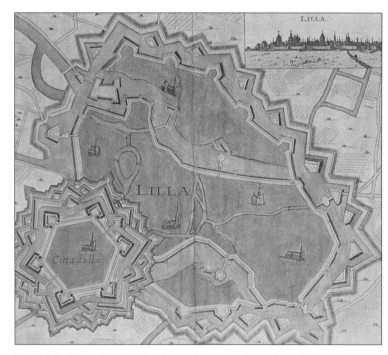

Fig. 22.2 Migraine aura. Fortification spectra showing progressive enlargement in 5 stages. Fixation is indicated by O. (Hubert Airey, 1870)

Fig. 22.3 Plan of the fortifications of the city of Lille, from Galeazzo Gualdo Priorato's *Teatro del Belgio*, 1673. (Courtesy of Dr Richard Peatfield, published in Peatfield R. *Headache*. [Dorchester: Springer–Verlag, 1986])

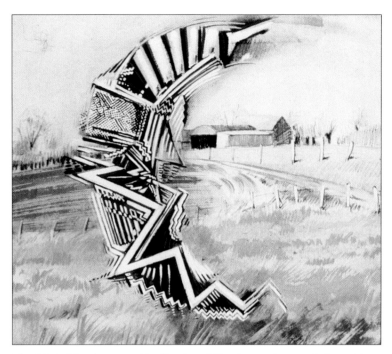

Fig. 22.4 Migraine aura. Fortification. (Migraine art by permission of the British Migraine Association and Boehringer Ingelheim)

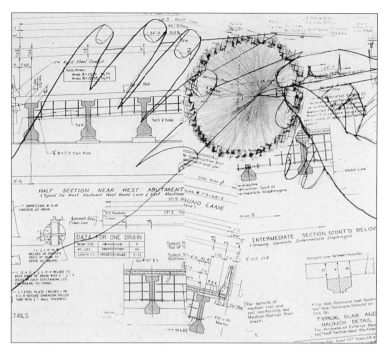

Fig. 22.5 Migraine aura. Scintillating scotoma drawn by a draftsman who developed the visual symptoms at work. (Courtesy of Dr H Stanley Thompson)

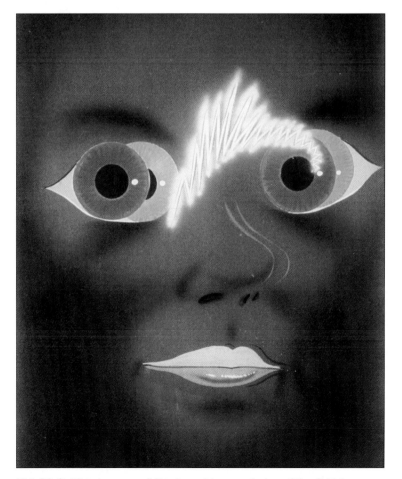

Fig. 22.6 Migraine aura. (Migraine art by permission of the British Migraine Association and Boehringer Ingelheim)

OTHER AURAS

In addition to visual auras some patients from the visual aura go on to develop paresthesia down the side of the face, the side of the tongue, and the ipsilateral arm and hand, which may be associated with aphasia. This is known as cherio-oral aura. In basilar migraine the patient may develop either positive or negative symptomatology in one or other or both hemifields, which then progresses to vertigo, tinnitus with impaired hearing, dysarthria, and ataxia, the whole episode lasting about 15–30 minutes. This is the only form of migraine which can be associated with an alteration in consciousness.

MIGRAINE AURA WITHOUT HEADACHE

Often referred to as acephalgic migraine or migraine equivalents, migraine aura without headache consists of the neurologic disturbances of aura but without any pain. Once again, visual phenomena are most commonly reported but any neurologic symptoms can occur. Although migraine aura without headache may occur at any age, it is most common above the age of 40 years. The majority of patients are aged between 50 and 70 years, hence the term 'late-life migrainous accompaniments' that has also been used. The major task in these patients is to rule out transient ischemic attacks, which are common in this age group.

OPHTHALMOPLEGIC MIGRAINE

A rare entity, ophthalmoplegic migraine consists of a migraine headache, followed by ophthalmoplegia. The third cranial nerve is

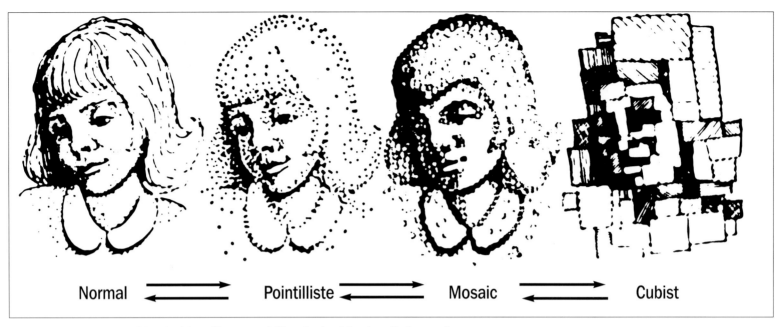

Fig. 22.7 Migraine aura. Mosaic vision. (Courtesy of Oliver Sacks. *Migraine: Understanding a Common Disorder*. Expanded and updated edition. [Berkeley: University of California Press, 1993])

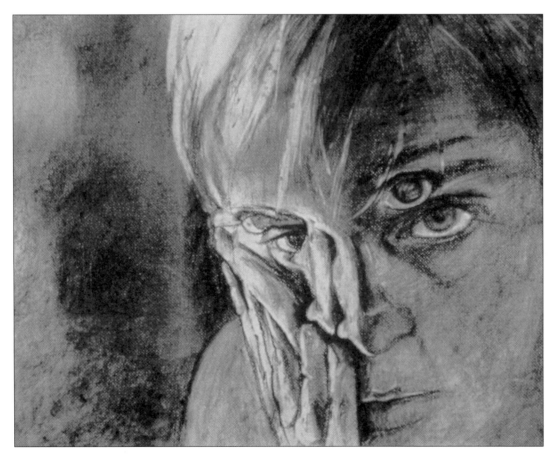

Fig. 22.8 Migraine aura. Diplopia. (*Through a Glass Darkly* by Janet Morgan Mol, from the *Through the Looking Glass* Headache Art Exhibition, courtesy of Sandoz Pharmaceuticals Corporation)

most frequently affected and the pupil is often dilated. Involvement of the sixth cranial nerve is less common, with the fourth cranial nerve being the least likely to be affected. The ophthalmoplegia usually resolves within several days but permanent paresis may occur. More common in children, it is unusual enough at any age to warrant further investigation. Diagnostic considerations include aneurysm, tumor, pituitary apoplexy, Tolosa–Hunt syndrome, cavernous sinus thrombosis, and diabetic ophthalmoparesis.

PUPILLARY DISTURBANCES

Both the sympathetic and parasympathetic innervation of the pupil can be involved in migraine. Mydriasis is usually associated with other signs of third cranial nerve involvement. Isolated mydriasis with migraine has been reported. Horner's syndrome with ptosis and miosis is often seen in cluster headache (see below) but is occasionally found in migraine patients. The 'tadpole pupil' is a segmental pupil enlargement that may be due to spasm of part of the pupil dilator muscle and may be seen in migraineurs.

MIGRAINE WITHOUT AURA

Previously referred to as common migraine, this condition is much more frequent than migraine with aura, accounting for approximately 85% of all migraine attacks. It consists of headache, and nausea or vomiting or both, and light and sound sensitivity (*Figs 22.9–22.11*).

Typically, the pain is unilateral (*Fig. 22.12*) but it can also be frontal, bitemporal, occipital, or on the vertex of the head (*Fig. 22.13*). The throbbing or pulsatile nature of the pain is usually present when the pain is severe. However, when mild, the pain may be a dull ache. Some patients complain of sharp pain or a pressure sensation, rather than throbbing (*Fig. 22.14*). The pain is often exacerbated by physical activity, such as climbing stairs.

Tenderness of the head and neck muscles is common and may be severe. Before a migraine attack (either with or without aura), there may be premonitory symptoms such as depression, euphoria, drowsiness, or cravings for certain foods. These symptoms should not be confused with an aura.

MIGRAINE PATHOPHYSIOLOGY

The mechanism of migraine was once thought to be relatively simple, with vasoconstriction causing the aura and vasodilatation causing the pain. This led to the term 'vascular headache' being introduced and used synonymously with migraine. Recently, however, extensive research has shown that migraine is much more complex. The changes in the cranial vasculature are very important but they are only one part of a much larger scheme and a multitude of events. The exact biology of migraine is still not fully understood but the pieces of the puzzle are beginning to come together.

Pathogenesis of the Aura

Both neuronal and vascular changes seem to be important in the aura of migraine. In animal brains, the phenomenon of spreading depression can be observed. This consists of neuronal activation, followed by suppression of the neurons and a shut-down of cortical activity. According to Leão this process spreads out across the cortex like a slow wave, at approximately 3 mm/min. According to Lashley this is about the speed of typical fortification spectra. Although this spreading depression of Leão has not been clearly

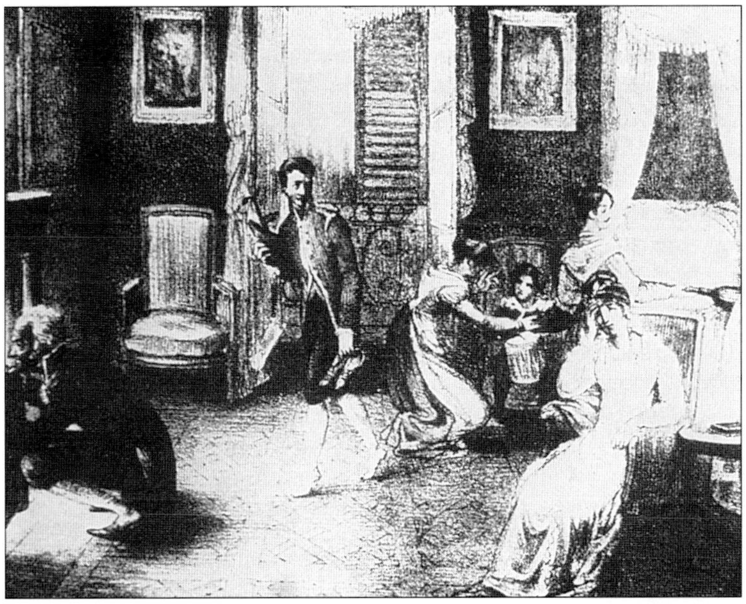

![La Migraine by Charles Aubry]

Fig. 22.9 *La Migraine* by Charles Aubry. This 19th-century French drawing shows a family creating a dark, quiet atmosphere to soothe the light and sound sensitivity of a migraine sufferer. (Courtesy of National Library of Medicine, Bethesda, Maryland)

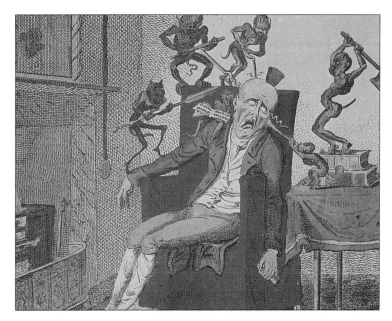

Fig. 22.10 *The Headache* by George Cruikshank (1792–1878). In this etching, the patient is tormented by demons inflicting pain and bombarding his sensitive ears with raucous noise. (Courtesy of Jean Loup Charmet, Paris, France)

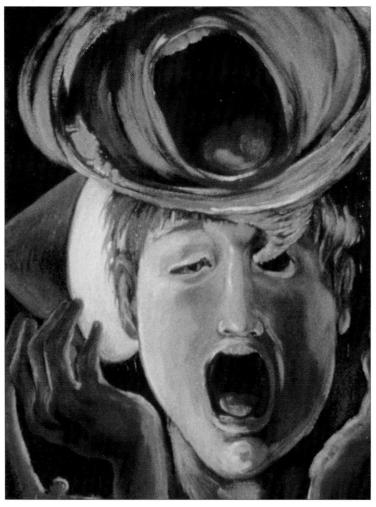

Fig. 22.11 Extreme photophobia is common with migraine. (*Roger Reacts to the Light* by Christine Lamb-Toubeau, from the *Through the Looking Glass* Headache Art Exhibition, courtesy of Sandoz Pharmaceuticals Corporation)

shown in humans, evidence supporting the theory has come from magnetoencephalography and MR spectroscopy.

In addition to the neuronal activity, changes in cerebral blood flow occur. There is a spreading oligemia, with cerebral blood flow dropping to ischemic levels in some areas. Neurologic symptoms may then appear. It is important to note that changes in cerebral blood flow have not been found in migraine without aura.

Headache Pathogenesis

As with migraine aura, current research indicates that both vascular and neuronal events are important in the pain of migraine. The locus ceruleus in the pons is the origin of the noradrenergic pain-control system. Ascending fibers innervate the brain's microcirculation and also project to the cerebral cortex. Descending fibers go to the spinal cord. The serotonergic system from the midbrain raphe is also involved. This system affects both intracranial and extracranial blood vessels and has connections to the thalamus, hypothalamus, and cerebral cortex. The descending serotonergic system originates in the midbrain periaqueductal gray matter, runs to the raphe magnus in the medulla, and then terminates in the spinal cord. These fibers are involved in pain regulation. Most of the medications used in migraine have effects on the serotonergic system.

In addition to these systems, the trigeminal nerve appears to play a large role in headache. The trigeminal nerve innervates the blood vessels of the pia mater and dura mater. Stimulation of the trigeminovascular system results in the release of vasoactive neuropeptides (substance P, neurokinin A, and calcitonin gene-related peptide). These chemical agents then interact with the blood vessel wall, resulting in vasodilatation, plasma protein extravasation, and sterile inflammation. This neurogenic inflammation may be responsible for the pain of a migraine headache.

Other changes that occur in migraine include platelet activation and aggregation, a decrease in platelet serotonin (5-hydroxytryptamine or 5-HT), an increase in urinary 5-HT and its major

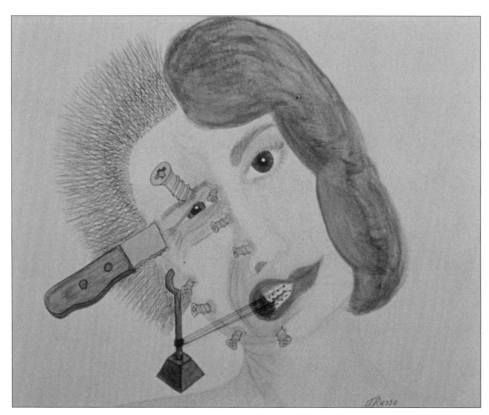

Fig. 22.12 The violent and violating intensity of a unilateral hemicrania is expressed in this painting. (*Pernicious Assault* by Terri Russo, from the *Through the Looking Glass* Headache Art Exhibition, courtesy of Sandoz Pharmaceuticals Corporation)

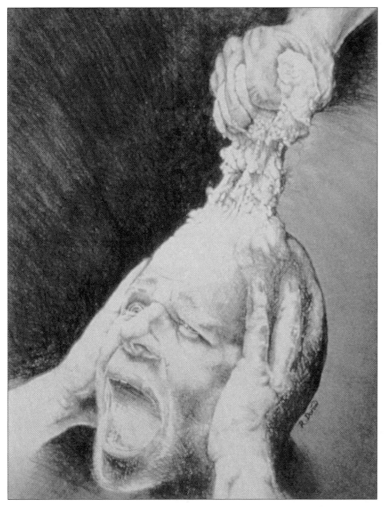

Fig. 22.13 The pain of migraine may be variable in location and is not always unilateral. (*Gripping Headache* by Raymond Dorow II, from the *Through the Looking Glass* Headache Art Exhibition, courtesy of Sandoz Pharmaceuticals Corporation)

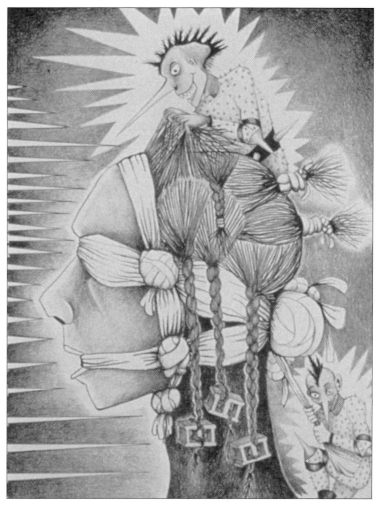

Fig. 22.14 Although throbbing pain is typical in a migraine headache, the pain can also be very sharp and stabbing as illustrated here. (*Fiorinal Calls* by Val Akula, from the *Through the Looking Glass* Headache Art Exhibition, courtesy of Sandoz Pharmaceuticals Corporation)

metabolite 5-hydroxyindoleacetic acid (5-HIAA), and an increase in free 5-HT in the plasma.

TRIGGERS OF MIGRAINE

It is not known why some people are prone to migraine and others are not. It may be that a migraineur's pain control system is defective, so that a certain stimulus, innocuous to most people, triggers the complicated events involved in migraine.

Many of the triggers for headache are listed in *Figure 22.15*. These factors can affect the cerebral cortex, thalamus, hypothalamus, or both internal and external carotid circulations, resulting in migraine.

EVALUATION OF THE MIGRAINE PATIENT

There are several questions the physician must consider. Is this a typical migraine? Is there an underlying medical condition that is triggering the migraine? Is there something present that is mimicking migraine?

A detailed history of the symptoms is mandatory. This should

be followed by a medical history, medication and allergy history, family and social history, and headache triggers. A general physical and neurologic examination should be carried out with all patients, with a thorough neuro-ophthalmic examination for patients with visual or ocular symptoms.

If the results of the examination are normal and the history is consistent with typical migraine, further work-up may not be needed. However, any abnormalities on examination or atypical features in the history should be investigated further. CT or MRI is necessary to exclude mass lesions, cerebral hemorrhage, and stroke. If subarachnoid hemorrhage is suspected, CT, followed by a lumbar puncture if the CT is normal, is indicated. Cerebral angiography may also be needed. Electroencephalography (EEG) is used if there is any history of coincident seizure. Other tests that are appropriate in certain situations include carotid ultrasound and echocardiography. Laboratory evaluation may include complete blood count with differential, chemistry profile, coagulation studies, erythrocyte sedimentation rate, antinuclear antibody titer, rheumatoid factor, and thyroid studies.

It is important to remember that migraine is a clinical diagnosis. There is no substitute for a careful history and physical examination. Any further work-up must be tailored to the individual patient based on the symptoms and clinical signs.

TREATMENT OF MIGRAINE

The first step in treatment is patient education. Identification and avoidance of headache triggers may be tremendously beneficial. If the patient has not kept track of the duration and frequency of headaches, or medication usage, a headache calendar will be helpful. The headache calendar will also alert the physician to possible overuse of analgesics (see Tension-type Headache).

Pharmacotherapy for migraines can be divided into symptomatic therapy and prophylactic therapy. Symptomatic treatment is aimed at the migraine attack as it occurs. Simple analgesics are tried first, followed by combination analgesics and non-steroidal anti-inflammatory drugs (NSAIDs). Antiemetics and sedatives can be used as adjunct therapy. Ergot alkaloids may be very useful in more refractory attacks but they do have significant side effects and may cause complications from the resulting vasoconstriction. Ergot alkaloids are contraindicated in coronary artery disease, hypertension, peripheral vascular disease, pregnancy, renal disease, and hepatic disease. Sumatriptan, a selective 5-HT[1]-receptor agonist, is a new migraine drug with fewer side effects than ergot alkaloids. Narcotics can be used with care in some patients. The various medications used in the symptomatic treatment of migraine are listed in *Figure 22.16*.

Prophylactic migraine therapy is used to decrease the frequency and severity of attacks. The medications used in headache prevention are listed in *Figure 22.17*. If analgesic overuse is present, preventative medications are ineffective and withdrawal of the analgesics must be dealt with first (see Tension-type Headache).

Non-pharmacologic treatment includes physical therapy, heat, ice, exercise, and biofeedback.

TENSION-TYPE HEADACHE

CHARACTERISTICS OF TENSION-TYPE HEADACHE

Previously, this type of headache was referred to as muscle contraction headache, tension headache, or psychogenic headache. Now classified as tension-type headache, both episodic and chronic forms are recognized by the International Headache Society. It is the most common headache type, affecting 60–70% of men and 90% of women.

The tension-type headache is characterized by a dull or aching pain, without any throbbing or pulsating. Patients may describe a pressure sensation or tight feeling around the head: 'my head feels like it is in a vice' or 'it's like a tight band around my head' (*Fig. 22.18*). The pain is usually bilateral and can involve any part of the head. As opposed to the severe pain in migraine, the pain of a tension-type headache is milder. The pain is not aggravated by exertion, unless the patient also has migraine headaches.

There is no associated nausea or vomiting but the appetite may be decreased. In general, photophobia and phonophobia are absent (although one, but not both, can be present). The muscles of the neck and head may be tender and show increased electromyogram activity. This is not required for diagnosis, however, and the muscle soreness is often less with tension-type headaches than it is with migraine headaches.

Headaches occurring on less than 15 days per month are episodic tension-type headaches. For chronic tension-type headaches to be diagnosed, a patient must have more than 15

Potential headache triggers					
Diet	Hormones	Life stresses	Changes in routine	Sensory stimulation	Iatrogenic
Alcohol	Menses	Activity	Weather	Bright light	Angiography
Caffeine	Ovulation	Marriage	Travel	Flickering lights	Histamine H_2 blockers
Aged cheese	Menopause	Divorce	Season	Strong odors	Nifedipine
Chocolate	Pregnancy	Birth	Altitude	Loud noises	Nitroglycerin
Nitrates and nitrites	Hormone replacement	Death	Sleeping patterns		Reserpine
Nuts	Oral contraceptives	Moving	Diet		Methyldopa
Home-made yeast breads		Job stress	Skipping meals		Estrogen
Monosodium glutamate (MSG)		Job loss or change			Progesterone
Aspartame		Let down from stress			
Other					

Fig. 22.15 Potential headache triggers.

headache days per month for at least 6 months. Many of these people have daily headaches. Patients may be affected by both tension-type headaches and migraines.

ANALGESIC-INDUCED OR REBOUND HEADACHES

Often overlooked or unknown to most healthcare providers is the condition of analgesic-induced or analgesic-rebound headaches. These occur in patients with frequent headaches, either migraine or tension-type headaches. As the headaches occur so often, the patient uses frequent, and many times daily, analgesics. The patient then develops a chronic daily headache, which is dependent on the pain medications and refractory to preventative drugs. The use of simple or combination analgesics on more than 3 days per week or the use of ergotamine tartrate on more than 2 days per week may lead to this condition. Stopping the analgesics usually leads to increased headache and withdrawal symptoms initially. However, cessation of the pain medications is mandatory for treatment and many patients do show improvement.

PATHOPHYSIOLOGY OF TENSION-TYPE HEADACHE

At one time it was thought that tension-type headaches were caused by sustained contraction of the head and neck muscles. Recent evidence does not support this and suggests a neuronal mechanism. In fact, the pathogenesis of tension-type headache

may be similar to migraine, with involvement of the trigemino-vascular system. Both types of headache can be triggered by the same stimuli (*Fig. 22.19*). The nucleus caudalis in the trigeminal complex may also be involved, receiving pain input from both cranial blood vessels and head and neck muscles.

Whether or not migraine and tension-type headaches are distinct entities is controversial. It is possible that some tension-type headaches are actually mild migraines, whereas others are a condition entirely separate from migraine.

TREATMENT OF TENSION-TYPE HEADACHE

As with any type of headache, triggering factors should be identified and altered if possible. Physical therapy, heat, ice, and biofeedback will be helpful in selected patients.

If the headaches are episodic and infrequent, symptomatic therapy with simple or combination analgesics is usually effective. To prevent analgesic rebound, ergotamine tartrate must be limited to 2 days per week and other analgesics limited to 3 days per week. Frequent headaches, in the absence of analgesic overuse, can be treated with prophylactic medications. Although antidepressants are often used as first-line therapy any of the migraine preventatives can be tried (see Treatment of Migraine).

If analgesic abuse is present, the patient must be weaned off pain medications and started on prophylactic drugs. The withdrawal from analgesics is often difficult given the physical and psychologic dependence that is usually present. In addition, the

Symptomatic migraine therapy					
Simple analgesics	Combination analgesics	NSAIDs	Ergot alkaloids	Severe, persistent pain	Adjunct therapy
Aspirin	Acetaminophen/ isomeptene/ dichlorophenazone	Ibuprofen	Ergotamine tartrate	Chlorpromazine	Antiemetics
Acetaminophen	Aspirin/caffeine/butalbital	Naproxen or naproxen sodium	Ergotamine tartrate/ caffeine	Prochloroperazine	Antihistamines
Aspirin/caffeine	Acetaminophen/caffeine/ butalbital	Diclofenac, ketoprofen	Dihydroergotamine (DHE)	Haloperidol	Benzodiazepines
Acetaminophen/ caffeine	Aspirin/caffeine/butalbital/ codeine	Flurbiprofen		Thiothixene	
	Acetaminophen/codeine	Diflunisol		Prednisone	
		Ketorolac		Dexamethasone	
		Sulindac		Meperidine	
		Piroxicam		Hydromorphone	
		Indomethacin		Nalbuphine	
		Meclofenamate		Morphine	
		Salsalate			

Fig. 22.16 Symptomatic migraine therapy.

Prophylactic migraine therapy			
Beta-blockers	Calcium-channel blockers	Anti-depressants	Miscellaneous
Propranolol	Verapamil	Amitriptyline	Valproate
Nadolol	Diltiazem	Nortriptyline	Phenytoin
Atenolol	Nifedipine	Doxepin	Methysergide
Timolol	Nimodipine	Trazadone	Cyproheptadine
Metoprolol	Flunarizine	Desipramine	Methylergonovine
		Paroxetine	
		Fluoxetine	
		Sertraline	
		Phenelzine	

Fig. 22.17 Prophylactic migraine therapy.

headaches get worse before they get better. Hospitalization may be required and repetitive intravenous dihydroergotamine (DHE) can be effective in breaking the rebound cycle.

CLUSTER HEADACHE

Although far less common than migraine or tension-type headache, cluster headache is an important cause of severe head pain. It is the only major headache type found predominantly in men, with a male to female ratio of about 6:1. The prevalence rate in men is 0.4–1%. In most patients the onset occurs in the late twenties, but cluster headache may start at any age.

CLINICAL FEATURES

Cluster headache derives its name from the stereotypical recurrence of the attacks. The headaches will come on in a 'cluster' or series of headaches that occur about once or twice a year. Each cluster period lasts, on average, 2–3 months. Although episodes seem to occur more in the spring and fall, seasonality has not been proven.

The pain in a cluster headache starts abruptly and builds to a peak in 10–15 min. The pain is excruciating and some patients become suicidal. The intense pain has a boring or stabbing quality and rarely throbs. The average length of a cluster headache is 45–60 min, with a range of 15 min to 3 h. Attacks occur every day or every other day and some patients have as many as eight attacks per day.

The pain is located primarily in the first division of the trigeminal nerve, in, behind, or around one eye (Fig. 22.20). There may be pain in the temple region and in the maxillary area (second division of the trigeminal nerve). There can also be pain in the posterior neck, around the carotid artery, and in the shoulder. The pain is typically unilateral and in most patients does not switch sides, even in different cluster periods.

Almost one-half of the cluster patients have a regularity to their attacks, with headaches occurring at a specific time of the day

or night (circadian accuracy). The headaches occur nocturnally in more than 50% of people, often awakening a patient from sleep. This generally occurs 90 min after the onset of sleep and coincides with the first rapid eye movement (REM) phase. Attacks during non-REM sleep have also been reported. Triggers for the headaches include alcohol, sublingual nitroglycerin, subcutaneous histamine and smoking.

In addition to the pain, the cluster headache attack has associated autonomic features. Overaction of the parasympathetic system produces lacrimation, conjunctival injection, and nasal congestion or rhinorrhea ipsilateral to the pain. Sympathetic dysfunction produces an ipsilateral Horner's syndrome with ptosis and miosis (Fig. 22.21). The Horner's pupil will show a dilatation lag in darkness (Fig. 22.22). The diagnosis of Horner's syndrome can be confirmed with cocaine eyedrops. A 10% cocaine solution, which blocks the re-uptake of noradrenaline, dilates the normal pupil. The Horner's pupil dilates minimally or not at all to the cocaine (Fig. 22.23). Some patients, after repeated attacks, may develop a permanent Horner's syndrome. Other findings include periorbital swelling, scalp and facial tenderness, and bradycardia.

Unlike the migraine patient who prefers to lie quietly in a dark room, the cluster patient is restless and would rather pace about and be active. The cluster patient may try to put pressure on the painful area or soothe the pain with something cold.

Cluster patients often have a history of heavy smoking and alcohol usage, as well as a high incidence of peptic ulcer disease. A characteristic 'lionine' facial appearance has been described with a ruddy, furrowed face and orange peellike skin.

TYPES OF CLUSTER HEADACHE

Cluster headache can be episodic or chronic. With episodic cluster, a cycle lasts from 1 week to 1 year and there must be at least 2 weeks before the next cycle begins. Chronic cluster is diagnosed if the cluster period lasts longer than 1 year without remission or if the remissions are shorter than 2 weeks.

Another form of cluster headache is chronic paroxysmal hemicrania. Unlike typical cluster headache, this condition is found mostly in women. The pain and associated features are identical to a typical cluster headache, but the attacks are very short in duration, lasting only 5–10 min. Patients have multiple (5–20) headache attacks per day. There is an absolute responsiveness of the headache to indomethacin, which is required for diagnosis.

CLUSTER-LIKE HEADACHES

Cluster variants include cluster–tic syndrome (with both cluster headaches and trigeminal neuralgia), cluster vertigo, and cluster migraine. In addition, some underlying conditions may mimic cluster headaches. Tumors (pituitary, nasopharyngeal, and high cervical), arteriovenous malformations, aneurysms, and head and facial trauma have all been reported to cause cluster-like headaches.

PATHOPHYSIOLOGY OF CLUSTER HEADACHE

As with migraine and tension-type headache, the specific etiology of cluster headache is not known. Extracranial vasodilatation does occur and vasodilators (alcohol, nitroglycerin, histamine) are

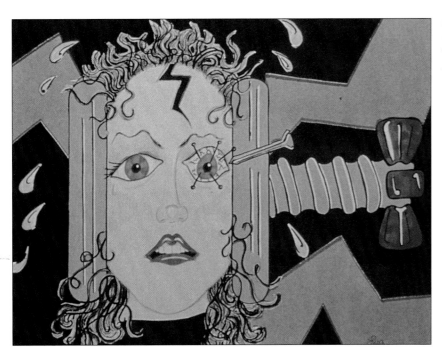

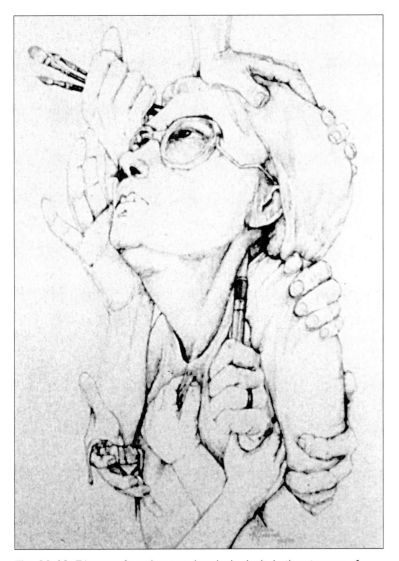

Fig. 22.19 Triggers of tension-type headache include the stresses of daily life, as shown in this picture with its play-on-words title of *Attention Headache*. (*Attention Headache* by Merana Cadorette, from the *Through the Looking Glass* Headache Art Exhibition, courtesy of Sandoz Pharmaceuticals Corporation)

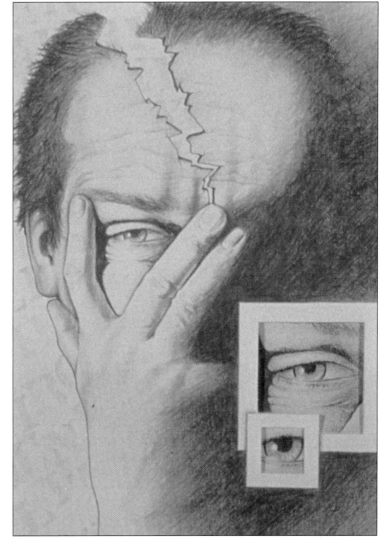

Fig. 22.20 The severe pain of cluster headache is located in or around one eye. (*The Eyes Have It* by Antonia Putman, from the *Through the Looking Glass* Headache Art Exhibition, courtesy of Sandoz Pharmaceuticals Corporation)

known to trigger cluster headaches. However, there is no evidence of intracerebral vasodilatation. The extracranial blood vessel changes may be secondary to neuronal causes.

Neuronal changes are important in the etiology of cluster headaches, with the trigeminal nerve and trigeminovascular system playing a pivotal role. Many of the clinical features of cluster headache could be caused by an abnormality around the cavernous portion of the carotid artery, where autonomic and pain fibers of the eye come together.

The most likely cause of the periodicity of cluster headaches is disruption of the normal biologic clock mechanism in the anterior hypothalamus. This central pacemaker is a serotonergic system. Changes in the posterior hypothalamus probably also occur, affecting autonomic function.

Other factors that may be involved in the pathogenesis of cluster headache include hypoxemia and dysfunctional chemoreceptors in the carotid body.

TREATMENT OF CLUSTER HEADACHE

The treatment of cluster headache can be divided into abortive therapy, prophylactic therapy, nerve blockades, and surgical therapy (*Fig. 22.24*). Lifestyle changes should also be encouraged, particularly the cessation of alcohol, tobacco, and caffeine.

Surgical therapy is indicated only in patients with chronic cluster headache who are totally refractory to medical therapy. Radiofrequency lesions of the trigeminal nerve are the most effective. Complications include anesthesia dolorosa and corneal injury due to the loss of corneal sensation.

The use of light treatment to reset the central pacemaker is a promising new therapy that is being investigated. Preliminary results with capsaicin in the nostril ipsilateral to the pain are also encouraging.

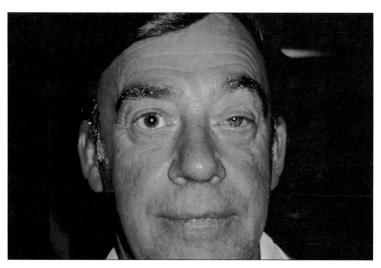

Fig. 22.21 Cluster headache patient with a left Horner's syndrome. Note the ptosis, miosis, and conjunctival injection of the left eye. (Courtesy of Dr Randy Kardon)

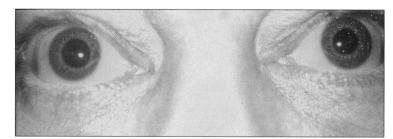
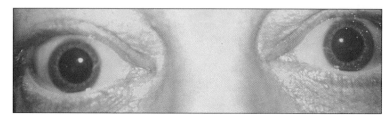

Fig. 22.22 Dilatation lag in a cluster headache patient with a left Horner's syndrome. The upper picture was taken after the patient was in the dark for 5 s, the lower picture after 15 s in the dark. Note how the left pupil dilates more slowly than the normal right pupil. (Courtesy of Dr Randy Kardon.)

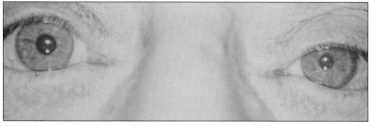

Fig. 22.23 Cocaine eyedrop testing in Horner's syndrome. The upper photograph shows a left Horner's syndrome with ptosis and miosis. The lower picture was taken 30 min after 10% cocaine in both eyes. Note the dilatation of the normal right pupil and the poor dilatation of the left pupil. (Courtesy of Dr Randy Kardon)

Treatment of cluster headache			
Abortive	**Prophylactic**	**Nerve blockade**	**Surgical procedures**
Oxygen inhalation	Verapamil	Sphenopalatine ganglion block	Radiofrequency trigeminal
Ergotamine	Nifedipine		Gangliorhizolysis
Dihydroergotamine	Diltiazem		
Sumatriptan	Nimodipine	Occipital nerve block	Retrogasserian glycerol injection
Dexamethasone	Lithium		
Intranasal lidocaine	Ergotamine		
	Prednisone		
	Indomethacin		
	Valproate		
	Methysergide		

Fig. 22.24 Treatment of cluster headache.

Further reading

Corbett JJ. Neuro-ophthalmic complications of migraine and cluster headaches. In: Smith CH, Beck RW, eds. Symposium on Neuro-Ophthalmology. *Neurol Clinics*. 1983;**1**:973–995.

Headache Classification Committee of the International Headache Society. Classification and diagnostic criteria for headache disorders, cranial neuralgias and facial pain. *Cephalalgia*. 1988;**8** (**suppl 7**):1–96.

Hupp SL, Kline LB, Corbett JJ. Visual disturbances of migraine. *Surv Ophthalmol*. 1989;**33**:221–236.

Lance JW, ed. Advances in biology and pharmacology of headache. *Neurology*. 1993; **43** (**suppl 3**):1–47.

Mathew NT, ed. Headache. *Neurol Clinics*. 1990;**8**:781–992.

Silberstein SD, ed. Intractable headache: inpatient and outpatient treatment strategies. *Neurology*. 1992;**42** (**suppl 2**):1–51.

Silberstein SD. Evaluation and emergency treatment of headache. *Headache*. 1992;**32**:396–407.

Silberstein SD. Tension-type and chronic daily headache. *Neurology*. 1993;**43**:1644–1649.

CHAPTER 23

Ocular and Facial Pain Syndromes

Patrick J M Lavin

INTRODUCTION

Facial and ocular pain are common and vexing problems, and are all the more challenging in the absence of clinical signs. Patients with facial or eye pain may consult specialists in internal medicine, neurology, ophthalmology, and otorhinolaryngology, but many eventually gravitate to the neuro-ophthalmologist.

The sensation of pain (Spiegel and Spiegel, 1978) is easily recognized but difficult to define and quantify. The International Association for The Study of Pain define it as '... an unpleasant sensory and emotional experience associated with actual or potential tissue damage ....' Pain may be divided into *nociceptive pain*, caused by external noxious environmental stimuli warning us of potential injury, and neuropathic pain, caused by dysfunction of the sensory nervous system. Neuropathic pain can occur spontaneously or be induced by external stimuli, including non-noxious stimuli such as touch (allodynia). Pain is processed by two largely separate systems in the cerebrum – a 'lateral pain system' involving the somatosensory cortex which deals with acute pain, and a 'medial pain system' involving the thalamus, anterior cingulate gyrus, and prefrontal cortex which deals with chronic pain.

Ocular pain is divided into four types:
- Pain of corneal origin mediated by non-myelinated C fiber endings, mainly in the midstromal and subepithelial plexus. These fibers transmit nociceptive sensation via the ophthalmic division of the trigeminal nerve and when stimulated also cause lacrimation, miosis, and release of substance P.
- Deep pain caused by inflammation of the anterior segment of the eye mediated by chemoreceptors (for kinins and substance P), mechanoreceptors, and thermal receptors. These receptors also transmit sensation via the ophthalmic division.
- Light-induced pain which is subdivided into *glare* caused by excessive light, and *photophobia* caused by 'normal' levels of light.
- Referred pain, which is discussed below.

ANATOMY AND PHYSIOLOGY

Pain-sensitive structures in the head are innervated by the trigeminal nerve, the nervus intermedius branch of the facial nerve, the glossopharyngeal and vagus nerves, and the upper three cervical sensory roots. Pain from the eyes, paranasal sinuses, scalp vessels, skin, teeth, and most of the periosteum is transmitted by the trigeminal nerve and referred to the appropriate dermatome. The intracranial pain-sensitive structures are the dura covering the floors of the anterior and posterior cranial fossae, the falx, the proximal cerebral and dural arteries, and the large cerebral veins

and venous sinuses. The brain itself, the bones of the cranium, the ependymal lining of the ventricles, the choroid plexuses, and much of the dura and pia-arachnoid are not pain sensitive. Pain from the anterior and middle cranial fossae, and from the superior surface of the tentorium, is transmitted by the first division of the trigeminal nerve and referred to the ocular and periocular region (*Fig. 23.1*). Pain from the inferior surface of the tentorium and the posterior fossa is transmitted mainly by the glossopharyngeal nerve, the vagus nerve, and the upper three cervical sensory roots, and referred to the occipital region and upper neck.

Distension of the middle meningeal artery causes retro-orbital pain. Distortion of the intracranial internal carotid artery, the proximal two centimeters of the middle cerebral artery, and the proximal anterior cerebral artery causes referred pain to the eye, forehead, or temple (Lance, 1993). Stimulation of the mid third of the middle cerebral artery causes retro-orbital pain, and of the distal third of the middle cerebral artery, pain above the eye. Stimulation of the vertebral artery causes ipsilateral, and occasionally bilateral, occipital pain. Superior sagittal sinus disease can cause frontoparietal pain.

Pain fibers descend through the brainstem in the spinal tract of the trigeminal nerve to the third or fourth cervical segments of the spinal cord (*Fig. 23.2*). Pain sensation from the upper three or four cervical sensory roots, and other sources, also converges on cells in the dorsolateral quadrant of the upper cervical cord. The nucleus of the trigeminal tract is continuous with the substantia gelatinosa of the posterior horn (see Fig. 23.2). This arrangement may explain why lesions in the posterior fossa and upper cervical cord can cause retro-orbital pain. The second order neurons, in the nucleus of the trigeminal tract, project across the midline and ascend through the brainstem as the trigeminothalamic (quintothalamic), or ascending, tract of the trigeminal nerve. These fibers project to neurons in the ventro-postero-medial nucleus (VPM) of the thalamus before relaying to the sensory cortex in the parietal lobe. There is also a parallel pathway to the cingulate gyrus in the limbic system, which contributes the emotional component of pain. The trigeminothalamic tract and thalamus may be involved in the pathogenesis of migraine and cluster headache, and could explain the occasional complaint of neck, upper limb, and even lower limb pain during headache attacks. Such complaints may be perceived by physicians as exaggerated or neurotic.

Convergence of cutaneous and vascular afferent input may explain why headaches of vascular origin are referred to the eye and forehead. The overlap between the trigeminal and cervical distribution, much greater than is commonly known, may also explain why both ocular and facial pain occur in disorders such as 'cervicogenic headache' (see below).

The principal descending pain modulating systems in the

Source and site of referred pain	
Source	**Site of referred pain**
Upper surface of tentorium	Periocular region
Lower (inferior) surface of tentorium	Occipital region, throat, and ear
Middle meningeal artery	Ipsilateral retro-orbital region
Intracranial internal carotid artery and proximal 2 cm of MCA	Eye, forehead, and temple
Anterior cerebral artery	Eye, forehead, and temple
Vertebral artery	Occiput
Superior sagittal sinus	Frontoparietal region
Distal internal carotid artery and proximal MCA	Lateral to the eye
Mid third of the MCA	Retro-orbital region
Distal third of the MCA	Above the eye
Frontal lobe hematoma	Frontal region
Temporal lobe hematoma	Pain in and anterior to the ear
Occipital hematoma	Ipsilateral eye pain (dense contralateral hemianopia)
Parietal lobe hematoma	Anterior temporal (temple)
Frontal sinus	Frontal region
Ethmoid sinus	Between, around, or behind eyes, parietal area
Sphenoid sinus	Frontal, bitemporal, behind or between eyes, mastoid, hemicranial, vertex, occipital region
Maxillary sinus	Cheek, temple, teeth (aggravated by stooping)
Mastoid	Ear, eye, hemicranial
Cluster headache	Peri- or retro-orbital, temple, frontal, jaw, teeth
Vascular headache	Eye and forehead
Temporomandibular joint (TMJ)	Periorbital, temple, jaw, ear, pre-auricular, neck
Pachymeningitis (plus cranial neuropathies)	Periorbital, face, frontal, parietal, temple
Dental	Teeth, mouth, ear, jaw, cheek
MCA = Middle cerebral artery	

Fig. 23.1 Source and sight of referred pain.

nervous system are: a) the serotonergic system which projects from the periaqueductal gray (PAG) in the midbrain to midline raphe nuclei in the medulla, and terminates in the spinal cord where it influences gabaminergic interneurons in the dorsal horn; and b) the noradrenergic system, in the locus ceruleus in the pons, which influences enkephalin-containing interneurons also in the dorsal horn (see Fig. 23.2).

The locus ceruleus, which projects to the cerebral cortex via the ascending noradrenergic system, also innervates the cerebral microcirculation. Similarly, the trigeminal nerve projects to cerebral blood vessels (Moskowitz, 1984). Trigeminal sensory C-fibers contain the pain transmitter substance P, and other neuropeptides, including calcitonin gene-related peptide (CGRP), neurokinin-A, and vasoactive intestinal polypeptide (VIP), which

are released by antidromic stimulation and can cause vasodilatation, plasma extravasation, sterile inflammation, and breakdown of the blood–brain barrier. Cerebral arteries contain predominantly 5HT-1 receptors, the superficial temporal artery contains 5HT-2 receptors, and meningeal arteries contain both. A detailed discussion of the central pain pathways, neurotransmitters, and neurovascular pain mechanisms may be found elsewhere (Lance, 1993).

Primary or 'central headache', such as migraine and cluster headache, may be generated by altered neurotransmission and modulation in the central pain pathways. Secondary, or symptomatic headache results from traction, displacement, inflammation or pressure on nociceptors in pain-sensitive structures.

APPROACH TO PATIENTS WITH OCULAR AND FACIAL PAIN

The physician's role is first, to identify the cause, or at least exclude the possibility of serious underlying disease; and second, to alleviate pain and suffering by explanation, reassurance, and appropriate management. A careful and detailed history is usually more revealing than an extensive physical examination, and certainly more productive, in the large majority of patients, than neuroimaging. It is important to establish at the beginning if the patient suffers from more than one type of headache, and to define each type, as in a migraineur with superimposed analgesic rebound headaches. A spontaneous history is preferable but the facts listed in *Figure 23.3* should be obtained, even if leading questions are necessary.

The physical examination is usually nonfocal but should include assessment of visual acuity, a neurologic evaluation with particular emphasis on cranial nerve function, palpation of the head and cervical region, assessment of neck mobility, auscultation for cardiac, carotid, and cephalic bruits, and blood pressure measurement. Features of special interest include anisocoria, corneal injection, facial asymmetry, ptosis, proptosis, periorbital swelling or ecchymosis, nodules or bumps about the head, pulsatility, and tenderness of the temporal arteries and other localized areas of sensitivity.

SPECIFIC CLINICAL SYNDROMES

In a retrospective review of 2000 patients with facial pain, an underlying tumor was found in only 16 (0.8%) (Bullitt *et al.*, 1986). Extracranial tumors frequently caused persistent burning or crawling facial pain, whereas posterior fossa tumors were more likely to cause typical trigeminal neuralgia (below), and were usually associated with subtle neurologic deficits such as ataxia, deafness, hypesthesia in the distribution of the trigeminal nerve, hyperreflexia, and tongue deviation. Middle fossa tumors usually caused either persistent pain with progressive neurologic deficits, or severe but otherwise typical trigeminal neuralgia (2 of 6 patients).

Patients with ocular or periorbital pain can be divided into those with an inflamed or *red eye* (*Fig. 23.4*) and those with an apparently normal or *white eye* (*Fig. 23.5*). Most causes of a painful red eye are ophthalmologic in nature. With the exception of those conditions listed below, 'a white eye is not the cause of a painful eye' (Daroff, 1995). However, patients with some of the disorders that

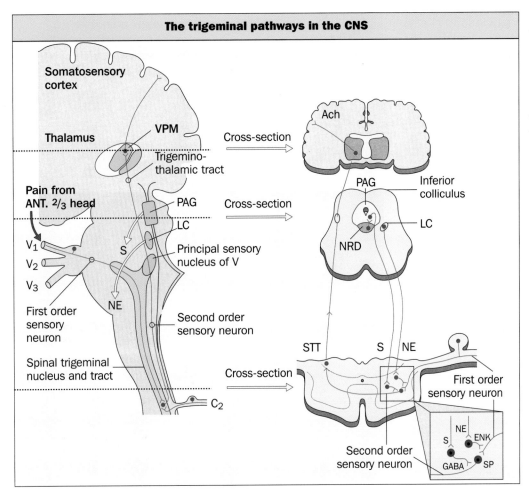

The trigeminal pathways in the CNS

Fig. 23.2 The trigeminal pathways in the CNS conveying pain sensation, and the central pain modulating pathways. (ACh, acetylcholine; ENK, enkephalin; GABA, gamma aminobutyric acid; LC, locus ceruleus; NE, norepinephrine; NRD, nucleus raphe dorsalis; PAG, periaqueductal gray; S, serotonin; SP, substance P; STT, spinthalamic tract; VPM, ventropostural medial nucleus of the thalamus)

Headache history
How many different types of headache?
Describe a typical headache
Age of onset?
Frequency and duration?
Mode of onset (sudden, first, or worst)?
Pattern (e.g. awakens patient or present on awakening)?
Premonitory symptoms or aura, or both?
Location and radiation?
Quality and nature of pain (stabbing, throbbing, burning, bursting, squeezing, etc.)?
Associated symptoms (nausea, vomiting, diarrhea, abdominal pain, photophobia, phonophobia, osmophobia, tearing or focal neurologic symptoms)?
Precipitating factors or triggers?
Aggravating factors?
Relieving factors?
Current medication and previous treatment (important for management)?
General health (system review), e.g. polymyalgia, jaw claudication, collagen vascular disease, infections, hypertension, malignancy, emotional state, sleep pattern?
Family history, especially of headache?
Social history (occupation, exposures, recreations, habits, marital status)?

Fig. 23.3 Headache history. Key questions in the evaluation of headache which must be answered, either spontaneously or by direct questioning.

Conditions associated with red eye
Carotid–cavernous fistula (high flow, low flow, dural shunt)
Conjunctivitis
Corneal disorders (abrasions, erosions, keratitis, ulcers)
Dry eye syndrome
Glaucoma (narrow angle, neovascular)
Infective processes
Orbital cellulitis
Ocular ischemia (carotid insufficiency)
Orbital pseudotumor
Trauma/foreign body
Scleritis/episcleritis
Uveitis

Fig. 23.4 Conditions associated with red eye.

usually result in an injected or red eye (see Fig. 23.4) may have an apparently normal (white) eye early in the course of their disease.

In certain situations a simple penlight test may be helpful when a slit lamp is not available. The 'tangential penlight test' for narrow angle glaucoma is particularly helpful as it may take a few days for the cornea to become cloudy: if the iris casts a shadow on part of the limbus when a beam of light is directed tangentially across the iris, normal to the line of gaze, then the angle is narrow and the anterior chamber shallow (*Fig. 23.6*). If the consensual light reflex causes discomfort in the symptomatic eye when a bright light is directed at the unaffected eye, then inflammatory

Conditions associated with white eye
Asthenopia
Adie's myotonic pupil
Brainstem disorders
Cavernous sinus disease
Tumor
Aneurysm
Fistula (high or low flow)
Thrombosis
Inflammation (Tolosa–Hunt syndrome)
Cervicogenic headache
Ciliary spasm
Corneal disorders (abrasions, erosions, keratitis,trichiasis, ulcers)
Cluster headache syndromes
Dry eye syndrome
Familial rectal pain
Frontal lobe hemorrhage
Greater occipital neuralgia
Hemicrania continua
HZO (pre- or noneruptive)
Ice-pick-like headache (cephalgia fugax)
Idiopathic (atypical) facial pain (see text)
Inferior orbital fissure syndrome
Increased intracranial pressure (eg Pseudotumor cerebri)
Iritis - early (see text)
Ischemic optic neuropathy
Isolated ocular motor nerve palsy
Migraine
Myocardial infarction
Narrow angle glaucoma – early
Optic neuritis/peri-optic neuritis
Orbital pseudotumor (usually conjunctiva injected)
Paranasal sinus disease
Infection
Mucocele
Tumor
Photo-oculodynia syndrome
Pituitary apoplexy
Posterior fossa lesions
Post-iritis pain cycle
Posterior scleritis (variant of orbital pseudotumor)
Postherpetic neuralgia
Pulmonary cancer
Psychogenic
Raeder's syndrome
Referred pain (TMJ, teeth, etc.)
Superior orbital fissure/orbital apex syndrome
Thalamic lesions
Thyroid orbitopathy
Trigeminal neuralgia (V^1)
Trochleitis (sup. oblique tendinitis)
Vascular disorders
Carotid dissection
Carotid stenosis (ocular ischemia)
Ischemic ocular motor palsy
Giant cell arteritis

Fig. 23.5 Conditions associated with white eye.

The penlight test for narrow angle glaucoma

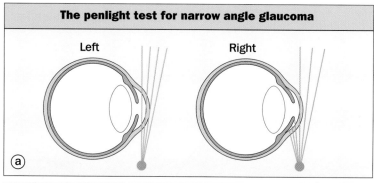
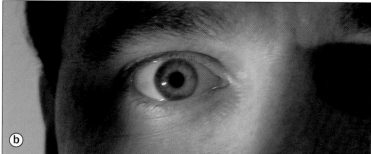
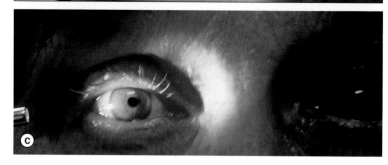

Fig. 23.6 The tangential penlight test for narrow angle glaucoma. (**a**) Left: the light is directed tangentially across the line of gaze of a normal eye and illuminates the iris. Right: the iris casts a shadow on itself when the corneal scleral angle is narrow. (**b**) A normal eye with the iris completely illuminated by a penlight. (**c**) The iris in a patient with narrow angle glaucoma showing a shadow on its medial aspect.

cells are likely, irritating the iris of the affected eye, i.e. iritis. The converse is not true; iritis may be painless, as in juvenile rheumatoid arthritis.

OCULAR AND FACIAL MIGRAINE SYNDROMES

Migraine is the most common cause of ocular, retro-orbital, and periocular pain in a patient with a 'white' eye. Migraine can also cause frontal, temporal, or facial (lower half headache) pain and is discussed elsewhere in this book. Ophthalmoplegic migraine causes transient ocular motor neuropathies, while retinal migraine causes transient visual disturbances.

CLUSTER HEADACHE

This condition, named because of its tendency to recur in 'clusters' lasting weeks to months, is one of the most painful (homicidal/suicidal) and stereotyped forms of headache syndrome. The average cluster duration is 6–8 weeks and most patients have one or two episodes per year. Typically the attack is characterized by severe unilateral non-throbbing, aching, or boring pain that is maximal behind the eye or in the cheek, but can involve the frontal, temporal, maxillary, vertex, or even occipital region. A warning pressure-like sensation sometimes precedes the severe pain. The ipsilateral nostril may burn or ache. The pain is associated with marked ipsilateral autonomic features that include lacrimation, conjunctival injection, a Horner's syndrome (in two-thirds of patients) which may be transient or persist between attacks, nasal congestion, and rhinorrhea. The autonomic symptoms may start before the pain. Ipsilateral photophobia is frequent and vision can be blurred because of tearing. Hyperalgesia of the face and scalp and occasionally photopsias may accompany the headache. Alcohol and vasodilators such as nitroglycerin may trigger an attack. The pain is virtually always on the same side during a cluster but, occasionally, may switch sides in a subsequent cluster.

Pain in the jaw or neck is atypical and suggests dissection of the carotid artery. Rarely, cluster headaches are reported in patients with pituitary tumors, parasellar lesions (meningiomas, aneurysms), clival epidermoids, arteriovenous malformations, sinusitis, vasculitis, whiplash injury, nasopharyngeal carcinoma, and following meningitis. The causality of these associations is not necessarily established and, for the most part, the etiology of cluster headache is unknown.

The pathogenesis of cluster headache is not well established. During an attack, ipsilateral vascular changes that may be associated are focal narrowing of the lumen of the internal carotid artery attributed to edema and spasm of the vessel wall, dilatation of the lumen of the ophthalmic artery, and increased diameter of both the internal carotid artery, in its course through the siphon, and the basilar artery. Idiopathic inflammation of the cavernous sinus, which is probably neurogenic in origin, and its associated venous connections, has been implicated by orbital phlebography. Appenzeller's group (1981) suggested that cluster headache was mediated by axonal reflex activity involving the trigeminal system following a viral infection; but Moskowitz (1984) implicated neurogenic inflammation in the superior pericarotid cavernous sinus. During an attack, a sterile inflammation of the ipsilateral internal carotid artery and its proximal

branches is associated with the release of vasoactive peptides and neurotransmitters. These vasoactive substances include CGRP and substance P from the trigeminovascular innervation, and VIP from the parasympathetic innervation of intracranial vessels, suggesting both the trigeminal and parasympathetic systems are active during the attack. Treatment with oxygen or sumatriptan, a 5HT-1$_D$ serotoninergic agonist, lowers CGRP levels to normal. Abnormalities of cortisol, gonadotrophin, growth hormone, melatonin, prolactin, testosterone, and thyrotropin release also occur, implicating the hypothalamus during an attack. Which structures are involved first is not established, but all are in some way linked to the biologic circadian and circannual regulating clocks in the hypothalamus.

Cluster headaches can be subdivided as follows:

• **Episodic cluster headaches** ('cluster vera') occur daily, usually in the early morning about 2 hours after going to sleep,

Synonyms for cluster headache
Alarm clock headache
Autonomic faciocephalgia
Ciliary neuralgia
Erythromelalgia of the head
Erythroprosopalgia
Greater superficial petros, neuralgia
Histamine cephalgia
Horton's histamine cephalgia
Migrainous neuralgia
Red migraine
Sluder's neuralgia
Sphenopalatine neurosis/neuralgia
Syndrome of hemicephalgic vasodilatation of sympathetic origin
Vidian neuralgia
Vail's neuralgia

Fig. 23.7 Synonyms for cluster headache.

Management outline of cluster headache
Acute attack (abortive therapy)
Compression of the superficial temporal artery
Oxygen 100% (7 liters/min for 15 mins)
Prednisone (50 mg b.i.d. for 5 days) and verapamil (40 mg t.i.d., increased to between 40 mg t.i.d. and 160 mg t.i.d. (JSW))
Sumatriptan (6 mg s.c.)
Sumatriptan (50–100 mg p.o.)
Ergot alkaloids (i.m. ors.c.)
Local anesthesia intranasally
Chlorpromazine (5–50 mg i.v.; 1 mg/kg i.m. up to 50 mg)
Promethazine (Phenergan; 25–75 mg i.m.)
Prochlorperazine (Compazine; 10 mg i.v.)
Somatostatin (10 μg/min i.v. over 20 min)
Diphenhydramine (50 mg i.v., slow push) followed by cimetidine (300 mg i.v., slow push)
Prophylaxis
Propranolol (to tolerance, approx. 480 mg)
Tricyclic antidepressants
Ergot alkaloids
Calcium channel blockers
Lithium
Methysergide
Chlorpromazine (50–700 mg/day)
Pizotifen (1.5–3 mg/day)
MAO inhibitors
Surgery (rarely necessary)
Section of nucleus intermedius
Section of greater petrosal nucleus
Sphenoplatine ganglionectomy
Preganglionic branch section of trigeminal ganglion
Trigeminal sensory rhizotomy
Percutaneous radio frequency trigeminal gangliorhizolysis
Stellate ganglion blockade

Fig. 23.8 Management outline of cluster headache.

hence the term 'alarm clock headache' (*Fig. 23.7*). Attacks last about 45 minutes, but can be as short as a few minutes or as long as 6 hours. The number of attacks in a 24-hour period varies from one to three, occasionally up to eight. Clusters last from a couple of weeks to a few months, and are more common in the spring and fall. Almost 90% of patients with episodic cluster are male and have their first attack between the first and sixth decade, although almost any age group can be affected. The diagnosis should be reevaluated in patients with an atypical history, a neurologic deficit other than Horner's syndrome, progression to chronic cluster headache, or failure to respond to appropriate therapy, as outlined in *Figure 23.8*.

- **Chronic cluster headache.** Attacks of episodic cluster headache that continue for a year or more without remission are termed chronic cluster. Such patients occasionally have sellar- or parasellar-region lesions and should be thoroughly evaluated, otherwise management is the same (see Fig. 23.8). A cluster that lasts for more than 3 months should be of particular concern to the physician.

- **Chronic paroxysmal hemicrania (CPH).** This condition differs from episodic cluster in several ways. It occurs mainly in middle-aged women, attacks last from 5–20 minutes (mean=15 minutes) and occur as many as 5–30 times a day. It is associated with photophobia and ipsilateral autonomic features. Chronic paroxysmal hemicrania responds dramatically to indomethacin, usually 12.5–300 mg/day (mean=50 mg, 3 times per day). If indomethacin fails or is contraindicated, lithium, verapamil, or acetazolamide may be beneficial. Attacks may be triggered by certain neck movements. Rarely, CPH may be caused by underlying lesion such as a pituitary tumor.

- **Episodic paroxysmal hemicrania.** This condition is similar to, and may precede, CPH, but remits after 3–16 weeks. It also responds exquisitely to indomethacin.

SUNCT SYNDROME

The SUNCT syndrome (Short-lasting, Unilateral, Neuralgiform headache attacks with Conjunctival injection, Tearing, sweating, and rhinorrhea) consists of 'cluster-like headaches where the duration becomes shorter but the name becomes longer' (paraphrased from Lance, 1993). Almost all patients are men over the age of 45 years. Brief attacks of pain in or around the eye, lasting 15 s to 2 minutes, occur with a frequency up to 30 times per hour. The pain is associated with sudden conjunctival injection and the autonomic features of cluster headache. Attacks may be precipitated by chewing, eating certain foods such as citrus fruits, touching the nose, lids, supraorbital area, or even hair, as well as by specific neck movements. Intraocular pressure may be elevated during attacks. SUNCT has been associated with an arteriovenous malformation in the cerebellopontine angle, an injury to the ipsilateral brow, and phlebographic abnormalities in the superior ophthalmic vein, and cavernous sinus. Response to medication is poor, but acetaminophen, carbamazepine, sumatriptan, verapamil, or tricyclic agents may be beneficial.

THE CLUSTER TIC SYNDROME

The cluster tic syndrome has features of both cluster headache and trigeminal neuralgia. The main feature is lancinating tic-like pain, which merges into or provokes a cluster headache. Control of the tic-like pain with carbamazepine also controls the cluster headache. The association is probably more than coincidental.

ICE-PICK-LIKE HEADACHE

Ice-pick-like headache (cephalgia fugax, 'needle in the eye' syndrome) is a brief sharp shooting or jabbing pain affecting the orbit, temple, parietal, or sometimes occipital region (O'Donnell and Martin, 1986). The episodes of pain last only a split second but may have an 'afterburn' for up to a minute, similar to the tic-like pain of trigeminal neuralgia. The frequency of attacks varies from several times a day to once a week. This benign condition is more common in migraineurs (42%) than the 'normal' population (3%), but also occurs in patients with tension headache, cluster headache, and hemicrania continua. Rarely, such 'jab headache' heralds vertebral artery dissection. Prophylactic non-steroidal anti-inflammatory agents, particularly indomethacin, are beneficial.

HEMICRANIA CONTINUA

Hemicrania continua is a rare disorder characterized by continuous unilateral headache that fluctuates in intensity but persists from morning till night, even awakening the patient. Autonomic features and photophobia may be associated. Precipitating features are not identified. Hemicrania continua may be associated with superimposed 'jabs and jolts' similar to 'ice-pick-like headache'. Pain is usually localized to the forehead and temple. Initially, the pain is sometimes paroxysmal (Newman *et al.*, 1994).

The mean age of onset is approximately 35 years, and the female to male ratio is 5:1. The essential feature of hemicrania continua is continuous, unilateral headache, which responds to indomethacin. If indomethacin does not relieve the pain, evaluation for structural disease should be performed.

ICE-CREAM HEADACHE

Migraineurs, and to a lesser extent patients with tension headache, are susceptible to transient mid-frontal, temporal, pharyngeal, and even ear pain when swallowing ice cream or a cold drink. Diving into cold water causes similar headache. Non-headache patients occasionally experience such phenomena.

EXTERNAL COMPRESSION HEADACHE

Tight-fitting hats, helmets, diving masks, swimming goggles, hair prostheses (particularly following craniotomy), and even certain 'tight' hairstyles can cause headache. Treatment is obvious.

TRIGEMINAL NEURALGIA

The onset of trigeminal neuralgia (tic douloureux) usually occurs in the fifth decade or later. The second division is affected more frequently than the third; the first division is affected in less than 5% of patients. Compression of the root entry zone of the trigeminal nerve by ectatic vessels, in the cerebellopontine angle, is a common cause. If the second or third division is involved the superior cerebellar artery may be responsible, whereas the inferior cerebellar artery is more likely to compress the first division. The onset of trigeminal neuralgia before the age of 40 years suggests multiple sclerosis, or a posterior fossa tumor. It may also occur in patients with Paget's disease and platybasia. Attacks of trigeminal neuralgia may be precipitated by dental malocclusion, temporomandibular joint (TMJ) dysfunction, such as a dental abscess infection, or injury involving the branches of the trigeminal nerve.

Trigeminal neuralgia is a clinical diagnosis based on a careful history; the examination is unrevealing except for mild hyperesthesia in the involved dermatome. The characteristic features are: a) sudden intense shock-like jabs of pain lasting a second or so, but with an 'afterburn' of up to a minute, typically along the upper or lower border of the maxillary division, but sometimes in the mandibular division (*Fig. 23.9*); b) touching trigger areas (such as the cheek, nostrils, teeth, lips, and brow), even lightly, may provoke a spasm of pain that makes brushing the hair or teeth, chewing, talking, sneezing, swallowing, and washing intolerable; c) attacks are usually worse in the morning. Bilateral involvement occurs in less than 6% of patients and is more likely in the rare familial form. However, patients with bilateral or persistent pain, objective sensory loss in the affected dermatome, or other cranial nerve deficit, should be evaluated for underlying disorders. The finding of a 'numb cheek' or 'numb chin' sign is ominous and should prompt aggressive evaluation, even to the extent of a nasopharyngeal biopsy. About one-third of patients with trigeminal neuralgia complain of photophobia; it is more common if the

first division is involved (Gutrecht and Lessell, 1994).

Painful spasms may occur many times a day, for weeks or months, but then remit for long periods of time. Carbamazepine suppresses the painful spasms in approximately 80% of patients. In older patients the initial dose of carbamazepine is 50 mg twice per day, which should be increased gradually to avoid side effects, particularly nausea and ataxia. The dose is increased to the maximum tolerable dose which controls symptoms without side effects. Alternative drugs include baclofen, clonazepam, gabapentin, and phenytoin. Misoprostol, a long-acting prostaglandin E_1 analogue, may be effective in MS patients when trigeminal neuralgia is refractory to conventional agents (Reder and Arnason, 1995). Patients who do not respond to medication should be considered for procedures such as trigeminal nerve decompression (the 'Jannetta procedure'), percutaneous radiofrequency gasserian thermocoagulation, glycerol rhizotomy, or alcohol blockade.

PRE-TRIGEMINAL NEURALGIA

Some patients develop a dull continuous aching pain in the upper or lower jaw days to years before the onset of classic trigeminal neuralgia. This prodromal discomfort, which is similar to a toothache or sinus-like pain and lasts several hours at a time, is sometimes triggered by jaw movement or by drinking hot or cold liquids. The pain may be suppressed by carbamazepine or baclofen.

GLOSSOPHARYNGEAL NEURALGIA

Severe lancinating paroxysmal pain in the distribution of the glossopharyngeal nerve is 100-times less common than trigeminal neuralgia. Episodic stabbing pain is experienced in the tonsilar region, deep in the ear, at the base of the tongue or under the jaw (pharyngeal or otologic neuralgia). It may be followed by a burning ache or pressure-like sensation lasting several minutes. The paroxysms are often provoked by swallowing, talking, or coughing. Glossopharyngeal neuralgia, like trigeminal neuralgia, is idiopathic except for rare cases of vascular compression of the nerve in the posterior fossa, tumors in the posterior fossa, or lesions in the oropharyngeal or jugular foramen region. Glossopharyngeal neuralgia has occurred in association with carotid aneurysms, parathyroid cysts, multiple sclerosis, an elongated styloid process, a calcified stylohyoid ligament (Eagle's syndrome), carcinoma of the nasopharynx and larynx with local spread, and with peripharyngeal abscess. It can also occur after injury to the throat during transesophageal echocardiography, and with herpetic aphthous ulceration of the pharynx.

Syncope and, rarely, vertigo are sometimes associated with paroxysms of pain, as a result of bradycardia, hypotension, or both; hence the term vagoglossopharyngeal neuralgia. The mechanism of bradycardia and hypotension is unclear, but may result from cross talk between the glossopharyngeal and vagus, or an abnormal communication between the nucleus of the tractus solitarius and the nucleus ambiguous. Spontaneous discharge in the glossopharyngeal nerve could then cause increased vagal tone, bradycardia, hypotension, syncope, or even asystole. Occasionally, this condition may be painless, presenting with pharyngeal paresthesias, or a tickling sensation, and syncope. Cardiac pacing may be necessary,

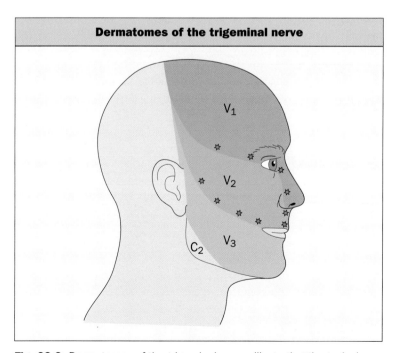

Fig. 23.9 Dermatomes of the trigeminal nerve, illustrating the typical pattern of pain distribution in trigeminal neuralgia.

otherwise the treatment is the same as for trigeminal neuralgia.

OTHER CRANIAL NEURALGIAS

- **Geniculate neuralgia and nervus intermedius neuralgia** cause pain within or just in front of the ear. Geniculate neuralgia may be caused by geniculate herpes (Ramsay Hunt syndrome). Both geniculate neuralgia and nervous intermedius neuralgia may be variants of glossopharyngeal neuralgia.

- **Superior laryngeal neuralgia** is characterized by severe pain in the throat, submandibular region, and under the ear. The pain is sometimes precipitated by swallowing, shouting, or turning the head. This rare condition may follow respiratory tract infections, tonsillectomy, or carotid endarterectomy. The diagnosis is confirmed by local anesthetic blockade of the superior laryngeal nerve. Neurectomy is beneficial when the pain does not respond to medications used in trigeminal neuralgia (Lance, 1993).

- **Charlin's nasociliary neuralgia** is a rare condition characterized by severe paroxysmal pain at the inner angle of the eye and nostril associated with corneal lesions, iridocyclitis, conjunctival injection, nasal congestion, and sweating of the nose or forehead. Pain is relieved by the intranasal application of cocaine (Lance, 1993).

Greater occipital neuralgia is discussed later in this chapter.

HERPES ZOSTER OPHTHALMICUS (HZO)

Herpes zoster (shingles) of the ophthalmic division of the trigeminal nerve causes severe burning pain. Occasionally, patients may have pain typical of 'shingles' but no rash, making the condition difficult to diagnose; this can occur in the uncommon noneruptive variant (zoster sine herpete) and the pre-eruptive stage which may exceed 100 days in duration. HZO is caused by reactivation of the dormant herpes zoster-varicella virus in the gasserian ganglion. Ocular inflammation occurs in 30–50% of patients, and ophthalmoplegia from involvement of one or more of the ocular motor nerves (Lavin *et al.*, 1984) in 5%. Treatment is outlined under 'post-herpetic neuralgia', below.

POST-HERPETIC NEURALGIA

Post-herpetic neuralgia is loosely defined as pain persisting 1 month after the onset of the rash. It occurs in 10% of patients with shingles, but the incidence is higher in older patients, reaching approximately 50% in those aged over 50 years. The pain, similar to that of shingles, is a spontaneous severe and persistent deep burning with increased painful sensitivity to the lightest touch (allodynia) and superimposed tic-like jabs. Post-herpetic neuralgia is difficult to prevent but an effort should be made to treat the initial shingles aggressively. Some recommend a regimen of acyclovir 800 mg 5 times per day for 7–10 days, and prednisone 60 mg daily tapered over 2 weeks (in those not immunocompromised); the efficacy of such a regimen remains unproven.

The initial treatment of post-herpetic neuralgia is with tricyclic agents. Amitriptyline, starting with 50 mg at bedtime and titrating the dose to effectiveness or tolerance, is suggested. Carbamazepine may be added for superimposed tic-like pain, starting at 50 or 100 mg and increasing slowly to effectiveness or tolerance. Mexilitine, clonazepam, phenytoin, and gabapentin are sometimes helpful in patients who do not respond to first line therapy. The efficacy of topical capsaicin is not established. Nonpharmacologic approaches in refractory patients include transcutaneous electrical nerve stimulation (TENS unit), nerve blocks, and a variety of surgical procedures.

GIANT CELL ARTERITIS (TEMPORAL ARTERITIS)

Commonly known as temporal arteritis, giant cell arteritis is a granulomatous disorder that affects medium-sized arteries and can cause myocardial ischemia, gastrointestinal claudication, as well as headache, visual disturbances, jaw claudication (virtually pathognomonic), and occasionally lingual claudication (tongue numbness and pain). It can also cause aortic aneurysms and aortitis by involving the vasa vasorum. Giant cell arteritis is a disease of the elderly (usually over 65 years) but is also reported in the fifth decade. It should be considered in all elderly patients with facial or head pain.

The headache may be localized to the frontal, temporal, or occipital regions, or become generalized. It is severe burning, intractable, and often worse at night. Nodules may be present along the extracranial vessels, particularly the temporal arteries, which can be tender and nonpulsatile. About 85% of patients have polymyalgia rheumatica and other systemic symptoms such as fever, night sweats, neck pain, and weight loss; they may also be anemic. Some may have ischemic radiculopathies, or a 'pseudo-malignant' presentation mimicking cancer. A high index of suspicion should be maintained in older patients with headache or ischemic visual loss, or both. The sedimentation rate is normal in up to 20% of patients.

Giant cell arteritis responds to systemic corticosteroids, though the initial dose is controversial. If visual symptoms are present, many physicians believe the patient should be admitted to hospital, but first given high dose intravenous corticosteroids (methylprednisolone in the range of 500–1000 mg) to avoid any therapeutic delay. A temporal artery biopsy should be performed within the next 48 hours or so, but it must not delay the initiation of treatment.

ASTHENOPIA (EYE STRAIN)

Headache caused by eye strain is over-diagnosed but not uncommon. It occurs in patients with accommodative or convergence insufficiency, or with a significant uncorrected or poorly corrected refractive error (Waltz and Lavin, 1993). Periorbital and retro-orbital aching or discomfort occurs with prolonged activity that requires concentrated visual effort. Eye strain can provoke a tension headache or migraine. Other asthenopic symptoms include blurring, itching, fatigue straining, and tearing. About 50% of patients have a dry eye syndrome.

Accommodative or *ciliary spasm* occurs in young patients, usually with myopia, with psychogenic overlay or conversion reactions. Ciliary spasm may also be triggered by eye strain in patients with hyperopia, presbyopia, ocular inflammation or injury, myotonic pupils (see below), and by topical cholinergic (muscarinic) agonists. Ciliary spasm can cause severe ocular and brow pain.

ADIE'S TONIC PUPIL

Patients with myotonic pupils often develop ocular discomfort due to photophobia because the pupil fails to constrict in bright light. They can also have ocular discomfort, ciliary spasm, or headache from accommodative insufficiency and induced astigmatism (Loewenfeld, 1993). These symptoms usually resolve spontaneously. Refraction, particularly for near work, sun glasses, and occasionally dilute pilocarpine solution (0.1% or less) are helpful.

CORNEAL AND CONJUNCTIVAL DISEASE

Relatively small lesions of the conjunctiva and cornea cause considerable pain because of their rich innervation by pain fibers. Such disorders include the dry eye syndrome, corneal abrasions and ulcers, foreign bodies, recurrent corneal erosion syndrome, blepharitis, and trichiasis.

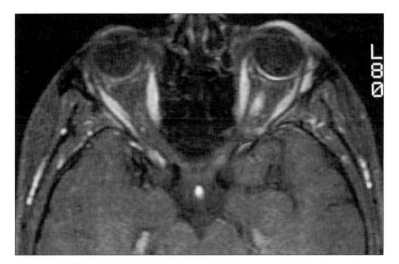

Fig. 23.10 Optic neuritis. Fat-suppressed axial orbital MRI scan demonstrating abnormal signal in the left optic nerve (arrow) in a patient with painful retrobulbar optic neuritis.

OPTIC NEURITIS

Sharp or aching pain above, around, or behind the eye, usually aggravated by ocular movement, was reported by 90% of patients in 'the optic neuritis treatment trial' (Beck *et al.*, 1992). There may also be associated ocular tenderness. Pain may precede visual loss by a couple of days. Ocular pain occurs with both papillitis and retrobulbar optic neuritis. The presumed mechanism is contiguous inflammation of the origins of the medial and superior rectus muscles, which are attached to the optic nerve sheath and the annulus of Zinn at the orbital apex. Tension produced by muscle contraction causes pain on eye movement. Inflammation of the optic nerve may occur with demyelinating optic neuritis (*Fig. 23.10*), inflammatory orbital pseudotumor, posterior scleritis (*Fig. 23.11a, b*), and perioptic neuritis.

OCULAR ISCHEMIC SYNDROME

Gradual occlusion or critical stenosis of the carotid artery, or of the ophthalmic artery or its branches, causes progressive ocular ischemia. This syndrome occurs with degenerative arterial disease and inflammatory disorders such as giant cell and Takayasu's arteritis. Ocular ischemia may cause a persistent ache over the brow, upper face, and temple. Pain and visual impairment may be worse when upright. Occasionally, visual loss increases on exposure to bright light or when a warm stimulus, such as a washcloth, is applied to the face.

The initial features of ocular ischemia mimic chronic uveitis but do not respond to topical anti-inflammatory agents. Other features include poorly reactive pupils, progressive ischemic optic neuropathy, ophthalmoplegia (occasionally), rubeosis iridis, and venous stasis retinopathy, which is occasionally mistaken for early diabetic retinopathy. Low ophthalmodynamometry readings support the diagnosis. Evaluation of the carotid circulation is indicated. Treatment is directed at the underlying disease.

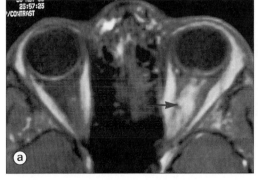
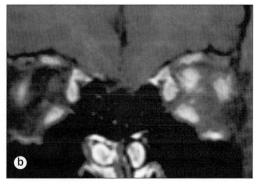
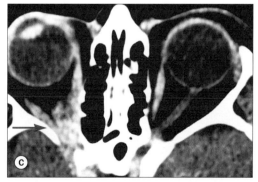

Fig. 23.11 Orbital pseudotumor. (**a**) Fat-suppressed axial orbital MRI scan of a 14-year-old boy with optic neuritis, showing enlargement and increased signal of the left optic nerve (arrow) and of the extraocular muscles. Despite fat suppression, the orbital fat also demonstrates increased signal. (**b**) Coronal view of the same patient, showing enlargement of the extraocular muscles and increased signal from the optic nerve and orbital fat on the left. (**c**) Uncontrasted axial orbital CT scan of a 52-year-old woman with painful ophthalmoplegia and decreased vision in the right eye. The extraocular muscles are enlarged, there is increased density at the apex of the right orbit (arrow), and the sclera is more dense on the right. Interestingly, the patient had a history of the Tolosa–Hunt syndrome affecting the same eye.

ISCHEMIC OPTIC NEUROPATHY

Although the nonarteritic form of anterior ischemic optic neuropathy (AION) is typically painless, some patients (up to 12% in one series – Swartz *et al.*, 1995) complain of ipsilateral head or eye pain. AION, however, is a clinical diagnosis and sometimes difficult to distinguish from demyelinating optic neuropathy.

If patients with AION complain of pain, particularly severe pain, underlying giant cell arteritis and the ocular ischemic syndrome should be considered. Rarely, migraine may be associated with AION.

PHOTOPHOBIA

Photophobia – an abnormal intolerance to light – may be accompanied by ocular discomfort or pain. It occurs in a wide variety of disorders including anterior segment disease, vitreoretinal disease, optic neuropathy, intracranial disease including trauma, infection, inflammation (meningitis and subarachnoid hemorrhage), and stroke. Photophobia is also frequent with migraine, cluster headache, and trigeminal neuralgia. Sometimes, no definite cause can be found (see 'Photo-oculodynia syndrome', below). Photophobia due to iritis or iridocyclitis can be relieved by cycloplegia; when corneal disease is the cause, topical anesthesia is effective. Painless photophobia, the so-called central dazzle syndrome, may occur with posterior circulation strokes, particularly those involving the thalamus, as well as in patients with achromatopsia, albinism, cone disorders, opacities in the ocular media, and even trigeminal sensory neuropathy.

POST-IRITIS PAIN SYNDROME

Patients with painful anterior uveitis may complain of severe photophobia and discomfort long after the active inflammation has cleared. No cause can be found. This may be a variant of the photo-oculodynia syndrome (see below), the deafferentation syndrome, or anesthesia dolorosa (see below). Treatment is controversial.

PHOTO-OCULODYNIA SYNDROME

The cause of the photo-oculodynia syndrome is not established. In some patients it is preceded by minor ocular trauma. Its clinical features are chronic eye pain with no evidence of ongoing tissue damage or inflammation, exquisite light sensitivity, dry eyes, a foreign body sensation, and blepharospasm. The mechanism may be sympathetically maintained pain, similar to reflex sympathetic dystrophy or causalgia in peripheral nerves; ipsilateral cervical sympathetic blockade may relieve symptoms (Fine and Digre, 1995).

REFLEX SYMPATHETIC DYSTROPHY OF THE FACE

This is a rare condition in which chronic facial pain follows injury to one of the branches of the trigeminal nerve, for example, after maxillofacial surgery, dental procedures, or gunshot wounds. The pain manifests as constant burning, tingling, or jabbing, and is exacerbated by minor tactile stimuli or emotional stress.

THYROID ORBITOPATHY (GRAVES' OPHTHALMOPATHY)

Thyroid orbitopathy (*Fig. 23.12*) often causes ocular discomfort and a foreign body sensation. Occasional patients have significant ocular pain that responds to systemic corticosteroids. Sometimes the pain of thyroid orbitopathy resembles trochleitis.

ORBITAL PSEUDOTUMOR

Idiopathic orbital inflammatory disease can affect most orbital tissues, alone or in combination. It causes myositis, dacryoadenitis, periscleritis, posterior scleritis, optic neuritis, optic perineuritis (perioptic neuritis), and diffuse disease involving orbital fat and connective tissue (see Fig. 23.11). Rarely, the disease may extend intracranially or into the paranasal sinuses; conversely, orbital pseudotumor may be exacerbated by concurrent sinus infection. Unlike thyroid ophthalmopathy, which is more common in

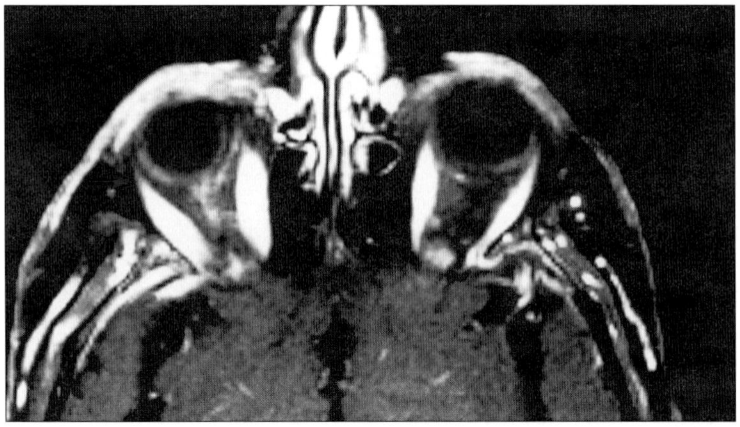

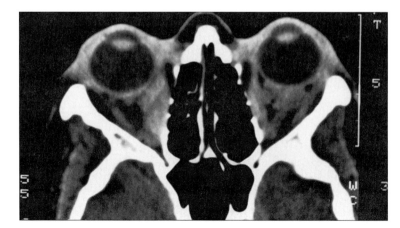

Fig. 23.12 Thyroid orbitopathy. Fat-suppressed axial MRI of the orbits, demonstrating enlargement of the extraocular muscles but sparing of the tendinous insertions (arrow).

Fig. 23.13 Metastases to the extraocular muscles. Contrasted axial CT scan of the orbits in a 51-year-old woman with bilateral involvement of the extraocular muscles and levator palpebral superiorus by metastatic adenocarcinoma from an unknown primary.

women, orbital pseudotumor has no gender preference, and can occur in any age group; it may be bilateral (40%). Orbital pseudotumor can have an acute, relatively short, monophasic course, be relapsing, or be indolent with a prolonged course. The typical features are periorbital, ocular or retro-ocular pain, ophthalmoplegia, proptosis, conjunctival injection, chemosis, and lid swelling. Vision may be decreased if the optic nerve is involved, or distorted (metamorphopsia) if the choroid or posterior sclera are affected. Conjunctival hemorrhage and orbital hematomas can occur. Occasionally, an underlying collagen vascular disease such as polyarteritis nodosa, Wegener's granulomatosis, or Crohn's disease may be responsible. Mollicute infection has been implicated in the chronic form of the disease, but remains controversial. The differential diagnosis of orbital pseudotumor includes real tumors, particularly lymphoma and metastases (*Fig. 23.13*), paraneoplastic orbital myositis (Harris *et al.*, 1994), thyroid orbitopathy, orbital vascular malformations, dural shunt fistulas, and infections such as orbital cellulitis, and, in diabetic patients, mucormycosis. Orbital pseudotumor and the Tolosa–Hunt syndrome (see below) have similarities and may overlap. Occasional patients develop one of these disorders, respond to treatment but later contract the other (see Fig. 23.11c).

A short course of systemic corticosteroid is usually effective. A regimen of prednisone 1 mg/kg daily for 2–4 weeks,

depending on the response, tapering the dose appropriately, is suggested. Some patients, however, require a longer course of prednisone, in which case the minimum effective dose should be used; side effects may prompt the use of more potent immunosuppressive agents such as azothiaprine or cyclophosphamide. Other immunosuppressive agents, nonsteroidal inflammatory agents, rifampin (for reputed mollicute infection), and high voltage orbital irradiation are also used.

PSEUDOTUMOR CEREBRI (IDIOPATHIC INTRACRANIAL HYPERTENSION)

Elevated intracranial pressure causes headache that may awaken, or be worse on waking. Retro-ocular pulsatile migraine-like headaches are common and occasionally facial pain may occur as a result of traction or compression of the trigeminal root over the petrous apex.

Causes of facial pain
All causes of eye pain (see Figures 23.4 and 23.5)
Anesthesia dolorosa
Bell's palsy
Brainstem lesions
Carotidynia
Cervical migraine (basilar migraine)
Dental (abscess, cracked tooth, etc.), neuralgic pain in V_1 and V_2
Eagle's syndrome
Ear disease
Facial reflex sympathetic dystrophy
Facial trauma
First bite syndrome
Glossopharyngeal neuralgia
Gradenigo's syndrome
Idiopathic (atypical) facial pain (suspect structural lesion)
Inferior orbital fissure syndrome
Intracranial hypertension
Lobar hemorrhage
Lower half headache (migraine variant)
Neck–tongue syndrome
Oral mucosal ulceration
Parotid gland disorders (infection, tumor, duct stone, or stricture)
Pre- or noneruptive herpes zoster (V_2 and V_3)
Retropharyngeal tendinitis
Thalamic lesions
Temporomandibular joint syndrome
Trigeminal neuralgia (V_2, V_3)

Fig. 23.14 Causes of facial pain.

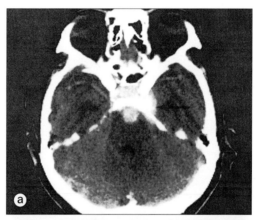

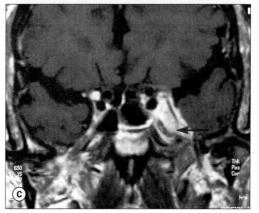

Fig. 23.15
Cavernous sinus tumors. (**a**) Contrasted axial CT scan, showing a meningioma enlarging the left cavernous sinus (arrow) in a middle-aged patient with painful ophthalmoplegia. (**b**) Uncontrasted axial CT scan showing involvement of the orbital apex (upper arrow) and cavernous sinus (lower arrow) by metastatic squamous cell carcinoma in an elderly patient with painful ophthalmoplegia. This neurotrophic tumor spread from the left temple along the branches of the trigeminal nerve, to involve the orbital apex and cavernous sinus. (**c**) Coronal MRI scan showing enlargement of the left cavernous sinus (arrow) in the same patient.

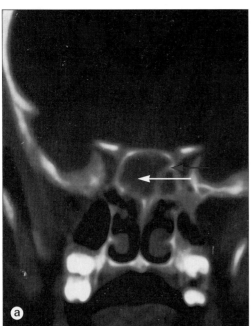

Fig. 23.16
Sphenoid sinusitis.
(a) Coronal CT scan
showing opacification
of the sphenoid sinus
(arrow) in a 16-year-
old boy who
developed cavernous
sinus thrombosis,
blindness, and
ophthalmoplegia.
(b) Axial T2-weighted
MRI scan showing
enlargement and
opacification of the
sphenoid sinus and,
to a lesser extent, of
the ethmoid sinuses
in the same patient.

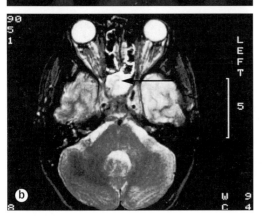

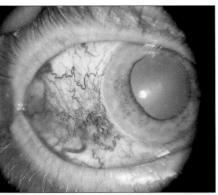

Fig. 23.17
Spontaneous
carotid–cavernous
dural shunt fistula.
(a) Arterialized
conjunctival and
episcleral veins.
(b) Axial MRI scan
showing proptosis
and enlargement of
the superior
ophthalmic vein
(arrow) in the same
patient.

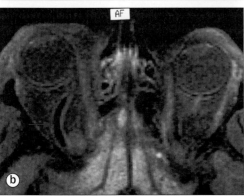

CAVERNOUS SINUS – ORBITAL APEX DISORDERS

Disorders of the parasellar region, cavernous sinus, superior orbital fissure, and orbital apex may be associated with ocular and facial pain (*Fig. 23.14*). Deficits of the ocular motor nerves, the ophthalmic and maxillary divisions of the trigeminal nerve, and the third order oculosympathetic innervation are frequently present. Disorders that occur in this region include tumors (*Fig. 23.15*), aneurysms, carotid–cavernous and dural-shunt fistulas (see below), cavernous sinus thrombosis, inflammation such as sarcoid, rheumatoid nodules, the Tolosa–Hunt syndrome or Wegener's granulomatosis, paranasal sinus disease, and syphilitic periostitis (*Fig. 23.16*).

CAROTID–CAVERNOUS SINUS AND DURAL SHUNT FISTULAS

Communication of the cavernous sinus system with the internal carotid artery, or one of its branches, results in increased pressure in the venous system. Such disorders fall into two major categories: a) direct- or high-flow carotid–cavernous fistulas caused by head injury (closed or penetrating), surgery, or rupture of an intracavernous carotid artery aneurysms; and b) indirect- or low-flow dural shunt fistulas which occur spontaneously, usually in middle-aged women, or following minor closed head injury. The pathogenesis is unclear, but thrombosis of small draining veins from the cavernous sinus may initially elevate the venous pressure and open up congenital connections with meningeal branches of the carotid artery.

The features of both disorders are essentially the same (*Fig. 23.17*), but direct fistulas are much more dramatic in onset and severity, whereas dural shunt fistulas are more insidious and of variable severity. Increased venous pressure causes congestion and progressive ischemia of the eye and other orbital contents, resulting in pain, proptosis, chemosis, arterialization of the conjunctival and episcleral vessels, ophthalmoplegia (ocular motor neuropathy or extraocular muscle congestion/ischemia), increased intraocular pressure, and venous stasis retinopathy. Rarely, an intracranial venous varix may rupture causing a catastrophic neurologic deficit.

Dural shunt fistulas may mimic thyroid ophthalmopathy, conjunctivitis (see Fig. 23.17), and orbital pseudotumor.

THE TOLOSA–HUNT SYNDROME

The clinical features of the Tolosa–Hunt syndrome (THS) are periorbital pain and ophthalmoplegia, in the absence of an identifiable cause. The THS, also called superior orbital fissuritis, is attributed to nonspecific granulomatous inflammation in the cavernous sinus–superior orbital fissure region (on the basis of a postmortem study of Tolosa's original patient in 1954). Phlebitis of the superior ophthalmic vein or anterior cavernous sinus has also been implicated.

The pain is described as severe gnawing and boring. Ophthalmoplegia is caused by involvement of one or more of the ocular motor nerves and can precede or be concurrent with the onset of pain. The concept that ophthalmoplegic migraine is a variant of THS is controversial (Daroff, 1995). Angiography may show narrowing of the carotid artery near the siphon and MRI

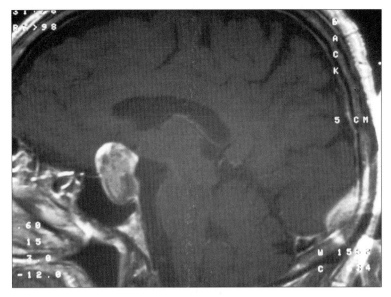

Fig. 23.18 Pituitary apoplexy. Sagittal MRI scan showing marked enlargement of the pituitary gland and sella with mixed signal, indicative of hemorrhagic infarction.

Raeder's paratrigeminal syndrome	
Type I	Postganglionic Horner's syndrome, pain, multiple cranial nerve deficit (III, IV, V, VI)
	suspect parasellar mass
Type IIA	Postganglionic Horner's syndrome, intermittent pain, no objective cranial nerve deficit
	cluster headache
	severe recurrent migraine
Type IIB	Postganglionic Horner's syndrome, persistent pain (weeks to months), with or without V^1 deficit
	carotid artery dissection
	carotid fibromuscular dysplasia
	idiopathic (possible Tolosa–Hunt syndrome variant)
	sphenoid sinusitis

Fig. 23.19 Approach to Raeder's paratrigeminal syndrome. (Modified from Grimson and Thompson, 1980)

may show abnormal signal in the cavernous sinus–superior orbital fissure region. The pain responds to systemic high-dose corticosteroids, usually within 48 hours. This response was once considered diagnostic, but is not specific. Aneurysms, fistulas, and tumors in the cavernous sinus region may mimic both the clinical features and corticosteroid responsiveness of THS, and must be excluded.

IDIOPATHIC CRANIAL PACHYMENINGITIS

Unexplained pachymeningitis associated with cranial neuropathies can cause periorbital pain or headache, or both. The mechanism of this condition is not established, but systemic corticosteroid therapy is beneficial (Masson *et al.*, 1993). Idiopathic cranial pachymeningitis may be one part of a larger inflammatory disorder such as Wegener's granulomatosis (Newman *et al.*, 1995), polychondritis, a variant of THS, or infections such as HTLV-1 infection, syphilis, or TB. Continued vigilance for infectious, granulomatous, or neoplastic disease must be maintained until the illness resolves.

PITUITARY APOPLEXY

Pituitary adenomas rarely cause headache unless they expand beyond the confines of the sella. Pituitary apoplexy can cause eye pain or headache when the tumor expands abruptly, as a result of infarction or hemorrhage (*Fig. 23.18*), into the adjacent cavernous sinus and impinges on pain-sensitive structures including the ocular motor and trigeminal nerves; it may also cause generalized headache as a result of chemical meningitis. Compression of the parasympathetic pupillomotor fibers in the oculomotor nerve is a rare cause of eye pain when mydriasis precipitates narrow angle glaucoma.

RAEDER'S PARATRIGEMINAL SYNDROME

The term Raeder's paratrigeminal syndrome is confusing because it is often applied loosely and incorrectly in clinical practice. It is discussed here for purposes of reference and for historic reasons.

In 1924 Raeder described five patients with varying degrees of facial pain and oculosympathetic paresis that spared facial sweating. Two patients did not have pain, one did not have ptosis, and some had other cranial nerve deficits. Raeder localized the clinical features to the paratrigeminal region. One patient had a meningioma, two had trauma to the base of the skull, one a presumed basal skull tumor, and one had no apparent cause. The original group of patients did not have a single disease or syndrome and the same is true of subsequent reports.

Raeder's syndrome has since been described with brain tumors, a carotid body tumor, aneurysms, migraine, inflammatory conditions including sinusitis, dental abscess, chronic otitis media, lobar pneumonia, syphilitic otitis, following trauma, and carotid dissection. Many patients with Raedar's syndrome have other identifiable disorders such as cluster headache, cavernous sinus tumors, hemicrania continua, and THS. The term Raedar's paratrigeminal syndrome is best discarded, but if used should fit the criteria provided in *Figure 23.19*.

GRADENIGO'S SYNDROME

In 1904, Gradenigo described the combination of ipsilateral facial pain and abducens palsy in patients with otitis media that extended medially to cause osteitis of the petrous temporal apex. The abducens nerve is injured where it crosses over the inferior petrosal sinus, presumably because of thrombophlebitis. Gnawing or throbbing pain, which is worse at night, is localized to the eye, ear, frontal, parietal, or temporal regions, or sometimes to the distribution of the whole trigeminal nerve. With the

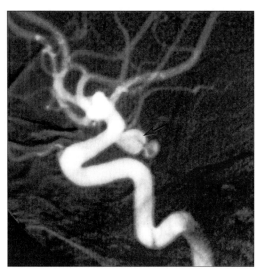

Fig. 23.20
Aneurysm. Lateral view of carotid arteriogram of a woman with a painful third nerve palsy and a dilated unreactive pupil demonstrating a lobulated aneurysm (arrow) of the internal carotid artery at the posterior communicating artery.

availability of effective antibiotics Gradenigo's syndrome has become less common; however, it may be mimicked by neoplasms, including clivus chordomas, nasopharyngeal carcinoma, and other tumors in the petrous temporal area. It can also occur when tumors, such as lymphoma, block the eustachian tube and cause secondary otitis media, or be mimicked by malignant external otitis in diabetic patients.

OCULAR MOTOR PALSIES

Isolated ocular motor neuropathies, whether a result of microvascular disease or compression by an aneurysm or tumor (*Fig. 23.20*), frequently cause ocular pain. The mechanism is believed to be involvement of either afferent trigeminal fibers in the affected ocular motor nerve, or involvment of the meninges, innervated by twigs from the first division of the trigeminal nerve, that cover the ocular motor nerves. Occasionally, a painful ocular motor palsy, with no signs of orbital congestion, may be caused by a posteriorly draining dural shunt fistula, the so-called 'white-eyed shunt'.

BELL'S PALSY

Bell's palsy is associated with pain in the ear, mastoid region, angle of the jaw, or occasionally the face. The pain is more severe when geniculate herpes (Ramsay Hunt syndrome) is responsible; vesicles may be seen in the external auditory canal, posterior auricle, or fauces.

TEMPOROMANDIBULAR JOINT SYNDROME (COSTEN'S SYNDROME)

Temporomandibular joint (TMJ) dysfunction is overdiagnosed as the cause of headache and facial pain. The characteristic features of the TMJ syndrome are jaw pain precipitated by movement, asymmetrical or limited jaw opening, joint tenderness, and crepitus over the TMJ during movement. The pain may also be experienced in the ear, face, periorbital region, or temple.

TMJ pain may be associated with bruxism and spasm of the temporalis and masseter muscles; the spasm may become more widespread and cause tension headache and even neck and upper limb pain. The incidence of malocclusion, bruxism, and TMJ derangement is high in patients who do not complain of such pain, suggesting other factors play a role.

TMJ syndrome may be mistaken for, or provoke, migraine or tension headache, and must be distinguished from the jaw claudication associated with giant cell arteritis (GCA), and other disorders such as tooth abscess and osteomyelitis, or neoplastic involvement of the jaw.

Management strategies include relaxation therapy, bite plates for malocclusion, physical therapy, tricyclic antidepressants, and avoidance of narcotics and of excessive use of nonprescription analgesics which often cause chronic daily (analgesic rebound) headache. If these measures fail, consultation with an oral surgeon or an appropriate specialist is suggested.

PAROTID GLAND REGION PAIN

Pain in the parotid region occurs with denervation, such as the first bite syndrome (see below), infection, stones, and tumors involving the gland. Treatment is directed at the cause.

FIRST BITE SYNDROME

A short, severe, spasm-like pain near the angle of the mandible, following the first bite of each meal, can occur in patients with sympathetic denervation of the parotid gland (Netterville *et al.*, 1994). The pain occurs a few seconds after the stimulus, particularly with strong sialagogues, and lasts about a half minute; it may occur with other salivary stimuli such as the sight or smell of food. Most patients in Netterville's series had ipsilateral cervical or skull-based surgery for resection of lesions including cervical paragangliomas, carotid body tumors, vagal paragangliomas, high cervical schwannomas, parapharyngeal space tumors, or a radical neck dissection; one patient had a Horner's syndrome following a gunshot wound injuring the ipsilateral carotid artery and sympathetic trunk. Netterville's group believe that the pain occurs when the parotid duct myoepithelial cells contract excessively on exposure to strong salivary stimuli, as a result of postganglionic sympathetic denervation hypersensitivity. They also found neurolysis of the preganglionic parasympathetic fibers to the tympanic plexus an effective treatment, although pain recurred in some patients after a year. Similar parotid pain occurs in patients with diffuse autonomic neuropathy; normal subjects may occasionally experience a mild form of such pain on exposure to strong sialagogues. Treatment of first bite syndrome includes dietary modification, carbamazepine, and surgery.

INFERIOR ORBITAL FISSURE SYNDROME

Pain, with or without sensory change, in the distribution of the second division of the trigeminal nerve, associated with an ipsilateral dry eye syndrome, may occur when the parasympathetic innervation of the lacrimal gland and maxillary nerve are injured by skull-based tumors (particularly those arising from the posterior maxillary sinus) in the inferior orbital fissure/pterygopala-

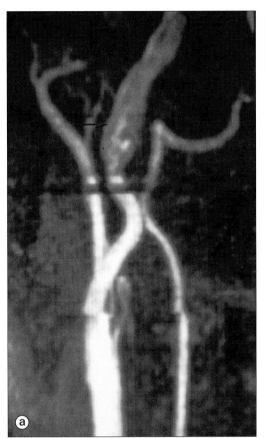 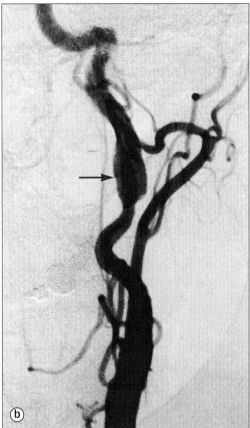 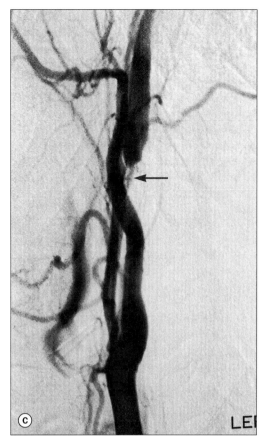

Fig. 23.21 Dissection of the internal carotid artery. (**a**) MR angiogram showing the dissection of the distal internal carotid artery and a false aneurysm (arrow). (**b**) Carotid arteriogram also showing the dissection and false aneurysm (arrow). (**c**) Arteriogram showing the 'string' sign (arrow) and the false aneurysm.

tine fossa region. The parasympathetic innervation to the lacrimal gland arises in the superior salivary nucleus and travels, via the facial nerve, geniculate ganglion, greater petrosal nerve, and vidian nerve, to synapse in the sphenopalatine ganglion in the pterygopalatine fossa. The course of the postsynaptic fibers is not established, but they probably reach the lacrimal gland via the maxillary and zygomaticotemporal nerves. Some fibers may extend through the inferior orbital fissure.

DENTAL PAIN

Dental disease, particularly in upper jaw teeth, can cause pain in the cheek, temple, or peri-orbital region. Periodontoid abscesses and cracked teeth may not be recognized, and the referred pain may prompt consultation with an ophthalmologist or neuro-ophthalmologist. Tenderness on tapping the suspected tooth, or sensitivity to cold or sweet foods, indicates the correct source of the pain.

CAROTID ARTERY DISSECTION

Arterial dissection – a separation of the layers of the vessel wall, usually between the internal elastic lamina and media – occurs following direct trauma or a traction injury. 'Spontaneous' dissection also occurs in patients with fibromuscular dysplasia, degenerative vascular disease, and disorders with defective collagen, such as Ehlers–Danlos and Marfan's syndromes.

Typically, the pain of carotid artery dissection is ipsilateral frontotemporal, orbital, and facial (particularly the lower jaw), and frequently involves the lower jaw, neck, and posterior auricular region. The pain usually clears within 72 hours, but can last months to years. Over half the patients have a postganglionic Horner's syndrome. Dysgeusia, pulsatile tinnitus, and involvement of the lower cranial nerves may occur; rarely, ocular motor nerves may be involved (Silbert *et al.*, 1995). The dissection narrows the lumen and may result in local thrombosis and embolism causing amaurosis fugax (25%) and hemispheric transient ischemic attacks (TIAs) or stroke (50%) which usually occur within 2 days of the onset of the pain. Sometimes, patients may present with eye pain alone.

The diagnosis of carotid artery dissection can be confirmed with ultrasound or angiography (MRA; *Fig. 23.21a*), but may require conventional angiography (*Fig. 23.21b,c*). Occasionally, when the dissection is subadventitial, conventional arteriography is normal but MRI/MRA of the skull base/upper neck region confirms the diagnosis (Mayville *et al.*, 1996). Management is controversial, but antiplatelet agents, anticoagulant therapy, and surgical intervention are options.

Vertebral artery dissection causes occipital headache, neck pain, and vertebrobasilar ischemic events, and has a higher risk of subarachnoid hemorrhage than carotid artery dissection.

CAROTIDYNIA

The features of carotidynia are unilateral, deep-seated neck pain associated with tenderness and/or swelling of the carotid artery. The pain can radiate to the ear and face, and may be aggravated by head movement, swallowing, chewing, coughing, yawning, and sneezing (Biousse and Bousser, 1994). Other criteria for the diagnosis include increased pulsations of the carotid artery, a duration of 2 weeks or less, and exclusion of other causes.

The symptom complex of neck pain and carotid artery tenderness may occur with several conditions, many of which benefit from specific treatment: lymphadenitis, giant cell arteritis, aphthous ulcers, dental infection, Eagle's syndrome, migraine, cluster headache, carotid occlusion, carotid dissection, carotid body tumors, malignant infiltration, and even muscle strain syndromes involving the neck. Biousse and Bousser (1994) have challenged the existence of 'carotidynia'; rather, the symptom complex should prompt the physician to consider the above disorders.

Rarely, acute idiopathic 'carotidynia' occurs in young or middle-aged adults and lasts 10–14 days. The only physical finding is carotid artery tenderness. The sedimentation rate is usually normal. A viral etiology is considered, but not established. Treatment is symptomatic, with simple analgesics, nonsteroidal anti-inflammatory agents, and occasionally corticosteroids.

One to 3 days after *carotid endarterectomy* some patients may complain of intense ipsilateral vascular headache in the frontotemporal area. The headache can recur intermittently for a number of months.

EAGLE'S SYNDROME

Eagle's syndrome, or stylalgia, is a cervicofacial pain caused by an elongated styloid process or mineralization of the stylohyoid complex. The clinical features are dysphagia and a dull, unilateral, nagging non-lancinating pain, which can radiate to the ear and is aggravated by swallowing. The elongated styloid process may be palpated below the angle of the mandible or in the posterior pharynx. The condition sometimes follows tonsillectomy. Treatment is usually surgical (Montalbetti *et al.*, 1995).

GREATER OCCIPITAL NEURALGIA

Greater occipital neuralgia (GON) causes pain in the occipital region that radiates to the eye. It is aggravated by stooping and reproduced by pressing on the greater or lesser occipital nerves just lateral to the midline under the occiput. The pressure may also cause pain in the eyebrow, orbit, temple, and occasionally down the back or arm. Lacrimation may cause blurring of vision. GON is more common in women with cervical spondylosis or following whiplash injury. 'Normal' tenderness should be distinguished from 'pathologic' tenderness by comparing each side. The diagnosis is confirmed by relief of pain following injection of 2% lidocaine into the area of maximal tenderness. Prolonged relief follows injection of lidocaine mixed with corticosteroids. The greater occipital nerve is usually located about 1.5 cm below the occipital ridge and 5 to 8 cm from the midline. Some patients obtain permanent relief by one injection, others require further injections.

NECK–TONGUE SYNDROME

Sudden rotation of the neck causes sharp pain in the upper neck or occipital region, sometimes accompanied by numbness or tingling in the same area and the ipsilateral half of the tongue (Lance, 1993). The pain and numbness last about 10 s, occasionally up to a minute. The hypothetical mechanism for this syndrome is as follows: afferent fibers from the tongue travel from the lingual nerve via the hypoglossal nerve to the second cervical root; symptoms occur when the ventral ramus of the second cervical root is stretched over the atlantoaxial joint during neck rotation. Subluxation of atlantoaxial joint can produce similar symptoms as the joint is innervated by the second cervical nerve. A comparable syndrome occurs in patients with cervical spondylosis, ankylosing spondylitis, or psoriatic arthropathy. The neck–tongue syndrome also occurs in patients with genetically predisposed ligament laxity.

CERVICOGENIC HEADACHE

Cervicogenic headache, similar to GON and *third occipital nerve headache*, causes a unilateral, continuous, boring, upper neck and occipital pain, which may radiate to the frontal, temporal, ocular regions or even upper limb. It is more common in women. Associated features are lacrimation, blurred vision, conjunctival injection, and lid edema, but not Horner's syndrome. The pain can be reproduced by neck movement. It does not respond to indomethacin, distinguishing it from hemicrania continua and chronic paroxysmal hemicrania (cluster). The pain is relieved by paracervical blockade of the second or third cervical root.

CERVICAL MIGRAINE

In 1925, Barré reported a syndrome of head and neck pain caused by injury to the cervical sympathetic system (the vertebral nerve) by cervical spondylosis. It was later called the *posterior cervical sympathetic syndrome of Barré–Liéou*. The pain may be unilateral or bilateral, and affects almost any part of the face, head, or neck. Its quality can be throbbing, burning, stinging, pricking, or creeping. Associated features are dizziness, tinnitus, blurred vision, and scintillations. The pain may be precipitated by sudden neck movements, coughing, sneezing, pressure on the neck muscles, or stress. This syndrome overlaps cervicogenic headache, GON, third occipital nerve headache, and vertebrobasilar migraine. Each patient should be managed accordingly.

RETROPHARYNGEAL TENDONITIS

This rare condition causes pain in the back of the neck or head that is aggravated by neck movement, particularly extension or rotation, and swallowing. It may be associated with pharyngeal swelling, fever, and sometimes an elevated sedimentation rate. Retropharyngeal tendonitis is self limited and responds to nonsteroidal anti-inflammatory agents. Osteomyelitis and retropharyngeal abscess must be excluded.

FACIAL TRAUMA

Cutaneous branches of the trigeminal nerve, particularly the supraorbital and infraorbital nerves, may be compressed by scar tissue following facial injury, causing chronic frontal headache or facial pain. Exacerbation of the pain by palpation over the scar confirms the diagnosis. Sensory loss may be present in the appropriate nerve distribution. When the inferior orbital nerve is injured in an orbital blow-out fracture, vertical diplopia may also be present as a result of extraocular muscle entrapment or contusion.

ANESTHESIA DOLOROSA

Anesthesia dolorosa results from injury to a sensory nerve, usually following a surgical procedure or trauma. Despite numbness of the deafferented area, the patient experiences severe, intractable burning pain similar to that of post-herpetic neuralgia. Pain management is comparable to that used for post-herpetic neuralgia. Deafferentation pain also occurs following central neural injury such as stroke.

BRAINSTEM AND THALAMIC PAIN

Injury to the nociceptive fibers in the trigeminal pathways of the brainstem or the VPM nucleus of the thalamus (see Fig. 23.2) can cause ocular or facial pain. Underlying disorders include stroke, tumor, syrinx, encephalitis, arteriovenous malformation (AVM), abscess, and demyelination. Thalamic stroke may be followed by persistent burning pain that is difficult to manage (Dejerine–Roussy syndrome). Tricyclic agents, carbamazepine, phenytoin, clonazepam, mexilitine, L-Dopa, and the combination of propranolol and doxepin, have been used with various degrees of success. Gabapentin may be helpful.

HEADACHE IN CEREBRAL LOBAR HEMORRHAGE

The usual features of intracranial hemorrhage are the abrupt onset of headache, vomiting, severe neurologic dysfunction, seizures, and obtundation that often progresses to coma. Patients with small lobar hematomas may complain only of focal headache (see Fig. 23.1).

CARDIAC PAIN

Pain of cardiac origin can be referred to a variety of areas including the neck, jaw, upper limb, back, epigastrium, and testes. It can also affect the bregma, brow, ear, nose, palate, tongue, mastoid or occipital regions, and, rarely, either eye. The mechanism is most likely referred pain via the shared autonomic nerve supply.

FACIAL PAIN AND LUNG CANCER

Patients with carcinoma of the lung occasionally complain of ipsilateral facial pain that is usually deep and aching and more often on the right side. The pain is typically severe, with paroxysmal worsening lasting minutes, and is located in or around the ear, but may involve the cheek, jaw, or eye. Some of these patients are diagnosed with 'atypical facial pain' (see below), particularly because neurologic investigations (MRI and CSF analysis) are usually normal; important clues are ear pain, recent weight loss, digital clubbing, and respiratory findings. Radiologic hypertropic osteoarthropathy is often present. Treatment of the tumor, either by surgery or irradiation, usually resolves the facial pain (Bongers, 1992). The pain is most likely referred to the face via the vagus nerve.

FAMILIAL RECTAL PAIN

In 1959, Hayden and Grossman described a family who suffered episodes of burning rectal pain followed by flushing of the legs. Ocular pain provoked by cold wind, or jaw pain triggered by the sight of food, can be associated (Schubert and Cracco, 1992). Carbamazepine may alleviate the paroxysms of pain.

IDIOPATHIC (ATYPICAL) FACIAL PAIN

The term atypical facial pain is used to describe persistent facial pain with no apparent cause in patients with a normal physical examination. It implies a psychogenic origin and should be abandoned in favor of idiopathic facial pain, or, more honestly, *facial pain of unknown origin*. A dental abscess, cracked tooth, nasopharyngeal carcinoma, or other tumor is eventually found in many patients with atypical facial pain.

Patients with early or mild organic brain disease, many of whom have affective or personality disorders, amplify symptoms to a distracting degree, with unfortunate consequences. Rare patients are encountered, usually with other features of mental illness, who have facial pain that is inexplicable, diffuse, persistent, of mixed character, crosses the midline, and may even involve other parts of the body. It may be associated with unusual odontalgia (continuous throbbing hypersensitivity) that improves with eating or drinking, a burning tongue (see below), a dry mouth, or intolerance to dentures. Psychogenic facial pain is not a diagnosis of exclusion; it requires positive psychiatric features.

Another variant of unexplained eye pain occurs in patients who may mutilate a seeing eye. The author examined two patients with apparently healthy eyes, who both successfully demanded enucleation for intractable but unexplained ocular pain following remote injury. The patients were believed to have deep-rooted psychiatric reasons for their demands (*'If thine eye offends thee, pluck it out.'*).

THE BURNING MOUTH SYNDROME

This is a poorly understood disorder in which patients complain of dysgeusia, and a burning or prickling sensation of the mouth and tongue, in the absence of an obvious cause (Lamey, 1996). Patients tend to be women and are usually post-menopausal. Irritants and allergic reactions may play a role. Tricyclic agents are often helpful.

Further reading

Appenzeller O, Becker WJ, Ragaz A. Cluster headache ultrastructural aspects and pathogenic mechanisms. *Archives of Neurology.* 1981;**38**:302–308.

Beck RW, Cleary PA, Anderson MA, *et al.* A randomized controlled trial of corticosteroids in the treatment of acute optic neuritis. *New Engl J Med.* 1992;**326**:581–588.

Biousse V, Bousser MG. The myth of carotidynia. *Neurology.* 1994;**44**:993–995.

Blau JN, Engel H. Episodic paroxysmal hemicrania: A further case and a review of the literature. *J Neurol Neurosurg Psychiat.* 1990;**53**:343–344.

Bongers KM, Willigers HMM, Koehler PJ. Referred pain from lung carcinoma. *Neurology.* 1992;**42**:1841–1842.

Bordino C, Antonaci F, Stovner LC, Schrader H, Sjaastad O. 'Hemicrania continua': A clinical review. *Headache.* 1991;**31**:20–26.

Bullitt E, Tew JM, Boyd J. Intracranial tumors in patients with facial pain. *J Neurosurg.* 1986;**64**:865–871.

Daroff RB. The eye and headache: The 1994 Cumings lecture. *Headache Quarterly Current Treatment and Research.* 1995;**6(2)**:89–96.

Fine PG, Digre KB. A controlled trial of regional sympatholysis in the treatment of photo-oculodynia syndrome. *J Neuro-Ophthalmol.* 1995;**15(2)**:90–94.

Grimson BS, Thompson HS. Raeder's syndrome. A clinical review. *Surv Ophthalmol.* 1980;**24(4)**:199–210.

Gutrecht JA, Lessell IM. Photophobia in trigeminal neuralgia. *J Neuro-Ophthalmol.* 1994;**14(2)**:122–123.

Harris GJ, Murphy ML, Schmidt EW, Hanson GA, Dotson RM. Orbital myositis as a paraneoplastic syndrome. *Arch Ophthalmol.* 1994;**112**:380–386.

Katusic S, Beard CM, Bergstralh E, Kurland LT. Incidence and clinical features of trigeminal neuralgia in Rochester, MN. 1945–1984. *Ann Neurol.* 1990;**27**:89–95.

Lamey PJ. Burning Mouth Syndrome. *Dermatologic Clinics.* 1996; **14**:339–354.

Lance JW. *Mechanism and management of headache, 5th edn.* (London: Butterworth-Heinemann, 1993)

Lavin PJM, Younkin SG, Kori SH. The pathology of ophthalmoplegia in herpes zoster ophthalmicus. *Neuro-Ophthalmology.* 1984;**4(2)**:75–80.

Lew D, Southwick FS, Montgomery WW, Weber AL, Baker AS. Sphenoid sinusitis. A review of 30 cases. *New Engl J Med.* 1983;**309**:1149–1154.

Loewenfeld IE. *The Pupil* (Ames: Iowa State University Press, 1993)

Masson C, Henin D, Hauw JJ, *et al.* Cranial pachymeningitis of unknown origin: A study of seven cases. *Neurology.* 1993;**43**:1329–1334.

Mayville CL, Warner JS, Lavin PJM. Case histories from the Vanderbilt Headache Clinic. *Headache Quarterly;* 1996 (in press).

Montalbetti L, Ferrandi D, Pergami P, Savoldi F. Elongated styloid process and Eagle's syndrome. *Cephalgia.* 1995;**15**:80–93.

Moskowitz MA. The neurobiology of vascular head pain. *Ann Neurol.* 1984;**16**:157–168.

Netterville JL, Charous SJ, Suen JY, Lavertu P, Armstrong WB. The first bite syndrome. Abstract: American Society for Head and Neck Surgery, 12, 1994.

Newman LC, Lipton RB, Solomon S. Hemicrania continua: Ten new cases and a review of the literature. *Neurology.* 1994;**44**:2111–2114.

Newman NJ, Slamovits TL, Friedland S, Wilson WB. Neuro-ophthalmologic manifestations of meningocerebral inflammation from the limited form of Wegener's granulomatosis. *Am J Ophthalmol.* 1995;**120**:613–621.

O'Donnell L, Martin EA. Cephalgia fugax: a momentary headache. *Brit Med J.* 1986; **292(6521)**: 663–664.

Reder AT, Arnason BGW. Trigeminal neuralgia in multiple sclerosis relieved by a prostaglandin-E analogue. *Neurology.* 1995;**45**:1097–1100.

Schubert R, Cracco JB. Familial rectal pain: A type of reflex epilepsy. *Ann Neurol.* 1992;**32**:824–826.

Silbert PL, Mokri B, Schievink WI. Headache and neck pain in spontaneous internal carotid and vertebral artery dissections. *Neurology.* 1995;**45**:1517–1522.

Spiegel ??, Spiegel ??. Trance and Treatment. (New York: Basic Books Inc., 1978) 251–262.

Waltz KL, Lavin PJM. Accommodative insufficiency. In: Margo CE, Mames RN, Hamed L, eds. *Diagnostic Problems in Clinical Ophthalmology* (Philadelphia: WB Saunders Co., 1993) 862–866.

CHAPTER 24

Cerebral Visual Dysfunction

Matthew Rizzo

INTRODUCTION

The human visual cortex includes Brodmann's areas 17, 18, and 19 of the occipital lobe, located above and below the calcarine fissure, and primarily on the mesial surface of the brain (*Fig. 24.1b*). The visual cortex also includes portions of occipital areas 18 and 19 and of the adjacent parietal and temporal cortex located in areas 5, 7, and 39, and area 37 on the lateral surface of the brain (*Fig. 24.1a*).

Damage to these areas produces a variety of complaints. A cerebrovascular lesion in the distribution of the posterior cerebral artery is the most common cause but tumors, trauma, Alzheimer's disease, and infectious conditions are also important. The resulting visual dysfunction can be considered in the light of recent concepts of primate vision, which postulate multiple cortical maps that process the inputs from 'parallel' subcortical pathways.

PARALLEL PATHWAYS

The parallel processing of visual information begins in the primate retina. Retinal ganglion cells with rapid response properties form the 'M' channel, which connects with the primary visual cortex (also known as the striate cortex, calcarine cortex, Brodmann's area 17, or area V_1) via magnocellular (M) layers 1 and 2 of the lateral geniculate nucleus (LGN). The 'P' channel arises from color-opponent ganglion cells and connects with area V_1 via parvocellular (P) layers 3–6 of the LGN.

Human M- or P-type defects have been postulated in developmental dyslexia, amblyopia, glaucoma, optic neuritis, and even Alzheimer's disease. M-pathway damage should impair flicker and motion perception but spare visual acuity and color, whereas P-pathway damage should affect acuity and color, sparing flicker and motion. However, these distinctions are rarely clean-cut. One factor is the distribution of pathologic lesions, and another is the likelihood of 'cross-talk' between parallel pathways (Merigan and Maunsell, 1993).

MULTIPLE MAPS IN THE VISUAL CORTEX

The monkey's visual cortex is thought to contain dozens of different specialized maps, as depicted in *Figure 24.2*.

Area V_1 is the direct recipient of the M and P pathways and connects with extrastriate areas V_2 and V_3 and surrounding regions in the visual association cortex. It also connects with area V_4 and the middle temporal (MT) area (also called V_5). The V_4 complex receives both M and P inputs, projects ventrally towards the inferotemporal cortex (IT) area, and operates in color and pattern perception. The MT complex receives a predominance of M inputs, projects dorsally toward the parieto-occipital regions, and plays a key role in the perception of movement (*Fig. 24.3*). Although there are differences in brain size and topography between monkeys and humans, human cortical visual disorders may be interpreted in terms of damage to homologous areas.

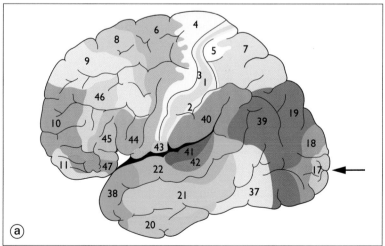

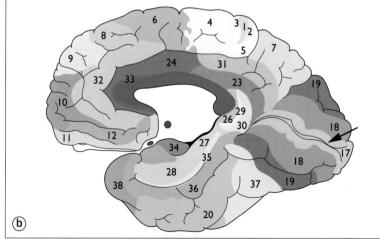

Fig. 24.1 Brodmann (1909) depicted the cytoarchitectural boundaries of the human brain on the lateral surface of the left hemisphere (**a**) and on the mesial surface of a corresponding right hemisphere (**b**). In each view, the calcarine fissure is indicated by an arrow. Area 17, the primary visual cortex (also known as functional area V_1), is almost entirely mesial. It is symmetrically distributed above and below the calcarine fissure and is concentrically surrounded by early visual association cortex areas 18 and 19. Visual areas on the lateral brain include functional maps in areas 5, 7, 39, 37, and superior 19.

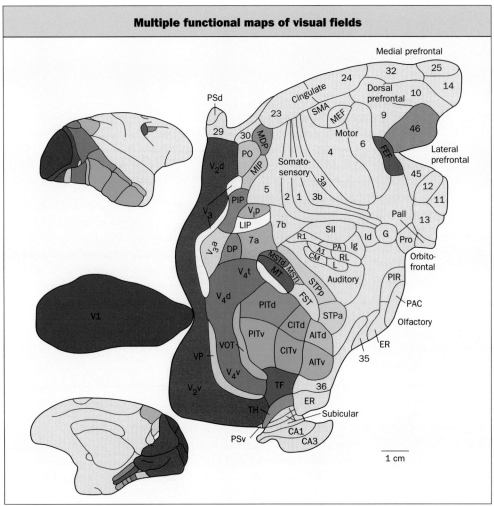

Multiple functional maps of visual fields

Fig. 24.2 In the main illustration the monkey's cortex is unfolded and splayed flat to reveal multiple functional maps of the visual fields in the monkey's brain. (Courtesy of Felleman DJ, Van Essen DC. *Cerebral Cortex* 1991;**1**:1–47) The insets on the upper and lower left show the location of these maps on the lateral and mesial hemispheric views. Human cortex is also likely to contain multiple maps but with differences related to brain size and topography. For example, area V_1, which corresponds to Brodmann's area 17, is much more laterally located in the monkey than in the human (see Fig. 24.1).

Deficit magnitude after PLGN, MLGN, V₄, and MT lesions

Function		PLGN	MLGN	V_4	MT
Color vision		severe	none	moderate	none
Texture perception		severe	none	mild	none
Pattern perception		severe	none	moderate	none
Shape perception:	fine	severe	none	mild	none
	coarse	mild	none	mild	none
Brightness perception		none	none		none
Coarse scotopic vision		none	none		none
Contrast sensitivity:	fine	severe	none	mild	mild
	coarse	mild	none	none	mild
Stereopsis:	fine	severe	none	none	none
	coarse	pronounced	none	none	none
Motion perception		none	moderate	none	moderate
Flicker perception		none	severe	none	pronounced

Fig. 24.3 Schiller and Logothetis (1990) summarized the different patterns of functional impairments caused by lesions of the P and M layers of the lateral geniculate nucleus (LGN), area V_4, and the middle temporal area (MT). An important research issue is whether lesions of homologous structures in the human brain produce similar patterns of impairment. (PLGN, parvocellular layer of the LGN; MLGN, magnocellular layer of the LGN; 'non' indicates no deficit.) (Courtesy of Schiller PH, Logothetis NK. *TINS.* 1990;**11**:392–398.)

DAMAGE TO AREA V₁

Focal damage to human area V_1 causes a scotoma: an area of visual loss surrounded by preserved vision. Patients have no conscious awareness of seeing in a V_1 scotoma, suggesting that human area V_1 functions as a critical bottleneck for ascending subcortical (M and P) inputs. There may be residual vision called 'blindsight' mediated by subcortical structures such as the superior colliculus, but this is rudimentary and uncommon.

V_1-type defects are 'homonymous' and 'congruent', meaning they occupy the same hemifield in each eye and the defects in the two eyes are nearly identical when superimposed. These visual defects fall opposite to the side of the V_1 lesion because the lens of each eye reverses the image cast on the retina and because the nasal fibers of the optic nerves subsequently cross (decussate) in the optic chiasm.

Damage to macular representation in area V_1 causes trouble at the fixation point, a 'central scotoma' (*Fig. 24.4a*), or nearby,

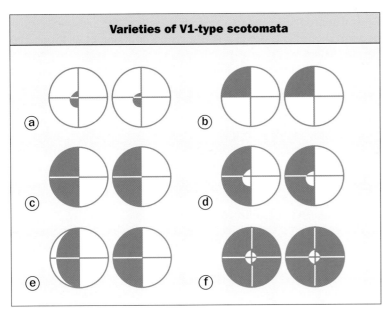

Varieties of V1-type scotomata

Fig. 24.4 Varieties of V_1-type scotomata are depicted. (**a**) Left homonymous central hemi-scotoma. (**b**) Left homonymous superior quadrantanopia. (**c**) Complete left homonymous hemianopia. (**d**) Left homonymous hemianopia with 'macular sparing'. (**e**) Left homonymous hemianopia with sparing of the 'monocular temporal crescent' of vision. (**f**) Double homonymous hemianopia with foveal and macular sparing and residual 'keyhole' vision. These patterns of impairment are often combined with visual deficits caused by lesions of the visual association cortex beyond V_1.

a 'paracentral scotoma'. Such defects may interfere with ocular fixation, scanning, and the ability to process visual details. A visual-field defect that is restricted to the upper or lower quadrant of a hemifield is known as a quadrantanopia. As the lens inverts the real-world image, a lesion of area V_1 below the calcarine fissure causes an upper quadrantanopia (*Fig. 24.4b*), whereas a V_1 lesion above the calcarine fissure results in a lower quadrantanopia.

A visual field defect that occupies both the upper and lower portions of the same hemifield of both eyes is a homonymous hemianopia (*Fig. 24.4c*). If the central 5–10° of the damaged hemifield is preserved it is called 'macular sparing' (*Fig. 24.4d*); foveal sparing refers to the central 1–3°. The most peripheral sector of the temporal visual fields of the eye opposite to an occipital lobe lesion

may also be spared. This 'monocular temporal crescent' of vision (*Fig. 24.4e*) depends on unpaired peripheral fibers of the nasal retina, which project to the portion of contralateral V_1 located in the anterior-most depths of the calcarine fissure. Its preservation may explain some reports of 'blindsight' and also of 'Riddoch's phenomenon', the ability to detect movement in the periphery of an otherwise blind hemifield. Homonymous hemianopias may be bilateral, leading to a severe loss of vision. If there is foveal sparing, a 'keyhole' of vision around fixation remains (*Fig. 24.4f*).

DAMAGE TO EXTRASTRIATE VISUAL AREAS

Striate area V_1 is usually not damaged in isolation. Damage to area V_1 generally also affects the adjacent white matter and extrastriate areas, yielding different combinations of V_1 and extrastriate dysfunction. Extrastriate dysfunction differs from subcortical M- or P-pathway type deficits and is less severe than that caused by a V_1 lesion. A possible exception to this rule is damage to Brodmann's areas 18 and 19 that spares both V_1 and the optic radiations. A lesion in this area (which should contain a human homolog of the monkey's areas V_2 and V_3) which may cause a dense, V_1-like quadrantanopia that splits the horizontal meridian, resembling Figure 24.4b. Beyond these early zones, the functional maps of human visual fields appear to segregate along a ventromesial–dorsolateral axis.

DAMAGE TO THE VENTROMESIAL VISUAL ASSOCIATION CORTEX

A ventromesial visual pathway in the human begins in the occipital lobe beneath the calcarine fissure, connects with adjacent temporal regions (see Fig. 24.1a), and may include human homologs of the monkey's areas V_4 and IT. Damage to this pathway is associated with three main syndromes: visual agnosia, central achromatopsia, and acquired alexia.

VISUAL AGNOSIA

Teuber defined visual agnosia as a recognition defect in which normal or near normal percepts are stripped of their meanings. Prosopagnosia is a restricted type of visual agnosia in which patients fail to recognize previously familiar faces or to learn new faces despite adequate visual acuity and spatial contrast sensitivity. Recognition usually relies on non-visual cues, such as a person's voice or the context of an encounter, or on special visual evidence, such as a person's gait, a scar, or paraphernalia such as beard and glasses. Associated lesions are often bilateral (*Fig. 24.5*) but when they are unilateral they tend to affect the right hemisphere.

Owing to the location of the lesions below the calcarine fissure, visual-field defects in one or both visual fields may result, especially in the upper quadrants (*Fig. 24.6*). Despite this, prosopagnosics can still recognize a face as a face and discriminate between faces they cannot recognize. Some may perceive the sex and emotion from faces. A weak form of unconscious face recognition is sometimes demonstrable by autonomic criteria. Patients with prosopagnosia may continue to inspect all portions of faces they cannot recognize (*Figure 24.7*).

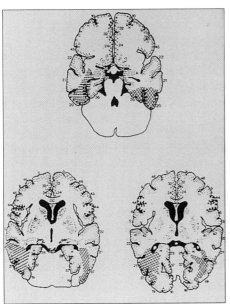

Fig. 24.5 Bilateral lesions of the visual cortex are depicted in transverse sections of the brain of a 65-year-old woman with prosopagnosia, achromatopsia, and acquired alexia. The CT-defined lesions are shown plotted on templates according to a standard neuroanatomic technique (Damasio and Damasio, 1989; courtesy of H Damasio) The right hemisphere is depicted on the left side of each section.

CENTRAL ACHROMATOPSIA (DYSCHROMATOPSIA)

Lesions of the ventral visual system may also cause central achromatopsia. Central achromatopsia can be defined as an acquired disorder of color perception involving all or part of the visual field. Patients report that colors appear 'washed out' or 'gray' in the affected field, yet they are still able to perceive form and motion (*Fig. 24.8*).

Central achromatopsia is associated with damage to areas 18 and 19 of the inferior visual association complex in the middle third of the fusiform and lingual gyri. Such lesions were depicted in red by Verrey (1888) in his depiction of the autopsy of a woman with right hemiachromatopsia and a left hemisphere lesion (*Fig. 24.9*).

Lesions located more anteriorly or in the superior visual association cortex above the calcarine fissure generally do not cause central achromatopsia. Area V_1 and the underlying radiations must be spared or else there is a dense visual-field defect in which the patient cannot even detect light.

The nature of the color deficit in central achromatopsia has not been well defined, probably because most patients cannot be studied with standard color tests. Standard tests are aimed at viewing near fixation, yet central achromatopsia typically affects a quadrant or hemifield and spares regions near fixation. Affected patients can bring these normal fields to bear on standard color tasks and achieve normal scores despite having a severe color vision defect. However, patients with bilateral cerebral lesions causing achromatopsia can be studied in detail, in central fixation, on a variety of color tasks (*Fig. 24.10*).

The results in these rare cases suggest that central achromatopsia spans a range of color defects that differs from the pro-

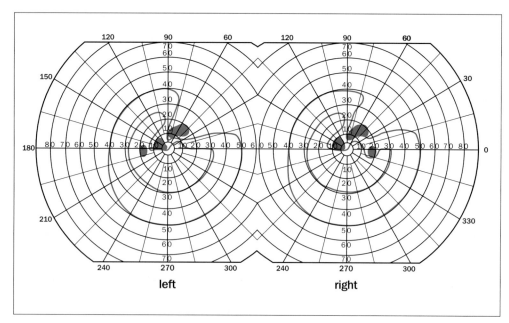

Fig. 24.6 The same patient as in Figure 24.5. The patient had bilateral upper quadrantic visual field defects, which spared fixation on the right and the peripheral fields on the left. The standard explanation for such defects is that the bilateral lesions that affected the ventromesial visual association cortex also undercut portions of the optic radiations to area V_1 (area 17) on both sides. However, Horton and Hoyt (1991) suggested that lesions of the early visual association cortex (human V_2/V_3 in Brodmann's areas 18 and 19) may produce similar defects.

left   right

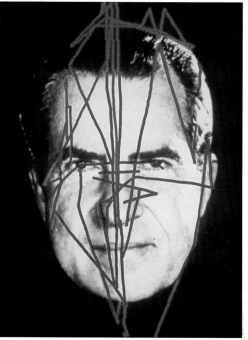

Fig. 24.7 The same patient as in Figure 24.5. The red lines represent the patient's eye movements to scan a famous face. The prosopagnosic patient scans all portions of a face she can no longer recognize.

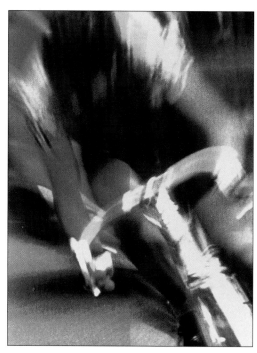

Fig. 24.8 Patients with central achromatopsia may report that colors appear 'washed out' or 'gray' in the affected field, yet their ability to perceive form and motion remains relatively intact, as simulated in this right hemiachromatopsic view of a bicycle racer.

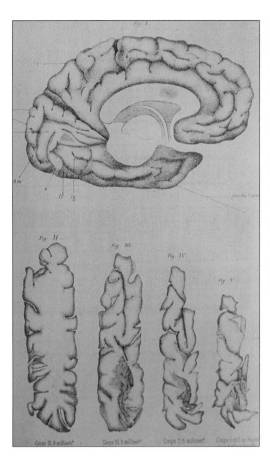

Fig. 24.9 From an 1888 case report by Verrey of a woman with a slight hemiachromatopsia. The location of the lesions in the patient's brain are marked in red. Damage to these areas (Brodmann's 18 and 19 in the ventromesial visual association cortex in the middle third of the fusiform and lingual gyri) still causes a cerebral ("central") hemiachromatopsia.

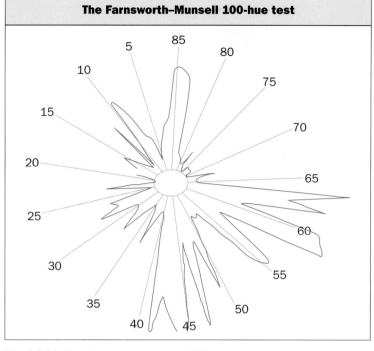

Fig. 24.10 The Farnsworth–Munsell 100-hue test requires an observer to order the hues in 88 isoluminant color tokens. Here the error scores are plotted in a man with full-field achromatopsia caused by bilateral cerebral lesions. The starburst appearance of the plot indicates widespread color confusions.

files of protanopia, deuteranopia, or tritanopia caused by hereditary retinal cone-cell deficiencies. The extent to which color can be dissociated from the processing of other visual cues by cerebral lesions remains a research issue.

ALEXIA

Achromatopsia and prosopagnosia are associated with acquired or 'pure' alexia. In this syndrome previously literate patients can still write but are unable to read what they have just written: alexia without agraphia. Dejerine marked with an 'X' the most economic lesion for causing this syndrome (*Fig. 24.11*). The lesion is locat-

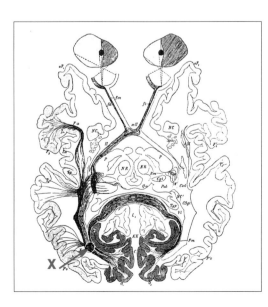

Fig. 24.11 Dejerine circled and marked with an 'X' the most economic lesion for causing pure alexia. The lesion is located near the left occipital horn and disrupts visual connections from both hemispheres with more anterior language areas.

ed near the left occipital horn, where it disrupts visual information from both the right and left hemispheres on its way towards more anterior language-related cortex.

The pattern-recognition defect in pure alexia differs from the much more subtle reading troubles found in developmental dyslexia. The latter has been associated with cortical heterotopias, loss of cells in the M pathway, and an inability to process 'transient' signals.

DAMAGE TO THE DORSOLATERAL VISUAL ASSOCIATION CORTEX

The dorsolateral visual association cortices are located above the calcarine fissure in areas 18 and 19 (see Fig. 24.1a) and extend onto adjacent parietal and temporoparieto-occipital regions of the human brain (see Fig. 24.1b). They occupy the lateral surface of the hemisphere, including human areas 5, 7, 39, 37, and superior 19, which may contain a homolog of the monkey's MT complex. Damage to these regions may affect motion perception, visually guided eye and hand control, and other visuospatial abilities, leading to aspects of the symptom complex reported by Bálint. V_1-type dysfunction may be associated with damage in this area, especially inferior homonymous quadrantic visual field defects.

BÁLINT'S SYNDROME

Bálint (1909) reported a triad of unusual defects in a man with posterior hemispheric lesions (*Fig. 24.12*).

First, Bálint's patient had 'optic ataxia', a defect of hand movements under visual guidance. The man would grope as if blind,

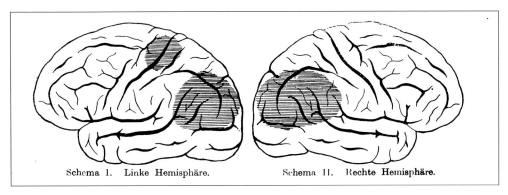

Fig. 24.12 Bálint idealized the lesions in his patient's brain on lateral views of the hemispheres. The calcarine cortex was supposedly preserved. Bálint emphasized damage to the angular gyri on both sides. The lesions affect the dorsolateral visual association cortices on both sides, including Brodmann's areas 5, 7, 37, 39, and superior 19 (see Fig. 24.1b).

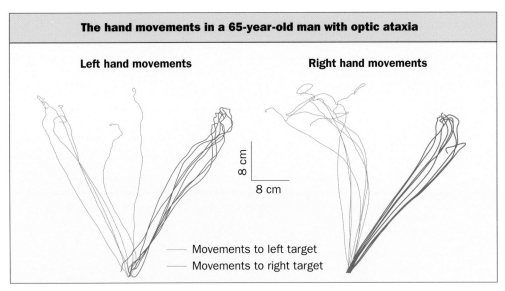

Fig. 24.13 The hand movements in a 65-year-old man with optic ataxia are shown. The patient had bilateral lesions of the dorsolateral visual association cortex resembling those in Bálint's patient. Here the patient is viewed from above as he reaches from a point directly in front of him to distal targets located to the left and right of the body midline. The performance for multiple reaches with the left hand and right hand are shown. Hand movement recordings depend on an infra-red technique. Head and eye movements are unrestricted. The hand-paths of both the left and right hands are wildly inaccurate, especially for reaches to the distal targets located to the left of midline. (Reproduced with permission from Rizzo M. In: Kennnard C, ed. *Visual Perceptual Defects: Baillière's Clinical Neurology*. London: Saunders, 1993.)

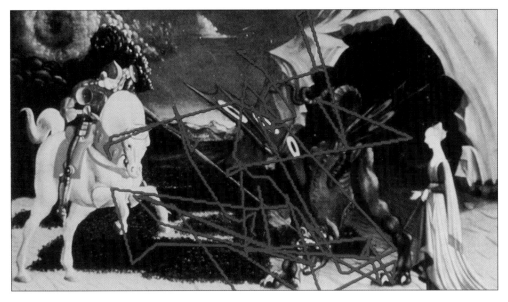

Fig. 24.14 The scan path (red lines) of a man with simultanagnosia viewing Uccello's St George and the Dragon. He scanned critical regions of the display, indicating he does not have the defect of voluntary gaze, known as ocular apraxia. However, he could not provide a coherent report on what he had viewed. Evidently ocular apraxia is not necessary to the development of simultanagnosia. (Reproduced with permission from Rizzo M, Hurtig R. *Neurology*. 1987;**37**:1642–1648)

even on reaching for targets that he could see and describe (*Fig. 24.13*). Somehow, visual information on the position of an object had become dissociated from position sense of the limb.

Second, Bálint's patient had a fragmentary view of the world and never seemed to see more than one object at a time. Bálint called this a 'spatial disorder of attention'. Holmes used the term visual disorientation. Wolpert called the defect simultanagnosia, although is not really an agnosia by Teuber's criteria. Simultanagnosia can be operationally defined by having patients view a picture of a complex scene; affected patients will fail to report all of the objects and object relationships depicted in the display. Aphasia, an acquired language defect in patients with left hemisphere lesions, must be excluded as the reason for a defective report.

Third, Bálint described an inability to move the eyes voluntarily to objects of interest despite unrestricted ocular rotations, which he called 'psychic paralysis of gaze', also known as 'spasm of fixation' or 'ocular apraxia'. (The latter should not be confused with the congenital defect, ocular motor apraxia.) However, ocular apraxia generally does not occur in the absence of severe visuoperceptive deficits. Moreover, severe perceptual deficits that meet operational criteria for simultanagnosia can occur in the face of relatively preserved eye-movement control (*Fig. 24.14*).

AKINETOPSIA

Cortical motion blindness, or central akinetopsia, was reported by Zihl *et al.* in 1983 in a patient (LM) who had bilateral lesions surrounding the temporoparieto-occipital junction. The patient has normal visual acuity and does not have prosopagnosia, achromatopsia, or alexia, which distinguishes LM from patients with lesions of the ventromesial structures.

The lesions reported in LM and subsequent patients generally include Brodmann's area 19 and adjacent area 37 (see Fig. 24.1b), the myelinogenesis of which resembles that of the monkey's area MT. It should be noted that similar areas were involved in Bálint's patients (see Fig. 24.12). The associated visual impairments include defective smooth pursuit eye movements (Morrow and Sharpe, 1993) (*Fig. 24.15*) and the inability to detect a directional motion signal in stimuli known as random-dot cinematograms (Newsome and Paré, 1988) (*Fig. 24.16*).

DIFFICULT-TO-CLASSIFY DISTURBANCES

Several visual cortical disturbances are difficult to classify under recent models of primate vision. Indeed, whether they exist in animals is difficult to prove because verbal complaints provide the main clues in affected individuals, and quantitative measurements are difficult. These disorders include hallucinations (seeing what is not there; *Fig. 24.17*), palinopsia (the persistence of visual afterimages), metamorphopsia (a carnival mirror-like effect), micropsia and macropsia (objects looking smaller or larger than they should), tilted vision, and even monocular polyopia (multiple images not caused by defects of the ocular surface or media, and not corrected by looking through a pinhole). The existence of these human disorders, which have concrete physiologic underpinnings (*Fig. 24.18*), together with other differences between man and primates, such as in brain size and topography, highlights the need to study humans to understand human vision.

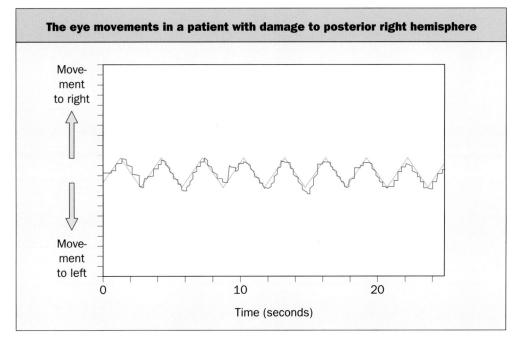

Fig. 24.15 The eye movements in a patient with damage to the posterior right hemisphere attempting to follow a moving visual target are shown. Eye movements and the target movements are superimposed. The patient successfully tracked the object over an excursion of 15° at 15° per second; however, the pursuit is saccadic. Such a pattern can result from defective motion perception caused by damage in the dorsolateral visual association cortex in patients with central akinetopsia.

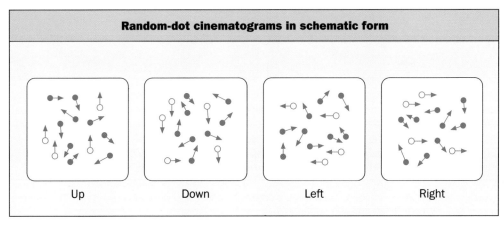

Fig. 24.16 Random-dot cinematograms are depicted in schematic form. The observer has to detect a global coherent motion direction signal (open circles) moving up, down, left, or right, from among background random noise resembling the 'snow' on a television screen. Monkeys with area MT lesions require a higher percentage motion signal at threshold, as should humans with lesions in homologous areas.

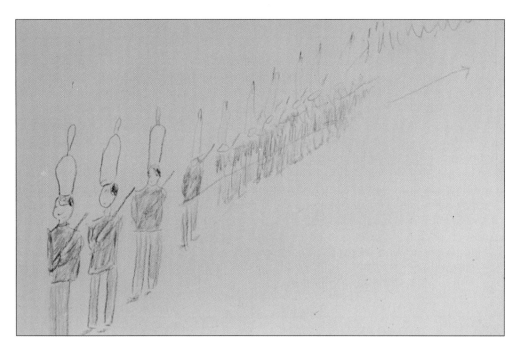

Fig. 24.17 A 79-year-old man suddenly began seeing objects coming out of his left visual field. The man was a reasonable artist and drew what he saw. Here, he depicted a procession of toy soldiers. He knew they were not real and he had no psychiatric disorder (Reproduced with permission from Anderson SW, Rizzo M, *J Clin Exp Neuropsychol* 1994;**16**: 651–663)

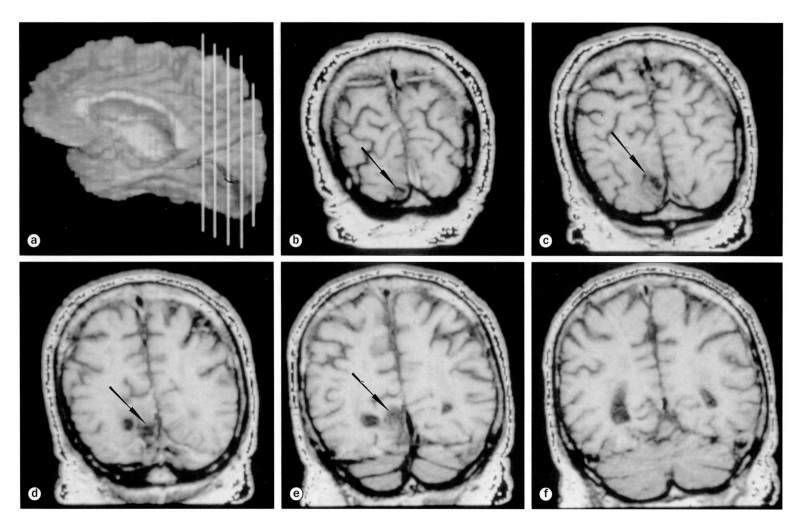

Fig. 24.18 A three-dimensional voxel reconstruction from the raw brain MR scan of the artist of Figure 24.17. (Damasio and Frank, 1992; courtesy of Damasio H and reproduced with permission from Anderson SW, Rizzo M. *J Clin Exp Neuropsychol.* 1994;**16**: 651–663) (**a**) The mesial surface of the left hemisphere is reconstructed in image. (**b–e**) The white lines through the reconstructed brain show the relative positions of the five coronal MR slices. The calcarine fissure is traced in red. The parieto-occipital fissure is traced in green. These tracings automatically transfer to the original MR slices to allow identification of these fissures. This patient had a unilateral right occipital lobe lesion surrounding the calcarine fissure and extending into the visual association cortex. The position of the lesion in the coronal sections is indicated by the black arrows. Goldmann perimetry (not shown) revealed an appropriate left visual-field defect. The point is that subjective visual phenomena, such as hallucinations, have physiological underpinnings. They reflect different patterns of damage or activation in the visual association cortex caused by stroke, tumor, trauma, infection, neurodegenerative disease, and drug or neurotransmitter effects at specific receptor sites.

Further reading

Anderson SW, Rizzo M. Visual hallucinations following occipital lobe damage: the pathological activation of visual representations. J Clin Exp Neuropsychol. 1994:16:651–663.

Bálint R. Seelenlahmung des 'Schauens', optische Ataxie, raumliche Storung der Aufmerksamkeit. *Monatsschrift fur Psychiatry and Neurology.* 1909;**25**:51–181.

Brodmann K. Vergleichende Lokalisationslehre der Grosshirnrinde in ihren Prinzipien dargestellt auf Grund des Zellenbaues. (Leipzig: JA Barth, 1909).

Damasio H, Damasio A. *Lesion Analysis in Neuropsychology* (New York: Oxford University Press, 1989).

Damasio H, Frank R. Three-dimensional in vivo mapping of brain lesions in humans. *Arch Neurol.* 1992;**49**:137–143.

Dejerine MJ. Différentes variétés de cécité verbale. *Memoires de la Société de Biologie.* 1892;**4**:61–90.

Felleman DJ, Van Essen DC. Distributed hierarchical processing in the primate cerebral cortex. *Cerebral Cortex.* 1991;**1**:1–47.

Horton JC, Hoyt WF. Quadrantic visual field defects. A hallmark of lesions in extrastriate (V2/V3) cortex. *Brain.* 1991;**114**:1703–1718.

Merigan WH, Maunsell JHR. How parallel are the primate visual pathways? *Ann Rev Neurosci.*1993;**16**:369–402.

Morrow MJ, Sharpe JA. Retinotopic and directional deficits of smooth pursuit initiation after posterior cerebral hemispheric lesions. *Neurology.* 1993;**43**:595–603.

Newsome WT, Paré EB. A selective impairment of motion perception following lesions of the middle temporal area (MT). *J Neurosci.* 1988;**8**:2201–2211.

Rizzo M. 'Bálint's syndrome' and associated visuo-spatial disorders. In: Kernnard C, ed. *Visual Perceptual Defects: Baillière's Clinical Neurology.* (London: WB Saunders, 1993) 415–437.

Rizzo M. The role of striate cortex. Evidence from human lesion studies. In: Peters A, Rockland KS, eds. *Cerebral Cortex, Vol 10.* (New York: Plenum Press, 1994) 505–540.

Rizzo M, Hurtig R. Looking but not seeing: attention, perception, and eye movements in simultanagnosia. *Neurology.* 1987;**37**:1642–1648.

Rizzo M, Smith V, Pokorny J, Damasio AR. Color perception profiles in central achromatopsia. *Neurology.* 1993;**43**:995–1001.

Schiller PH, Logothetis NK. The color-opponent and broad-based channels of the primate visual system. *TINS.* 1990;**11**:392–398.

Verrey D. Hemiachromatopsie droite absolue. *Arch Ophthalmol (Paris).* 1888;**8**:289–300.

Zihl J, von Cramon D, Mai N. Selective disturbance of movement vision after bilateral brain damage. *Brain.* 1983;**106**:313–340.

CHAPTER 25

Functional Visual Loss

T A S Buchanan

Patients with functional visual loss complain of visual impairment even though the visual system is normal. Symptoms are imagined and are caused by a loss of visual function rather than an organic disease along the visual pathways. Although patients describe blurring or deterioration of vision or loss of visual field, they are usually relatively undisturbed by their symptoms. Detection requires a high index of suspicion and the diagnosis is often initially overlooked but it should always be considered in any patient presenting with visual symptoms when the media, pupil light reflexes, and fundi are normal. The diagnosis should be made early to avoid unnecessary investigations (e.g. CT or MRI) as these serve only to increase patients' anxiety and encourage additional functional complaints.

HISTORY

Taking the patient's history is important because it usually provides valuable clues to the true nature of the patient's symptoms by indicating a disproportion between symptoms and objective findings on subsequent examination. Functional visual symptoms are observed in both children and adults but they form two distinct groups. In children, difficult relationships with parents or peers at school or poor academic performance may precipitate functional visual loss as an attention-seeking device. Symptoms are usually bilateral and restricted to the visual system. In contrast, adults develop visual symptoms for financial gain after injury at work, a road traffic accident, or an assault, or to support a claim for disability benefit. Adults may have additional functional symptoms, such as headache or back pain. Historically, clinicians have attempted to distinguish between patients with hysteria and malingering but a clear separation between these groups is often difficult. Patients with hysterical visual loss have little or no insight into their illness and display a lack of concern about their symptoms. A malingerer, in contrast, deliberately and consciously exaggerates any complaints and is often agitated and frightened to undergo examination. A truly blind person remains cooperative and usually accepts the blindness, especially if it is long standing. There is a high incidence of visual problems in relatives of patients with functional visual loss but most do not require psychiatric assessment or suffer from psychiatric disease.

EXAMINATION

Clinical examination should initially rule out organic disease (*Fig. 25.1*) and then obtain evidence of good visual function.

RULE OUT ORGANIC DISEASE

Assessment begins as the patient enters the office: the ability to avoid obstacles and sit down gives a good indication of visual function. The hysterical individual avoids objects; the malingerer, in contrast, may require assistance or deliberately walk into things but avoids serious injury. A blind patient moves with caution, feeling the way with hands and feet but often attempts to underplay the significance of the disability.

The hysterical or truly blind person cooperates fully during the examination. A malingering patient may complain that lights induce photophobia, headaches, or dizziness, and these symptoms may be used as excuses to terminate the examination.

Visual Assessment and Refraction
It is tempting to begin examination by having the patient read a Snellen chart but the examiner is often frustrated when the patient reads the same large letters as on previous occasions for other physicians and reads no further. The Snellen chart has an inbuilt safeguard so that a patient correctly reading all the letters in one line should always be able to read one or more letters on the next line; patients, therefore, should not stop abruptly at the end of one line and go no further. Vision in suggestible patients may improve if encouraged by the examiner pointing to letters but it is often more productive to delay Snellen testing until after the examination, when the patient has been reassured that the symptoms are not related to organic disease.

If visual acuity is reduced for distance, the patient should be refracted and the best corrected acuity established. The near vision should be tested with an appropriate presbyopic correction if needed. Distance and near vision should correlate closely (*Fig. 25.2*). Uncorrected refractive error has a predictable detrimental effect on distance acuity and this is useful in evaluating patients with functional visual symptoms. For example, the uncorrected 2.00 diopter sphere myope should achieve a distance acuity of approximately 6/36 (20/120), whereas an uncorrected 2.00

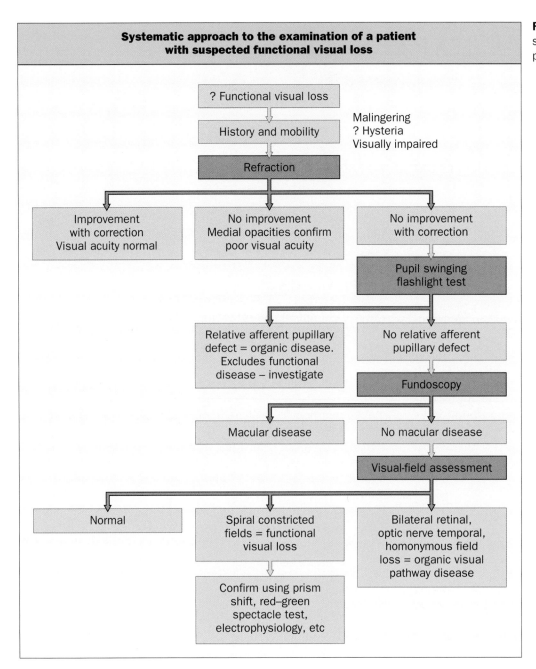

Fig. 25.1 Flow chart used to provide a systematic approach to the examination of a patient with suspected functional visual loss.

Correlation between distance and near visual acuity at 25 cm

Corrected visual acuity	Equivalent LogMar acuity	Near equivalent	
3/60 20/400	–	N48	J18
6/60 20/200	1.0	N24	J17
6/36 20/120	0.8	N12	J12
6/24 20/80	0.6	N8	J9–J11
6/12 20/40	0.3	N6	J4–J5

Fig. 25.2 Correlation between distance and near visual acuity at 25 cm with equivalent of +4.00 DS near spectacle addition and approximate relation of visual acuity and power of correcting sphere for myopia or hypermetropia.

diopter sphere hypermetrope will use any accommodative reserve to overcome a distance blur and thereby optimize acuity. In young adults, accommodation defects are rare and suspicion should be raised when, after achieving a corrected distance acuity of 6/12 (20/40), the patient fails to read N6 (J4–J5) sized print. Visual acuity can be assessed at differing working distances and by using low- and high-contrast test types.

Pupil Assessment and Fundoscopy

If acuity fails to improve after refraction the pupil should be examined using the swinging flashlight test. This is an objective assessment and a very helpful test in patients with functional visual loss because the patient has no input into and cannot modify the pupil response. A normal pupil reaction in a symptomatic eye strongly suggests functional disease. An afferent pupillary defect (APD), if present, excludes functional visual loss and indicates unilateral or bilateral but asymmetric visual pathway disease. A relative afferent pupillary defect (RAPD) with normal visual function is rare. Macular disease produces an APD only if extensive and easily seen by the ophthalmoscope. Subtle macular disease due to centroserous retinopathy, cystoid macular edema, cone rod dystrophy, retinitis pigmentosa, or Stargardt's disease may affect vision but leave the pupil intact and should be excluded by fundus examination in patients with suspected functional visual loss. Color saturation and light brightness tests are useful 'back up' investigations to confirm an APD if the swinging flashlight test is equivocal. Confirmatory evidence of an APD is a 25% or greater difference in light brightness between the eyes. If after pupil and fundus assessment the eyes appear normal, the patient should undergo visual-field assessment.

Visual-Field Assessment

Visual-field testing in a patient with functional visual symptoms is helpful because the field loss does not usually simulate defects

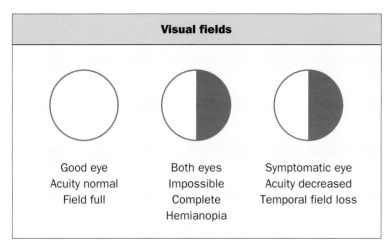

Fig. 25.3 Visual fields showing the 'missing half' hemianopia in a patient with functional visual loss.

caused by organic disease. Functional bitemporal, bi-nasal, and central field defects are unusual and indicate organic visual pathway disease. The type of field defect may vary, depending on the examiner's field technique and use of suggestion. Confrontation methods encourage a hemianopic pattern of visual-field loss, 'the missing half visual-field defect', in the 'affected' eye. The field is full in the other eye. A complete hemianopia is observed towards the affected side with both eyes open. The incompatibility of the monocular and binocular fields confirms the functional nature of the patient's visual loss (*Fig. 25.3*). When computerized perimetry is used it is much more difficult with random, rapid, and short duration stimuli to create consistently and deliberately an abnormal visual field and the high numbers of false-positive and false-negative responses and fluctuations in performance will alert the perimetrist to the true nature of the patient's visual-field loss. The most common visual-field abnormalities in patients with functional visual loss are bilateral and concentric constriction or tunnel visual-fields (*Fig. 25.4*). Unilateral constriction is uncommon. These field defects show steep margins and remain the same regardless of the size of the test object or the test distance from the screen. Patients with organic disease always demonstrate expansion of the visual-field defect when the test distance is increased. The degree of functional constriction may vary in the same patient from one examination to the next. This may be demonstrated in a malingering patient using the tangent screen. Marks used to outline the patient's visual field are moved to new positions closer to fixation when the patient is absent. When the test is repeated the new field will often conform to the new pin arrangement.

Spiral fields may also be observed and reflect variation in patient response to stimuli. Although the patient does not fully understand what is going on, he or she reacts to successive stimuli by waiting longer intervals until quite sure of seeing the target before responding , leading to a spiral field. Moving the test object from the periphery towards fixation, the stimulus is initially identified in the normal position but, as each successive meridian is examined, the test object moves closer to fixation, producing a

Fig. 25.4 Concentric constriction or tunnel visual field in hysteria. The field in each eye was the same size at both 1 and 2 meters.

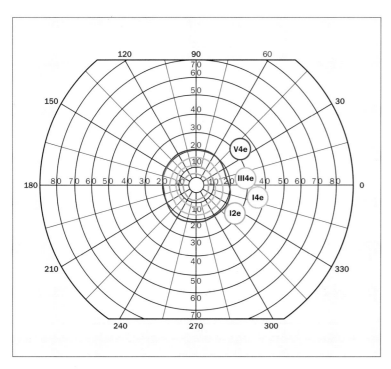

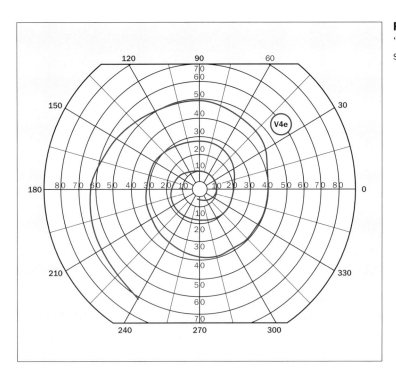

Fig. 25.5 Visual field in a suggestible patient with 'somatic concerns' or 'hysterical' symptoms showing a typical spiral visual field resulting from systematically testing each meridian in sequence.

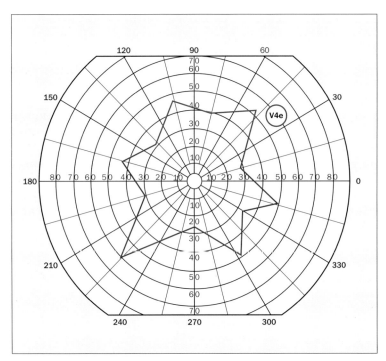

Fig. 25.6 Fields showing star-shaped fatigue resulting from alternately testing opposite ends of various meridians in a patient inclined towards concentric constriction of visual fields. This field, and the field in Figure 25.5, is an artefact of the perimetric technique; it can be obtained only if the perimetrist is not sensitive to what is happening, or is deliberately setting out to demonstrate the patient's suggestibility.

contracting spiral (*Fig. 25.5*). Moving the test object outwards from fixation into the peripheral field produces an expanding spiral and when opposite ends of a meridian are tested the resultant visual field may be star shaped (*Fig. 25.6*).

Having confirmed clinically normal visual pathways and excluded organic disease by pupil, fundus, and field examination, the examiner should then obtain evidence of normal visual function. It is not sufficient for the examiner to suspect functional visual disease; the tests should be able to confirm the diagnosis and obtain evidence of normal visual function so that the patient's family, teachers, or employers may be reassured about the true nature of the visual symptoms.

OBTAIN EVIDENCE OF GOOD VISUAL FUNCTION

Subjective tests that rely on the patient's cooperation are used to trick the patient into using the symptomatic eye without his or her knowledge and to confirm good visual function. These tests should be performed rapidly and accurately to manipulate the patient successfully.

TESTS TO CONFIRM BILATERAL FUNCTIONAL VISUAL LOSS

Complete functional visual loss is unusual because it is difficult to sustain for more than a short period. Unilateral visual loss is more common and may persist indefinitely.

Fixation Targets

Asked to look at his or her hand, the malingerer interprets this request as an assessment of vision and looks everywhere but at the hand. The patient may also be unable to sign his or her name, not realizing that with normal proprioception it should be possible to carry this out accurately even if blind.

Appreciation of Light

Sudden strong illumination of a slit lamp beam usually produces blinking or photophobia, indicating vision even in the difficult malingerer.

Optokinetic Nystagmus

An optokinetic drum will often elicit normal pursuit and saccadic movements and indicate a visual acuity of at least 6/60 (20/200). Difficult patients may look to the side of the drum or suppress the optokinetic stimulus unless the drum is held close to the eyes.

TESTS FOR UNILATERAL FUNCTIONAL VISUAL LOSS

Distance Acuity

The 6/24 (20/80) letters on a Snellen chart read at 6 m are equivalent to 6/12 (20/40) targets read at 3 m. Performance in the symptomatic eye may be compared with the good eye and functional visual loss is confirmed if vision fails to improve at half the distance.

Near Acuity

Testing with a +4.00 diopter sphere in front of the symptomatic eye and holding the near chart at the appropriate distance (25 cm) should provide unit magnification and improve near acuity in this eye. Increasing the near addition in +4.00 diopter sphere steps increases magnification by a factor of two and normally enables the individual to read print twice as small.

Prism Shift Test

If a 4 diopter base out prism is placed before the symptomatic eye as the patient fixes on a light or reads the Snellen chart, fixation is not interrupted if vision in the eye is poor. However, if the eye retains vision, the patient will experience diplopia, the eye will move medially, re-adjust and the patient will continue to read. When the prism is removed the eye deviates outwards to regain binocular vision.

Fogging Tests

A +3.00 diopter sphere placed in the trial frame can be used to fog vision in the normal eye and trick the patient into reading with the symptomatic eye. Combinations of +3.00 and −3.00 diopter cylinders placed in a trial frame along the same axis and before both eyes allow the patient to read with the normal eye. Rotating one cylinder in the good eye through 90° fogs vision in this eye and further reading is carried out with the symptomatic eye.

Red–Green Spectacle Test

With a green filter before the symptomatic eye the patient is asked to identify red numbers on a white card. These numbers are invisible to the normal eye and near vision in the symptomatic eye can be directly quantified by varying the size of the letters presented. Some patients may deny seeing the red print irrespective of which eye is viewed through the green filter, making assessment impossible.

TESTS OF FUNCTIONAL VISUAL LOSS IN CHILDREN

Titmus Stereopsis Test

A child correctly identifying all nine circles in this test must have good visual function in each eye. Reduction in stereo acuity may be directly correlated with the degree of visual loss on Snellen or near assessment.

Electrodiagnostic Testing

A normal pattern visual-evoked response, although strongly suggestive of non-organic disease, does not exclude cortical blindness. One-third of patients suspected of hysteria or malingering may alter or obliterate the visual-evoked response by making subtle convergence movements, which may not be detected by the examiner, or by daydreaming, thus limiting the usefulness of this method of examination.

THERAPY

Patients with functional visual loss should be reassured that their eyes are healthy and working normally. They should be told that their symptoms are temporary, that they do not require further investigations or treatment, and that they do not have serious organic disease. If the positive aspects of examination are emphasized, the hysterical patient is usually pleased and reassured. The malingerer may react differently, become hostile towards the examiner, and question the examiner's ability to understand his or her difficulties. Arguments about test performance in front of patients and relatives are generally unproductive because family members usually support the patient. Children should be told that stress is responsible for their complaint and reassured that vision will return once this stress is relieved. It is helpful to discuss the child's problem with the parents alone and offer advice. Psychiatric or neurologic referral is generally unhelpful, resented by the patient, and serves only to increase the patient's view that something serious is wrong. The findings should always be reviewed if new symptoms present to avoid overlooking organic disease.

A follow-up study in patients with functional visual loss years after the initial visit showed that constricted or spiral visual-field defects persisted in 50% of patients but few patients were impaired either socially or economically by their deficit. Patients with other types of visual-field loss or reduced visual acuity were more likely to improve and their symptoms resolve.

'Dealing with these patients is not without its satisfactions; there is an opportunity to do some good doctoring, to apply knowledge, experience, and goodwill to the patient's problem and to offer an effective treatment. The patient is trusting and naive; what he needs is a thorough examination from a confident physician who sends clear messages and who gives him a large dose of unadulterated reassurance' (Thompson, 1985).

Further reading

Bumgartner J, Epstein CM. Voluntary alteration of visual evoked potentials. *Ann Neurol.* 1982;**12**:475–478.

Celesia GG, Archer CR, Kuroina Y, Goldfader PR. Visual function of the extrageniculo-calcarine system in man. *Arch Neurol.* 1980;**37**:704–706.

Forman S, Beherns MM, Odel JG, Spector RT, Hilal S. Relative afferent pupillary defect with normal visual function. *Arch Ophthalmol.* 1990;**108**:1074–1075.

Kardon R, Thompson HS. The Pupil. In: Rosen E, Thompson HS, Eustace P, Cumming K, eds. *Color Atlas and Text of Neuro-Ophthalmology* (London: Mosby, 1994)

Kathol RG, Cox TA, Corbett JJ, Thompson HS, Clancy J. Functional visual loss: 1. A true psychiatric disorder? *Psychol Med.* 1983;**13**:307–314.

Kathol RG, Cox TA, Corbett JJ, Thompson HS, Clancy J. Functional visual loss. Follow-up of 42 cases. *Arch Ophthalmol.* 1983:**101**:315–324.

Keane JR. Hysterical hemianopia. The 'missing half' field defect. *Arch Ophthalmol.* 1979;**97**:865–866.

Levy NS, Glick EB. Stereoscopic perception and Snellen visual acuity. *Am J Ophahalmol.* 1974;**78**:722–724.

Thompson HS. Functional visual loss. *Am J Ophthalmol.* 1985;**100**:209–213.

CHAPTER 26

Is My Child Blind?

Michael O'Keefe

INTRODUCTION

There is a wide variation between infants in the rate of visual development, and some normal infants show significant delay. Although visual fixation is usually present at birth, it becomes well developed by 6 weeks of age and fixation and following are usually well established between 6 and 12 weeks (*Fig. 26.1*). In the Western world, infants with suspected disorders of vision are referred between 6 and 12 weeks of age as a result of routine neonatal screening policies. Some infants have medical problems, following premature birth, whereas others have eye movement disorders that can be confused with blindness, such as ocular motor apraxia.

The first interview with parents of such a child is often an emotional one. They usually have three questions to which they require answers:
'What can my child see now?'
'Will my child see in the future?'
'How well can my child see?'
In many situations, a multidisciplinary approach is necessary, and the ophthalmologist involves the neonatologist, electrophysiologist, and radiologist. A proper history and a thorough eye examination are of course the first requirements. Parental observations of the child's eyes and visual behavior, and a medical history, including details of exposure to drugs or radiation and complications during pregnancy or at the time of delivery, are elicited. Growth and development of the child are evaluated and the existence of any hereditary, medical, or neurologic abnormalities is established. Events that may cause central nervous system damage, such as fetal distress, seizures, respiratory arrest, and low Apgar scores, are also of interest, as is any family history of ocular disorders, particularly those commencing early in life.

VISUAL ASSESSMENT

Assessment of vision in the pre-verbal child begins with evaluation of fixation and following ability of each eye under both monocular and binocular conditions. The three most important questions to ask the parents are:
Does the child turn towards light?
Does the child follow the mother's face?
Does the child follow objects?
For young infants, a human face, hand-held light, or suitable fixation target is an appropriate object for this assessment. For older infants, toys, movie pictures, cards, or other targets that require accommodation, are appropriate. A pacifier or bottle, which the child can suck during the accommodation, is helpful. To evaluate fixation and following, one eye is covered and the examiner's thumb is offered for the child to follow. A thumb seems to be less threatening than other hand movements. The position of the corneal light reflex relative to the centre of the cornea is noted. If it is centrally located, the fixation is assumed to be foveal and the letter 'C' (for 'central') is recorded. If the eye maintains alignment with both a stationary and moving object, the alignment is steady, and the letter 'S' (for 'steady') is recorded. The occluder is then removed and the examiner determines whether, under binocular conditions, the previously fixing eye continues to fixate or whether the previously occluded eye takes up fixation. This maintenance in denoted by the letter 'M'. This method of assessment is, however, by no means perfect, especially in infants with small angle esotropia. It also correlates poorly with Snellen acuity.

More specialized methods of assessment are also available, including preferential looking, optokinetic nystagmus, and visual-evoked potential tests. Preferential looking takes advantage of the fact that the infant or young child prefers to look at a patterned

Human visual development	
Function	**Age**
Visual fixation	Birth
Visual fixation fully developed	6 weeks
Visual following	6–12 weeks

Fig. 26.1 A guide to visual development in the new-born.

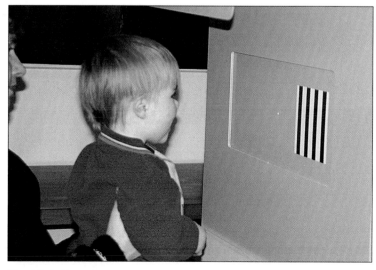

Fig. 26.2 The infant is held in front of a screen with grating patterns and homogenous test objects in the preferential looking vision test.

stimulus rather than an homogenous field (*Fig. 26.2*). The infant is presented with two simultaneous stimuli and his or her visual behavior observed. If he can see movement the child will turn his eyes to look at the target that is moving. Smaller targets are naturally harder to see. One of the drawbacks to preferential looking is that the child has a 50% chance of correctly identifying the patterned stimulus by chance alone. It may also give false-high acuities in the child with amblyopia. Note that preferential acuity should not be equated with recognition acuity: they represent different brain functions.

Optokinetic nystagmus (OKN) is the eye movement that occurs when the child fixates on a moving target such as the stripes on a rotating drum. Slow following eye movements and fast restorative eye movements occur. The slow following eye movements have the same velocity as the target, whereas the fast restorative eye movements are independent of the speed of the moving target. The combination of slow following movements in one direction and fast restorative movements in the opposite direction constitutes a jerk type of nystagmus known as OKN. A motor response is required for this movement and the combination of sensory and motor function can be measured.

Normal infants under 3 months of age have an asymmetrical OKN response; that is, OKN can be driven monocularly if the motion of the patterned field is in the temporal to nasal direction but not if the direction is reversed. If an infant or young child responds to OKN testing, some vision must be present; on the other hand, a lack of response to OKN does not mean that vision is not present. Most OKN drums and tapes take up only a small portion of an infant's visual field. Some infants have difficulty moving their eyes, which may be interpreted as reduced vision.

Visual evoked potential (VEP) tests can be performed in two ways. The 'flash VEP' generates a wave with amplitude and latency, and can be used to assess conditions that affect visual pathways. Patterned VEPs measure visual acuity by stimulating the macula. This method, however, requires steady gaze fixation and good attentiveness, so that children with nystagmus and seizures, or those who are uncooperative, are unsuitable.

EYE EXAMINATION

In the first 6 weeks of life, the position of the eye can vary, so that diagnosing abnormal eye movements during this time is not advisable. Examination of the pupils, however, is very important in infants. Pupillary responses to light first appear between 29 and 31 weeks' gestation. In a darkened room, an infant's pupil should respond to light regardless of his or her state of mind. If the pupillary response is absent or abnormal, the size and appearance of the optic nerve should be carefully evaluated. By moving the light from one eye to the other and watching the illuminated eye, the pupil in the more normal eye can be seen to react faster than the affected eye, which may even dilate in response to light. A paradoxical pupil response, in which the pupil constricts rather than dilates in response to darkness, occurs in achromatopsia and congenital stationary night blindness (see below). A cortically blind child can have normal pupil responses to light, and blink in a very natural way in response to light. These are both brainstem reflexes.

Assessment of the refractive error can also be helpful. Myopia in the first year of life is unusual and signals the possibility of a congenital retinal disorder or retinopathy of prematurity. Severe

hyperopia is often associated with Leber's congenital amaurosis (see below).

Congenital nystagmus often goes unnoticed until 8–12 weeks of age and may not manifest itself until 20 weeks after birth. It is a common feature in infants with congenital ocular or anterior visual pathway disorders but is absent in infants with cortical visual loss. Slow pendular nystagmus indicates poor vision, whereas faster frequency, small amplitude nystagmus is indicative of better vision. Roving eye movements with nystagmus may be associated with very low vision. Nystagmus that occurs when the other eye is occluded is more pronounced in the eye with the worst vision.

Nystagmus in an apparently blind infant is a valuable sign of anterior visual pathway disease. Patients with bilateral disorders of the eye and anterior visual pathway may display roving eye movements if the vision is extremely poor. Many children with nystagmus will adopt a head turn to dampen the nystagmus. The head turn allows the child to find the so-called null position, which is usually eccentric visual fixation (*Fig. 26.3*).

Monocular nystagmus occurs in conditions such as spasms nutans, chiasmal disorders, and congenital unilateral loss of vision. Spasms nutans refers to a constellation of nystagmus, head nodding, and torticollis. The nystagmus is usually fine, rapid, and horizontal in direction but may also be vertical or rotatory. It is often monocular or asymmetrical.

It is important to realize that the ocular fundus of the infant eye differs significantly from that of the adult, in that the optic disk appears pale and the fundus is pale and speckled. This can cause diagnostic problems.

SIGNS

Children with low vision from any cause hold objects close to their eyes, because of the increased magnification. Eye pressing occurs with bilateral retinal disease such as cicatricial retinopathy of prematurity, hereditary retinal dystrophies, and congenital retinal infections. This is a specific sign and should be distinguished from eye poking or eye rubbing. Many normal children rub their eyes, whereas those with severe mental retardation and self-injurious behavior poke their eyes. It is postulated that eye pressing stimulates the visual cortex by mechanically triggering ganglion cells to release phosphenes. Absence of eye pressing in children with blockade of the visual pathways, due to optic nerve or cortical damage, supports this hypothesis.

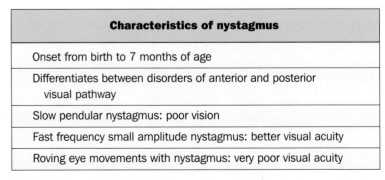

Characteristics of nystagmus
Onset from birth to 7 months of age
Differentiates between disorders of anterior and posterior visual pathway
Slow pendular nystagmus: poor vision
Fast frequency small amplitude nystagmus: better visual acuity
Roving eye movements with nystagmus: very poor visual acuity

Fig. 26.3 Important clinical features of congenital nystagmus and their relationship to visual prognosis.

Some infants display the phenomenon of over looking; that is, instead of looking at the object of regard directly, the infant looks above the object. This is thought to be a sign of bilateral cortical scotoma and the majority of patients who display this sign have congenital retinal disorders.

Head thrusting occurs in a condition called oculomotor apraxia. This is a condition with normal eyes but there is an inability to move them in the desired field of gaze. By thrusting the head, the infant drags the eyes to the desired location.

Some congenital retinal disorders, such as achromatopsia and rod-cone dystrophy, are associated with various degrees of photophobia. Photophobia can also arise with dominant optic atrophy, corneal or lenticular opacities, and a variety of neurologic disorders, including cortical visual impairment. Conversely, some patients with cortical visual impairment have a tendency to gaze at room lights, bright lights, or the sun (*Figs 26.4, 26.5*).

CAUSES OF VISUAL IMPAIRMENT

DELAYED VISUAL MATURATION

Delayed visual maturation (DVM) is diagnosed when a baby shows reduced or absent visual input for its age but later improves. In some infants there is a history of prematurity or of being small for dates. The causes are speculative but it is postulated that there is a delay in myelination, affecting both the visual pathway and visual association areas. Follow-up studies of children with this condition reveal a tendency to developmental problems, including global developmental delay and, later, a tendency towards autism.

Signs of visual impairment
Nystagmus
Head nodding
Head thrusting
Over looking
Photophobia
Holding objects close to eye
Variable vision
Paradoxical pupil response
Visual findings

Fig. 26.4 Some important findings that point to visual impairment.

Differentiating disorders of anterior and posterior visual pathways	
Anterior visual pathway	Posterior visual pathway
Visual acuity decreased	Variable acuity
Nystagmus	No nystagmus
Fundal findings	Normal fundus
Eye (poking) pressing	Over looking
Paradoxical pupil response	

Fig. 26.5 Visual findings differentiating disorders of the anterior and posterior visual pathways.

Type 1 is an isolated anomaly and complete recovery occurs within 6 months. Type 2 is diagnosed when the infant has an associated systemic disease, mental retardation, or other neurodevelopmental disorder, with limited visual improvement over time. Type 3 is diagnosed when the child has an associated ocular disease such as cataract or albinism, the visual improvement depending on the cause. Type 4 describes severe congenital or structural abnormalities, with little if any improvement of vision.

VISUAL PATHWAY DAMAGE

The visual pathways can be damaged by asphyxia, injury, infection, tumors, and toxins, and degenerative, neurologic, and metabolic disorders. It is possible to differentiate the visual findings into those that affect the anterior or posterior visual pathway. The neurological signs and visual behavior can differ in both (see *Figs. 26.4, 26.5*). The eye examination usually uncovers ocular abnormalities when the anterior visual path is damaged (opacities of cornea and/or lens with refractive errors. Retinal damage may reveal disc pallor and pupillary abnormalities.).

Optic nerve hypoplasia (*Fig. 26.6*) is a significant cause of blindness. Risk factors include maternal age, maternal diabetes, and pre-natal abuse of alcohol and cocaine. It is sometimes associated with endocrine and multiple structural (*Fig. 26.7*), chiasmal, or vascular disorders of the brain. Before 32 weeks, gestation, the optic disc may appear gray or pale and may be surrounded by a peripapillary halo bordered by a ring of increased or decreased pigmentation (double ring sign). The major retinal vessels are often tortuous. Once the optic nerve is fully developed, insults resulting from asphyxia, hydrocephalus, tumors, infections, cranial synostosis, and cerebral hemorrhage, produce optic atrophy. More obvious causes of absent vision are albinism, cicatricial retinopathy of prematurity (*Fig. 26.8*), and anophthalmos (*Fig. 26.9*).

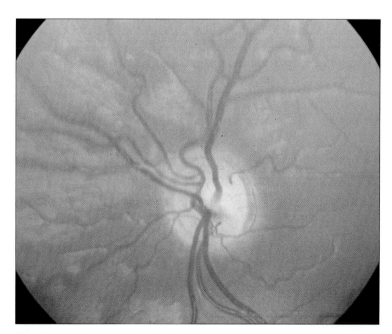

Fig. 26.6 Optic nerve hypoplasia. Shows a small nerve with diminished number of axons and a peripapillary halo known as a double ring sign.

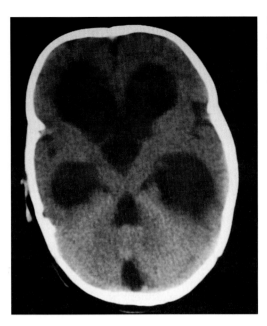

Fig. 26.7 CT scan showing a dilated fourth ventricle and absence of vermis associated with optic nerve hypoplasia.

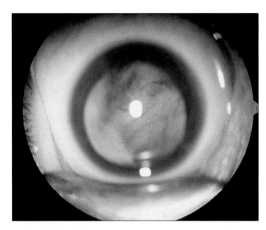

Fig. 26.8 A blind eye from stage IV retinopathy of prematurity in a premature infant born at 27 weeks' gestation.

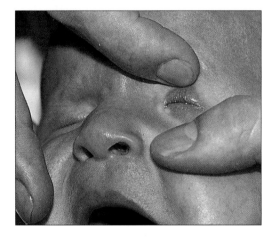

Fig. 26.9 Full-term infant with bilateral anophthalmos showing absent eyes and shallow sockets.

RETINAL DISORDERS

Children with retinal dystrophies have characteristic features that indicate this diagnosis. Leber's congenital amaurosis, a recessive condition involving rods and cones, is associated with blindness at birth and an initially abnormal fundus picture, later leading to a variable pigmentary retinopathy, including colobomata and disc abnormalities. Infants show nystagmus, poorly reactive or unreactive pupils, hyperopia, and oculo-digital signs such as eye pressing. Leber's disease may be associated with other systemic abnormalities such as retinal disease, cardiac abnormalities, and hypoplasia of the cerebellum.

Joubert's syndrome is an autosomal recessive disorder with cerebullar vermis hypotoria and is associated with episodic tachypnoea, apnoea, rhythmic protrusion of the tongue, ataxia, and hypotonia. A retinal dystrophy, with similar appearance to Leber's amaurosis, occurs in 50% of patients with this disorder.

Achromatopsia is an autosomal recessive disorder that affects the cones and rods. Children with this disorder show fast frequency, small amplitude, binocular nystagmus, photopsia, and better visual function in the dark than in the light. A paradoxical pupil response may also be present. In achromatopsia and congenital stationary night blindness, the pupils often constrict when the lights are turned out. Therefore on seeing this odd pupillary behavior, the examiner should consider retinal disease. These children do not see well in the dark, but see much better under well-lit conditions. They show nystagmus, night blindness, and myopia. It may be inherited as autosomal dominant, recessive, or X-linked.

Many neurodegenerative conditions, such as neuronal ceroid lipofuscinosis and peroxisomal disorders such as Refsum's disease, Zellweger's, and neonatal adrenoleukodystrophy, also cause retinal as well as neurologic changes.

CORTICAL VISUAL IMPAIRMENT

Diseases of the posterior visual pathway are associated with cortical visual impairment. This is defined as a loss of vision caused by a disturbance of the posterior visual pathway and/or occipital cortex. In some patients there may be co-existing disorders of the anterior visual pathway but the pupillary response to light may be completely normal. Optic atrophy may also be present due to either anterior pathway disease or trans-synaptic degeneration of the retrogeniculate pathway.

There are many causes of cortical visual impairment, including perinatal hypoxic ischemia, postnatal hypoxic ischemia, periventricular hemorrhage, head trauma, cerebral malformations such as encephaloceles, malformations, perencephalic cysts, infection, and hydrocephalus.

The most common cause of cortical visual impairment, however, is asphyxia. The resulting ischemia damages different regions of the brain in premature infants than it does in full-term infants because certain areas in premature brains have a very tenuous blood supply. In premature infants a meningeal anastomosis bridges the zone between the major cerebral arteries. The periventricular region thus provides a transient watershed zone in premature brains, between ventriculopetal and vetriculofugal branches of penetrating arteries, involving the optic radiations. Periventricular leukomalacia thus affects both the geniculocalcarine tract and the visual cortex.

In full-term infants the watershed areas between the two major circulating vessels lie in the regions between the anterior and middle, and the middle and posterior cerebral arteries. The resulting watershed area is termed the parasagittal area. Damage to the radiation thus carries a worse prognosis than damage to the cortical areas.

HYDROCEPHALUS

Patients with hydrocephalus (*Fig. 26.10*) may show a mixture of anterior and posterior visual damage. Damage to the anterior visual pathway may cause papilledema, optic atrophy, and strabismus. Damage to the posterior visual pathway affects vision due to compression of the posterior cerebral arteries against the tentorium, causing necrosis of the visual cortex. Patients with cortical visual impairment show no nystagmus, an important finding in differentiating anterior from posterior visual pathway disorders.

DIAGNOSIS

Although clinical examination reveals significant information about the level of visual impairment and its etiology, a number of infants require further investigations. CT or MRI scanning demonstrates changes in the posterior visual pathways and brain itself and provides clues to the likelihood of visual recovery. Children with intraventricular hemorrhage associated with severe periventricular leukomalacia demonstrated on imaging have a poorer prognosis than infants with cortical visual impairment and a normal or mildly abnormal CT scan. The VEP is helpful in establishing that vision is present and for monitoring visual recovery. Taylor (1991) reported that flash VEPs have prognostic value in infants with acute cortical blindness because an intact flash VEP in a previously normal child with cortical visual loss carries a favorable prognosis for visual recovery. Conversely, an absent VEP signal carries a poor prognosis.

The electroretinogram (ERG) is particularly useful in retinal disorders. It is flat in Leber's and Joubert's syndromes and in achromatopsia. In congenital stationary night blindness, the ERG shows diminished or absent cone responses and a normal rod response.

The electroencephalogram (EEG) is also a valuable diagnostic tool. Jeavons (1964) reported that the most common EEG pattern in blind children with ocular lesions was similar to that of sighted children with their eyes open. There is no posterior slowing or occipital spikes, which are signs of occipital lobe disturbance. The presence of normal alpha rhythm rules out central visual impairment and infants who appear totally blind but have alpha rhythm will have enough vision to read print. An absent alpha rhythm and multifactorial epiliptiform activity indicate that the neurons in the occipital cortex are substantially reduced in number and do not function normally. The prognosis for vision is, therefore, poor.

Infants with suspected glaucoma, those who require retinal examination, or those requiring management of retinoblastoma require examination under anesthesia. A sequence of steps is useful, beginning with insertion of a speculum in each eye, followed by measurement of corneal diameter, slit-lamp examination of the anterior chamber, fundoscopic examination, refraction, and finally assessment of intraocular pressure. Pupil dilatation is achieved by using a sympathomimetic agent combined with a parasympatholytic agent. The sympathomimetic agent of choice is 2.5% phenylephrine and the parasympatholytic agent is 0.5–1.0% cyclopentolate.

CONCLUSION

The understanding of infant vision has improved greatly over the past decade. Those who work regularly with visually impaired children claim that certain techniques in stimulating vision result in improved vision. This is based on the view that vision is a learned skill and results from the recruitment of neurons increasing the synapses. There is evidence of an extra-geniculate visual system that facilitates a different form of visual stimulation known as 'blindsight'. This is believed to be an integrated geniculo-striate pathway which mediates the unconscious awareness of motion in the peripheral field spatial localization. It is estimated that 20% to 30% of optic nerve fibers terminate in structures outside the lateral geniculate body.

Many visually impaired children have associated medical problems such as mental retardation, cerebral palsy, and epilepsy. The approach to the apparently blind infant is, therefore, multidisciplinary, relying on clinical observation and special investigations to arrive at an accurate diagnosis and prognosis, and to plan rehabilitation.

Further reading

Aroyo HA, Jan JE, McCormack AQ, Farrell K. Permanent visual loss after shunt malfunction. *Neurology.* 1985;**35**:25–29.

Atkinson J. Development of optokinetic nystagmus in the human infant and monkey infant: An analogue to development. In: Freeman RD, ed. *Developmental Neurobiology of Vision.* (New York: Plenum Publishing Corp, 1979)

Barricks ME, Flynn JT, Kushner BJ. Paradoxical pupillary response in congenital stationary night blindness. *Arch Ophthalmol.* 1977;**33**:722.

Burke JB, Bowell R, O'Keefe M. Optic nerve hypoplasia, encephalopathy and neurodevelopmental handicap. *Br J Ophthalmol.* 1991;**75**:236–239.

Celesia GG, Archer CR, Kuroiwa Y. Visual function of the extrageniculate-calcarine system in man. Relationship to cortical blindness. *Arch Neurol.* 1980;**37**:704–706.

Chan T, Bowell R, O'Keefe M. Ocular manifestations of the fetal alcohol syndrome. *Br J Ophthalmol.* 1991;**75(8)**: 524–526.

Cogan DG. Congenital ocular motor apraxia. *Can J Ophthalmol.* 1966;**1**:53.

Cogan DG. *Neurology of the Ocular Muscles.* 2nd edn. (Springfield IL: Charles C Thomas, 1956)

De Morsier G. Etudes sur les dystrophies cranioencephaloques III. Agenesis, du septum fucidum avec malformation du tractus optique. La dysplasie septo-optique Schwelzer. *Arch Fur Neurologic und Psychiatric.* 1956;**77**:267–292.

Donin JF. Acquired monocular nystagmus in children. *Can J Ophthalmol.* 1967;**2**:212–215.

Fielder AR, Mayer DL. Delayed visual maturation. *Semin Ophthalmol.* 1991;**6**:182–193.

(*Continued overleaf*)

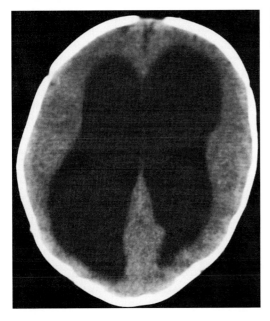

Fig. 26.10 Child with hydrocephalus and dilated ventricles.

Celesia GG, Archer CR, Kuroiwa Y. Visual function of the extrageniculate-calcarine system in man. Relationship to cortical blindness. *Arch Neurol.* 1980;**37**:704–706.

Chan T, Bowell R, O'Keefe M. Ocular manifestations of the fetal alcohol syndrome. *Br J Ophthalmol.* 1991;**75(8)**: 524–526.

Cogan DG. Congenital ocular motor apraxia. *Can J Ophthalmol.* 1966;**1**:53.

Cogan DG. *Neurology of the Ocular Muscles.* 2nd edn. (Springfield IL: Charles C Thomas, 1956)

De Morsier G. Etudes sur les dystrophies cranioencephaloques III. Agenesis, du septum fucidum avec malformation du tractus optique. La dysplasie septo-optique Schwelzer. *Arch Fur Neurologic und Psychiatric.* 1956;**77**:267–292.

Donin JF. Acquired monocular nystagmus in children. *Can J Ophthalmol.* 1967;**2**:212–215.

Fielder AR, Mayer DL. Delayed visual maturation. *Semin Ophthalmol.* 1991;**6**:182–193.

Flodmark O, Jan JE, Wong KHP. Computerized tomography of the brains of children with cortical visual impairment. *Dev Med Child Neurol.* 1990;**32**:611–620.

Flynn JT, Cullen RF. Disc oedema in congenital amaurosis of Leber. *Br J Ophthalmol.* 1975;**59**:497–502.

Foxman SG, Wirtchafter JD, Letson RD. Leber's congenital amaurosis and high hypermetropia. A discrete entity. In: Henkins P, ed. *Acta XXIV International Congress of Ophthalmology, Vol. I.* (Philadelphia: JB Lippinott, 1983) 55–58.

Frisén L, Holmegoaad L: Spectrum of optic nerve hypoplasia. *Br J Ophthalmol.* 1975;**62**:627–635.

Gelbart SS, Hoyt CS. Congenital nystagmus: A clinical perspective in infancy. *Graefe's Arch Clinical Exp Ophthalmol* 1988;**226**:178–180.

Good WV. Behaviours of visually impaired children. *Semin Ophthalmol.* 1991;**6**:158–160.

Good WV, Crain CS, Quint RD, Koch TK. Overlooking a sign of bilateral central acotoma in children. *Dev Med Child Neurol.* 1992;**34**:69–73.

Good WV, Koch TS, Jan JE. Monocular nystagmus caused by unilateral anterior visual pathway disease. *Dev Med Child Neurol.* 1993;**35**:1106–1110.

Goodman R, Ashby L. Delayed visual maturation and autism. *Dev Med Child Neurol.* 1990;**32**:814–819.

Harris SJ, Hansen RM, Fulton AB. Assessment of acuity of amblyopic subjects using face grating and recognition stimuli. *Invest Ophthalmol Vis Sci.* 1986;**27**:1184.

Hoernagee D, Biery B. Spasms nutans. *Dev Med Child Neurol.* 1968;**10**:32–35.

Hoyt CS, Billson FA. Optic nerve hypoplasia changing perspectives. *Aust N. Z J Ophthalmol.* 1986;325–331.

Hoyt CS, Jastrzebski G, Marg E. Delayed visual maturation in infancy. *Br J Ophthalmol.* 1983;**67**:127.

Hoyt CS, Mousel DK, Uleber AA. Transient supranuclear disturbance of gaze in healthy neonates. *Am J Ophthalmol.* 1980;**87**:708.

Jan JE, Farrell K, Wong PK, McCormack AQ. Eye and head movements of visually impaired children. *Dev Med Child Neurol.* 1986;**28**:285–293.

Jan JE, Freeman RD, McCormack AQ, Scott EP, Robertson WD, Newman DE. Eye pressing by visually impaired children. *Dev Med Child Neurol.* 1983;**25**:755–762.

Jan JE, Groenveld M, Sykanda AM, Hoyt CS. Light gazing by visually impaired children. *Dev Med Child Neurol.* 1990;**32**:755–759.

Jan JE, McCormack AQ, Hoyt CS. The unequal nystagmus test. *Dev Med Child Neurol.* 1988;**30**:441–443.

Jan JE, Wong PK. Behaviour of the alpha rhythm in electro-encephalograms of visually impaired children. *Dev Med Child Neurol.* 1988;**30**:444–450.

Jan JE, Wong PKH, Groenveld D. Travel vision: Collicular visual system? *Paediatr Neurol.* 1986;**2**:359–362.

Jeavons PM. The electro-encephalogram in blind children. *Br J Ophthalmol.* 1964;**48**:83–101.

Joubert M, Eisenberg J, Robb JP. Familial agenesis of the cerebellar vermis. *Neurology.* 1969;**19**:823–825.

King MD, Dudgeon J, Stephenson JBP. Joubert's syndrome with retinal dysplasia: neonatal tachypnoea as a clue to the genetic brain eye malformation. *Arch Dis Child.* 1984;**59**:709–718.

Lambert SR. Degenerative retinal diseases in childhood. *Semin Ophthalmol.* 1991;**6**:219–226.

Lambert SR, Hoyt CS, Jan LE, Barkovica J. Visual recovery from hypoxic cortical blindness during childhood. Computerized tomographic and magnetic resonance imaging predictors. *Arch Ophthalmol.* 1987;**105**:1371–1377.

Lambert SR, Kriss A, Taylor D. Delayed visual maturation. A longitudinal clinical and electrophysiological assessment. *Ophthalmology.* 1989;**96**:524–529.

Lee DS, Yee RD, Singer HS. Congenital ocular motor apraxia. *Brain.* 1977;**100**:581–599.

Mayer DL, Fulton AB, Rodier D. Grading and recognition acuities of pediatric patients. *Ophthalmology.* 1984;**91**:447.

McDonald MA, Dobson V, Sebris SL. The acuity card procedure, a rapid test of infant acuity. *Invest Ophthalmol Vis Sci.* 1985;**26**:1158.

Moore AT, Taylor DS, Harden A. Bilateral macular dysplasia and congenital retinal dystrophy. *Br J Ophthalmol.* 1985;**69**:691–699.

Nickel BL, Hoyt CS. Leber's congenital amaurosis in mental retardation. A frequent associated defect? *Arch Ophthalmol.* 1982;**100**:1089–1092.

Norton EWD, Cogan DG. Spasms nutans: A clinical study of twenty cases followed two or more years since onset. *Arch Ophthalmol.* 1954;**52**:442–446.

Preston KL, McDonal M, Sebris SL. Validation after acuity card procedure for assessment of infants with ocular disorders. *Ophthalmology.* 1987;**94**:644.

Robertson R, Jan LE, Wong PK. Electroencephalograms of children with permanent cortical visual impairment. *Can J Neurol Sci* 1986;**13**:256–261.

Robinson GC, Kinnis C. Congenital ocular blindness in children. *Am J Dis Child.* 1987;**141**:1321–1324.

Robinson RJ. Assessment of gestational age by neurological examination. *Arch Dis Child.* 1966;**41**:437.

Russell-Eggitt I, Taylor DSI, Clayton PT, et al. Leber's congenital amaurosis: A new syndrome with cardiomyopathy. *Br J Ophthalmol.* 1989;**73**:250–254.

Senior B, Friedmann AI, Brando JL. Juvenile familial nephropathy with tapetoretinal degeneration. *Am J Ophthalmol.* 1961;**64**:726–732.

Sonksen PM. Promotion of visual development in severely visually impaired babies. Evaluation of a developmentally based programme. *Dev Med Child Neurol.* 1991;**33**:320–335.

Stromland K. Ocular abnormalities in foetal alcohol syndrome. *Acta Ophthalmol.* 1985;**1719(suppl)**:1–50.

Taylor D. Congenital tumours of the anterior visual system with dysplasia of the optic discs. *Br J Ophthalmol.* 1982;**66**:455–463.

Taylor MJ, McCulloch DL. Prognostic value of VEPs in young children with acute onset of cortical blindness. *Pediatr Neurol.* 1991;**7**:111–115.

Taylor MJ, McCulloch DL. Visual evoked potentials in infants and children. *J Clin Neurophysiol.* 1992;**9**:357–372.

Wilcox LM, Sokol S. Changes in the binocular fixation patterns and the visually evoked potential in the treatment of esotropia with amblyopia. *Ophthalmology.* 1980;**87**:1273.

Yee RD, Balch RW, Honrubin V. Eye movement abnormalities in rod monochromacy. *Ophthalmology.* 1981;**88**:1010–1018.

Zipf RF. Binocular fixation pattern. *Arch Ophthalmol.* 1976;**94**:401.

CHAPTER 27

Metabolic Neurodegenerative Diseases

Lois J Martyn

INTRODUCTION

Intensive research and crucial technologic developments in recent years have elucidated the metabolic and genetic bases underlying a broad spectrum of disease processes. There have been attendant changes in methods of diagnosis and exciting advances in approaches to treatment, prevention, and genetic counseling.

With this progress has come increased interest in the ophthalmic manifestations of inborn metabolic defects. Readily accessible to clinical examination by ophthalmoscopy, biomicroscopy and electrophysiologic techniques, the eye can provide significant clues to the detection and differentiation of a wide array of metabolic disorders and their mode of inheritance. Biopsy of the conjunctiva can be used for ultrastructural, biochemical and cytogenetic study. Tears can be analyzed to detect certain enzyme defects. In addition, the eye can be used to monitor the effects of specific treatment regimens.

As the body of knowledge concerning inborn errors of metabolism is massive, this chapter is designed to: 1) summarize the salient features of the metabolic disorders that have significant effects on the eye and nervous system; and 2) review the major neuro-ophthalmic signs of inborn metabolic defects, with emphasis on clinical presentation and differential diagnosis.

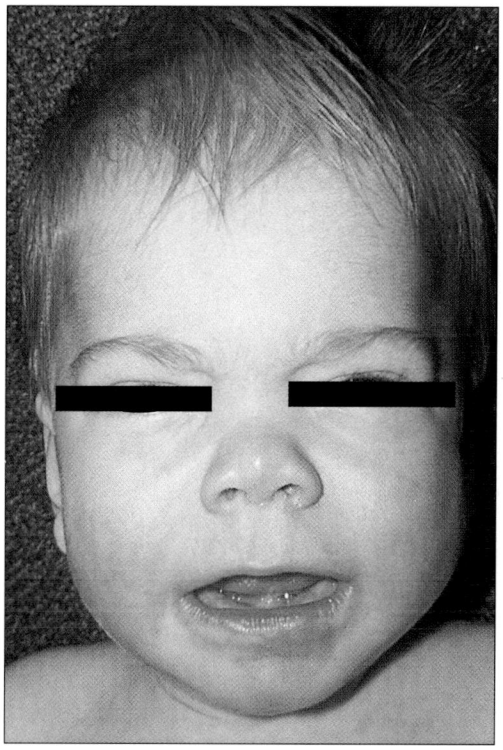

Fig. 27.1
Characteristic dysmorphism of Hurler syndrome.

MUCOPOLYSACCHARIDOSES

The mucopolysaccharidoses (MPS) are a group of hereditary disorders caused by deficiency of lysosomal enzymes involved in the catabolism of the glycosaminoglycans (mucopolysaccharides) dermatan sulfate, heparan sulfate, and keratan sulfate, singly or in combination; chondroitin sulfate may also be affected. The undegraded or partially degraded glycosaminoglycans are stored in lysosomes and accumulate in various tissues throughout the body, and are excreted in the urine. Ten enzyme deficiencies that give rise to MPS have been identified. Clinical similarity between different enzyme deficiencies, and clinical variability within individual enzyme deficiencies occur. Multiple allelism has been proposed to explain the latter. With the exception of MPS type II (Hunter syndrome), the MPS are autosomal recessive disorders; MPS II is X-linked recessive.

As a group the MPS are characterized by a rather distinctive spectrum of clinical manifestations. Bone abnormalities (dysostosis multiplex), joint contractures, skeletal deformity and dwarfing are prominent findings in most of the syndromes. Varying degrees of visceromegaly, cardiovascular disease, respiratory problems, hearing impairment and mental deficiency occur within the group. There is a characteristic facies with

coarse features (*Fig. 27.1*). Hypertrichosis is common. The familiar prototype is Hurler syndrome (MPS I H).

The principal ocular manifestations of the various MPS are progressive corneal clouding (*Fig.27.2*), pigmentary retinal degeneration, optic atrophy, sometimes papilledema, and in certain cases glaucoma. Diagnosis of the various MPS is made on the basis of the distinguishing clinical features, including the ocular signs, identification of excessive mucopolysaccharide substances in tissues and urine, and demonstration of specific enzyme defects (*Fig. 27.3*). Enzyme assays for the diagnosis of MPS, using serum, leukocytes, and cultured fibroblasts are available. Prenatal diagnosis by amniocentesis and chorionic villus biopsy is possible for some MPS. Identification of the carrier state can be difficult and is not always reliable. Enzyme replacement therapy is being investigated; some encouraging results have been achieved with bone marrow transplantation.

GANGLIOSIDOSES

Gangliosides are sialic acid-containing glycosphingolipids that are normally present in the neural and extraneural tissues throughout the body; they are found in highest concentration in the gray

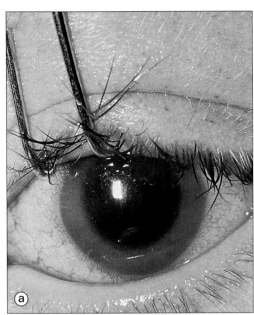

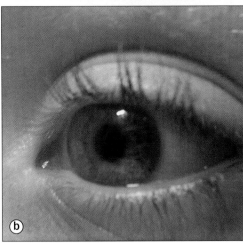

Fig. 27.2 (**a**) Generalized corneal clouding of Hurler syndrome. (**b**) Mild corneal haze of Morquio syndrome.

matter of the brain. A number of defects in lysosomal degradation of gangliosides can result in abnormal accumulation of these lipids and related products in the brain and other tissues, producing a wide spectrum of clinical manifestations. Two major types of ganglioside storage disease occur: G_{M1} gangliosidoses and G_{M2} gangliosidoses (*Figs 27.4 & 27.5*).

G_{M1} GANGLIOSIDOSES

The G_{M1} gangliosidoses are due to deficiency of acid β-galactosidase activity. There is storage of G_{M1} ganglioside in the nervous system, and abnormal accumulation of galactose-containing oligosaccharide and keratan sulfate degradation products in somatic cells.

Infantile, juvenile and adult variants of G_{M1} gangliosidoses occur (see *Fig. 27.4*). The acute infantile form (type 1), commonly referred to as *generalized gangliosidosis*, is characterized by dysmorphism, severe bony abnormalities, visceromegaly, and rapidly progressive neurologic deterioration in infancy, leading to early death usually by age 2 years. The juvenile variant (type 2) is characterized by motor weakness, mild somatic and bony abnormalities, and slowly progressive psychomotor deterioration. The adult variant (type 3) is characterized by dysarthria, choreoathetosis, and mild if any bony abnormalities; intellectual impairment, if present, is mild and survival is prolonged.

The mucopolysaccharidoses

Designation	Metabolic Features
MPS I H: Hurler Syndrome	Profound deficiency of α-L-iduronidase
	MPS accumulation in virtually every system of the body, producing marked somatic and visceral abnormalities
	Urinary excretion of dermatan sulfate and heparan sulfate
	Autosomal recessive
MPS I S : Scheie Syndrome	α-L-iduronidase deficiency
	Urinary excretion of dermatan sulfate and heparan sulfate
	Autosomal recessive
MPS I H/S: Hurler–Scheie Compound	α-L-iduronidase deficiency
	Urinary excretion of dermatan sulfate and heparan sulfate
	Autosomal recessive
MPS II: Hunter Syndrome	Iduronate sulfatase deficiency
	Urinary excretion of dermatan sulfate and heparan sulfate
	X-linked recessive
MPS III: Sanfilippo Syndrome	Four biochemically different forms:
	Type A: Heparan N-sulfatase deficiency
	Type B: α-N-Acetylglucosaminodase deficiency
	Type C: Acetyl-CoA: α-glucosaminide acetyl transferase deficiency
	Type D: N-Acetylglucosamine 6-sulfatase deficiency
	Urinary excretion of heparan sulfate in all four forms
	Autosomal recessive
MPS IV: Morquio Syndrome	Two biochemically different forms:
	Galactose 6-sulfatase deficiency in classic form (MPS IV A)
	β-Galactosidase deficiency in milder form (MPS IV B)
	Urinary excretion of keratan sulfate in both forms
	Autosomal recessive
MPS V: No longer used	
MPS VI: Maroteaux–Lamy Syndrome	N-acetylgalactosamine-4-sulfatase (arylsulfatase B) deficiency
	Urinary excretion of dermatan sulfate
	Autosomal recessive
MPS VII: Sly Syndrome	β-glucuronidase deficiency
	Urinary excretion of dermatan sulfate and heparan sulfate
	Autosomal recessive

Fig. 27.3 The mucopolysaccharidoses. ERG, Electroretinograph

The mucopolysaccharidoses (cont.)	
General Clinical Manifestations	**Ophthalmologic Manifestations**
MPS prototype. Large misshapen head, abnormal facies, coarse features. Wide-set prominent eyes, prominent supraorbital ridges, heavy brows. Broad nose, wide nostrils, flat bridge. Patulous lips, large protuberant tongue. Stubby wide-spaced teeth, hyperplastic gums. Short neck, often low-set large ears. Hypertrichosis. Moderate dwarfism: short extremities and phalanges, broad hands and feet. Joint stiffness, flexion contractures, clawhand deformity, kyphoscoliosis, gibbus. Semi-crouching posture, awkward gait. Prominent radiologic abnormalities (dysostosis multiplex). Vertebral bodies wedge shaped with anterior hook-like projections (beaking). Medullary cavity of tubular bones expanded, cortex thinned. Ribs spatulate or saber-shaped. Often shoe-shaped deformity of sella and enlargement of optic foramina. Protuberant abdomen, marked hepatosplenomegaly. Diastasis recti, umbilical and inguinal hernias. Chest large and wide. Cardiovascular and respiratory disease. Mental deficiency. Sometimes hydrocephalus. Hearing impairment. Progressive physical and mental deterioration. Death usually by age 10 years, frequently from cardiac or respiratory problems.	Shallow orbits. Hypertelorism. Prominent corneal clouding, usually evident by age 2 to 3 years, often present at birth, progressing from generalized haziness to dense, milky ground-glass opacification. Keratoplasty usually not recommended. Evidence for retinal degeneration, including arteriolar attenuation, decreased foveal reflex, pigmentary changes. ERG usually reduced. Optic atrophy. Sometimes papilledema. In some cases megalocornea. Occasionally glaucoma. Corresponding histopathologic changes and evidence of MPS accumulation in ocular tissues well documented. Progressive impairment of vision secondary to corneal clouding, retinal degeneration, optic atrophy, glaucoma, cerebral changes, hydrocephalus, singly or in combination.
Minimal to moderate somatic and visceral signs of MPS, less severe than in Hurler prototype. Somewhat coarse facial features. Stature, habitus relatively normal. Prominent manifestations are joint stiffness, clawhand deformity, carpal tunnel syndrome, aortic valve disease. Hearing impairment common. Intellect normal or nearly normal. Psychiatric disturbances in some cases. Life span relatively normal.	Progressive corneal clouding, diffuse or more dense peripherally, developing early in life, sometimes present at birth, and worsening with age. Little success with keratoplasty. Retinitis pigmentosa-like retinal degeneration with retinal pigmentary changes, progressive night blindness and visual field changes. ERG (Electroretinograph) reduced or extinguished. Glaucoma in some cases. Possibly reduced corneal sensitivity.
Clinical manifestations intermediate between those of Hurler and Scheie syndromes. Dwarfing, progressive joint stiffness, clawhand deformity, hypertelorism, progressive coarsening of facial features, micrognathia. Hepatosplenomegaly. Cardiovascular disease. Intellectual impairment. Hearing impairment. Survival into teens or twenties.	Progressive corneal clouding. Keratoplasty may be helpful. Possibly disc swelling; documented increased intracranial pressure in one such case.
Coarse facial features. Dwarfing, skeletal deformities, joint stiffness similar to but less severe than in Hurler prototype. Hepatosplenomegaly, cardiac, and respiratory disease. Hernias. Hydrocephalus. Motor paralysis in some. Hearing impairment. Nodular or pebbly ivory colored skin lesions. Rapid physical and psychomotor deterioration, and early death, often by age 15 years, in severe form. Fairly normal mental development and longer survival into 20s to 60s in milder form.	Corneas grossly clear; occasionally microscopic changes. Progressive retinal degeneration (R–P-like), usually severe, with retinal pigmentary changes, arteriolar attenuation, optic disc pallor, night vision problems, and field changes. Abnormal ERG. Sometimes optic disc swelling.
Clinical manifestations similar in all four forms. Early and severe progressive mental deterioration. Less severe somatic changes. Coarse facial features. Megalocephaly. Hypertelorism. Moderate skeletal changes. Hepatosplenomegaly. Survival into third decade.	Corneas grossly clear; some microscopic changes reported. Attenuation of retinal arterioles, some retinal pigmentary changes documented. ERG subnormal in some cases. Possibly optic atrophy.
In **classic form,** severe dwarfing, skeletal dysplasia, with kyphosis, sternal bulging. Joint laxity rather than stiffness. Odontoid hypoplasia, atlantoaxial instability, spinal cord and medullary compression, long tract signs, and respiratory paralysis may occur. Prominent joints, knock-knees. Semi crouching stance, waddling gait. Somewhat coarse facial features. Hypoplastic dental enamel. Occasionally hepatomegaly. Protuberant abdomen. Cardiopulmonary complications. Hearing impairment. Intellect normal or mildly impaired. In **milder form,** findings similar to those of classic form, but less severe dwarfism, less tendency to atlantoaxial instability, and usually normal dental enamel.	Corneal clouding in A and B; usually mild or fine haze rather than dense opacification. Subcortical lens opacities noted in type A. Arteriolar attenuation noted in adult. ERG normal or reduced. Possibly optic atrophy or disc blurring.
Morphologic changes similar to those of Hurler syndrome. Coarse features, dwarfing, kyphosis, joint stiffness, visceromegaly, cardiac disease. Hydrocephalus. Atlantoaxial subluxation, spinal cord compression. Hearing impairment. Normal intellect. Milder forms occur.	Progressive corneal clouding, usually evident within first few years of life. Graft may reaccumulate MPS. Papilledema and abducent palsy secondary to hydrocephalus in some cases. Retinal vascular tortuosity. Typically no signs of retinal degeneration, but pigmentary and ERG–VER (Visual Evoked Response) changes noted in mild variant.
Variable, often moderate, clinical manifestations. Coarse features, short stature and skeletal deformity, gibbus, visceromegaly, cardiovascular and respiratory problems. Intellectual impairment.	Corneal clouding in some patients

The G$_{M1}$ gangliosidoses			
Designation	**Metabolic and Genetic Features**	**General Manifestations**	**Ophthalmic Manifestations**
Type 1: Infantile G$_{M1}$ gangliosidosis (generalized gangliosidoses: familial neurovisceral lipidosis)	Profound deficiency of acid β-galactosidase activity. Prominent accumulation of G$_{M1}$ ganglioside throughout nervous system. Accumulation of galactosyl oligosaccharides and keratan sulfate degradation products in somatic cells. Autosomal recessive.	Signs evident at birth or soon thereafter. Dysmorphism: frontal bossing, depressed nasal bridge, large low-set ears, coarse features. Sometimes gingival hyperplasia and mild macroglossia. Skin may be thick and hirsute. Often facial and peripheral edema. Prominent skeletal abnormalities resembling those of Hurler syndrome: dysostosis multiplex, joint stiffness, contractures, dorsolumbar kyphoscoliosis, non-tender enlargement of epiphyseal joints. Hepatomegaly, splenomegaly. Macrocephaly may develop. Severe psychomotor retardation. Hypotonia, hyper-reflexia. Poor appetite, weak suck, poor weight gain. Tonic clonic convulsions after 1 year. Progressive neurologic deterioration regressing to a state of decerebrate rigidity, spastic quadriplegia, blindness, and deafness after age 16 months or so. Death usually by age 2 years.	Macular cherry-red spots in 50% of cases, usually by 6 months or so. Retinal vascular tortuosity, retinal hemorrhages also reported. Optic atrophy. Early loss of vision. Strabismus and nystagmus common. Mild diffuse corneal clouding in some cases. Occasionally tortuosity and saccular microaneurysms of conjunctival vessels. Evidence for ganglioside accumulation in retina and mucopolysaccharide accumulation in cornea well documented.
Type 2: Juvenile G$_{M1}$ gangliosidosis	Deficiency of acid β-galactosidase activity. Moderate accumulation of G$_{M1}$ ganglioside throughout nervous system. Accumulation of galactosyl oligosaccharides and keratan sulfate degradation products in somatic cells less prominent than in infantile form (type 1). Autosomal recessive.	Onset later, coarse slower, skeletal abnormalities milder than those of infantile G$_{M1}$ gangliosidosis (type 1). Coarsening of facial features usually not present. Hepatosplenomegaly usually not evident. Psychomotor development often normal in first year. Neurologic manifestations beginning at about 1 year of age, including lethargy, dulling of sensorium, locomotor ataxia, choreoathetoid movements, moderate generalized weakness of extremities, loss of speech, hyper-reflexia, progressive spasticity. Major motor seizures after age 16 months. In time, deterioration to a state of decerebrate rigidity. Recurrent infections, especially bronchopneumonia. Average life span only 3 to 10 years.	Fundi usually appear normal clinically. Macular cherry-red spot not a feature of this variant. Microscopic evidence of retinal lipidosis and optic atrophy reported. Corneas usually clear. Strabismus and nystagmus may be present. Blindness may occur in later stages of disease.
Type 3: Adult G$_{M1}$ gangliosidosis	Deficiency of acid β-galactosidase activity. Neuronal accumulation of G$_{M1}$ ganglioside predominantly in basal ganglia, less in cortex and white matter. Accumulation of galactosyl oligosaccharides and keratan sulfate degradation products in somatic cells less prominent than in infantile form (type 1). Autosomal recessive.	Gait disturbance and dysarthria, beginning in teens, sometimes earlier. Slowly progressive ataxia, spasticity. Dystonia affecting face and limbs eventually incapacitating. Seizures uncommon. Absence of dysmorphism and organomegaly. Mild if any bony abnormalities; occasionally minimal radiologic changes such as flattening of vertebral bodies. Slow course. Intellectual impairment mild, if present. Survival prolonged into adult years.	Ocular changes not a feature of this variant. Absence of cherry-red spot. Corneas usually clear. Vision usually not impaired.

Fig. 27.4 The G$_{M1}$ gangliosidoses.

Significant ocular manifestations occur in the infantile form. Macular cherry-red spots (see below) are found in approximately 50% of patients with generalized gangliosidosis. Tortuosity of the retinal vessels, retinal hemorrhages, and optic atrophy also have been noted. Mild corneal clouding has been reported in some patients. Loss of vision occurs early in the course of the disease. Strabismus and nystagmus are common. Evidence for ganglioside accumulation in the retina and mucopolysaccharide accumulation in the cornea has been well documented. Ocular findings are more variable in the juvenile form and are not a feature of the adult variant.

The G$_{M1}$ gangliosidoses are autosomal recessive disorders. The diagnosis is confirmed by acid β-galactosidase assays of leukocytes, cultured skin fibroblasts, and amniotic cells. The enzyme defect also can be detected in tears.

G$_{M2}$ GANGLIOSIDOSES

Three enzymatic variants of G$_{M2}$ gangliosidosis occur. There may be deficiency of hexosaminidase A, deficiency of hexosaminidase isoenzymes A and B, or deficiency of the G$_{M2}$ activator protein that is needed for degradation of G$_{M2}$ by hexosaminidase A.

A wide range of severity is seen among patients with hexosaminidase deficiency disorders. Clinically these disorders are usually classified according to age of onset and course as infantile, juvenile, chronic and adult types (see *Fig. 27.5*). Generally the later the disease manifests, the slower its progression and the more variable its symptomatology.

The prototype of the G$_{M2}$ gangliosidoses is Tay-Sachs disease, the severe infantile form of hexosaminidase A deficiency. The clinical picture is one of progressive psychomotor deterioration

G_{M2} Gangliosidoses			
Designations	**Metabolic and Genetic Features**	**General Manifestations**	**Ophthalmologic Manifestations**
Infantile G_{M2} Gangliosidosis: Tay–Sachs Disease	Profound deficiency of hexosaminidase A activity due to hexosaminidase α-subunit defect or deficiency. Hexosaminidase B unaffected. Abnormal accumulation of G_{M2} ganglioside throughout central, autonomic, and peripheral nervous system. Autosomal recessive. Most common in infants of Ashkenazi Jewish descent.	Clinical prototype of the severe early onset G_{M2} gangliosidoses. Onset in infancy with listlessness, hypotonia, weakness, feeding difficulties, or irritability. Psychomotor retardation. Exaggerated extensor startle response to sharp sound. Progressive mental and motor deterioration, decreasing responsiveness by age 6 to 10 months. Seizures after first year. Megancephaly by age 1.5 to 2 years. Rapid deterioration in second year, leading to decerebrate rigidity, blindness, deafness. Death usually by age 2 to 4 years.	Classic macular cherry-red spots in virtually all cases, usually present by the time other neurologic manifestations appear in infancy. Optic atrophy. Vision loss commencing early, usually complete by 1 to 2 years of age; of both central and peripheral origin. Pupil responses may be retained until late in disease. ERG may not become abnormal until late in disease. VEP may be extinguished. Progressive deterioration of eye movements. Dysconjugate eye movements and nystagmus common. Pathologic changes throughout retina similar to those in brain. Demyelination and degeneration of optic nerves, chiasm, and tracts documented.
Juvenile G_{M2} Gangliosidosis: Bernheimer–Seitelberger Disease	Hexosaminidase A deficiency due to hexosaminidase α-subunit defect or deficiency. Neuronal accumulation of G_{M2} ganglioside. Autosomal recessive. Most patients of Ashkenazi Jewish or mixed Jewish/non-Jewish parentage.	Locomotor ataxia beginning between age 2 to 6 years. Progressive dementia, loss of speech, increasing spasticity and seizures by end of first decade. Deterioration to a state of decerebrate rigidity by age 10 to 12 years. Death usually by age 10 to 15 years.	Vision loss in later stages of disease. Macular cherry-red spot may develop, but is not a constant feature. Pigmentary retinal changes may develop. Optic atrophy may develop. There may be strabismus.
Chronic G_{M2} Gangliosidosis	Hexosaminidase A deficiency due to hexosaminidase α-subunit defect or deficiency. Neuronal storage of G_{M2} predominantly in subcortical structures in cerebellum. Autosomal recessive. Usually in Jewish or mixed Jewish/non-Jewish families.	Onset by age 2 to 5 years with abnormalities of gait and posture. Clinical picture of atypical spinocerebellar degeneration with spasticity, dysarthria, ataxia of limbs and trunk, progressive muscle wasting and weakness. Mentation and sensory modalities intact. Indolent course. Survival into third or fourth decade.	Normal fundus findings. Vision unimpaired. ERG, VEP normal. Disturbances of horizontal pursuit movements and varying defects of voluntary up-gaze. Diminished OKN (Opticokinetic Nystagmus). Decreased convergence.
Adult-onset G_{M2} Gangliosidosis	Hexosaminidase A deficiency due to hexosaminidase α-subunit defect or deficiency. Neuronal accumulation of G_{M2} ganglioside. Autosomal recessive.	Clinically variable. Manifestations in adult years, sometimes childhood. Signs of spinocerebellar and lower motor neuron dysfunction, muscle weakness or tremor. Psychosis in one-third of cases. Sometimes dementia. Prolonged survival.	Vision usually unaffected.
Infantile Sandoff Disease	Deficiency of both hexosaminidase A and hexosaminidase B activity due to hexosaminidase β-subunit defect or deficiency. Neuronal storage of G_{M2} ganglioside and visceral accumulation of globoside. Autosomal recessive.	Neurologic manifestations similar to those of Tay–Sachs disease, with psychomotor retardation, progressive deterioration, hyperacusis, megancephaly. Also liver, spleen, renal, and cardiac involvement. Death usually by age 2 to 4 years.	Macular cherry-red spot. Optic atrophy. Progressive vision loss leading to early blindness. Cornea opalescent in one case. Evidence of ganglioside storage in retina and optic nerves well documented.
Juvenile Sandoff Disease	Profound but not total deficiency of hexosaminidase A and virtual absence of hexosaminidase β, due to hexosaminidase β-subunit defect or deficiency. Neuronal storage of G_{M2} ganglioside. Autosomal recessive.	Onset at 3 to 10 years with slurred speech, cerebellar ataxia, and progressive psychomotor retardation, followed by increasing spasticity, hypertonia, and mental deterioration.	Vision and fundi normal.
G_{M2} Activator Deficiency	Hexosaminidase A and hexosaminidase B isoenzymes are present, but degradation of G_{M2} by hexosaminidase A does not occur due to G_{M2} activator protein defect or deficiency. Neuronal accumulation of G_{M2} ganglioside. Autosomal recessive.	Phenotype identical to that of infantile Tay–Sachs disease.	

Fig. 27.5 The G_{M2} gangliosidoses.

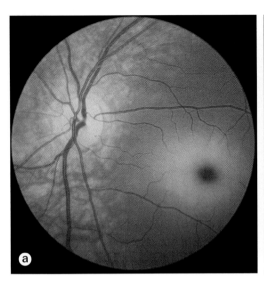
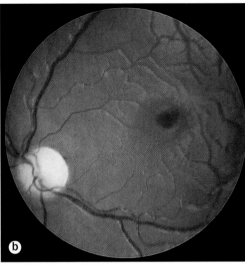

Fig. 27.6 (**a**) Typical cherry-red spot of Tay–Sachs disease. (**b**) Degenerated cherry-red spot of Tay–Sachs disease.

beginning early in infancy. The onset is often insidious with listlessness, hypotonia, feeding difficulties, or irritability. Increasing weakness and decreasing attentiveness become evident in the early months. Spasticity and seizures develop. In time there is regression to a state of decerebrate rigidity, deafness and blindness with death usually occurring by age 3 to 4 years. Macular cherry-red spots develop in virtually all patients with Tay-Sachs disease. With accumulation of lipid, there is loss of transparency of the multilayered macular ganglion cells, producing a creamy white, yellow or grayish halo around the fovea, accentuating the red blush of the ganglion cell-free central region (*Fig. 27.6a*). The macular sign is usually evident by the time other neurologic manifestations appear in infancy. As cell destruction proceeds, the cherry-red spot may become less distinct (*Fig. 27.6b*). Optic atrophy is common. Vision loss commences early, leading to blindness usually by age 2 years. Pathologic changes of the retina similar to those in the brain have been well documented, and deficiency of hexosaminidase A in the retina and nerves has been demonstrated.

The G_{M2} gangliosidoses are autosomal recessive disorders. Heterozygotes are asymptomatic. The diagnosis is confirmed by specific enzyme assay techniques. Hexosaminidase A deficiency variants can be diagnosed prenatally using amniotic fluid, amniotic fluid cells, and chorionic villus biopsy. Specific therapy for the G_{M2} gangliosidoses is not available.

MUCOLIPIDOSES

The mucolipidoses (ML) are a group of lysosomal storage diseases having features in common with both the mucopolysaccharidoses and the sphingolipidoses. Included in this classification are galactosialidosis (ML I), I-cell disease (ML II), pseudo-Hurler polydystrophy (ML III), and sialolipidosis (ML IV) (*Fig. 27.7*). The diagnosis of these disorders can be suspected clinically on the basis of the phenotype in the absence of mucopolysacchariduria. Definitive diagnosis depends on enzyme assays and ultrastructural morphology.

It should be noted that four other lysosomal storage disorders, namely mannosidosis, fucosidosis, mucosulfatidosis, and generalized gangliosidosis, which have clinical features in common with the mucolipidoses, were previously grouped as ML; however, on the basis of the enzyme defects these disorders have been re-classified out of the mucolipidoses (*Fig. 27.8*).

ML I: GALACTOSIALIDOSIS (SIALIDOSIS III)

In ML I, deficiency of the glycoprotein-specific lysosomal enzymes N-acetyl-neuraminidase and β-galactosidase, results in intracellular accumulation of sialic acid-containing oligosaccharides. Hepatocytes, macrophages, hepatic and splenic sinusoidal lining cells, neurons, and renal glomerular and collecting tubular epithelial cells are most affected.

Congenital, infantile, juvenile and adult forms of ML I occur. Diagnostic features include mild Hurler-like manifestations, moderate mental retardation, absence of mucopolysacchariduria, and the presence of cellular inclusions similar to those found in ML II (I-cell disease). Macular cherry-red spot (see p. 27.16) is the major ocular finding in ML I. Vision loss and optic atrophy have been documented. Corneal clouding occurs in the congenital form.

Galactosialidosis is a recessive disorder. Definitive diagnosis is based on measurement of neuraminidase and β-galactosidase activity in skin fibroblasts or white blood cells. Prenatal diagnosis is possible by enzyme assay of cultured amniotic fluid cells.

ML II: I-CELL DISEASE

This is a disorder of lysosomal phosphorylation and localization. In I-cell disease there is deficiency of N-acetylglucosamine phosphotransferase, a key enzyme in the pathway by which mannose-6-phosphate, a recognition marker, is added to lysosomal enzymes. Newly synthesized lysosomal enzymes are secreted into the extracellular medium, instead of being targeted correctly to lysosomes. In affected patients, there is deficiency of multiple lysosomal enzymes in cultured fibroblasts, with increased levels of lysosomal enzymes in culture medium, serum, and other body fluids. A characteristic feature of the disease is the presence of numerous membrane-bound vacuoles containing electron-lucent or fibrillogranular material in the cytoplasm of mesenchymal cells, especially fibroblasts. It is these inclusions for which the disease is named. The storage material includes oligosaccharides, mucopolysaccharides and lipids.

The mucolipidoses			
Designation	**Metabolic Defect**	**General Clinical Manifestations**	**Ophthalmic Manifestations**
ML I: Galactosialidosis (Sialidosis III) Formerly lipomucopoly-saccharidosis.	Combined deficiency of β-galactosidase and N-acetyl-neura-minidase in all forms.	**Congenital Form.** Phenotype similar to G_{MI}. Facial dysmophism, skeletal dysplasia. Psychomotor retardation. Hepatosplenomegaly, cardiomegaly, renal failure. Hydrops. Lethal within first 2 years of life.	Corneal clouding. Macular cherry-red spots.
	All forms autosomal recessive.	**Late Infantile Form.** Normal or minimally abnormal at birth. Signs by age 6–12 months. Coarse facies, dysostosis multiplex. Hepatosplenomegaly. Mild mental retardation. Motor retardation with axial hypotonia and peripheral hypertonicity. Progressive neurologic deterioration. Recurrent infections. Occasional renal involvement ('nephrosialidosis'). Death in early childhood.	Macular cherry-red spots.
		Juvenile Form. Onset in late infancy or early childhood. Progressive neurologic degeneration. Mental retardation, ataxia, myoclonus. Hearing impairment. Mild Hurler phenotype. Coarse facies, small stature, dysostosis multiplex, joint contractures. Hepatosplenomegaly. Angiokeratomatous rash in bathing suit area. Survival into adulthood.	Macular cherry-red spots. Corneal opacities. Vision loss.
		Adult Form (previously cherry-red spot–myoclonus syndrome). Onset in adolescence. Progressive myoclonus. Insidious vision loss. Mild coarsening of features. Hepatosplenomegaly. Normal or only slightly impaired intelligence. Survival into 4th decade.	Macular cherry-red spots. Vision loss.
ML II: I-Cell Disease	Deficiency of N-acetylglucosamine phosphotransferase.

Autosomal recessive. | Early onset, sometimes evident at birth. Coarse facial features, high forehead, puffy eyelids, prominent epicanthal folds, flat nasal bridge, anteverted nostrils, gingival hyperplasia, macroglossia. Progressive impairment of joint mobility. Severe skeletal abnormalities including kyphoscoliosis, lumbar gibbus, claw-hand deformity. Anterior breaking and wedging of vertebral bodies, widening of ribs, proximal pointing of metacarpals. Congenital hip dislocation, congenital fractures in some cases. Abdominal protuberance with hepatomegaly. Minimal splenomegaly. Commonly umbilical and inguinal hernias. Psychomotor retardation. Failure to thrive. Cessation of lineal growth during 2nd year. Frequent respiratory infections. Cardiomegaly, murmurs; aortic insufficiency in some. Rapidly progressive coarse. Death usually by age 5–8 years. Sometimes survival into teens. | Corneal haziness: fine granular stromal opacities. Glaucoma in some case, also megalocornea in the absence of glaucoma. |
| ML III: Pseudo-Hurler Polydystrophy | Deficiency of N-actylglucosamine phosphotransferase.

Autosomal recessive | Onset about age 2–4 years. Slowly progressive skeletal dysplasia. Stiffness of hands and shoulders early. Claw-hand deformity, scoliosis, short stature by age 4–6 years. Progressive destruction of hip joint, often leading to waddling gait; sometimes disabling. Carpal tunnel syndrome common. Moderately severe dysostosis multiplex. Mild coarsening of facial features, thickening of skin after 6th year. Some degree of learning disability or mental retardation in approximately 50% of cases. Cardiac valvular involvement. May survive to 4th or 5th decade. | Progressive corneal clouding: fine stromal opacities. Retinal venous tortuosity, surface wrinkling macul-opathy, mild retinal pigmentary changes. Papilledema or peripapillary elevation. Hyperopic astigmatism. |
| ML IV: Sialolipidosis | Deficiency of ganglioside sialidase proposed. | Psychomotor retardation by age 6–12 months. Motor and language development rarely progresses beyond 12–15 months level. Hypotonia in infancy, followed by development of spastic quadriparesis. Physical growth also retarded. Mild coarsening of facial features and puffiness of eyelids in some cases. Protracted coarse. Survival into 2nd or 3rd decade. | Corneal clouding of variable course, prominent opithelial involvement, sometimes with bouts of pain, tearing, photophobia.

Retinal degeneration, optic atrophy.

Visual impairment, usually in infancy. Strabismus. Nystagmus. Occasionally cataracts. Sometimes severe myopia. |

Fig. 27.7 The mucolipidoses.

Patients with I-cell disease exhibit many of the clinical features and radiologic abnormalities that are seen in Hurler syndrome, including a characteristic facies, skeletal dysplasia, visceromegaly, and psychomotor retardation, but they do not exhibit mucopolysacchariduria.

The principal ocular manifestation of I-cell disease is corneal haziness. Slit lamp examination shows fine granular stromal opac-ities. Glaucoma, and megalocornea in the absence of glaucoma, also have been reported. Macular cherry-red spots are not a feature of I-cell disease. The typical inclusions have been demonstrated in the cornea, sclera, and other tissues of the eye. Conjunctival biopsy may be useful in the diagnosis of the disease.

I-cell disease is an autosomal recessive condition. Biochemically, the diagnosis is made by measurements of serum lysosomal enzyme

Conditions formerly classified with mucolipidoses	
Mannosidosis	**Mucosulfatidosis**
Disorder of glycoprotein degradation (autosomal recessive). Deficiency of lysosomal enzyme α-D-mannosidase. Tissue accumulation and increased urinary excretion of oligosaccharides. Psychomotor retardation, facial coarsening, dysostosis multiplex. Also recurrent infections, deafness, hepatomegaly, hernias. Severe infantile form (type I), onset 3–12 months, rapidly progressive, leading to death between 3 and 10 years. Milder juvenile–adult form (type II), onset 1–4 years, with survival into adulthood. Lenticular opacitics: spoke-wheel pattern composed of small vacuoles in posterior lens cortex in some cases, and other patterns including scattered cortical opacities reported. Superficial corneal opacities.	A sulfatide lipidosis (autosomal recessive). Deficiency of multiple sulfatases. Increased urinary sulfatide and mucopolysaccharide excretion. Combined features of metachromatic leukodystrophy and mucopolysaccharidosis. Progressive psychomotor deterioration, skeletal changes, facial dysmorphism. Signs in 1st or 2nd year of life. Death in 1st or 2nd decade. Pigmentary retinal degeneration, macular grayness or cherry-red-like changes, optic atrophy. Peripheral circumferential opacitites of anterior lens capsule. Occasionally corneal clouding.
	Generalized gangliosidosis
Fucosidosis	Type I G$_{MI}$ gangliosidosis (autosomal recessive). Deficiency of acid β-galactosidase activity. Storage of ganglioside in nervous system, abnormal accumulation of oligosaccharide and keratan sulfate degradation products in somatic cells. Dysmorphism, severe bony abnormalities, visceromegaly, progressive neurologic deterioration. Onset in infancy. Death usually by age 2 years. Macular cherry-red spot in 50% of patients. Also tortuosity of retinal vessels, retinal hemorrhages, optic atrophy. Early loss of vision. Mild corneal clouding in some patients.
Disorder of glycoprotein degradation (autosomal recessive). Deficiency of lysosomal enzyme α-L-fucosidase. Vacuolation of cells of brain, peripheral nerves, liver, pancreas, skin, conjunctiva, cultured fibroblasts. Increased urinary excretion of oligosaccharides. Retardation and progressive psychomotor deterioration, mild coarsening of facial features, dysostosis multiplex, growth retardation. Angiokeratoma corporis diffusum. Also visceromegaly, cardiomegaly, recurrent infections, seizures. Onset 3 months (fatal infantile form) to 1 or 2 years (milder form with survival into 2nd decade). Tortuosity and saccular dilatation of conjunctival vessels and retinal veins. Pigmentary retinopathy. Corneal opacities in region of Bowman's membrane and epithelium.	

Fig. 27.8 Conditions formerly classified with mucolipidoses.

levels. Phosphotransferase activity also can be measured in white blood cells or in cultured fibroblasts. Homozygotes have very low or undetectable levels of phosphotransferase activity. Heterozygotes have intermediate levels of phosphotransferase activity. Prenatal diagnosis of the disease can be made using cultured amniotic cells. There is no specific treatment for I-cell disease.

ML III: Pseudo-Hurler Polydystrophy

This is a rare genetic disorder biochemically related to I-cell disease. As in I-cell disease, there is abnormal lysosomal enzyme transport in cells of mesenchymal origin associated with deficiency of N-acetylglucosamine phosphotransferase. Affected cells contain dense inclusions filled with storage materials, and the level of lysosomal enzymes in serum and body fluids is elevated, while levels of lysosomal enzymes are deficient within cultured fibroblasts. Pseudo-Hurler polydystrophy and I-cell disease are differentiated on the basis of clinical criteria.

Manifestations of pseudo-Hurler polydystrophy are milder, appear later and progress more slowly than those of I-cell disease. Patients with ML III share many clinical features with those having mild to moderately severe forms of MPS I and MPS VI, but they do not exhibit mucopolysacchariduria.

The ocular manifestations of pseudo-Hurler polydystrophy include progressive corneal clouding, retinal and optic nerve abnormalities, and hyperopic astigmatism. Slit lamp examination reveals fine stromal opacities that increase with age. Faint ground-glass haziness of the cornea may be grossly evident by age 7 or 8 years, but the changes are not as striking as those of MPS I or MPS VI. Retinal venous tortuosity, surface wrinkling maculopathy, retinal haze, and mild retinal pigmentary changes have been reported. There may be papilledema or peripapillary elevation, and possibly progressive visual field loss.

Like ML II, ML III is an autosomal recessive disorder. Biochemical diagnosis of the disease, carrier detection and prenatal diagnosis are made as in ML II. No definitive treatment is available.

ML IV: Sialolipidosis

This lysosomal storage disease is characterized by profound psychomotor retardation and vision impairment of early onset, with corneal clouding and retinal degeneration, but without skeletal dysplasia or organomegaly.

The exact metabolic defect is unknown, though deficiency of ganglioside sialidase has been proposed. Ultrastructural examination reveals striking lysosomal storage inclusions in the cells of almost every organ and tissue of the body. Biochemically, ML IV is characterized by accumulation of gangliosides, particularly polysialylated gangliosides, phospholipids, and acid mucopolysaccharides.

Corneal clouding is an early and prominent feature of ML IV. Its onset varies from infancy to age 5 years; it may be evident at birth. The severity varies from slight haziness to dense clouding. The course also is variable; it may remain stable, worsen or in some cases improve. Slit lamp examination shows prominent epithelial involvement without stromal opacities. There may be marked corneal surface irregularities. Some patients experience bouts of pain, tearing, photophobia and conjunctival injection, possibly related to recurrent corneal erosions. Lubrication may be helpful. Keratoplasty has been tried in ML IV, but with re-epithelialization the clouding may return. Retinal degeneration is present to some degree in most patients. Pigmentary changes, arteriolar attenuation, optic atrophy, and reduced ERG responses have been documented.

Visual impairment usually is evident in infancy. It may be apparent before other signs. Strabismus is an early manifestation in many children. Nystagmus may develop. Some patients are severely myopic. Cataracts also have been reported.

Ultrastructural examination of the eye has confirmed the presence of storage material in the corneal epithelium with relative sparing of the stroma and endothelium, and in conjunctival epithelial cells, in ciliary epithelial cells, and within retinal ganglion cells. Conjunctival biopsy showing the characteristic inclusions can be helpful in diagnosis.

The disorder is autosomal recessive. Its frequency is relatively greater in Jews of Ashkenazic origin than in non-Jews. Prenatal diagnosis has been accomplished by identifying the storage inclusions in amniocytes and chorionic villus cells.

NIEMANN–PICK DISEASE

A number of biochemically and clinically distinct conditions are classified under the eponym *Niemann–Pick disease* (NPD) (*Fig. 27.9*).

TYPES A AND B NPD

Types A and B NPD are sphingomyelin lipidoses. There is deficiency of acid sphingomyelinase activity resulting in lysosomal accumulation of sphingomyelin, cholesterol and other metabolically related lipids. The histopathologic hallmark of the disease is the large lipid-laden foam cell, referred to as the Niemann-Pick cell, found particularly in tissues and organs of the monocyte-macrophage system.

Type A NPD is characterized by failure to thrive, hepatosplenomegaly, and rapidly progressive neurologic degeneration in infancy, leading to death by age 2 to 3 years. Type B NPD is characterized primarily by hepatosplenomegaly in childhood with little or no neurologic involvement, and survival into adulthood. Progressive pulmonary infiltration can be a major problem in more severely affected type B NPD patients.

The principal ocular finding is the macular cherry-red spot (see above), occurring in approximately 50% of patients with type A NPD, and less than 10% of patients with type B NPD (*Fig. 27.10*). In some cases there is milder grayness of the macular ring or a granular perifoveal halo. Corneal and lenticular changes also may occur in type A NPD. Histologic studies have documented evidence of lipid storage in the eye, including the presence of lipid-laden retinal ganglion cells, vacuolated cells in the choroid, and lamellar deposits in corneal and lens epithelium.

Types A and B NPD are autosomal recessive conditions. The diagnosis is readily made by enzymatic determination of acid sphingomyelinase activity in cells or tissue extracts. Heterozygote detection requires molecular studies. Prenatal diagnosis by enzymatic or molecular analysis of cultured amniocytes and chorionic villus cells is possible. Currently there is no specific effective treatment for types A and B NPD.

TYPE C NPD

Type C NPD is an autosomal recessive lipidosis distinguished by a unique disorder in cellular cholesterol processing associated with abnormal lysosomal accumulation of unesterified cholesterol. The primary molecular defect has not yet been identified. Characteristic foam cells are present in affected tissues.

The 'classic' phenotype of type C NPD is characterized by hepatosplenomegaly, progressive ataxia, dystonia, dementia, and progressive supranuclear vertical gaze palsy. Manifestations appear

Niemann–Pick disease			
Designation	Metabolic Features	General Manifestations	Ophthalmologic Manifestations
Type A NPD	Profound deficiency of acid sphingomyelinase activity (less than 5% of normal). Sphingomyelin lipidosis. Characteristic foam cells in affected tissues and organs. Autosomal recessive. More common in patients of Ashkenazic Jewish descent.	Onset in infancy, with hypotonia, weakness, feeding difficulties, failure to thrive. Hepatosplenomegaly. Psychomotor retardation evident age 6 months. Progressive neurodegeneration and debilitation. Sometimes respiratory involvement. Osteoporosis common. Occasionally xanthomas. Death by age 2–3 years.	Macular cherry-red spot in 30–50% of cases, often with extension of retinal opacification beyond the peripheral region, even mild generalized retinal haze. Diffuse stromal haze of cornea in some cases. Lens changes including brownish granular 'deposits' on or in anterior lens capsule, and scattered white spots on or in posterior lens capsule. ERG abnormal. Vision loss late in course. Widespread distribution of lipid inclusions in the eye.
Type B NPD	Deficiency of acid sphingomyelinase (5–10% of normal). Sphingomyelin lipidosis. NP foam cells in affected tissues and organs. Autosomal recessive. Panethnic.	Onset in childhood to adolescence. Phenotypic variability. Usually diagnosed by presence of hepatosplenomegaly. Little or no neurologic involvement in most patients. Progressive pulmonary involvement in more severely affected patients. Death in childhood or adulthood.	Macular cherry-red spot in less than 10% of cases. Macular changes ranging from grayness of macular region to perifoveal halo of punctate or granular opacities.
Type C NPD	Abnormality of cholesterol transport. Primary metabolic defect not yet identified. Secondary reduction in acid sphingomyelinase activity. Lysosomal accumulation of cholesterol and sphingomyelin. Characteristic inclusions; NP foam cells. Autosomal recessive. Panethnic (includes those of Nova Scotia descent previously classified as type D).	Presents in childhood. Slowly progressive variable neurodegenerative course with ataxia, dysarthria, dysphagia, drooling, dystonia, seizures. Hepatosplenomegaly less than in types A and B NPD. May present with jaundice. Death in teens, commonly from inanition, aspiration. May survive into adulthood.	Progressive supranuclear vertical gaze palsy affecting upward and downward gaze; blinking and head thrusting may be noted on attempted vertical gaze. Horizontal gaze also may be affected. Occasionally opalescence of perifoveal retina.

Fig. 27.9 Niemann–Pick disease.

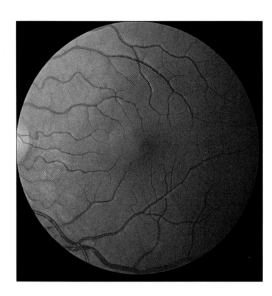

Fig. 27.10 Mild cherry-red-like macular changes in Neimann–Pick disease.

in late childhood. Death occurs in the teens. Other type C NPD presentations include neonatal liver disease with death in infancy, early infantile onset with hypotonia and delayed motor development, and slowly progressive adult variants in which psychosis and dementia predominate.

The diagnosis of type C NPD requires demonstration of abnormal intracellular cholesterol processing and intralysosomal accumulation of unesterified cholesterol by specific testing. Heterozygote identification and prenatal diagnosis can be accomplished in some cases. No specific treatment for type C NPD is available, though strategies to reduce intracellular cholesterol accumulation have been formulated.

GAUCHER DISEASE

This is a lysosomal storage disease characterized by abnormal accumulation of glucosylceramide (glucocerebroside). The underlying metabolic defect is impaired intracellular hydrolysis of the glycolipid glucosylceramide and related glucosphingolipids due to deficiency of acid β-glucosidase. A hallmark of the disease is the presence of distinctive lipid-laden cells of the monocyte-macrophage system throughout the body; these so-called *Gaucher cells* are distinguished by cytoplasmic inclusions having a twisted tubular appearance.

Based primarily on the absence or presence and severity of neurologic involvement, three major types of Gaucher disease have been delineated (*Fig. 27.11*). Hepatosplenomegaly and skeletal lesions occur in all three. Involvement of other organs is variable. Type 1, the nonneuronopathic form, is characterized primarily by hepatosplenomegaly and bone lesions. Type 2, the acute neuronopathic form, is characterized by early onset with severe neurologic involvement and extensive visceral involvement. In type 3, the subacute neuronopathic form, neurologic involvement is of later onset than in type 2 and the course is more chronic; there is usually marked visceral involvement.

A variety of ocular manifestations occur in Gaucher disease. Lesions resembling pingueculae have been noted in patients with type 1 disease. These appear as brownish wedge-shaped

Gaucher disease: glucosylceramide lipidosis		
Designation	**Principal Features**	**Ophthalmic Manifestations**
Type 1: Nonneuronopathic form (previously 'adult' form)	Onset in childhood or adult years. Broad spectrum of severity. Splenomegaly, frequently with thrombocytopenia, anemia, leukopenia, bleeding tendencies. Hepatomegaly; varying degrees of liver dysfunction. Skeletal involvement, often debilitating. Osteolytic lesions, painful episodic 'bone crises' (sometimes with fever), infarctions, pathologic fractures. Pulmonary infiltration, pulmonary failure in some cases. Occasionally yellow-brown pigmentation of the skin. Variable progression – rapid or protracted course. Normal life span in most. Sometimes death in 1st or 2nd decade secondary to complications. Absence of primary neurologic manifestations. Occasionally secondary neurologic signs due to vertebral collapse, fat emboli, coagulopathies. Increased incidence of neoplastic disease.	Brownish triangular or cuneiform areas of thickening of bulbar conjunctiva, nasal and temporal to limbus, resembling pingueculae. Occasionally, retinal hemorrhage, edema. Possibly macular, perimacular changes.
Type 2: Acute neuronopathic form ('infantile' form)	Onset usually early infancy, sometimes later. Neurologic involvement by age 6 months. Signs of cranial nerve nuclei and extrapyramidal tract involvement. Progressive spasticity, dysphasia. Classic triad of trismus, strabismus, retroflection of head. Seizures. Sometimes choreoathetoid movements. Hepatosplenomegaly. Osseous lesions. Rapidly progressive course. Death usually by age 2 years, often from apnea or aspiration pneumonia.	Paralytic strabismus; often a presenting sign. Progressive impairment of conjugate gaze movements.
Type 3: Subacute neuronopathic form (so-called 'juvenile' form)	Variable age of onset. Severity intermediate between that of types 1 and 2. Hepatosplenomegaly, usually preceding neurologic signs. Osseous lesions. Neurologic involvement usually beginning in childhood or adolescence. Ataxia, spastic paraparesis, seizures, slowly progressive dementia. More chronic course than type 2.	Ocular motor abnormalities often the first manifestation. Progressive impairment of conjugate gaze. Supranuclear ophthalmoplegia. Signs of ocular motor apraxia. Paralytic strabismus. Multiple discrete small white spots of retina posteriorly. Grayness of macular region.

Fig. 27.11 Gaucher disease: glucosylceramide lipidoses.

areas of thickening of the bulbar conjunctiva adjacent to the corneoscleral junction (limbus) nasally and temporally. Some have been reported to contain Gaucher-like cells. Macular or perimacular changes also may occur in type 1 disease and the presence of Gaucher cells in the choroid has been reported. In addition, with anemia and thrombocytopenia retinal hemorrhages and edema may develop. Paralytic strabismus is the principal ophthalmic manifestation of type 2 Gaucher disease. Progressive impairment of conjugate gaze movements may occur. Patients with type 3 disease also may show progressive impairment of conjugate gaze movements. Findings may simulate those of congenital ocular motor apraxia with impairment of horizontal saccades, and compensatory head movements. Patients with type 3 Gaucher disease also may exhibit multiple discrete white spots of the retina. There may be grayness of the macular area, but true cherry-red spots are not a feature of Gaucher disease.

Gaucher disease is an autosomal recessive disorder. The disease is most common in the Ashkenazi Jewish population, though all types are panethnic. The diagnosis can be established by enzyme assay of leukocytes, cultured skin fibroblasts, amniotic fluid cells and chorionic villi. DNA analysis also can be helpful.

The quality of life can be improved with a variety of treatment modalities including splenectomy and joint replacement. Accumulation of glucosylceramide and associated clinical manifestations can be reversed by repeated infusions of modified acid β-glucosidase (alglucerase). Response to marrow transplantation has been encouraging in some cases.

SULFATIDE LIPIDOSIS: METACHROMATIC LEUKODYSTROPHY

Sulfatide lipidosis is an inherited disorder of myelin metabolism characterized by abnormal accumulation of galactosyl sulfatide (cerebroside sulfate), a major lipid of the nervous system. The lipid accumulates predominantly in the white matter of the central nervous system and in peripheral nerves. It also accumulates within the kidney, gallbladder and other visceral organs, and is excreted in excessive amounts in the urine. In histologic preparations the accumulated lipid granules stain metachromatically, giving rise to the descriptive term *metachromatic leukodystrophy* (MLD). Clinically the major manifestations of the disorder are progressive mental and motor deterioration.

Several variants of metachromatic leukodystrophy are described (*Fig. 27.12*). A congenital form of MLD may occur, based on histologic findings in two cases, but further documentation is lacking. The late infantile form of MLD presents within the second year of life and is fatal within a few years. Developmental delay, weakness and ataxia are followed by progressive spasticity and quadriparesis. The juvenile forms of MLD manifest between age 4 and 12 years. Early signs include behavioral changes, intellectual deterioration, slurring of speech, and gait disturbances. The course may be protracted, lasting 20 years or more, but most patients with juvenile MLD do not live beyond their teens. The adult form of MLD may begin in the teens or adult years. Behavioral disturbances and dementia are the major presenting signs. The course may be rapid or progress slowly over

Sulfatide lipidosis: metachromatic leukodystrophy variants		
Designation	Principal Features	Ophthalmic Manifestations
Congenital form	Metabolic defect unknown. Signs at birth. Apnea, cyanosis, generalized weakness, seizures. Death in newborn period or early infancy.	
Late infantile form	Arylsulfatase A deficiency. Elevated urinary sulfatide excretion. Insidious onset between age 1 and 2 years. Developmental delay, weakness, ataxia, loss of speech, bulbar palsies, progressive spastic quadriparesis, mental regression. Occasionally seizures. Relatively rapid course. Death in 1–7 years.	Optic atrophy. Macular grayness or cherry-red-like spot. Vision loss. Nystagmus. Strabismus.
Juvenile form	Arylsulfatase A deficiency. Elevated urinary sulfatide excretion. Onset between age 4 and 12 years. Mental regression, abnormal behavior, clumsiness, ataxia. Incontinence. Progressive spastic quadriparesis. Speech impairment. Seizures. Protracted course; survival sometimes 20 years or more.	Vision loss. Optic atrophy. Nystagmus.
Adult form	Arylsulfatse A deficiency. Elevated urinary sulfatide excretion. Onset from age 14–62 years. Changes in mentation, behavior, performance. Clumsiness, ataxia, progressive spastic quadriparesis. Peripheral neuropathy. Incontinence. Seizures. Progressive corticobulbar, corticospinal, cerebellar signs. Survival of 5–10 years or more.	Optic atrophy. Vision loss. Delayed VEP. Nystagmus.
Multiple sulfatase deficiency: mucosulfatidosis	Arylsulfatase A, B, and C deficiency, and other sulfatase deficiencies. Elevated urinary mucopolysaccharide excretion. Evident in 1st or 2nd year of life. Manifestations like those of late infantile MLD, plus features of MPS. Course facial features, skeletal changes, joint stiffness, growth retardation, hepatosplenomegaly. Also ichthyosis. Intellectual and motor regression. Seizures. Death usually toward end of 1st decade, or early in 2nd or 3rd decade.	Macular grayness, cherry-red-like spot. Retinal degeneration. Optic atrophy. Vision loss, blindness. Nystagmus. Strabismus. Occasionally corneal clouding. Lenticular changes.
Mild variant without arylsulfatase deficiency	Deficiency of cerebroside sulfate activator factor (saposin B). Arylsulfatase A normal or mildly reduced. Elevated urinary sulfatide excretion. Signs by age 4–6 years. Clinically similar to juvenile MLD. Behavior changes and psychomotor deterioration.	Possibly optic atrophy.

Fig. 27.12 Sulfatide lipidosis: metachromatic leukodystrophy variants.

several decades. In the late infantile, juvenile and adult forms of MLD, there is profound deficiency of arylsulfatase A in all tissues. A number of patients having features of MLD without deficiency of arylsulfatase A have also been reported.

Multiple sulfatase deficiency (MSD) is a rare form of MLD that includes features of mucopolysaccharidosis. In this disorder there is deficiency of arylsulfatase A as well as deficiency of other sulfatases involved in the degradation of mucopolysaccharides. In addition to progressive mental and motor deterioration, patients develop skeletal changes, facial dysmorphism and visceromegly.

The ophthalmologic manifestations of MLD are significant. In late infantile MLD, optic atrophy is common. Progressive vision loss and impairment of the pupillary light response have been documented. There may be grayness of the macular region, and in some cases a cherry-red-like spot has been described. Strabismus and nystagmus may develop. Optic atrophy is also common in juvenile MLD, but macular changes are not a clinical feature of the juvenile forms. In patients with adult MLD, progressive vision loss, optic atrophy and nystagmus have been documented.

Reported ocular findings in MSD include pigmentary retinal degeneration, grayness or cherry-red-like macular changes, optic atrophy, and occasionally corneal clouding. Circumferential opacity of the peripheral region of the anterior lens capsule also has been noted.

Corresponding histopathologic changes of the eye, particularly degenerative changes of the optic nerve and retina, and the presence of metachromatic material have been well documented in the infantile, juvenile and adult forms of MLD. Similar changes have been found in MSD, along with evidence of mucopolysaccaride accumulation. It is also of interest that arylsulfatase deficiency can be detected in tears.

These disorders are autosomol recessive conditions. Enzyme assay is important in delineation of these MLD variants and in detection of the carrier state, using peripheral leukocytes or cultured skin fibroblasts. Prenatal diagnosis is based on arylsulfatase A activity in cultured amniotic fluid or chorionic villus cells. Several modes of therapy are being investigated. As yet there is no specific effective treatment for MLD, though bone marrow transplantation may slow the progress of the disease.

GALACTOSYLCERAMIDE LIPIDOSIS: GLOBOID-CELL LEUKODYSTROPHY

Also called *Krabbe disease*, globoid-cell leukodystrophy is a rare metabolic degenerative disease of the nervous system. It affects predominantly the white matter, leading to progressive mental and motor deterioration and early death.

The underlying defect is deficiency of galactosylceramidase (galactocerebroside β-galactosidase). This enzyme normally catalyzes degradation of galactosylceramide (galactocerebroside), a constituent of myelin and oligodendroglia. The disease process is characterized by widespread loss of myelin and oligodendrocytes, infiltration by multinucleated macrophages (globoid cells) that contain undegraded galactosylceramide, axonal degeneration, and astrocytic gliosis in the white matter of the brain; peripheral nerves also are commonly affected.

Clinical manifestations usually appear by age 3 to 6 months, sometimes later. Three clinical stages have been described. The early stage is characterized by irritability and hypersensitivity to external stimuli, episodic fevers of unknown origin, some stiffness of the limbs, slight retardation or regression of psychomotor development, feeding difficulties, vomiting, and seizures. The next stage is marked by rapid and severe mental and motor deterioration, hypertonicity and hyper-reflexia, and tonic or clonic seizures. In the final or 'burnt-out' stage the infant is decerebate, often blind and deaf. Affected infants rarely survive beyond age 2 years.

The major ophthalmic manifestations of globoid-cell leukodystrophy are optic atrophy, attendant impairment of the pupillary light response, and progressive loss of vision leading to blindness. Loss of the foveal reflex may be evident. Histopathologic studies of the optic nerve have shown loss of axons, loss of myelin, gliosis, and the presence of globoid cells. Degenerative changes of the retinal nerve fiber and ganglion cell layers also have been documented. Concurrent cerebral changes may contribute to vision loss in this disease.

Globoid-cell leukodystrophy is an autosomal recessive disorder. Diagnosis is confirmed by assay of galactosylceramidase activity in leukocytes or cultured fibroblasts, or by brain biopsy demonstrating the characteristic globoid cells. Carrier detection by enzyme assay is possible but not always reliable. Prenatal diagnosis by enzyme assay of amniotic fluid cells or chorionic villus biopsy can be accomplished. There is no effective specific treatment for this disease.

FABRY DISEASE

Fabry disease, also referred to as *angiokeratoma corporis diffusum universale*, is an X-linked disorder of glycosphingolipid catabolism resulting from deficient activity of the lysosomal hydrolase, α-galactosidase A. There is profound deficiency of enzymatic activity in the tissues and fluids of affected hemizygous males; most heterozygous females have intermediate levels of enzymatic activity.

The enzymatic defect leads to progressive systemic accumulation of neutral glycosphingolipids with terminal α-galactosyl moieties, predominantly trihexosylceramide globotriaosylceramide and, to a lesser extent, galabiosylceramide and blood group B substances, in most tissues, organs and fluids of the body. Birefringent lipid crystals are found primarily in the lysosomes of blood vessel cells, in reticuloendothelial, connective tissue and myocardial cells, and in epithelial cells of the kidney, adrenal gland and cornea. Lipid also accumulates in ganglion cells of the brain and in cells of the peripheral and autonomic nervous system, and vascular changes are prominent throughout the nervous system.

In hemizygous males, clinical manifestations usually develop during childhood or adolesence. Flat or elevated angiectatic lesions of the skin, referred to as angiokeratomas, develop early and increase in number and size with age. The lesions tend to be most numerous in distribution between the umbilicus and knees. Mucosal areas, particularly the oral mucosa and conjunctiva, are commonly involved. Paroxysomal episodes of severe burning pain in the extremities are typical. These crises may last minutes to days and may be accompanied by low-grade fever. Hypohidrosis is common. With increasing age there is progressive cardiovascular and renal involvement. Angina, myocardial infarction, arrythmias, valvular disease, heart failure and cardiac enlargement may develop. Albuminuria, uremia, and systemic hypertension are common. Cerebrovascular complications including aneurysms, thrombosis and hemorrhage are frequent; patients may develop seizures, hemiplegia, aphasia, and personality changes. Death usually occurs in adult life from renal failure, or from cardiovascular or cerebrovascular complications.

Heterozygous females may have an attenuated form of the disease; they are usually asymptomatic but can have significant manifestations.

Distinctive corneal opacities resulting from accumulation of lipid in the corneal epithelial cells are the ocular hallmark of Fabry disease. The typical appearance is that of a fine stippling of intra- or subepithelial opacities arranged in a whorl-like pattern of radiating lines, often more prominent inferiorly. These corneal changes are seen in almost all affected males and in many carrier females. The opacities do not seem to interfere with vision.

Lenticular opacities also occur in Fabry disease. Granular anterior capsular or subcapsular opacities arranged in a radiating wedge-shaped or 'propeller' pattern may be seen in affected males. Fine whitish opacities arranged in a linear spoke-like pattern on or near the posterior lens capsule also may be seen in affected males and in some carrier females.

Ocular signs of vascular involvement may also develop. Some patients develop orbital and lid edema. Conjunctival changes, including tortuosity, aneurysmal dilatation, sludging and telangiectasis are common. There may may tortuosity and segmental dilatation of retinal vessels, retinovascular signs of systemic hypertension, retinal edema, and even papilledema. Central retinal artery occlusion also may occur as a serious complication of Fabry disease. In addition, neuro-ophthalmic manifestations, including internuclear ophthalmoplegia, oculomotor palsy, strabismus, nystagmus and optic atrophy, have been reported. The presence of lamellar intracytoplasmic lipid inclusions has been documented in the eye, particularly in the cornea and conjunctiva, sclera, lens, uvea and retina.

The diagnosis of Fabry disease is confirmed by demonstration of defective α-galactosidase A activity in plasma, leukocytes or tears, or increased levels of globotriaosylceramide in plasma or urinary sediment. Conjunctival biopsy and enzyme analysis of tears also can be useful in diagnosis. Heterozygote identification and prenatal diagnosis can be accomplished. The possibility of enzyme replacement is being investigated.

FARBER LIPOGRANULOMATOSIS

A rare disorder of lipid metabolism, Farber disease is characterized by abnormal accumulation of ceramide due to deficiency of the lysosomal enzyme acid ceramidase. Ceramide plays a key role in sphingolipid metabolism; it is an intermediate in the synthesis and degradation of gangliosides, myelin constituents such as galactosylceramide and sulfatide, and membrane components such as sphingomyelin and the complex glycolipids.

Pathologic studies show accumulation of lipid-laden macrophages and granulomatous infiltrations in many organs and tissues. There is usually prominent involvement of joints, skin and larynx, with variable involvement of lungs, heart, liver, spleen, and other sites. In addition there may be accumulation of ceramide and ganglioside in neurons of the central and peripheral nervous system.

The principal clinical manifestations of Farber disease are painful swelling and progressive deformity of the joints, subcutaneous nodules, particularly around affected joints and tendon sheaths and over pressure points, and progressive hoarseness. Feeding and respiratory problems, poor weight gain and intermittent fever are common. There may be generalized lymphadenopathy, moderate enlargement of the liver or spleen, or cardiac involvement. In some cases there are neurologic manifestations, including mild to severe psychomotor retardation or

deterioration, seizures, peripheral neuropathy and myopathy. Signs usually develop in infancy. The disease is progressive, often leading to death early in childhood, although in some cases the course is protracted. There is considerable phenotypic variability and several subtypes have been described.

A number of ocular abnormalities have been reported in patients with Farber disease, particularly xanthoma-like conjunctival lesions, parafoveal grayness and mild cherry-red-like macular changes. Disc pallor, retinal pigmentary changes, vision loss, punctate corneal opacities and lenticular opacities have also been documented. Pathologic studies have confirmed lipid accumulation in the retina and other tissues of the eye.

Farber disease is autosomal recessive. Specific diagnosis depends on demonstration of the enzyme deficiency in cultured skin fibroblasts or in white blood cells. Obligate heterozygotes show reduced acid ceramidase activity. Prenatal diagnosis has been accomplished by demonstrating acid ceramidase deficiency in cultured amniotic cells. There is no specific therapy for this disease.

NEURONAL CEROID-LIPOFUSCINOSES: BATTEN DISEASE

The term *neuronal ceroid-lipofuscinosis* (NCL) is used to describe a group of hereditary progressive encephalopathies in which the characteristic pathologic finding is marked accumulation of lipopigments in neural and non-neural cells. The eponym commonly applied to this group of disorders is *Batten disease*. The major NCL syndromes of childhood are the infantile, late infantile and juvenile forms, referred to respectively as *Santavuori–Haltia disease* (INCL), *Jansky–Bielschowsky disease* (LINCL), and *Spielmeyer–Sjögren disease* (JNCL). There is also an adult form of NCL, referred to as *Kufs disease*. Occurring worldwide, the neuronal ceroid-lipofusinoses are probably the most frequent of the hereditary progressive neurodegenerative disorders of childhood. All are autosomal recessive.

The principal neurologic manifestations of the childhood forms of NCL are developmental retardation and progressive psychomotor deterioration, ataxia, seizures, and progressive vision loss, with signs of retinal degeneration and optic atrophy (*Figs 32.13 & 32.14*). Atrophy of the brain is often evident on CT and MRI scanning.

The biochemical pathogenesis of NCL is not yet known. Pathologic studies show severe neuronal atrophy, particularly of the cerebral cortex and cerebellum, and demyelination of the white matter, with reactive gliosis. A characteristic ultrastructural finding is the presence of distinctive cytoplasmic inclusions; these storage cytosomes may have a curvilinear, fingerprint or rectilinear profile or contain granular osmophilic dense bodies.

Confirmation of the diagnosis of NCL is often dependent on examination of biopsy material, particularly skin or conjunctiva, for the distinctive cytosomes. Preclinical and prenatal diagnosis can be accomplished in some cases. An important diagnostic finding in JNCL is the presence of vacuolated lymphocytes in peripheral blood. There is no specific treatment for these disorders.

WILSON DISEASE

Also referred to as *hepatolenticular degeneration*, Wilson disease is an autosomal recessive disorder of copper metabolism in which both biliary excretion of copper and incorporation of copper into ceruloplasmin are severely impaired. Intestinal absorption of

Neuronal ceroid – lipofuscinoses – Batten disease
Infantile NCL: Santavuori–Haltia disease
Onset age 8–14 months. Retardation, phsychomotor regression with hypotonia, ataxia, myoclonus, often micrenephaly. Seizures, usually by 3rd years of life. Vision loss early, progressing to blindness usually by age 2 years. Retinal degeneration characterized by pigmentary changes (hypopigmentation and/or pigment aggregation), attenuation of vessels, and optic atrophy. ERG and VEP reduced or extinguished early in course. Occasionally stellate posterior lens opacities. Progression vegetative state. Death usually between ages 6 and 15 years.
Late Infantile NCL: Jansky–Bielschowsky disease
Onset between 2 and 4 years of age. Seizures an early manifestation, followed by dementia, myoclonia, ataxia. Rapidly progressive psychomotor deterioration. Visual failure, evident by age 4–6 years. Signs of retinal degeneration may be evident, including pigmentary changes, attenuation of vessels, optic atrophy. ERG often diminished early, extinguished later in course. VEP, pathologically high early, may be abolished late in course. Regression to vegetative state in 2–4 years. Death usually by age 8–12 years.
Juvenile NCL: Spielmeyer–Sjögren disease
Onset between 5 and 10 years of age. Insidious intellectual deterioration, behavior changes. Progressive dementia, often profound later in course. Progressive motor dysfunction. Seizures later in course, often by age 10 years. Vision loss a prominent sign, usually evident between 4 and 7 years of age, ultimately progressing to blindness. Maculopathy, often described as bull's eye maculopathy, an important sign. Other sings of retinal degeneration, including pigmentary changes (granularity, clumping, spicule formation), vessel attenuation, and optic altropy may develop. ERG and VEP reduced or extinguished. In some cases, keratoconus, cataracts, possibly related to rubbing and poking of eyes. Course rapidly progressive or protracted.
Adult NCL: Kufs disease
Mental and motor changes in 2nd or 3rd decade. Personality changes, ataxia, myoclonus common. Vision loss is not a prominent feature of this form, but evidence for retinal degeneration has been documented.

Fig. 27.13 Neuronal ceroid-lipofuscinoses: Batten disease.

copper is normal. The defective biliary excretion leads to abnormal accumulation of copper in the liver with progressive liver damage. Subsequently the level of nonceruloplasmin copper in plasma increases, resulting in increased renal excretion of copper and abnormal deposition of copper in extrahepatic sites, particularly in the brain, eye and kidney, and in skeletal and heart muscle, bones and joints. Patients with Wilson disease most often present with liver disease or with neurologic symptoms.

The liver disease may produce signs at any age beyond 6 years, but this form of presentation is most frequent between age 8 and 16 years; it can manifest as late as 60 years without associated neurologic or ocular signs. Episodes of jaundice, vomiting and malaise are common. Often the course is chronic with progressive hepatic insufficiency, portal hypertension, splenomegaly, gastroesophageal varices and ascites. In some cases the onset is acute. There may be fulminant hepatic failure with rapidly progressive jaundice, coagulopathy and encepholopathy.

Neurologic manifestations are unusual before age 12 years; they may appear in adolescence but are more frequent in the adult years, and can develop as late as 60 years. The most frequent neurologic

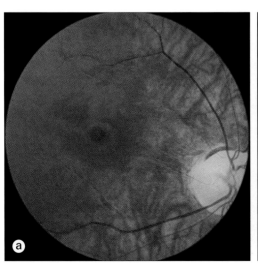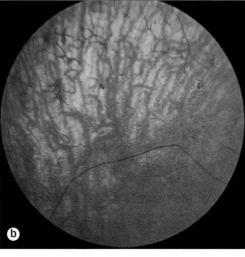

Fig. 27.14 (**a**), (**b**) Pigmentary retinal degeneration of Batten disease.

signs are dysarthria and incoordination of voluntary movements, often accompanied by involuntary movements and by disorders of posture and tone. Pseudobulbar palsy may develop and can lead to death in untreated cases. Cognitive and sensory functions are usually preserved, but intellectual and behavioral deterioration may occur. The neurologic manifestations are attributed to involvement of the basal ganglia (lenticular degeneration), deep cerebral cortical layers, cerebellum, and less commonly, the brainstem.

Renal tubular malfunction is common. Poor growth and acidosis, or renal stones may be presenting features. Many patients have bone and joint involvement; frequent findings are osteomalacia, osteoporosis, and spontaneous fractures, osteoarthritis, osteophytes, ligamentous laxity and joint hypermobility. Cardiac involvement may lead to arrythmias and congestive heart failure. Some patients develop hypoparathyroidism.

The characteristic ocular sign of Wilson disease is the *Kayser–Fleischer (K–F) ring* of the cornea (*Fig. 27.15*). Of dull golden to greenish-brown hue, this ring is due to copper-containing granular deposits in the periphery of Descemet's membrane. The ring may be complete, forming a circumferential band (typically 1 to 3 mm in width) near the limbus, or involve only the superior and inferior crescents of the cornea. When advanced, the ring may be detected with the naked eye or ophthalmoscope, but slit lamp biomicroscopy is usually required for diagnosis, particularly in the early stage. The K–F ring is present in virtually all patients with Wilson disease who have neurologic signs, and is commonly present in those with non-neurologic signs, though it is often lacking in children who present with acute liver disease. It should be noted that a similar ring can be seen in patients with non-Wilsonian liver disease.

Another important ocular manifestation of Wilson disease is the *sunflower* cataract, a central pigmented lens opacity with tapering petal-like extensions, occurring in 15 to 20% of cases.

Remarkably, ocular motor functions generally are spared in Wilson disease; jerking oscillation of the eyes, involuntary upward gaze, impairment of upward gaze, impairment of accomodation and convergence, and infrequent blinking have occasionally been noted. Night blindness and signs of retinal degeneration have been reported in some cases.

Wilson disease can be effectively treated with penicillamine, a chelating agent, which reduces body stores of copper. However, neurologic improvement takes weeks, and it may be months before improvement in liver function is seen. Both the K–F ring

and sunflower cataract may regress with treatment. Treatment alternatives are triethylene tetramine (trientine) and orally administered zinc salts. Liver transplantation has a place in the treatment of patients with advanced liver damage and can be successful in fulminant cases.

MENKES DISEASE: TRICHOPOLIODYSTROPHY

In Menkes disease, there is widespread disturbance in the cellular transport of copper. There is defective intestinal absorption leading to copper deficiency, and defective synthesis of copper enzymes, with neurologic and connective tissue consequences. Major features of the disease are abnormal hair, a characteristic facies, hypopigmentation, progressive neurologic degeneration, lax skin and arterial degeneration, bone changes, urinary tract diverticulae, and hypothermia.

Manifestations develop in infancy; some may be evident in the newborn period. The hair is typically pale, brittle, often stubbly, giving rise to the descriptive terms *kinky hair* or *steely hair syndrome*; microscopic examination shows pili torti, with twisting, segmental narrowing and fracture of the hair shaft. The facies is distinguished by pudgy cheeks and sagging jowls. By age 3 months, affected infants show developmental delay and regression. Seizures develop. The course is one of progressive psychomotor deterioration, the result of widespread neuronal destruction and associated gliosis, especially in the cerebral cortex and cerebellum. Vascular complications (thrombosis, rupture) occur; subdural hematomas are common. Arteriograms show segmental narrowing and dilatation of arteries in the brain, viscera and limbs. Osteoporosis and fractures are common. Diverticule of the bladder or ureters may predispose to infection or rupture. In most cases, death occurs between ages 3 months and 3 years, though some patients may live for years, severely incapacitated.

The eyes may appear sunken owing to paucity of orbital fat. The eyebrows typically are pale and 'steely', often broken and sparse. The eyelashes are sometimes better preserved and slightly more pigmented, and may be long and straight, or curly. The irides usually are light blue or grayish with a delicate stromal pattern, but do not transilluminate like those of an albino. In most cases there is generalized hypopigmentation of the fundi, often more marked peripherally (*Fig. 27.16*). In some cases there is attenuation or tortuosity of the retinal arteries. Often the maculae are poorly

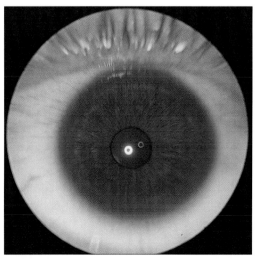

Fig. 27.15
Kayser–Fleischer ring of Wilson disease.

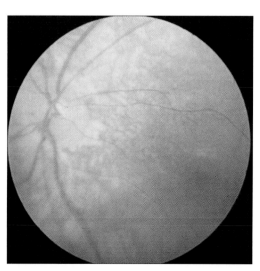

Fig. 27.16
Generalized fundus hypopigmentation in Menke disease.

defined, the discs somewhat pale. Visual function deteriorates with progression of the disease. The ERG and VEP become diminished. Nystagmus and strabismus are common. There may also be signs of blepharitis, dacryostenosis, possibly tear deficiency.

Histopathologic examination of the eyes has shown attenuation of the retinal ganglion cells and nerve fiber layer, demyelination and partial atrophy of the optic nerve with an increase in glial elements, and multiple microcysts in the pigment epithelium of the iris.

Menkes disease is inherited as an X-linked disorder, typically affecting hemizygous males, though occasionally heterozygous females may show manifestations. Heterozygote detection and prenatal diagnosis are possible. Presymptomatic treatment with copper histidinate injections can modify the disease, but treatment has not yet been found to significantly alter the course of the disease once brain damage has occurred.

OCULAR SIGNS OF NEUROMETABOLIC DISEASE: A REVIEW

Although a great variety of ophthalmic changes occur within the spectrum of metabolic disease, those most prominently associated with the neurometabolic diseases are cherry-red spots, pigmentary retinal degeneration, optic atrophy, vision loss and ocular motor dysfunction. Also of major importance in the differential diagnosis of many neurometabolic disorders are corneal opacities, cataracts, glaucoma, and vascular signs.

MACULAR CHERRY-RED SPOT

A cherry-red spot is the distinctive fundus sign produced when transparency of the macular ganglion cells is lost, usually as the result of edema or lipid storage. On ophthalmoscopic examination, the multilayered ganglion cell ring of the macula appears pale and thickened, forming a hazy gray to creamy white or yellow perifoveal halo. In contrast to the pallor of the halo, the normal vascular blush of the ganglion cell-free foveola is accentuated, forming a well defined bright to dark red spot at the center of the macula (see *Fig.27.6*).

The cherry-red spot is a major feature of many neuronal storage diseases (*Fig. 27.17*). It is especially common in the gangliosidoses, occurring in virtually all cases of Tay–Sachs disease (G_{M2} type 1), the Sandhoff variant (G_{M2} type 2), and approximately 50% of cases of generalized gangliosidoses (G_{M1} type 1). As a rule, the macular changes are evident by the time psychomotor retardation and neurologic deterioration become apparent in infancy. The spot usually is striking early in the course, but may fade as ganglion cell destruction progresses (see *Fig.32.6a*). Classic cherry-red spots like those seen in the gangliosidoses are also associated with galactosialidosis (sialidosis III) and may occur in some cases of sphingomyelin lipidosis (Niemann–Pick disease) and lipogranulomatosis (Farber disease).

A variety of less striking macular changes ranging from subtle 'cherry-red-like' spots to mild haziness of the perifoveal region also may occur in many neuronal storage diseases. A cherry-red-like spot or just perifoveal grayness can be seen in patients with sulfatide lipidosis (metachromatic leukodystrophy). In glucosylceramide lipidosis (Gaucher disease) there is usually just grayness of the macular area; discrete white spots of the retina also have been noted in some cases. Some patients with sphingomyelin lipi-

Cherry-red spots and related macular changes in neurometabolic disorders	
Gangliosdoses	
G_{M1} type 1: Generalized Gangliosidosis	Cherry-red spot like that of Tay–Sachs disease in approximately 50% of cases, usually evident by age 6 months.
G_{M2} type 1: Tay–Sachs disease	Cherry-red spot in virtually all cases of infantile form, in some cases of juvenile form. Classic prototype: opacification of the macular ganglion cell ring producing white or grayish halo around the fovea, accentuating reddish blush of the ganglion-cell-free central region. Appearance may change with progressive degeneration of ganglion cells.
G_{M2} type 2: Sandhoff variant	Cherry-red spot in most if not all cases of infantile form.
Sphingomyelin Lipidosis: Niemann–Pick Disease	
Type A NPD	Cherry-red spot in 30–50% of cases, often with extension of retinal haze beyond the macula.
Type B NPD	Cherry-red spot in less than 10% of cases. Sometimes just grayness of macular region, or perifoveal halo of punctate or granular opacities
Type C NPD	Occasionally opalescence of perifoveal retina.
Sulfatide Lipidosis: Metachromatic Leukodystrophy	
Late infantile form MLD	Macular grayness or cherry-red-like spot.
Multiple sulfatase deficiency	Macular grayness or cherry-red-like spot.
Glucosylceramidosis: Gaucher Disease	
Type I: Nonneuro-nopathic (adult) form	Macular, perimacular changes in some cases.
Type III: Subacute neuro-nopathic (juvenile) form	Grayness of macular region. Sometimes discrete white retinal spots posteriorly.
Mucolipidoses	
ML I: Galactosialidosis (Sialidosis III)	Cherry-red spots in all forms.
Ceramide Lipidosis: Farber Disease	
	Gray opacification of perifoveal area in some cases, or mild cherry-red-like changes.
Neuronal Ceriod-Lipofuscinosis: Batten Disease	
Juvenile NCL: Speil-meyer–Sjögren disease	Bull's eye maculopathy in some cases; brownish pigmentation of macula.

Fig. 27.17 Cherry-red spots and related macular changes in neurometabolic disorders.

dosis (Niemann-Pick disease), lipogranulomatosis (Farber disease), and (sialidosis II) may have only perifoveal grayness. In some patients with lipofuscinosis (juvenile type) there may be 'bull's eye' maculopathy, characterized by pigmentary changes of the macula, with or without a dull red spot in the center.

The cherry-red spot that occurs with retinal ischemia secondary to central retinal artery occlusion or the edema that follows ocular contusion should be differentiated from the macular changes of neuronal storage disease.

PIGMENTARY RETINAL DEGENERATION: RETINITIS PIGMENTOSA AND ITS VARIANTS

Retinitis pigmentosa (RP) is a progressive retinal degeneration affecting both the neuroretina (particularly the photoreceptors) and the retinal pigment epithelium. It is characterized by retinal pigment dispersion and aggregation, arteriolar attenuation, optic atrophy, and impairment of visual function with corresponding ERG changes. Changes in the retinal pigmentation vary from fine granularity or coarse mottling, to the formation of distinctive focal pigment aggregates having the configuration of bone corpuscles or 'spicules'. Pigment changes usually appear first in the mid-to far periphery, though in some cases the central or macular region is affected first (*inverse* type); there is usually progression to generalized retinal involvement. Depending on the site of predominant involvement, there may be impairment of dark adaptation (nyctalopia or *night blindness*), loss of peripheral vision (field defects), loss of central vision (decreased acuity), or impairment of color vision (dyschromatopsia), singly or in various combinations; commonly there is progression to blindness.

Retinitis pigmentosa may occur as a primary ocular disorder, unassociated with other defects or diseases. It can be inherited as an autosomal dominant, autosomal recessive or X-linked recessive condition. Alternatively, retinitis pigmentosa or RP-like retinal degeneration may occur in association with a variety of diseases and morphologic defects of other organ systems (see *Fig. 27.14*). It is a major clinical manifestation of several neurometabolic diseases; in particular it is a prominent feature of the mucopolysaccaridoses and ceroid lipofuscinoses, but may also occur in certain of the gangliosidoses, mucolipidoses, and lipoprotein disorders (*Fig. 27.18*).

It should be noted that in certain disorders, signs of retinal degeneration can be obscured by concurrent corneal clouding (e.g. MPS I H and IS). In such cases, ERG changes can be helpful in the diagnosis of retinal involvement.

OPTIC ATROPHY

When injury or disease results in irreparable damage to the optic nerve, with resultant degeneration of nerve fibers and attendant loss of function, optic atrophy occurs. Pathologic features such as the degree of axonal loss, demyelination, vascular change, cellular reaction and gliosis vary with the disease process. Clinically the principal signs of optic atrophy are diminished vascularity of the disc, pallor and loss of substance of the nerve head; there may be enlargement or excavation of the disc cup; in some cases there is glial proliferation on or around the disc. Signs of visual impairment range from mild to severe, and include diminished acuity, altered color perception, and visual field defects. Often there is a detectable afferent pupillary defect.

Optic atrophy is a common manifestation of numerous metabolic neurodegenerative diseases. In many, such as the mucopolysaccharidoses and various sphingolipidoses, there is direct involvement of the optic nerve with accumulation of stor-

Retinitis pigmentosa and related retinal degenerations: associated neurometabolic disorders
Mucopolysaccharidoses
Particularly MPS I H (Hurler), MPS I S (Scheie), MPS II (Hunter), and MPS III (Sanfilippo); possibly in mild variant of MPS IV (Maroteaux–Lamy).
Ceroid Lipofuscinoses
Particularly infantile NCL (Santavouri–Haltia), late infantile NCL (Jansky–Bielschowsky), and juvenile NCL (Spielmeyer–Sjögren).
Gangliosidoses
Juvenile G_{M2} (Bernheimer–Seitelberger).
Mucolipidoses
Possibly ML III (Pseudohurler polydystrophy) and ML IV (Sialolipidosis).
Others
Abetalipoproteinemia (Bassen–Kornzweig). Phytanic acid deficiency (Refsum). Congental adrenoleukodystrophy (Zellweger and variants).

Fig. 27.18 Retinitis pigmentosa and related retinal degenerations: Associated neurometabolic disorders.

age material and attendant cellular changes. Often concurrent retinal degeneration contributes to the optic atrophy, as in the mucopolysaccharidoses, gangliosidoses, and neuronal ceroid-lipofuscinoses. Hydrocephalus and increased intracranial pressure, particularly in the mucopolysaccharidoses, can also cause secondary optic atrophy. Occasionally, glaucoma can also play a role in producing optic atrophy, as in Hurler syndrome.

OCULAR MOTOR DYSFUNCTION

Whereas nystagmus (abnormal oscillation of the eyes) and strabismus (misalignment of the eyes) are frequent and often nonspecific findings common to many metabolic neurodegenerative disorders, ophthalmoplegia and gaze disturbances are findings of special significance, important in the differential diagnosis of a limited number of neurometabolic diseases.

In classic infantile Tay–Sachs disease (G_{M2} gangliosidosis) there is progressive deterioration of eye movement. First there is loss of voluntary movements, then followingmovements, optokinetics and vestibular responses. Patients with chronic G_{M2} gangliosidosis may develop prominent disturbances in horizontal pursuit movements, and varying defects of voluntary upgaze, diminished optokinetics and decreased convergence. Supranuclear paralysis of vertical gaze is also a principal feature of type C Niemann–Pick disease; in addition, horizontal gaze can be affected. In Gaucher disease, the key ocular motor signs are progressive ocular motor apraxia and nuclear ophthalmoplegia. In diseases associated with hydrocephalus, such as Maroteaux–Lamy, abducent palsy can be the presenting sign of increased intracranial pressure. It should be noted that eye movement disorders are not a major feature of Wilson disease, though jerky eye movements, involuntary upward gaze, impairment of upward gaze, and impairment of convergence have been reported.

Corneal manifestations of neurometabolic disease	
Mucopolysaccharidoses	
Hurler syndrome (MPS I H)	Progressive corneal clouding a prominent feature. Fine generalized haze to opaque ground-glass appearance. Usually evident by age 2–3 years, some times at birth.
Scheie syndrome (MPS I S)	Corneal clouding evident early in life, worsening with age. Diffuse or more dense peripherally.
Hurler–Scheie Compound (MPS I H/S)	Progressive corneal clouding.
Morquio syndrome (MPS IV)	Corneal clouding in both forms. Relatively mild to fine haze rather than dense opacificaton. May not be evident to unaided eye in early years, but usually apparent before age 10 years.
Maroteaux–Lamy syndrome (MPS VI)	Progressive corneal clouding usually evident within first few years of life. Marked opacification, sometimes more dense peripherally.
Sly syndrome (MPS VII)	Corneal clouding only in some cases.
Sphingolipidoses	
Generalized Gangliosidosis (Infantile G_{MI} gangliosidosis)	Mild diffuse corneal clouding in some cases.
Niemann–Pick Disease (Sphingomyelin lipidosis)	Diffuse stromal haze in some cases of type A NPD.
Fabry Disease	Whorl-like pattern of epithelial or subepithelial corneal opacities in affected males and in some carrier females. Usually evident in early years.
Mucolipidoses	
Galactosialidosis (ML I)	Corneal clouding may occur in infantile and juvenile forms. Generally of mild degree.
I-Cell disease (ML II)	Mild corneal clouding may occur, often as a later finding.
Pseudo-Hurler Polydstrophy (ML III)	Progressive corneal clouding a prominent feature, usually evident in 1st decade.
Sialolipidosis (ML IV)	Corneal clouding evident early. Mild to dense haze. Prominent epithelial involvement often with episodes of pain, photophobia, tearing.
Other	
Mannosidosis	Superficial corneal opacities.
Fucosidosis	Superficial corneal opacities.
Mucosulfatidosis	Occasionally corneal clouding.
Wilson disease	Kayser–Fleischer ring of peripheral cornea.

Fig. 27.19 Corneal manifestations of neurometabolic disease.

Cataracts in neurometabolic diseases
Wilson Disease
'Sunflower cataract' in 15–20% of patients: discoid opacity of anterior lens capsule, with petal-like fronds that radiate peripherally, composed of green, golden-brown, or gray granular deposits. Also spoke-like changes of posterior cortex.
Fabry Disease
Granular wedgelike or propeller-shaped anterior subcapsular lens opacities, in approximately 35% of hemizygotes; also linear spoke-like granular opacities under posterior capsule in hemizygotes. Lens opacities (posterior) in only 14% of heterozygotes.
Niemann–Pick Disease Type A
Brownish granular deposits of anterior lens capsule and scattered white opacities of posterior lens capsule.
Mannosidosis
Spoke-wheel pattern composed of small vacuoles in posterior cortex in some cases. Punctuate cortical opacities.
Galactosialidosis
Posterior spoke-like opacities.
Mucosulfatidosis
Peripheral circumferential opacities of anterior lens capsule.
Morquio Syndrome Type A
Subcortical lens opacities.
Farber Disease
Lenticular opacities in some cases.
Infantile Neuronal Ceroid-Lipofuscinosis
Occasionally stellate posterior lens opacities.

Fig. 27.20 Cataracts in neurometabolic diseases.

CORNEAL OPACITIES

Corneal manifestations of neurometabolic disease range from generalized corneal clouding, as in certain mucopolysaccharidoses, sphingolipidoses, and mucolipidoses, to distinctive patterns of corneal deposits, as in Fabry disease and Wilson disease (Fig. 32.19). The primary corneal signs in these diseases are caused by abnormal accumulation of specific storage substances and attendant cellular changes within the cornea. In some disorders, particularly the mucopolysaccharidoses, there can also be corneal clouding of edema secondary to glaucoma.

Whereas corneal signs of neurometabolic disease are often apparent to the unaided eye, in most cases careful slit lamp biomicroscopy is essential to precise diagnosis.

CATARACTS

By definition, a cataract is any opacity of the lens. The causes are protean, including anomalies of development, chromosomal aberrations, trauma, toxic insults, infections and inflammatory processes, and numerous systemic and metabolic disorders. The list of diseases and syndromes associated with lens changes is seemingly endless. Only a few of the metabolic neurodegenerative diseases included here are associated with significant lens opacities (*Fig. 27.20*). Most distinctive are the spoke-like lens opacities of Fabry disease, and the so-called sunflower cataract of Wilson disease.

GLAUCOMA

The term glaucoma encompasses a complex group of ocular disorders in which the intraocular pressure is too high for the health of the optic nerve. Uncontrolled, the disease results in atrophy of the optic nerve, often with enlargement and excavation of the disc cup, and progressive loss of visual field that can ultimately lead to blindness.

Although glaucoma is not regularly associated with the neurometabolic diseases, it has been reported in mucopolysaccharidoses I-H (Hurler syndrome), I-S (Scheie syndrome), and I H/S (Hurler-Scheie syndrome). Glaucoma has also been reported in some cases of I-cell disease.

It should be noted that corneal edema, an important sign of increased intraocular pressure, can be masked by the corneal clouding of these storage processes.

VASCULAR SIGNS

In the differential diagnosis of nerometabolic disease, the most important ocular vascular signs are those of Gabry disease. Tortuosity and aneurysmal dilatation of the conjuntival vessels, sludging , and telangiectasias are common. There may also be tortuosity and segmental dilatation of the retinal vessels. Central retinal artery occlusion can occur.

Tortuosity of the conjunctival and retinal vessels has also been described in generalized gangliosidosis (G_{M1} type 1). Retinal vascular tortuosity occurs in Maroteaux–Lamy syndrome (MPS VI), and conjunctival vascular changes have been documented in sialidosis and fucosidosis.

Attenuation of the retinal arteriole is and important feature of neurometabolic disease associated with pigmentary retinal degerneration (RP-like changes).

Further reading

Beaudet AL, Thomas GH. Disorders of glycoprotein degradation: mannosidosis, fucosidosis, sialidosis, and aspartylgylycosaminuria. In: Scriver CR, Beaudet AL, Sly WS, Valle D, eds. *The Metabolic Basis of Inherited Disease*. (New York: McGraw-Hill Inc., 1989):1603–1621.

Beutler E, Grabowski GA. Gaucher disease. In: Scriver CR, Beaudet AL, Sly WS, Valle D eds. *The Metabolic and Molecular Bases of Inherited Disease*. New York: McGraw-Hill Inc.; 1995:2641–2670.

Danks DM. Disorders of copper transport. In: Scriver CR, Beaudet AL, Sly WS, Valle D, eds. *The Metabolic and Molecular Bases of Inherited Disease*. New York: McGraw-Hill Inc.; 1995:2211–2235.

Desnick RJ, Ioannou YA, Eng CM. α-Galactosidase A deficiency: Fabry disease. In: Scriver CR, Beaudet AL, Sly WS, Valle D, eds. *The Metabolic and Molecular Bases of Inherited Disease*. New York: McGraw-Hill Inc.; 1995:2741–2784.

Gilbert-Barness EF, Barness LA: The Mucolipidoses. In: Landing BH, Haust MD, Bernstein J, Rosenberg HS, eds. *Genetic Metabolic Diseases. Perspectives in Pediatric Pathology*. Basel: Karger; 1993:148–184.

Gravel RA, Clarke JTR, Kaback MM, Mahuran D, Sandhoff K, Suzuki K. The G_{M2} gangliosidoses. In: Scriver CR, Beaudet AL, Sly WS, Valle D, eds. The Metabolic and Molecular Bases of Inherited Disease. New York: McGraw-Hill Inc.; 1995:2839–2879.

Kolodny EH, Fluharty AL. Metachromatic leukodystrophy and multiple sulfatase deficiency: sulfatide lipidosis. In: Scriver CR, Beaudet AL, Sly WS, Valle D, eds. *The Metabolic and Molecular Bases of Inherited Disease*. New York: McGraw-Hill Inc.; 1995:2693–2739.

Kornfeld S, Sly WS. I-cell disease and pseudo-Hurler polydystrophy: disorders of lysosomal enzyme phosphorylation. In: Scriver CR, Beaudet AL, Sly WS, Valle D, eds. *The Metabolic and Molecular Bases of Inherited Disease*. New York: McGraw-Hill Inc.; 1995:2495–2508.

Moser HW. Ceramidase deficiency: Farber lipogranulomatosis. In: Scriver CR, Beaudet AL, Sly WS, Valle D, eds. *The Metabolic and Molecular Bases of Inherited Disease*. New York: McGraw-Hill Inc.; 1995:2589–2599.

Nelson LB, Martyn LJ. Metabolic diseases affecting the eyes. In: Duane TD, ed. *Biomedical Foundations of Ophthalmology*. Philadelphia: Harper & Row; 1989: :54,1–52.

Neufeld EF, Muenzer J. The Mucopolysaccharidoses. In: Scriver CR, Beaudet AL, Sly WS, Valle D, eds. *The Metabolic and Molecular Bases of Inherited Disease*. New York: McGraw-Hill Inc.; 1995:2465–2494.

O' Brien JS: β-galactosidase deficiency (G_{M1} gangliosidosis, galactosialidosis, and Morquio syndrome type B); ganglioside sialidase deficiency (mucolipidosis IV). In: Scriver CR, Beaudet AL, Sly WS, Valle D, eds. *The Metabolic Basis of Inherited Disease*. New York: McGraw-Hill Inc.; 1989:1797–1896.

Pentchev PG, Vanier MT, Suzuki K, Patterson MC. Niemann-Pick disease type C: a cellular cholesterol lipidosis. In: Scriver CR, Beaudet AL, Sly WS, Valle D, eds. *The Metabolic and Molecular Bases of Inherited Disease*. New York: McGraw-Hill Inc.; 1995:2625–2639.

Rapola J. Neuronal ceroid-lipofuscinoses in childhood. In: Landing BH, Haust MD, Bernstein J, Rosenberg HS, eds. *Genetic Metabolic Diseases. Perspectives in Pediatric Pathology*. Basel: Karger; 1993:**17**:7–14.

Sandhoff K, Conzelmann E, Neufeld EF, Kaback MM, Suzuki K. The G_{M2} gangliosidoses. In: Scriver CR, Beaudet AL, Sly WS, Valle D. *The Metabolic Basis of Inherited Disease*. New York: McGraw-Hill Inc.; 1989:1807–1839.

Schuchman EH, Desnick RJ. Niemann-Pick disease types A and B: acid sphingomyelinase deficiencies. In: Scriver CR, Beaudet AL, Sly WS, Valle D, eds. *The Metabolic and Molecular Bases of Inherited Disease*. New York: McGraw-Hill Inc.; 1995:2601–2624.

Suzuki K, Suzuki Y, Suzuki K. Galactosylceramide lipidosis: globoid-cell leukodystrophy (Krabbe disease). In: Scriver CR, Beaudet AL, Sly WS, Valle D, eds. *The Metabolic and Molecular Bases of Inherited Disease*. New York: McGraw-Hill Inc.; 1995:2671–2692.

Suzuki Y, Sakuraba H, Oshima A. β-Galactosidase deficiency (β-galactosidosis): G_{M1} gangliosidosis and Morquio B disease. In: Scriver CR, Beaudet AL, Sly WS, Valle D, eds. *The Metabolic and Molecular Bases of Inherited Diseases*. New York: McGraw-Hill Inc.; 1995:2785–2823.

CHAPTER 28

Molecular Biology in Ophthalmology

W J K Cumming

INTRODUCTION

The most rapidly expanding field in medicine at present is that of molecular biology. As with all such explosions of knowledge, the language and terminology employed have become increasingly specialized and less intelligible to the non-specialist. The aim of this chapter is to give a background to the principles of molecular genetics and to provide an interpretation of the terminology used in this important branch of medicine.

BASIC MOLECULAR BIOLOGY

In any cell that contains a nucleus (eukaryotic cell), DNA exists as a double strand, each strand consisting of purine (adenine and guanine) and pyrimidine (cytosine and thymine) bases (or nucleotides) which are linked linearly. The basic unit of a DNA molecule is a base pair (bp), the pair of nucleotides that bond to each other.

The two strands are complementary and run in opposite directions, the so-called antiparallel arrangement. One strand runs from the 5 prime (5') end to the 3 prime (3') end, the other from the 3' end to the 5' end. By convention, the 5' end refers to the left end of a DNA fragment, whereas the 3' end refers to the right end (*Fig. 28.1*).

The genomic DNA molecules (chromosomes) occur in pairs, except for the X and Y chromosomes. The two chromosomes that pair are said to be homologous because they carry the same genes. However, as a result of mutations, a pair of homologous chromosomes may have genes with slightly different sequences at particular points (loci) and these are known as alleles.

Transcription of the DNA to RNA starts at the 5' end with promoter sequences that are upstream from the coding sequences. If the protein from a specific coding sequence is expressed in multiple types of cells, there may be different promoters for each cell type. Some of the coding sequences may be many thousands of base pairs away from the promoter region and are found along the length of the DNA; these are known as enhancer sequences.

Most of the DNA in the genome is required for the structural integrity of the chromosome. Only a small percentage is required for protein-coding expressing regions. These latter are known as exons and are interrupted by, frequently much longer, stretches of non-coding sequences called introns (see Fig. 28.1).

Initially, when the DNA molecule is transcribed, both exons and introns are produced in the primary transcript. Subsequent post-transcriptional regulatory processes remove the introns by a process known as splicing (see Fig. 28.1).

In the majority of protein transcripts the exons are spliced consecutively; however, in some instances non-consecutive exons are joined together, producing an alternative pattern of RNA that will encode related but different protein isoforms. This can result in a significant increase in the phenotypic variability and diversity arising from a single gene.

MOLECULAR TECHNIQUES

Bacteria protect themselves from invading DNA by producing a series of enzymes, restriction endonucleases which split the DNA into fragments. This produces a series of different-sized restriction fragments of the foreign DNA.

These fragments can be labeled or stained and co-incubated with single-stranded (host) DNA that is derived by splitting normal double-stranded DNA. The restriction fragment finds its complementary sequence on the single-stranded host DNA , which can then be recognized either by electrophoresis or by Southern blotting (a technique named after its inventor).

Many bacteria have the ability to acquire circular mini chromosomes known as plasmids as a supplement to their normal genomic material. Short segments of DNA, which have been created by restriction endonucleosis, can be inserted into these bacteria and a large number of copies of the fragment can be made. This copied DNA (complementary DNA) can then be inserted into single-stranded DNA and used as a probe to find a particular gene sequence using electrophoresis and Southern blotting.

The polymerase chain reaction (PCR) can be used to increase the amplification of DNA fragments and mimic natural DNA replication. Up to 1 megabase (Mb) can be produced by this technique. The plasmid system cannot cope with this amount of DNA and therefore the yeast artificial chromosome (YAC) was developed.

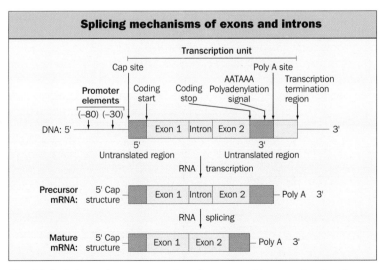

Fig. 28.1 Schematic representation of exons and introns showing the mechanism of splicing.

This has allowed up to 1 Mb of DNA to be cloned at a given time.

These techniques can be used to identify a possible area of a chromosome where a gene may be located. The technique of linkage analysis is then used to look for a marker (a previously identified sequence of DNA), at either a clinical or molecular level, which co-segregates with the cDNA. The degree of linkage is measured by the lod score: the logarithm of the odds of two loci being within a measurable distance of one another. The lower the lod score the tighter the linkage.

To these techniques has now been added analysis of tandem repeats. Tandem repeats are short lengths of DNA which are stably inherited, but exist in a wide variety of isoforms within the population through variation in the repeat number. These can be identified and used as markers against the cDNA.

When a possible 'disease region' has been identified, various techniques can be used to identify the gene itself. cDNA libraries from tissues likely to express the gene can be screened with genomic probes from the isolated region to obtain a number of candidate genes. These candidate genes can then be sequenced to identify the structural protein or other tissue abnormality.

These techniques have shown that in the majority of genetically defined diseases the mutations that occur fall into six categories (*Fig. 28.2*).

- Deletions of DNA disrupt the production of the appropriate protein. Depending on the degree of the deletion, either no protein will be produced (as in Duchenne muscular dystrophy) or an aberrant form of the protein will be produced (as in Becker muscular dystrophy). This is the basis of the so-called reading frame hypothesis, by which, if the deletion is such that downstream from it only non-sense codons are produced, then consequently no protein will be produced. If, however, the deletion is such that it simply removes a single codon and the subsequent downstream codons are intact, then an aberrant protein will be produced. This accounts for the phenotypic variability seen, for example, in abnormalities at Xp21, the gene locus for the Duchenne and Becker dystrophy (see chapter 29).
- Single codon deletions.
- Point mutations within the genome. An increasing number of diseases are now recognized as being due to
- expansion or
- contraction of tandem repeats; and finally
- duplications of the gene may occur. Each of these abnormalities

will disrupt the normal replication of DNA and hence messenger RNA and protein products.

In some cases it is obvious from the loss of protein that this is causative of the disease process. In other diseases, although abnormalities have been detected in terms of deletions and so on, their relevance to the physiology of the underlying disease has not yet been established.

THE MITOCHONDRIAL GENOME

In addition to the nuclear genome, mitochondria contain their own DNA (mtDNA). This occurs in a circular form and is about 16 kb in length (*Fig. 28.3*). Mitochondria contain anywhere between two and 10 circular DNA molecules. Unlike the nuclear genome, virtually all of the mitochondrial genome is sequenced, that is there is very little intronic material.

Mitochondrial DNA encodes about one-third of the subunits in the mitochondrial respiratory chain and oxidative phosphorylation enzyme system; subunits of complex 1, cytochrome B, three subunits of cytochrome oxidase, and two subunits of ATP synthetase. The remainder of the polypeptides and respiratory chain enzymes are encoded by the nuclear genome, as is replication, transcription, and translation of the mitochondrial genome.

Mitochondrial DNA is exclusively maternally transmitted although the male preponderance, for example, in Leber's hereditary optic neuropathy, indicates that nuclear genomic influences must play a part.

Mitochondrial DNA replicates rapidly and the surveillance mechanisms that are in place for nuclear genomic replication, which ensure that atypical or damaged DNA is removed, do not appear to be either in place or as effective in mtDNA. This leads to more frequent abnormalities in mtDNA than in the nuclear DNA. For example, single deletions and duplications in mtDNA underlie Kearns Sayer syndrome and sporadic progressive external ophthalmoplegia. Point mutations in mtDNA underlie some forms of progressive external ophthalmoplegia and Kearn Sayers syndrome. As yet unidentified nuclear DNA mutations underly autosomal dominant progressive external ophthalmoplegia.

Although the complete mtDNA genome has been sequenced the genotype–phenotype correlations in this group are less well established than those for nuclear DNA (see chapter 29).

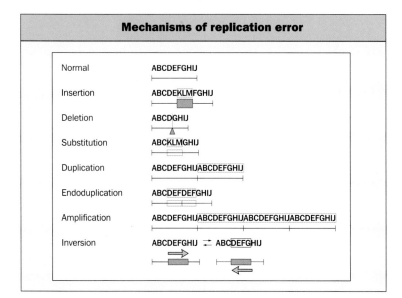

Fig. 28.2 The mechanisms by which abnormalities occur in DNA replication leading to mutation and consequent disease.

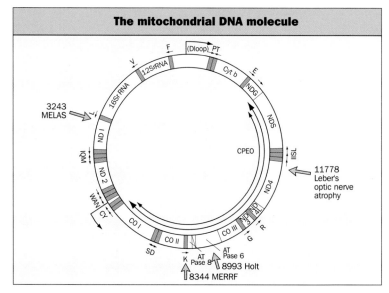

Fig. 28.3 Schematic representation of the circular mitochondrial DNA molecule.

CHAPTER 29

Neuromuscular Disease in the Eye

W J K Cumming

INTRODUCTION

The neuromuscular system is comprised of the anterior horn cell, the nerve emanating from it, the myoneural junction, and the muscle fiber itself. Disorders of the individual nerves supplying the ocular muscles are described elsewhere and will not be considered here. This chapter is concerned with primary disorders of muscle that have an ocular component, with disorders of the myoneural junction, and with aberrant nerve function.

PRIMARY MUSCLE DISORDERS

Irrespective of the insult applied to a muscle fiber, whether it be an abnormality of the membrane or a disorder of the cytoplasm, the end result is muscle weakness. Only four patterns of muscle weakness are commonly seen. In order of frequency these are: the limb girdle syndrome (LG syndrome, 80% of patients), the fascioscapulohumeral syndrome (FSH syndrome, 10–15% of patients), the scapuloperoneal syndrome (SP syndrome, approximately 5% of patients), and the distal syndrome (1–2% of patients). These 'syndromes' are simply a shorthand way of describing the muscle involvement in a given patient. Hence, in limb girdle syndrome, the proximal upper and lower limb girdles are affected. In the fascioscapulohumeral syndrome, the facial muscles are weak, with weakness in the proximal upper limb girdle. In the scapuloperoneal syndrome, the weakness is proximal in the upper limb girdle and distal in the lower limbs, and in the distal syndrome, the weakness is from the elbows to the hands and from the knees to feet.

With the passage of time, virtually all of these initial presentations merge into a generalized weakness involving all muscle groups. Progression to this state is extremely variable and depends on the underlying etiology of the neuromuscular condition. This cannot be deduced from the pattern of weakness and requires investigation, including estimation of the serum creatinine kinase, electromyography studies, and muscle biopsy, to determine the underlying cause for the condition. Increasingly in the era of molecular biology, specific testing of muscle biopsies for the presence or absence of the protein product of a gene abnormality is becoming routine.

This application of molecular techniques to muscle disorders has shown that a single deficiency may lead to a variety of clinical syndromes, depending on the degree of that deficiency. Hence, for example, with Xp21 deletional myopathies, in which the abnormality relates to the protein dystrophin, complete absence of that protein results in classic Duchenne muscular dystrophy; partial absence may produce a milder form of muscle weakness but in the same distribution as Duchenne dystrophy (Becker dystrophy) or may simply cause unilateral muscle hypertrophy or exercise-induced muscle pain and cramp. Similar variations in clinical expression are seen in the mitochondrial disorders (vide infra).

LIMB GIRDLE SYNDROME

It is unusual for LG syndrome to involve the eye in terms of abnormalities of extraocular movement. The presence of an ocular movement disorder in a patient with an otherwise typical LG syndrome should alert the attending physician to the possibility of alternate diagnoses. However, the major abnormality in the genetically determined disorders is in Duchenne dystrophy with absence of dystrophin. Dystrophin has been localized to the outer plexiform layer in the normal retina, and in the vast majority of patients with Duchenne dystrophy electroretinography will be abnormal. This indicates that in addition to the muscle isoforms, the retinal isoform of dystrophin is abnormal in Duchenne dystrophy. Given that dystrophin acts as a stabilizing protein to the otherwise flexible muscle membrane, a similar role may be deduced for the retinal isoform in the outer plexiform layer.

FASCIOSCAPULOHUMERAL SYNDROME

As the name suggests, involvement of the facial muscles is an integral part of fascioscapulohumeral (FSH) syndrome. The extraocular muscles are preserved but ptosis, which is often

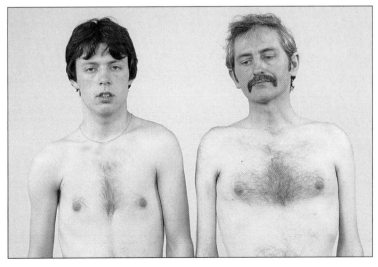

Fig. 29.1 Father and son with FSH, showing asymmetric involvement.

asymmetrical, is a typical feature (*Fig. 29.1*). As in other forms of muscle disease, muscle biopsy is required to define the underlying etiology of FSH syndrome; however, the majority of cases are due to fascioscapulohumeral dystrophy.

The age of onset of FSH syndrome is very variable, with some patients presenting in pre-puberty, the majority between puberty and the mid-twenties, and a few presenting as late as the mid-forties. The onset of weakness is very slow and many patients do not realize they have the disorder until, for example, the ptosis has progressed to the point where it is interfering with vision. The weakness around the mouth, in the early stages, simply produces a transverse smile and does not interfere with eating. Scapular winging due to weakness in the serratus anterior is more often thought to be an abberation and sometimes a 'party trick' rather than an abnormality.

As it is commonly the ptosis that brings a patient to clinical attention, the majority of new patients present via ophthalmology departments. Hence, when a young patient presents with ptosis (particularly if this is asymmetric), it is important to enquire specifically about family history not only of facial involvement but also of limb involvement. About 50% of patients with FSH dystrophy will become wheelchair-confined by their fifties due to proximal lower limb weakness. In addition to testing their obicularis oculi, it is important to test for function of the obicularis oris. Patients will often give a history of never being able to whistle or having difficulty in using a straw. Asking patients to elevate their arms will show evidence of over riding of the scapula (*Fig. 29.2*).

Molecular genetics revealed a locus on the long arm of chromosome 4 at site 4.5 where there is a repeat-DNA sequence. Deletions in this area have been identified in FSH dystrophy.

It has previously been suggested that Coats syndrome is ubiquitous in families with FSH dystrophy. However, most series indicate that this occurs in only about 10% of families.

SCAPULOPERONEAL SYNDROME

Individuals with SP syndrome only rarely show any ocular abnormality. The ocular movements are typically normal and any deviation should lead to re-assessment of the diagnosis. A very small subset of patients show a mild facial weakness, resulting in ptosis, in addition to their scapuloperoneal peripheral weakness. It has

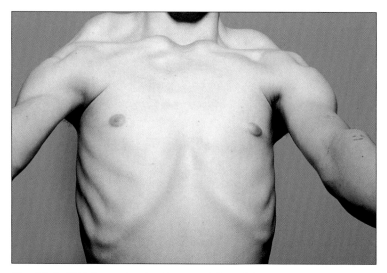

Fig. 29.2 FSH dystrophy showing over riding of the scapula above the clavicular line.

been suggested that these patients are intermediate between FSH syndrome and SP syndrome; it is possible, however, that this subgroup of patients is allelic to FSH dystrophy.

DISTAL SYNDROME

The majority of patients whose presentation is initially distal have neurogenic weakness of muscle and represent rare forms of spinal muscular atrophy. Involvement of facial or extraocular muscles has not been described.

ION CHANNEL DISORDERS

Myotonia is defined as an uncontrolled temporary stiffness of muscle due to transient hyperexcitability in the muscle fiber surface membrane. The hereditary myotonias are divided into four groups: myotonia congenita; paramyotonia congenita (see Periodic paralyses below); dystrophia myotonica; and Schwartz Jampel syndrome. The most important of these, in respect to ophthalmology, is dystrophia myotonica, which will be considered first.

DYSTROPHIA MYOTONICA

Dystrophia myotonica (DM; myotonic dystrophy) is the commonest form of adult muscular dystrophy, with a prevalence of 1:20 000 per population. In addition to peripheral myotonia and weakness, involvement of the facial muscles, the extraocular muscles, and the eye is characteristic of the disorder.

One of the characteristic features of DM is 'anticipation', with the disease appearing earlier in succeeding generations. This is accounted for by the molecular genetics of the condition. The gene defect has been identified as being an unstable triplet repeat on the long arm of chromosome 19, at position 13.3. At that site, in a normal individual, there are some 15–30 copies of the cytosine–thiamine–guanine (CGT) triplet repeat. In patients with DM there is amplification of the repeat, with 50 to thousands of copies being present. There is some correlation between the size of the triplet repeat and the severity of the clinical manifestation. There is also evidence that the expansion of the triplet repeat increases in succeeding generations. This provides the molecular basis for anticipation, with increase in the size of repeats from generation to generation leading to earlier and more severe clinical manifestation.

The situation, therefore, where a grandmother with mild myotonia, mild weakness, and cataract has an offspring with early onset of cataract, more marked facial weakness, myotonia, and peripheral weakness, who in turn has a child with an even earlier presentation of cataract and more severe clinical involvement, is relatively common (*Fig. 29.3*).

Facial Weakness
Facial weakness is one of the earliest and most constant features of DM and old family photographs may show its presence many years before the diagnosis was established. The ptosis associated with DM is usually symmetrical and less severe than that seen in FSH. It is rarely sufficiently severe to warrant surgical intervention, although it may occasionally cause compensatory head tilting.

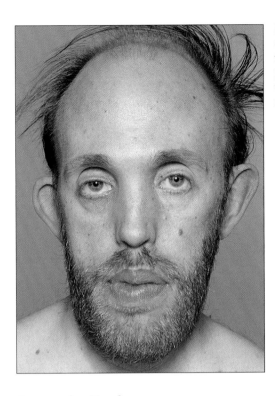

Fig. 29.3 Myotonic dystrophy, showing frontal balding, ptosis, facial weakness, and masseter wasting.

Extraocular Muscles
This is rarely sufficiently severe to cause diplopia but abnormalities in extraocular muscle function are found in some 10–20% of patients with DM.

Iris Abnormalities
Using anterior segment fluoroscein angiography, abnormal vascular 'tufts' are seen in some patients.

Intraocular Pressure
The intraocular pressure is consistently low in patients with DM, with the pressure tending to fall further with increasing age. This is thought to be due to a degeneration of the ciliary muscle.

Corneal Lesions
These have not been systematically studied in patients with DM. However, the paucity of eye closure may lead to considerable corneal damage, to the degree that corneal grafting may be required.

Cataract
The cataract in DM is characteristic and is seen in virtually all patients. Abnormalities are rare in pre-puberty and are most common in the 30–50-year-old age group. Evolution of the cataract has been divided into four stages:
Stage 1: A slit lamp examination shows scattered dust-like opacities in the posterior subcapsular regions. The opacities are iridescent, glinting blue or red as the angle of the lamp is changed. In some patients whitish opacities are seen.
Stage 2: Cortical spokes may be present and the iridescence opacities are increased in size and number, and anterior and posterior subcapsular plaques are visible.
Stage 3: Diminution of visual acuity is usually present. Star-shaped opacities and spokes are seen with the ophthalmoscope. The slit lamp examination shows numerous opacities throughout the lens. The iridescent opacities tend to be less conspicuous as general clouding increases before the cataract matures. At this stage the cataract is usually indistinguishable from any other form of cataract.

Stage 4: Mature cataract. It is important that young people presenting with cataract should be screened for the presence of DM, given the known anesthetic hazards of the disorder (i.e. prolonged paralysis after depolarizing agents). If cataract removal is undertaken via general anesthesia, severe complications, which are preventable, may occur.

Retinal Changes
Peripheral pigmentary retinopathy is commonly seen, and on some occasions may spread to involve the macula.

MYOTONIA CONGENITA

Myotonia congenita exists in two forms, autosomal dominant and recessive. Involvement of the facial and extraocular muscles is rare, although myotonic lid-lag is occasionally seen and can be precipitated by cooling the eyelid with ice.

SCHWARTZ JAMPEL SYNDROME

Schwartz Jampel syndrome is a rare disorder characterized by myotonia, small stature, multiple skeletal deformities, unusual facial features, and myopia. Patients develop the full syndrome within the first few years of life. Blepharophimosis, myopia, and cataracts are common; strabismus and nystagmus may be present.

PERIODIC PARALYSES

In this small group of uncommon diseases attacks of muscle weakness occur at irregular intervals. Weakness can progress to paralysis in virtually all skeletal muscle. The attacks subside spontaneously with time. During an attack of paralysis, the muscle membrane is not excitable. Although hypokalemic periodic paralysis, hyperkalemic periodic paralysis, and paramyotonia congenita have different molecular origins, they all share common clinical features. The paralytic attacks can vary from 1 h to days with features being localized or generalized. The cranial muscles are typically spared but occasionally can become paralyzed. The attacks are frequently precipitated by cold and, with progressive attacks over years, a degree of fixed muscle weakness may develop.

HYPOKALEMIC PERIODIC PARALYSIS

In this condition, it is unusual for facial or extraocular muscles to be affected. The classic situation is a patient who, although completely flaccid peripherally, is able to move his or her face and eyes at will.

HYPERKALEMIC PERIODIC PARALYSIS

This condition exists in two forms. Most patients have only flaccid weakness which, like hypokalemic periodic paralysis, rarely affects the facial and extraocular muscles. There are a subgroup of patients, however, who, in addition to their flaccid weakness, display myotonic stiffness characteristically affecting facial muscles and leading to myotonic lid-lag, again provoked by cold.

PARAMYOTONIA CONGENITA

This disease is allelic to hyperkalemic periodic paralysis, both diseases sharing an abnormality of the muscle sodium channel. Unlike the other periodic paralyses, however, paramyotonia congenita has a predilection for involvement of the face and the neck. Typically, symptoms are induced by cold; it is not unusual in adolescents to find a history of an inability to open the eyes for several seconds when the face is cold, for example due to wind or rain. The same is seen in affected newborn infants when their face is washed with a cold cloth.

OROPHARYNGEAL MUSCULAR DYSTROPHY

Oropharyngeal muscular dystrophy (OPMD) is a relatively rare dystrophy, first described in French-Canadian families. It presents in an autosomal dominant manner, with progressive ptosis and dysphagia. It usually becomes manifest between the ages of 50 and 60 years, initially with ptosis and the coincident development of dysphagia. These symptoms progress slowly and eventually there is a complete loss of all extraocular muscle function and the limb muscles slowly become involved.

Although this is usually a disorder of late onset, where there is an obvious family history the ptosis may be described in patients in their thirties. To compensate for the loss of visual field that is a consequence of the ptosis, there is overaction of the frontalis muscles so that the head is thrown back ('Hutchinson's posture' or the 'Astrologer's posture'). Clearly this posture can aggravate the dysphagia, which may be improved by surgical correction of the ptosis. With the evolving loss of extraocular function the patient often complains of diplopia. The dysphagia is first for solids but progresses insidiously to involve liquids, often leading to undernutrition. Pathologically, the disorder is characterized by a dystrophic process with an associated rimmed vacuolar change.

RARE CONGENITAL DYSTROPHIES

WALKER, WARBURG, CONGENITAL MUSCLE DYSTROPHY: MUSCLE, EYE, BRAIN DISEASE

This is a rare condition, first described in 1942 by Walker. Children are born blind, they have difficulty in swallowing and sucking, have a weak cry, and are hypertonic. The ocular abnormalities include fixed pupils, central corneal opacities, shallow anterior chamber, posterior synechiae, retinal detachment and retinal dysplasia, microphthalmia, and hypoplasia of the optic nerves and anterior segment.

SANTAVUORI CONGENITAL MUSCULAR DYSTROPHY: MUSCLE, EYE, BRAIN DISEASE

This disorder has been described in Finnish patients. Motor development is slow during the first few years of life but most children do eventually walk. By the age of 5 years, however, mental retardation is severe. There is marked spasticity with contractures of multiple joints, and proximal weakness is usually present. The eye signs are those of severe myopia and retinal dysplasia, followed by progressive failure of vision and uncontrolled eye movements.

CONGENITAL MYOPATHIES

The congenital myopathies are a heterogeneous group of disorders in which arrest occurs at various stages of muscle development, leading to internal abnormalities within the muscle fiber. These typically form the basis of the nomenclature of the disease.

The congenital myopathies share a common feature of hypotonia, particularly in infancy, and disorders of ocular movement have been described in about 50% of these myopathies. It is probable that as more patients are described, ocular movement disorders will be found to be increasingly frequent and their absence in any particular patient should not lead to a diagnostic classification, which remains on the basis of muscle biopsy and molecular genetics.

CENTRAL CORE DISEASE

In this condition (*Fig. 29.4*), weakness throughout early childhood is common, although some patients do not present until their late teens or early adult life. The predominant effect is in the peripheral musculature. Occasionally, facial muscle involvement, with ptosis, is seen and very rarely there are abnormalities of extraocular movement.

NEMALINE MYOPATHY

Nemaline myopathy (*Fig. 29.5*) has been described in three forms, a severe neonatal myopathy, a mild non-progressive or slowly progressive myopathy, and an adult-onset form. The severe neonatal myopathy is incompatible with life beyond the first few weeks or months and the facial musculature is profoundly affected. The most common form is the mild non-progressive or slowly progressive myopathy, often with a mild to moderate proximal myopathy. Involvement of the extraocular muscles is highly unusual but ptosis has been described in a few patients.

CENTRONUCLEAR MYOPATHIES

Centronuclear myopathies (*Fig. 29.6*) can be divided into early onset and late onset patients. The early onset patients have the most common form of the disease. Weakness presents very early

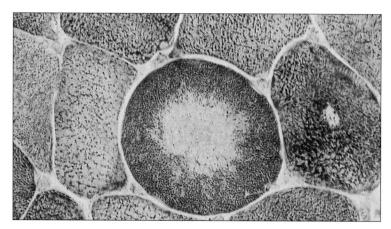

Fig. 29.4 A central core lacking mitochondrial enzyme activity, surrounded by a dense-staining rim. Central cores are usually restricted to type I fibers. (NDH-Tr ×732)

in life, sometimes with respiratory distress at birth. Ptosis, strabismus, and facial weakness are frequent early clinical manifestations. Total or subtotal ophthalmoplegia is common. In late onset patients, ptosis and limitation of eye movements are less frequent and less marked than in the early onset patients.

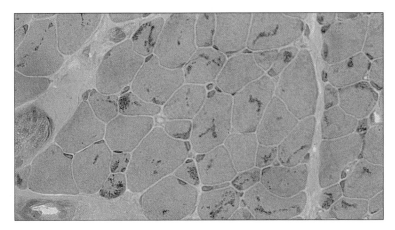

Fig. 29.5 Nemaline myopathy illustrating nemaline rods. These thread-like rods are present in most fibers of this biopsy and are easily recognized by their dark-staining appearance. (Modified Gomori trichrome, ×378)

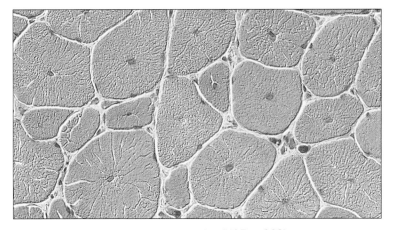

Fig. 29.6 Adult centronuclear myopathy. (H&E, ×263)

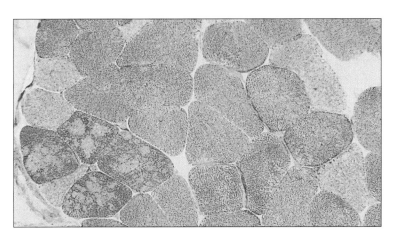

Fig. 29.8 Central cores (multi-cores or mini-cores), in this case of central core disease, are shown as areas devoid of staining in this section. (NADH-TR, ×293)

X-LINKED MYOTUBULAR MYOPATHY

X-linked myotubular myopathy (*Fig. 29.7*) is a severe condition presenting with marked hypotonia at birth. There is usually bilateral ptosis, facial diplegia, and moderate to severe limitation of eye movement.

MULTI-CORE DISEASE

The clinical presentation of multi-core disease is variable (*Fig. 29.8*). The majority of patients present in infancy and have delayed motor development but late onset patients have been described. Facial weakness is common and ptosis with extraocular muscle weakness, progressing to complete external ophthalmoplegia, is relatively common.

CONGENITAL FIBER TYPE DISPROPORTION

As the name suggests, there is an abnormal population of muscle fibers in this condition (*Fig. 29.9*), which is associated with facial weakness but not with disturbance of ocular muscles.

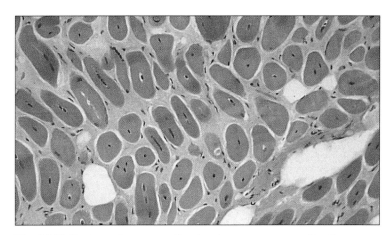

Fig. 29.7 Centronuclear myopathy showing excess connective tissue and small rounded muscle fibers with centrally located chains of nuclei. (H&E, ×175)

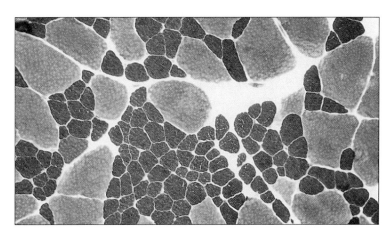

Fig. 29.9 Congenital fiber type disproportion, showing marked hypotrophy and excess of Type I fibers. (Myofibrillar ATPase, pH 4.35, ×236)

MITOCHONDRIAL DISORDERS

The mitochondrial myopathies and encephalomyopathies have proved a major challenge to diagnostic acumen over the years. With the advent of sophisticated methods of investigating mitochondrial function, including histopathology, biochemical assays, and molecular genetic analysis, however, the situation is becoming somewhat clearer. Given that the same abnormality (either deletional or substitutional) at the molecular level results in different clinical phenotypes, there is, as yet, some considerable way to go before these diseases are finally phenotypically distinct.

Mitochondria are intracellular organelles involved in the aerobic production of energy (in the form of ATP). The mitochondrium is small (approximately 1–2 μm × 0.5–1 μm, about the size of a bacterium) and is composed of two membranes, an external (or outer) membrane and an internal (or inner) membrane. The outer membrane separates the mitochondrium from the cytoplasm. The mitochondrial matrix is enclosed within the inner membrane (*Fig. 29.10*).

Defects of each of the major processing steps (*Fig. 29.11*) have been identified. However, not all mitochondrial encephalomyopathies fit precisely into the biochemical classification.

Mitochondria have distinct genetic properties in that they derive their DNA from two sources, the nucleus and the mitochondrium itself. Mitochondrial genetics indicate that mitochondrial DNA (mtDNA) is transmitted exclusively from the mother through the ovum; the inheritance is thus strictly maternal. Each mitochondrium has several copies of mtDNA and each cell contains multiple mitochondria. The ratio therefore of normal to mutant mtDNA can vary widely; the co-existence of mutant and normal mtDNA in the same cell is called heteroplasmy (*Fig. 29.12*).

For a mutation in mtDNA to be expressed it has to be above a certain threshold or percentage relative to normal mtDNA, the so-called threshold effect. It is probable that this threshold depends on the metabolic requirements of the particular tissue.

Given that there is a contribution from nuclear DNA to the mitochondria, nuclear factors may influence the expression of mutations in mtDNA. This is seen particularly in Leber's optic atrophy, in which there is a distinct male predominance thought to be due to a nuclear factor.

The histopathologic characteristic of mitochondrial disorders is the presence of an abnormal mitochondria seen with the Gomori trichrome stain, producing groups of so-called 'ragged red fibers' (RRFs) (*Fig. 29.13*; see also chapter 5).

In the appropriate clinical situation the finding of such fibers on muscle biopsy can be considered diagnostic. RRFs are not unique to mitochondrial disorders, however, and are seen in other myopathies as well as in aging muscle. Specific enzymes and defects can be demonstrated by the SDH (cytochrome oxidase stain) (*Fig. 29.14*).

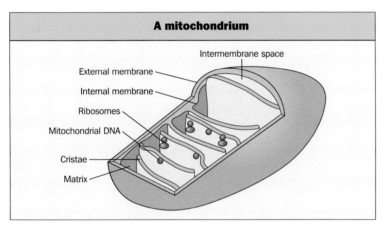

A mitochondrium

- Intermembrane space
- External membrane
- Internal membrane
- Ribosomes
- Mitochondrial DNA
- Cristae
- Matrix

Fig. 29.10 Schematic representation of a mitochondrium.

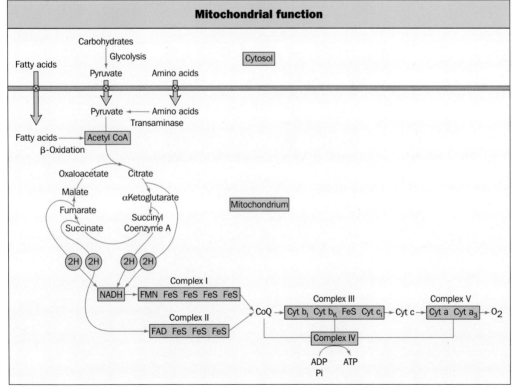

Mitochondrial function

Cytosol

Carbohydrates
Glycolysis
Fatty acids   Pyruvate   Amino acids

Mitochondrium

Pyruvate ← Amino acids
Transaminase
Fatty acids → Acetyl CoA
β-Oxidation
Oxaloacetate   Citrate
Malate   αKetoglutarate
Fumarate   Succinyl
Succinate   Coenzyme A

2H 2H   2H 2H

Complex I
NADH → FMN FeS FeS FeS FeS
Complex II
FAD FeS FeS FeS
CoQ → Complex III Cyt b$_I$ Cyt b$_K$ FeS Cyt c$_I$ → Cyt c → Complex V Cyt a Cyt a$_3$ → O$_2$
Complex IV
ADP   ATP
Pi

Fig. 29.11 Schematic representation of mitochondrial function. There are five steps in mitochondrial processing: 1) Substrate Transport. In this process, substrates such as fatty acids are transported across the mitochondrial membranes into the matrix. 2) Substrate Utilization. The energy substrates are further metabolized to form Acetyl CoA. 3) Krebs' Cycle. Carbon dioxide is produced with NAD$^+$ and FAD. 4) Oxidation Phosphorylation Coupling. In this NAD$^+$ and FAD are reduced to NADH and FADH$_2$. 5) Respiratory Chain. NADH and FADH$_2$ enter the respiratory chain and pass through a series of four complexes (I – IV) arriving at complex V, which uses the energy generated by the respiratory chain to generate ATP from ADP, and inorganic phosphate.

CLINICAL FEATURES

The general clinical features of the mitochondrial encephalomyopathies clearly include abnormalities of muscle. With respect to ophthalmology (*Figs 29.15, 29.16*), these represent an external ophthalmoplegia with exercise intolerance, limb weakness, and marked loss of muscle bulk. An elevated creatinine kinase is observed.

Within the central nervous system acute optic neuropathy or atrophy, or both, may occur as may pigmented retinopathy associated with mental retardation and dementia, seizures, ataxia, hearing loss, leukodystrophy, myoclonus, stroke-like episodes at a young age, migraine, and extrapyramidal signs. In the peripheral nervous system, sensory motor neuropathy has been described.

Abnormalities of the endocrine system have been reported, including diabetes mellitus, hypothyroidism, infertility, and growth hormone deficiency with a short stature. In the heart, cardiac conduction block and a hypertrophic cardiomyopathy can occur. Abnormalities are also seen in the kidneys, pancreas, gastrointestinal tract, skin, and blood. It is the combination of these abnormalities that leads to the clinically defined syndromes.

As mentioned above, the identification of abnormalities in mtDNA has allowed some progress in defining these syndromes. Point mutations, duplications, and multiple deletions of mtDNA have all been identified. Point mutations are seen in MERRF, MELAS and MHON (see below), whereas single deletions are seen in Kearns Sayre syndrome and progressive external ophthalmoplegia (PEO).

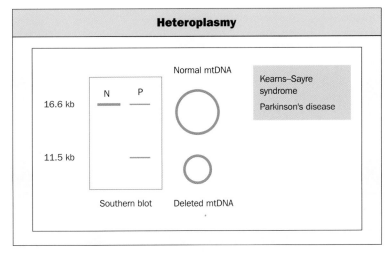

Fig. 29.12 Schematic representation of heteroplasmy.

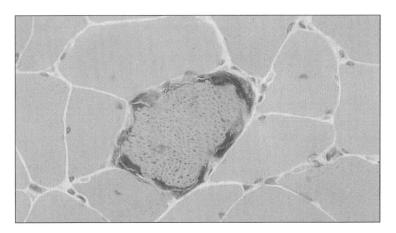

Fig. 29.13 A ragged red fiber with characteristic red peripheral staining can be seen. Such fibers are often 'cracked' in appearance. (Modified Gomori trichrome, ×543)

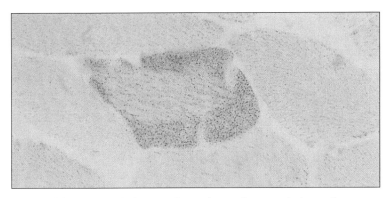

Fig. 29.14 Abnormally dense subsacrolemmal accumulations of mitohondria from the same biopsy as Fig.29.13. (SDH,×560)

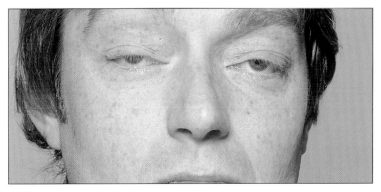

Fig. 29.15 Chronic progressive external ophthalmoplegia, attempted upgaze.

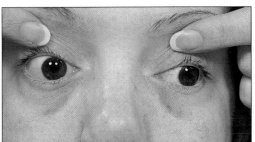
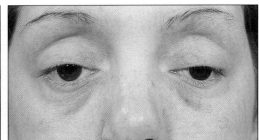
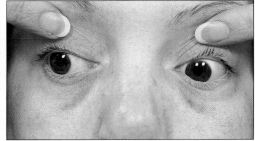

Fig. 29.16 Chronic progressive external ophthalmoplegia showing restriction of eye movement on right and left lateral gaze.

MITOCHONDRIAL DNA DELETIONS AND DUPLICATIONS

KEARNS SAYRE SYNDROME

Kearns Sayre Syndrome (KSS) was originally described as a combination of retinitis pigmentosa, external ophthalmoplegia, and complete heart block (*Fig. 29.17*). There is an invariant triad of ophthalmoplegia, pigmentary retinopathy, and onset under the age of 20 years, and at least one of the following should be present:
• Cerebrospinal fluid protein greater than 100 mg/dl.
• Cardiac conduction block.
• Cerebellar syndrome.
In KSS, large scale mtDNA heteroplasmic deletions are identified, although a few cases have been associated with a duplication of mtDNA. Apart from these required symptoms, hearing loss and limb weakness have been described as has diabetes mellitus, hypoparathyroidism, irregular menses and growth hormone deficiency, and renal tubular dysfunction (usually in the form of De Toni Fanconi Debré). Occasionally, patients have had stroke-like disease as a clinical feature of MELAS (mitochondrial encephalopathy, lactic acidosis, and stroke-like episodes). Virtually all cases of KSS are sporadic.

Usually patients with KSS are normal at birth and develop normally but then slowly accumulate their abnormalities. It is possible that the deleted, and hence shorter, mtDNA replicates more rapidly; serial assessment has shown that the amount of deleted mtDNA increases with time.

PROGRESSIVE EXTERNAL OPHTHALMOPLEGIA

Progressive external ophthalmoplegia (PEO) and ptosis typically present in childhood and adolescence, when the patient rarely has diplopia. There is frequently associated limb weakness. The majority of patients are sporadic.

Progressive External Ophthalmoplegia⁺

Progressive External Ophthalmoplegia+
As it has not been possible to classify (on the basis of either a mitochondrial or biochemical disorder) all patients who have the same clinical phenotype, the concept of PEO⁺ has arisen. These are patients who do not fulfill the classic criteria for the diagnosis of KSS or the progressive form of PEO, or have unusual features associated with their ophthalmoplegia. It is possible but not yet proven that this group of patients may have a lower percentage of mutant mtDNA.

A rare autosomal dominant PEO is characterized by age of onset in the late twenties with ptosis, dysphagia, dysphonia, facial and limb weakness, cataracts, and exercise intolerance, leading to death in the mid-forties to late fifties. In families with this disorder, multiple deletions of mtDNA, as opposed to the single deletion shown in KSS and sporadic PEO, have been shown to occur.

MITOCHONDRIAL DNA POINT MUTATIONS

MYOCLONIC EPILEPSY WITH RAGGED RED FIBERS (MERRF)

The majority of patients with this disorder present with myoclonus and generalized epilepsy and are shown to have RRFs on muscle biopsy. Optic atrophy is not infrequent, however, occurring in some 40% of patients; an ophthalmoparesis occurs in about 12% of patients.

MITOCHONDRIAL ENCEPHALOMYOPATHY, LACTIC ACIDOSIS AND STROKE-LIKE EPISODES (MELAS)

This disorder is defined by stroke under the age of 40 years, an encephalopathy characterized by seizures, dementia, or both, lactic acidosis, RRFs, and limb weakness; ophthalmoparesis is unusual but optic atrophy can affect up to 20% of patients.

PEO WITHOUT MITOCHONDRIAL DNA DELETIONS

In a significant number of patients with this disorder, there is a point mutation at site 2343 [PEO⁺²³⁴³]. Most of these patients, unlike those with deletions (PEO), have a history of an affected relative.

NUCLEAR DNA MUTATIONS

AUTOSOMAL DOMINANT PEO (SEE ABOVE)

Mitochondrial neuropathy, gastrointestinal encephalomyopathy (MNGIE), or mitochondrial pseudo-obstruction, ophthalmoplegia, and polyneuropathy (MEPOP), are rare autosomal recessive disorders and are associated with an ophthalmoparesis and evidence of gastrointestinal dysfunction; patients may also have a polyneuropathy. Some patients have been found to have deletions in mtDNA.

It is evident that a patient presenting with ophthalmoplegia may fall into any of the categories described above and it is often associated features that help to delineate the condition. However, investigation with at least a muscle biopsy and analysis of mitochondrial DNA is now routine in attempting to unravel the pathophysiology of the phenotype.

MYONEURAL JUNCTION DISORDERS

These disorders represent a disturbance of the neuromuscular transmission between the terminal nerve fiber and the muscle

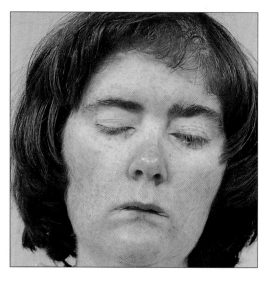

Fig. 29.17 Kearns Sayre syndrome.

end plate. They are divided into two major categories: acquired autoimmune myasthenia gravis and the myasthenic syndromes.

ACQUIRED AUTOIMMUNE MYASTHENIA GRAVIS

There are two populations of patients with myasthenia gravis (MG). In the younger age group, with onset between the ages of 20 and 30 years, women predominate. In this group of patients, the classic presentation is of ocular symptomatology, spreading via oculopharyngeal involvement to the limbs, and subsequently ventilatory involvement.

In the second group, in which patients present between the ages of 45 and 65 years, the male to female ratio is almost one. In this group of patients, ocular disease is less likely to be the initial presentation. The patient more typically presents with limb weakness, then develops oropharyngeal weakness, and lastly ocular weakness.

The cardinal symptomatology of MG is weakness and abnormal fatiguability on exercise. The disease either selectively involves the external ocular muscles or it may be generalized. The pathophysiology is of an autoimmune attack on the postjunctional acetylcholine receptor. Whereas only 80–90% of patients show the presence of circulating acetylcholine receptor antibodies, all patients show evidence of immune deposits of immunoglobulin G and complement components on the postsynaptic membrane of the neuromuscular junction.

The muscle weakness associated with MG increases with repeated or sustained exertion and is improved by rest. The weakness is usually increased if the core temperature is elevated; conversely, it is improved by cold. Intercurrent illness, emotional upset, and menses often increase the symptoms; ocular symptoms are increased by exposure to bright light.

The extraocular muscles are eventually involved in virtually all patients. The voluntary muscles innervated by the cranial nerves (facial, masticatory, lingunopharyngeal), and the proximal limb girdles, are frequently affected, distal limb involvement being common. There are no objective sensory signs. The symptoms tend to fluctuate on a daily, weekly, or yearly basis and spontaneous remission is sometimes seen within the first 3 years of the disease.

The ocular signs are those of ptosis, which is unilateral or bilateral. The extraocular muscles are, again, affected either unilaterally or bilaterally but more typically bilaterally. The ocular palsies are usually asymmetric and predominantly affect convergence and vertical gaze. Variable diplopia on testing extraocular movement is a classic finding. It must be emphasized, however, that a patient who presents with a complaint of diplopia that is not present at the time of examination (almost certainly due to the length of the outpatient waiting time) should be exercised to the point where symptoms develop.

The disease is classified according to the Osserman classification, Osserman Class 1 being purely ocular disease, Osserman Class 2 being involvement of pharyngeal musculature, Osserman Class 3 being involvement of limb musculature, and Osserman Class 4 being involvement of ventilation. In patients in whom the disease remains confined to the eyes for a period of 2–3 years, the likelihood of developing generalized disease becomes exceedingly limited.

Investigation

The single most important part of the investigation is that of clinical examination of a symptomatic patient. Examination when the patient is symptom free and at rest is worthless. If a patient presents with diplopia, it is of immense importance to establish what factors induce or exacerbate the symptoms.

Acetylcholine receptor antibodies are present in only about 40% of patients with purely ocular disease, probably reflecting the difference in the acetylcholine receptor epitopes present in the eye musculature compared with the limb musculature. At present, the antibody test is based on the use of acetylcholine receptors gathered from limb musculature usually from patients who have undergone amputations for vascular disease. It is probable that the epitope in elderly limb muscle differs considerably from that present in the much more active eye muscle.

It may be possible to make use of the acetylcholine receptor antibody test to distinguish between those patients who have an ocular onset but will eventually develop generalized disease, from those with purely ocular disease. In the vast majority of patients whose disease will become generalized, there will be an acetylcholine receptor antibody present from the outset.

Electromyograph studies, with repetitive stimulation, provided they involve the ocular muscles, are diagnostic in the vast majority of patients.

Treatment

Treatment of generalized electromyography is by stabilization of the disease preferably by plasmapheresis with early thymectomy. On this basis, the majority of patients are soon rendered asymptomatic.

Treatment of purely ocular disease is much more difficult. The majority of patients will respond to a course of oral steroids (40–60 mg daily for a period of 4–6 weeks, reducing to zero over a period of 3–4 months). The relapse rate after such a course is high and the side effects of steroids are considerable, necessitating gastric protection and potentially treatment of associated side effects. The majority of patients will respond to azathioprine in the long term. It is the author's preference to prescribe a single course of oral steroids, with the coincident introduction of azathioprine, and to continue the azathioprine for a period of some 3 years. Patients who relapse at that stage are further treated with azathioprine. Only a small percentage (1–2%) of patients with purely ocular disease require thymectomy to bring their disease under control.

LAMBERT EATON MYASTHENIC SYNDROME (LEMS)

In this condition, the autoimmune reaction is directed at the presynaptic voltage-sensitive calcium channels (VACCs). The resulting loss of VACCs decreases the dose of calcium into the motor nerve terminal during activity, thus reducing quantum release. Hence, patients present with fatiguability.

A large proportion of patients with LEMS (approximately two-thirds) have an underlying malignancy, particularly small cell carcinoma of the lung. In contrast to acquired MG, LEMS occurs more frequently in elderly people and has a strong male preponderance. Characteristically, the weakness initially involves the trunk and lower limb musculature. Some 70% of patients, however, will have mild or transient ocular symptomatology involving the autonomic systems, with decreased salivation and decreased lacrimation; sweating, hypotension, impotence, and abnormal pupillary light responses can occur.

On examination there is a characteristic initial decrement in muscle strength; the peak of exercise leads to an improvement in contraction. Investigation is with repetitive stimulation which shows an incremental response. Antibodies to VACCs can be determined by specialist laboratories but this is not commonly available as a routine diagnostic test.

In patients with carcinoma-associated disease there is usually clinical improvement with treatment of the underlying tumor. Otherwise 3–4 mg di-aminopyridine with or without immunosuppression is the therapy of choice. The benefit of anticholinesterase drugs is limited.

CONGENITAL MYASTHENIC SYNDROMES

Certain syndromes have been described in which the abnormality in transmission of acetylcholine (either in its release or uptake) at the neuromuscular junction does not have an autoimmune basis. Typically, such patients present in the neonatal period with ocular, bulbar, or respiratory symptomatology, worsened by crying or activity. Symptoms persist through childhood and adolescence and there may be a degree of developmental delay.

The assessment, therefore, of a patient with ocular symptomatology that is fatiguable, is directed to determining the underlying cause. Age is an important factor in terms of MG: disease from early childhood is suggestive of a congenital disorder, whereas onset in the late teens to early twenties indicates the presence of acquired autoimmune MG; the development of the disease in middle to late life suggests LEMS. Investigations with electromyograph studies and testing of the appropriate antibodies can usually delineate these syndromes.

TICS AND OTHER MOVEMENT DISORDERS

A tic is an abrupt jerking type of movement which involves a discrete muscle group. It mimics the normal movement of the muscle and can vary markedly in intensity. Acute transient tics are frequently seen in childhood and tend to involve a single muscle group, often the eyelid; these tics usually remit within a year. Persistent or multiple tics can occur in childhood and persist for several years before disappearing in adolescence or adult life. Chronic tic, either single or multiple, can persist throughout life and vary little in frequency or intensity.

With respect to the eye, the common tics are those of eye winking, eye rolling, curling in of the eyelids, staring, and eyebrow raising. All tics are affected by anxiety, anger, and self-consciousness, and hence are more evident in public places or unusual situations. They are suppressed by pleasurable pastimes and alcohol and disappear with sleep.

Parents can be reassured that in the majority of cases their child's tic will disappear with the passage of time. In adult life the tic may be very embarrassing and treatment with anxiolytics is sometimes of benefit. Only rarely will tic disorders require treatment with *Botulinum* toxin.

ADULT ONSET FOCAL DYSTONIAS

Meige Syndrome

Meige syndrome is described as an idiopathic focal dystonia which affects the facial musculature symmetrically, causing blepharo-spasm, grimacing, and oromandibular dystonia. It has in the past been described as 'cranial dystonia', 'Breueghel's syndrome', 'blepharospasm/oromandibular dystonia syndrome', 'idiopathic orofacial dystonia', 'orofacial cervical dystonia,' and 'mental trismus'.

The peak age of incidence is the sixth decade but about 20% of patients will present before the age of 40 years. It is probable that blepharospasm occurring in isolation is a restrictive form of MEIGE syndrome. The vast majority of patients with MEIGE syndrome have no underlying pathology but it can be seen in association with Wilson's disease and essential blepharospasm is not infrequent in the late stages of Parkinson's disease. There may be associated torsion dystonias of other segments in the body, for example, spasmodic torticollis and writer's cramp.

Two-thirds of patients present with blepharospasm and progress to oromandibular involvement. The onset tends to be gradual but the forced eye closure increasingly interferes with vision.

Most patients find that their attacks are provoked by reading, watching television, driving, bright sunlight, emotional stress or embarrassment, fatigue, cold winds, depression, and crowded places. They usually have a history of adopting mannerisms to relieve their symptoms, although these tend to become less effective with the passage of time. Often drinking water or alcohol will help, as will gentle pressure to the eyeball. Some patients get relief by yawning or singing. Eventually these relieving factors become less constant. Many patients become withdrawn and depressed as they find outside contact or excitement increases their symptoms. However, solitary pastimes such as reading or watching television may also stimulate their attacks and many patients become socially isolated as a result.

In some 20% of patients the condition is confined to the eyelids (essential blepharospasm) but in the majority the facial muscles become involved with the passage of time. In the majority of patients there is a steady progression from onset to maximum severity and thereafter the disorder tends to remain static. The time course is variable but the majority of patients have achieved their maximum dysfunction within 10 years.

Treatment of MEIGE syndrome has been revolutionized by the use of *Botulinum* toxin.

INDEX